DIAGNOSTIC CYTOLOGY AND HEMATOLOGY OF THE HORSE

Second Edition

DIAGNOSTIC CYTOLOGY AND HEMATOLOGY OF THE HORSE

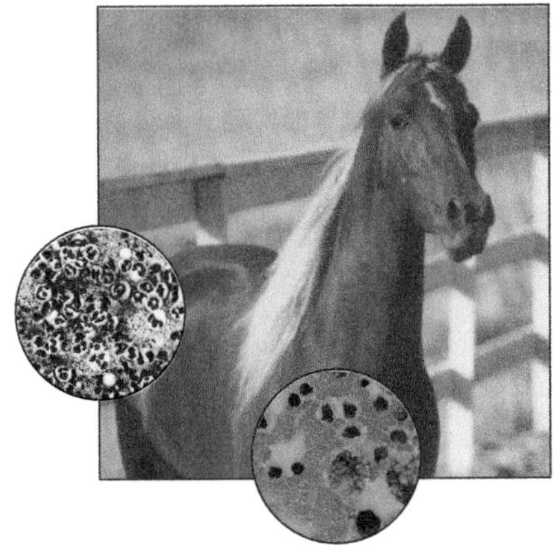

Rick L. Cowell, DVM, MS, Dipl ACVP

Professor, Veterinary Clinical Pathology
Director, Clinical Pathology Laboratory
Department of Veterinary Pathobiology
College of Veterinary Medicine
Oklahoma State University
Stillwater, Oklahoma

Ronald D. Tyler, DVM, PhD, Dipl ACVP and ABT

Vice-President, Medicines and Safety Evaluations, USA
Glaxo-Wellcome, R&D
Research Triangle Park, North Carolina
Adjunct Professor
Department of Veterinary Pathobiology
College of Veterinary Medicine
Oklahoma State University
Stillwater, Oklahoma

with 392 illustrations

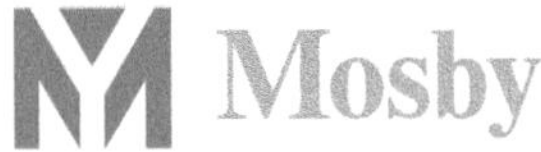

A Harcourt Health Sciences Company

St. Louis London Philadelphia Sydney Toronto

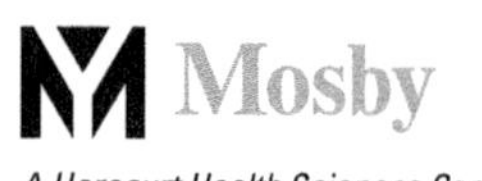

A Harcourt Health Sciences Company

Editor-in-Chief: John A. Schrefer
Editorial Manager: Linda L. Duncan
Senior Development Editor: Teri Merchant
Project Manager: Peggy Fagen
Designer: Judi Lang
Cover Design: Michael Warrell

SECOND EDITION

Mosby, Inc.
A Harcourt Health Sciences Company
11830 Westline Industrial Drive
St. Louis, Missouri 63146

International Standard Book Number 0-323-01317-1

Transferred to digital print 2012

Contributors

Claire B. Andreasen, DVM, MS, PhD
Interim DEO and Associate Professor
Veterinary Clinical Pathology
Department of Veterinary Pathology
College of Veterinary Medicine
Iowa State University
Ames, Iowa

Sylvie Beaudin, DVM
Resident, Veterinary Clinical Pathology
Department of Veterinary Pathobiology
College of Veterinary Medicine
Oklahoma State University
Stillwater, Oklahoma

Kimberly J. Caruso, DVM
Resident, Veterinary Clinical Pathology
College of Veterinary Medicine
Oklahoma State University
Stillwater, Oklahoma

Kenneth D. Clinkenbeard, PhD, DVM
Professor and Head
Department ofVeterinary Pathobiology
College of Veterinary Medicine
Oklahoma State University
Stillwater, Oklahoma

Rick L. Cowell, DVM, MS, Dipl ACVP
Professor, Veterinary Clinical Pathology
Director, Clinical Pathology Laboratory
Department of Veterinary Pathobiology
College of Veterinary Medicine
Oklahoma State University
Stillwater, Oklahoma

Heather L. DeHeer, DVM
Instructor, Clinical Pathology
Department of Microbiology, Pathology, and Parasitology
North Carolina State University
College of Veterinary Medicine
Raleigh, North Carolina

Wynne A. Digrassie, DVM, PhD
SW Equine Medical and Surgical Center
Scottsdale, Arizona

Karen E. Dorsey, DVM
Senior Resident, Veterinary Clinical Pathology
Department of Veterinary Pathobiology
Oklahoma State University
Stillwater, Oklahoma

Elizabeth A. Giuliano, DVM
Ophthalmology Section
Department of Veterinary Medicine and Surgery
University of Missouri-Columbia
Columbia, Missouri

Carol B. Grindem, DVM, PhD, Dipl ACVP
Professor
Department of Microbiology, Pathology, and Parasitology
College of Veterinary Medicine
North Carolina State University
Raleigh, North Carolina

M.A. Guglick, DVM, Dipl ACVIM
Associate Professor
Department of Clinical Studies
School of Veterinary Medicine
St. George's University
St. George, Grenada, West Indies

G. Reed Holyoak, DVM, PhD, Dipl ACT
Boren Veterinary Medical Teaching Hospital
College of Veterinary Medicine
Oklahoma State University
Stillwater, Oklahoma

Kenneth S. Latimer, DVM, PhD, Dipl ACVP
Professor
Department of Veterinary Pathology
College of Veterinary Medicine
University of Georgia
Athens, Georgia

William B. Ley, DVM, MS, Dipl ACT
Head, Department of Veterinary Clinical Sciences
College of Veterinary Medicine
Oklahoma State University
Stillwater, Oklahoma

Charles G. MacAllister, DVM, Dipl ACVIM
Professor
Department of Veterinary Clinical Sciences
College of Veterinary Medicine
Oklahoma State University
Stillwater, Oklahoma

Peter S. MacWilliams, DVM, PhD, Dipl ACVP
Professor of Clinical Pathology
Department of Pathobiological Sciences
School of Veterinary Medicine
University of Wisconsin
Madison, Wisconsin

Edward A. Mahaffey, DVM, PhD, Dipl ACVP
Associate Dean for Public Service and Outreach
College of Veterinary Medicine
University of Georgia
Athens, Georgia

James H. Meinkoth, DVM, PhD, Dipl ACVP
Associate Professor
Department of Veterinary Pathobiology
College of Veterinary Medicine
Oklahoma State University
Stillwater, Oklahoma

Cecil P. Moore, DVM, MS, Dipl ACVO
Chairman
Department of Veterinary Medicine and Surgery
University of Missouri-Columbia
Columbia, Missouri

Rebecca J. Morton, DVM, PhD, Dipl ACVM
Associate Professor
Department of Veterinary Pathobiology
College of Veterinary Medicine
Oklahoma State University
Stillwater, Oklahoma

Bruce W. Parry, BVSc, PhD, Dipl ACVP
Professor, Clinical Pathology
Department of Veterinary Science
University of Melbourne
Werribee, Victoria, Australia

Pauline M. Rakich, DVM, PhD, Dipl ACVP
Associate Professor
Department of Veterinary Pathology
Athens Diagnostic Laboratory
College of Veterinary Medicine
University of Georgia
Athens, Georgia

Steven H. Slusher, DVM, MS, Dipl ACT
Dubai, United Arab Emirate

Ronald D. Tyler, DVM, PhD, Dipl ACVP
Vice-President, Medicines and Safety Evaluations, USA
Glaxo-Wellcome, R&D
Research Triangle Park, North Carolina;
Adjunct Professor
Department of Veterinary Pathobiology
College of Veterinary Medicine
Oklahoma State University
Stillwater, Oklahoma

Joseph G. Zinkl, DVM, PhD, Dipl ACVP
Professor
Department of Pathology, Microbiology, and Immunology
College of Veterinary Medicine
University of California–Davis
Davis, California

Preface

Cytologic evaluation of blood, fluid, and tissue specimens is a valuable diagnostic aid in veterinary medicine. This textbook is intended to provide the basic and practical information required for veterinary students and practitioners to collect, prepare, and interpret cytologic specimens from blood, fluid, and tissue. It is also intended to aid students and practitioners in integrating cytologic findings from these samples with hematologic and other clinical pathology results, clinical signs, and other relevant information to arrive at the most specific diagnosis possible.

Diagnostic Cytology and Hematology of the Horse is a practical reference that presents common clinical findings in an easy-to-use text/atlas format. Following a general chapter on sample collections and techniques, the remainder of the book takes a "systems" approach. Within systems chapters, normal findings are presented first. Then abnormal findings are presented by "class" of problems, such as bacterial lesions, fungal lesions, parasitic lesions, and so on, as in the case of the eye. Algorithms (flow charts) on sample evaluations enhance text discussions by guiding readers to the most likely cytologic diagnosis. In addition, there is a color plate section featuring 64 illustrations for quick viewing and comparing cell types and infectious agents. The detailed index will aid utilization of this edition as a quick photographic and textual reference.

Many improvements have been incorporated in this edition, including:

- Completely revised/rewritten chapters on gastrointestinal tract, cerebrospinal fluid, and synovial fluid, reflecting new tests and methods of collection
- New tests and techniques
- Completely revamped art program, with hundreds of new full-color slides
- Updated terminology reflects current language used in the field (e.g., new bacterial/viral/protozoal species names)

We thank our families for their support and understanding. Many other people deserve sincere thanks and acknowledgment also. Two of these are Linda Duncan of Harcourt Health Sciences for her help and patience and Sherl A. Holesko for her typing and artistic skills.

It was a privilege to work with each of the many excellent authors and we thank them for sharing their time, talent, and expertise.

Rick L. Cowell
Ronald D. Tyler

Contents

DIAGNOSTIC CYTOLOGY AND HEMATOLOGY OF THE HORSE

CHAPTER 1

Introduction

Ronald D. Tyler, Rick L. Cowell, Charles G. MacAllister, Rebecca J. Morton, and Kimberly J. Caruso

When properly applied, cytologic examination can be an extremely powerful diagnostic aid.[1-11] Generally, cytologic samples can be collected quickly, easily, and inexpensively, with little or no risk to the patient. The cytologic interpretation often is valuable in establishing a diagnosis, identifying the disease process (neoplasia vs inflammation), directing therapy, forming a prognosis, and/or determining what diagnostic procedure should be performed next. Frequently, the samples can be prepared, stained, and interpreted while the client waits in the examination room. This allows other diagnostic procedures to be performed or therapy to be altered based on cytologic findings at the initial visit. As a result, the patient receives better and/or more expeditious care, and the client is more satisfied.

Risk vs. Value

The accuracy of cytologic examination as a diagnostic tool has been studied and reviewed in human and veterinary literature.[5,12-17] Most studies have compared cytologic results to histopathologic results and/or biologic behavior of the lesion. Some studies indicate that properly performed fine-needle aspiration biopsy (FNAB) is more accurate than conventional core needle biopsy or fine-aspirate core biopsy.[12,13,16] FNAB also poses very little risk to the patient. Complications subsequent to FNAB of abdominal organs (eg, liver, spleen, pancreas, prostate) or abdominal masses are much less than those expected for conventional core biopsy techniques.[17,19] In a study of 11,700 human patients, Livraghi et al concluded that *some* serious complications (peritonitis through the crossing of the digestive tract, fistula formation, bacteremia, tumor seeding), theoretically possible with FNABs, have either never occurred or occurred in such a tiny percentage of cases as to be regarded as negligible for practical purposes.[19] Implantation of malignant cells along the aspiration tract and induction of hematologic metastasis subsequent to FNAB of malignant tumors are extremely rare and pose no practical danger to the patient, especially when the aspiration tract is removed during excision of the malignant tumor.[12,14,19,20] However, some contraindications do exist and will be discussed in the relevant chapters.

Terminology

To facilitate the following discussions, some of the terms used throughout the text are briefly discussed here.

Hypertrophy refers to an increase in cell size and/or functional activity in response to a stimulus.

Hyperplasia refers to an increase in cell numbers, via increased mitotic activity, in response to a stimulus. If a tissue is capable of mitotic division, hyperplasia will occur in concert with hypertrophy.

Neoplasia refers to increased cell replication that is not dependent on a stimulus external to the neoplastic tissue.

Metaplasia refers to a reversible process in which one mature cell type is replaced by another mature cell type. It often represents the adaptive replacement of cells sensitive to a stimulus by cells less sensitive to the stimulus.

TABLE 1-1

Selected Chromatin Patterns

Pattern	Description	Schematic
Smooth (sometimes referred to as a "fine" chromatin pattern	Finely etched, uniform pattern of thin chromatin strands; no aggregates of chromatin	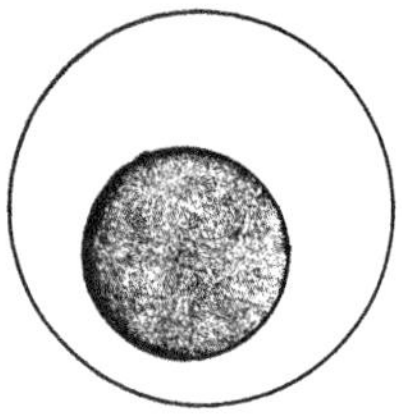
Finely stippled	Smooth chromatin pattern with small discrete aggregates of chromatin scattered throughout nucleus	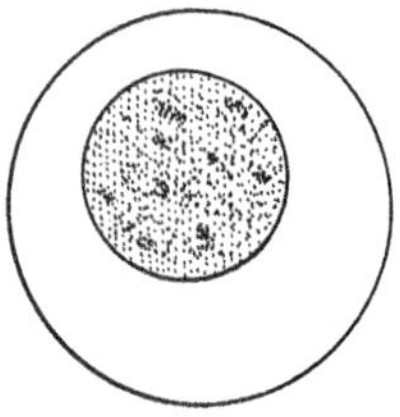
Lacy (reticular)	Uniform pattern of medium-sized chromatin strands; no significant aggregates of chromatin; sometimes "reticular" used to imply pattern with slightly thicker chromatin strands than in lacy patterns	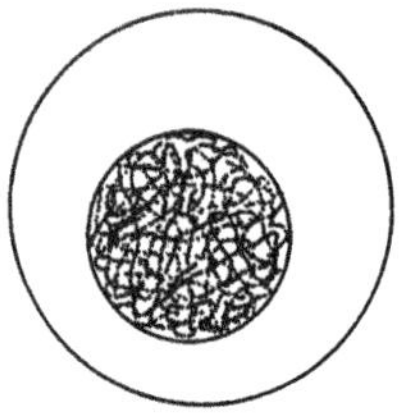
Coarse (ropy or cordlike)	Pattern of very thick chromatin strands	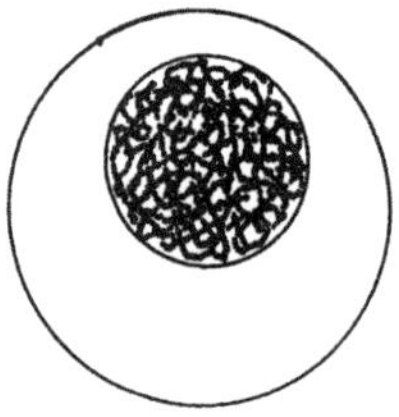
Clumped	Large aggregates of chromatin scattered throughout nucleus; may occur with lacy or coarse chromatin patterns	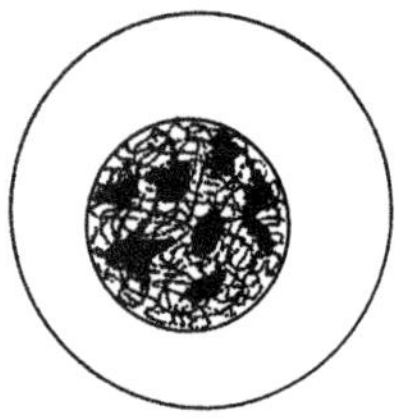
Smudged	Chromatin pattern not discrete; outlines of chromatin strands and/or clumps vague; usual pattern for small lymphocytes	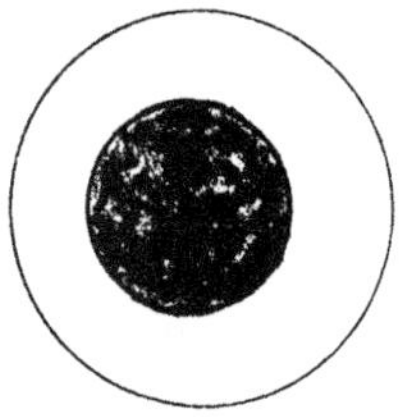

For example, chronic irritation of the ciliated columnar epithelial cells of the trachea and bronchi results in their focal or widespread replacement by stratified squamous epithelial cells.

Dysplasia, in common medical usage, refers to reversible, irregular, atypical, proliferative cellular changes in response to irritation or inflammation.

Anaplasia refers to a lack of differentiation of tissue cells. The less differentiated a tumor is, the more anaplastic it is and, generally, the greater its malignant potential.

Dyscrasia refers to an increase or decrease in the numbers of one or more cell components or maturational stages of a tissue out of proportion to the other cell components or maturational stages.

Chromatin pattern refers to the microscopic appearance of the nuclear chromatin. In general, the chromatin pattern coarsens as malignant potential increases. Some commonly used terms for chromatin patterns are listed, briefly described, and schematically depicted in Table 1-1.

Romanowsky-type stains, in this text, refers to hematologic stains (Wright's, Giemsa, Diff-Quik, etc) commonly used to perform differential WBC counts on peripheral blood smears.

Hematologic stains can refer to those stains commonly used in hematologic examination and include Romanowsky-type stains and supravital stains, such as new methylene blue, or may refer only to Romanowsky-type stains. The context of the discussion in which it is used generally makes its meaning obvious.

Collection and Smear Preparation

Cytologic samples can be collected by swabbing, scraping, or aspirating a lesion. The anatomic location and characteristics of the tissue being sampled and characteristics of the patient (eg, tractability) influence the choice of collection technique. The aim is always collection of an adequate quantity of representative material with minimal stress to the animal and danger to attendants. When possible, sufficient material should be collected to allow preparation of several slides so that some can remain unstained and available for special stains as necessary.

Specific techniques and preparation procedures will be discussed in the chapter dealing with the tissue for which they are used. General considerations for collection and preparation of cytologic samples are discussed in the following material.

Imprints

Imprints for cytologic evaluation can be prepared from external lesions or from tissues removed during surgery or necropsy. They are easy to collect but yield fewer cells than scrapings and contain greater contamination (bacterial and cellular) than FNABs. As a result, imprints from superficial lesions often only reflect a secondary bacterial infection and/or inflammation-induced tissue dysplasia. This markedly hinders their use in diagnosis of neoplasia.

Ulcers should be imprinted before they are cleaned. The lesion should then be cleaned with a saline-moistened surgical sponge and reimprinted or scraped. A FNAB of the tissue underlying the surface of the lesion should be collected also. In some conditions, such as *Dermatophilus congolensis* infection (streptothrichosis) and *Coccidioides immitis* infection, impressions from the uncleaned lesion contain far more organisms than impressions from cleaned lesions and samples collected by FNAB. Imprints of the underside of the scabs from *Dermatophilus congolensis*–produced lesions are usually most rewarding. In the healing phase of the disease (dry crusts), direct smears are rarely positive, and slides prepared from crusts that have been minced and soaked are preferred. Other conditions may yield more information on the imprints from cleaned lesions than the imprints from uncleaned lesions.

To collect imprints from tissues collected during surgery or necropsy, one must first cut the tissue so there is a fresh surface for imprinting. Next, remove excess blood and tissue fluid from the surface of the lesion being imprinted by blotting with a clean absorbent material. Excessive blood and tissue fluids inhibit tissue cells from adhering to the glass slide, producing a poorly cellular preparation. Also, excessive fluid inhibits cells from spreading and assuming the size and shape they usually have in air-dried smears. Blot excess blood and tissue fluids from the surface of the lesion, then touch (press) the surface of the lesion against the middle of a clean glass microscope slide and lift directly up. Do not slide the tissue around on the glass surface, since this causes cells to rupture. When possible, imprint several slides so that a few can be retained in case special stains are necessary.

Scrapings

Scrapings can be collected from tissues during necropsy or surgery or from external lesions on the living animal. Scraping a lesion generally collects more cells than does imprinting or aspirating. However, scrapings are generally more painful to the animal than imprints and do not collect cells as deeply as do FNABs. As a result, scrapings from superficial lesions often only reflect a secondary bacterial infection and/or inflammation-induced tissue dysplasia. This hinders their use in diagnosis of neoplasia. Scrapings are prepared by holding a scalpel blade perpendicular to the lesion's cleaned and blotted surface and pulling the blade toward oneself several times. The material collected on the blade is transferred to the middle of a glass microscope slide and spread by one or more of the techniques described for preparation of smears from aspirates of solid masses.

Swabs

Generally, swab smears are collected only when imprints, scrapings, and aspirates cannot be made, as with fistulous tracts. The lesion or area of interest is swabbed with a sterile cotton swab moistened with isotonic fluid, such as 0.9% NaCl. Moistening the swab helps minimize cell damage during sample collection and smear preparation. If the lesion is very moist, the swab need not be moistened. After sample collection, the swab is gently rolled along the flat surface of a clean glass microscope slide. *Do not rub the swab across the slide surface; this causes excessive cell damage.*

Aspiration of Masses

Fine-needle aspiration biopsies (FNAB) can be collected from raised cutaneous lesions, external and internal masses (including lymph nodes), and internal organs. They collect fewer cells than scrapings but avoid the superficial contamination that plagues imprints and scrapings.

Selection of Syringe and Needle: Fine-needle aspiration biopsies are collected with a 21- to 22-gauge needle and a 3- to 20-ml syringe. The softer the tissue, the smaller the needle and syringe used. It is seldom necessary to use a needle larger than 21 gauge for aspiration, even for firm tissues such as fibromas. When needles larger than 21 gauge are used, tissue cores tend to be aspirated, resulting in a poor yield of free cells. Also, larger needles tend to cause greater blood contamination.

The size of syringe used is influenced by the consistency of the tissue being aspirated. Softer tissues, such as lymph nodes, usually can be aspirated with a 3-ml syringe. Firm tissues, such as fibromas and squamous cell carcinomas, require a larger syringe to maintain adequate negative pressure (suction) for collection of a sufficient number of cells. A 12-ml syringe is a good choice if the texture of the tissue is unknown.

Preparation of the Site for Aspiration: If microbiologic tests are to be performed on a portion of the sample collected or if a body cavity (peritoneal and thoracic cavities, joints, etc) is to be penetrated, the area of aspiration is surgically prepared. Otherwise, skin preparation is essentially that required for a vaccination or venipuncture. An alcohol swab can be used to clean the area.

Aspiration Procedure: Hold the mass to be aspirated firmly; introduce the needle, with syringe attached, into the center of the mass; and apply strong negative pressure by withdrawing the plunger to about three-fourths

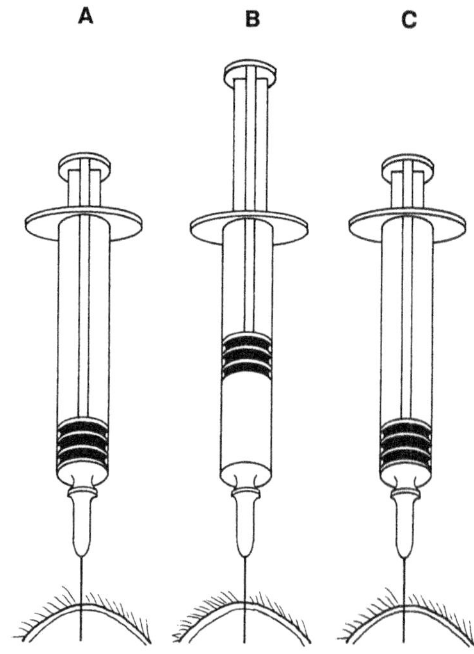

Fig. 1-1 Fine-needle aspiration from solid mass. After needle is in mass **(A)**, apply negative pressure to syringe by rapidly withdrawing plunger **(B)** one-half to three-fourths volume of syringe barrel. Redirect needle several times while maintaining negative pressure, if this can be accomplished without needle's point leaving mass. Before removing needle from mass, release plunger, relieving negative pressure on syringe **(C)**.

the volume of the syringe (Fig. 1-1). Sample several areas of the mass. Take care not to aspirate the sample into the barrel of the syringe or to contaminate the sample by aspirating tissue surrounding the mass. Therefore, maintain negative pressure during redirection and movement of the needle only when the mass is large enough to allow the needle to be redirected and moved to several areas within it without danger of the needle leaving the mass. When the mass is too small for the needle to be moved without danger of it leaving the mass, relieve negative pressure during movement of the needle. Often, high-quality collections do not have aspirated material visible in the syringe and sometimes not even in the hub of the needle.

After sampling several areas, relieve the negative pressure and remove the needle from the mass and skin. Remove the needle from the syringe and draw air into the syringe. Replace the needle onto the syringe and expel some of the tissue in the barrel and hub of the needle onto the middle of a glass microscope slide by rapidly depressing the plunger. When possible, make several preparations, as described below.

Nonaspiration Procedure (Capillary Technique, Stab Technique): A nonaspiration technique has been described for collection of cytology samples.[21] This technique works well for most masses, especially in highly vascular tissues. The technique described here is a modification of the nonaspiration technique that is used at Oklahoma State University. This technique is similar to the standard fine-needle aspiration technique except that no negative pressure is applied during collection.

Perform the procedure by placing a small-gauge needle (21 or 22 gauge) on a 5- to 12-cc syringe. Draw a few cubic centimeters of air into the syringe barrel prior to the collection attempt (to allow rapid expulsion of material onto a glass slide). Grasp the syringe at or near the needle hub with the thumb and forefinger to allow for maximal control. Or, as some clinicians prefer, grasp the syringe as if holding a throwing dart. Stabilize the mass to be aspirated with a free hand, and insert the needle into the mass. Move the needle rapidly back and forth in a stabbing motion, trying to stay along the same tract. This allows cells to be collected by cutting and tissue pressure. Take care to keep the needle tip within the mass to prevent contamination with surrounding tissue. Withdraw the needle and rapidly expel the material in the needle onto a clean glass slide, and then make a smear using one of the techniques listed later in this chapter. Having air already in the syringe saves time and allows the person collecting the sample to make the smear more quickly, thereby helping to avoid desiccation (drying-out) of the collected cells.

Generally, material sufficient for only one smear is collected. If possible it is optimal to perform multiple collection attempts at various sites within the mass to increase the chance of obtaining diagnostic material and to ensure a representative sampling of the lesion.

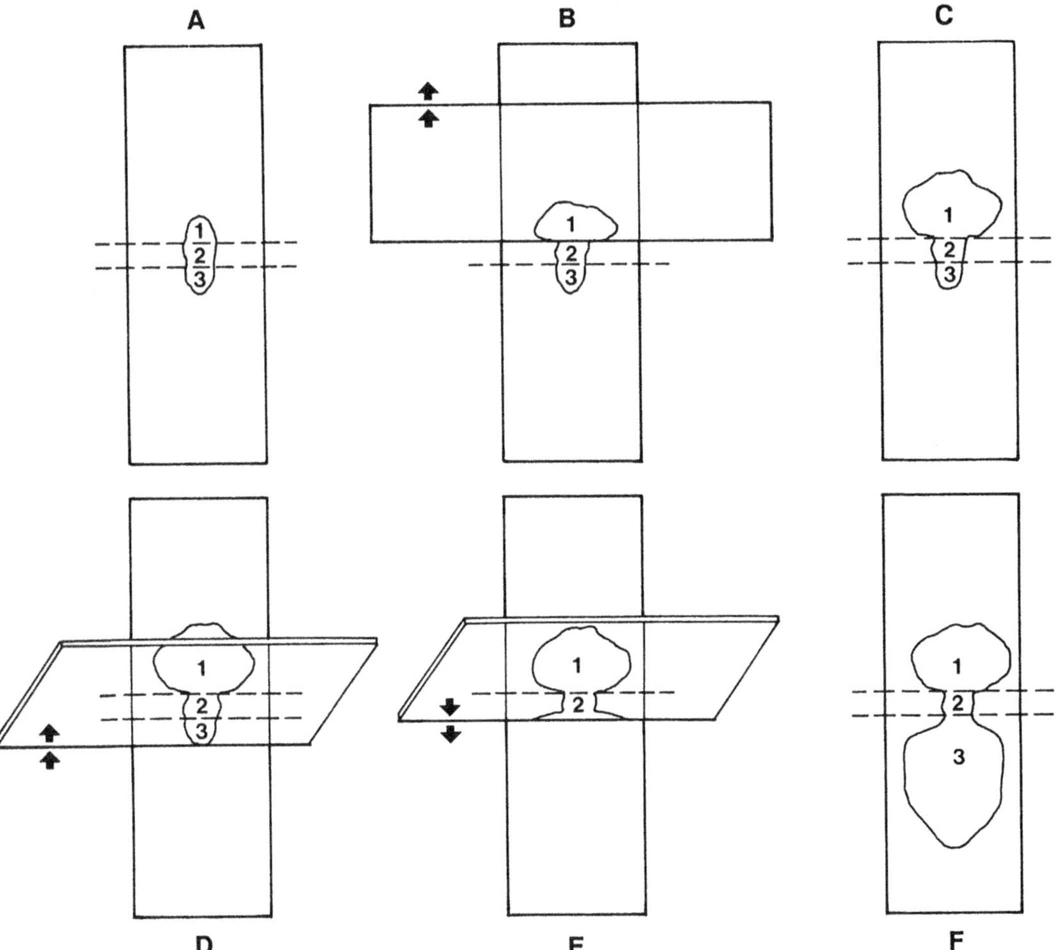

Fig. 1-2 Combination cytologic preparation.
A, Expel portion of aspiration onto glass microscope slide (prep slide). **B,** Place another glass microscope slide over about one third of preparation. Avoid excessive pressure. Slide spreader slide forward smoothly. **C,** This makes a squash preparation of about one third of aspirate (*area 1*). Spreader slide also contains a squash prep (not depicted). **D** and **E,** Slide edge of a tilted glass microscope slide (second spreader slide) backward from end opposite squash prep until it contacts about one third of expelled aspirate. Then slide second spreader slide rapidly and smoothly forward. **F,** This produces an area (*3*) that is spread with mechanical forces like those of blood smear preparation. Middle area (*2*) is left untouched and contains high concentration of cells.

Preparation of Smears from Aspirates of Solid Masses

Several methods can be used to prepare smears for cytologic evaluation of solid masses, including lymph nodes. The experience of the person preparing the smears and characteristics of the sample influence the choice of smear preparation technique. We suggest a combination of slide preparation techniques. Some cytologic preparation techniques are described here.

Combination Technique: One combination procedure involves spraying the aspirate onto the middle of a clean glass microscope slide (prep slide), which is held firmly on a flat, solid, horizontal surface. Place the edge of a second slide (spreader slide) onto the flat surface of the prep slide in front of the sample at a 45-degree angle to the prep slide and pull backward about one third of the way into the aspirate (Fig. 1-2). Slide the spreader slide forward smoothly and rapidly, as if making a blood smear. Next, place the flat surface of the spreader slide horizontally over the back third of the aspirate at a right angle to the prep slide. Allow the weight of the spreader slide (top slide) to spread the material, resisting the temptation to compress the slides. Keeping the spreader slide flat and horizontal, quickly and smoothly slide it across the prep slide.

This makes a squash prep of the back third of the aspirate. The front third of the aspirate is gently spread and the middle third is untouched. This accommodates all potential sample characteristics. The back third (squash prep area) will spread clumps of cells that are difficult to spread, the front third (gently spread area) will spread fragile cells without excessive damage, and the middle third (untouched) will allow best evaluation if the sample is of very low cellularity.

Squash Preps: In expert hands, the squash prep technique can yield excellent cytologic smears. However, in less experienced hands, it often yields smears that are unreadable because too many cells are ruptured or the sample is not sufficiently spread. Make a squash prep by expelling the aspirate onto the middle of one slide and then placing a second slide over the aspirate horizontal with and at right angles to the first slide (Fig. 1-3). Quickly and smoothly slide the second slide across the first slide. A modification of the squash prep that has less tendency to rupture cells is to lay the second slide over the aspirate, then rotate the second slide 45 degrees and lift it upward (Fig. 1-4).

"Starfish" Preps: Another technique for spreading aspirates is to drag the aspirate peripherally in several directions with the point of a syringe needle, producing a starfish shape (Fig. 1-5). This technique tends not to damage fragile cells, but it allows a thick layer of tissue fluid to remain around the cells. Sometimes the thick layer of fluid prevents the cells from spreading well and interferes with evaluation of cell detail. Usually some acceptable areas are present, however.

Preparation of Smears from Fluids

Cytologic smears should be prepared immediately after fluid collection. When possible, fluid samples for cytologic examination should be collected in ethylenediamine tetra-acetic acid (EDTA) tubes. Smears can be prepared directly from fresh, well-mixed fluid or from the sediment

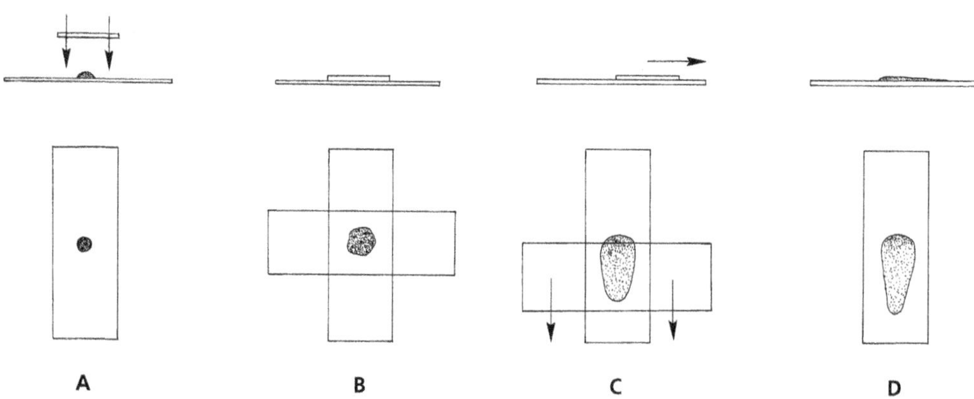

Fig. 1-3 Squash preparation.
A, Expel portion of aspirate onto glass microscope slide and place another slide over sample. **B,** This spreads sample. Take care not to place excessive pressure on slide, causing cells to rupture. **C,** Smoothly move slides apart. **D,** This usually produces well-spread smears but may result in excessive cell rupture.

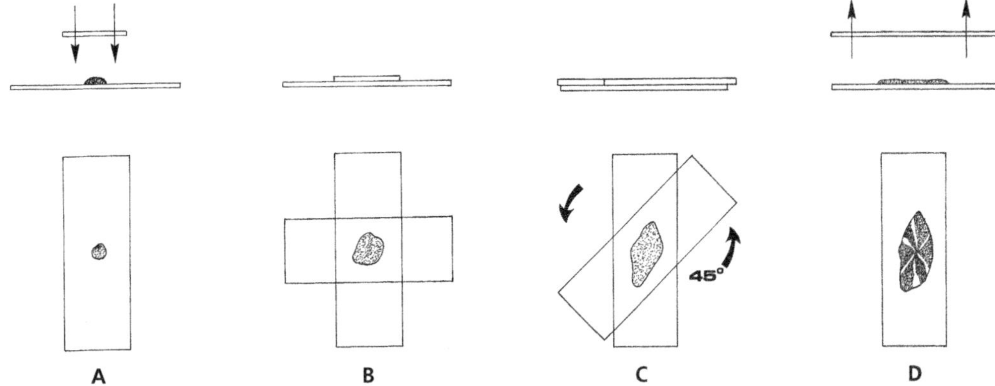

Fig. 1-4 Modification of squash preparation.
A, Expel portion of aspirate onto glass microscope slide and place another slide over sample. **B,** This spreads sample. Take care not to place excessive pressure on slide, causing cells to rupture. **C,** Rotate top slide about 45 degrees and lift directly upward, producing spread preparation with subtle ridges and valleys of cell **(D)**.

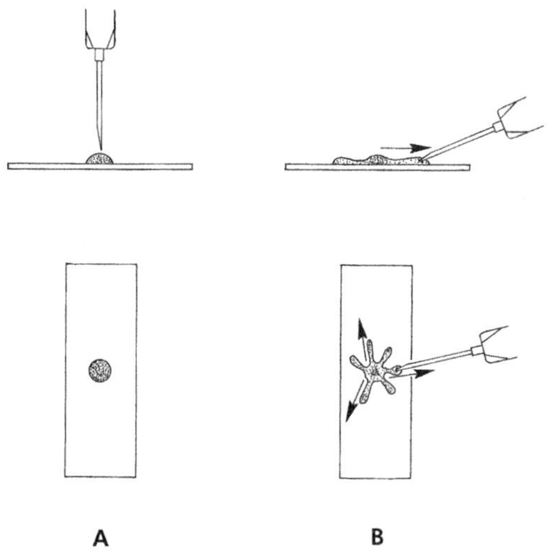

Fig. 1-5 Needle spread or "starfish" preparation.
A, Expel portion of aspirate onto glass microscope slide. **B,** Place tip of needle in aspirate and move peripherally, pulling trail of sample with it. Repeat procedure in several directions, creating preparation with multiple projections.

of a centrifuged sample using blood smear (Fig. 1-6), line smear (Fig. 1-7), and squash prep (see Fig. 1-3) techniques. The cellularity, viscosity, and homogeneity of the fluid influence the selection of smear technique.

The squash prep technique often spreads viscous samples and samples with flecks of particulate material better than the blood smear and line smear techniques. The blood smear technique usually produces well-spread smears of sufficient cellularity from homogeneous fluids containing ≥5000 cells/μl but often produces smears of insufficient cellularity from fluids containing <5000 cells/μl. The line smear technique can be used to concentrate fluids of low cellularity, but often it does not sufficiently spread cells from highly cellular fluids. In general, translucent fluids are of low to moderate cellularity, whereas opaque fluids are usually highly cellular. Therefore, translucent fluids often require concentration, either by centrifugation or by the line smear technique. When possible, concentration by centrifugation is preferred. To prepare a smear by the blood smear technique, place a small drop of the fluid on a glass slide about 1.0 to 1.5 cm from the end (see Fig. 1-6). Slide another slide backward at a 30- to 40-degree angle until it contacts the drop. When the fluid flows sideways along the crease between the slides, quickly and smoothly slide the second slide forward until the fluid has all drained away from the second slide. This makes a smear with a feathered edge.

To concentrate fluids by centrifugation, centrifuge the fluid for 5 minutes at 165 to 360 G. This is achieved by operating a centrifuge with a radial arm length of 14.6 cm (the arm length of most urine centrifuges) at 1000 to 1500 rpm. After centrifugation, separate the supernatant from the sediment and analyze for total protein concentration. Resuspend the sediment in a few drops of supernatant by gently thumping the side of the tube. Place a drop of the resuspended sediment on a slide and make a smear using the blood smear or squash prep technique. When possible, make several smears by each technique.

When the fluid cannot be concentrated by centrifugation or the centrifuged sample is of low cellularity, use the line smear technique (see Fig. 1-7) to concentrate cells in the smear. Place a drop of fluid on a clean glass slide and use the blood smear technique, except raise the

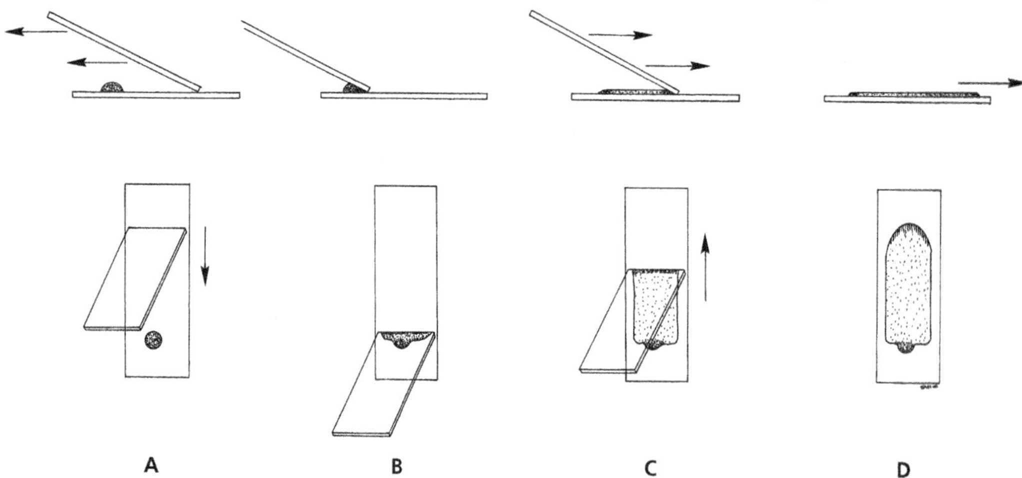

Fig. 1-6 Blood smear technique.
A, Place drop of fluid sample on glass microscope slide close to one end, then slide another glass slide backward to contact front of drop. **B,** When drop is contacted, it rapidly spreads along juncture between both slides. **C** and **D,** Slide spreader slide smoothly and rapidly forward along length of prep slide, producing smear with feathered edge.

spreading slide directly upward about three fourths of the way through the smear, yielding a line containing a much higher concentration of cells than the rest of the slide. Unfortunately, an excessive amount of fluid may also remain in the line and prevent the cells from spreading well.

Staining

Types of Stains

Several types of stains have been used for cytologic preparations. The two general types most commonly used are the Romanowsky-type stains (Wright's stain, Giemsa stain, Diff-Quik) and Papanicolaou stain and its derivatives, such as Sano's trichrome. The advantages and disadvantages of both types of stains are discussed later. However, because the Romanowsky-type stains are more rewarding, practical, and readily available in practice situations, the remainder of the text will deal predominantly with Romanowsky-type stained preparations.

Romanowsky Stains: Romanowsky-type stains are inexpensive, readily available to the practicing veterinarian, and easy to prepare, maintain, and use. They stain organisms and the cytoplasm of cells excellently. Though nuclear and nucleolar detail cannot be perceived as well with Romanowsky-type stains as with Papanicolaou-type stains, nuclear and nucleolar detail usually is sufficient for differentiating neoplasia and inflammation and for evaluating neoplastic cells for cytologic evidence of malignant potential (criteria of malignancy). Smears to be stained with Romanowsky-type stains are first air dried. Air drying partially preserves (*fixes*) the cells and causes them to adhere to the slide so they do not fall off during the staining procedure.

There are many commercially available Romanowsky-type stains, including Diff-Quik, DipStat, and other quick Wright's stains. Most, if not all, Romanowsky stains are acceptable for staining cytologic preparations. Diff-Quik does not undergo the metachromatic reaction. As a result, granules of some mast cells do not stain. When mast-cell granules do not stain, the mast cells may be misclassified as macrophages. This can lead to confusion in examination of some mast-cell tumors. The variation between different Romanowsky-type stains should not cause a problem once the evaluator has become familiar with the stain he or she uses routinely.

Each stain usually has its own unique recommended staining procedure. These procedures should be followed in general but adapted to the type and thickness of smear being stained and to the evaluator's preference. The thinner the smear and the lower the total protein concentration of the fluid, the less time needed in the stain. The thicker the smear and the greater the total protein concentration of the fluid, the more time needed in the stain. As a result, fluid smears with low protein and low cellularity, such as some abdominal fluid samples, may stain better using half or less of the recommended time. Thick smears, such as smears of neoplastic lymph nodes, may need to be stained twice the recommended time or longer. Each person tends to have a different technique that he or she prefers. By trying variations in the recommended time intervals for

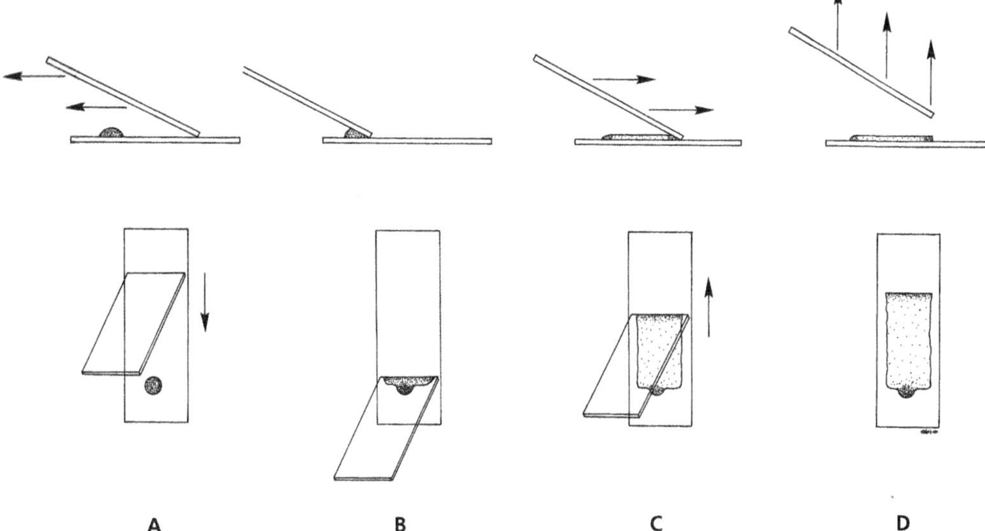

Fig. 1-7 Line smear concentration technique.
A, Place drop of fluid sample onto glass microscope slide close to one end, then slide another glass slide backward to contact front of drop. **B,** When drop is contacted, it rapidly spreads along juncture between both slides. **C,** Slide spreader slide smoothly and rapidly forward. **D,** After spreader slide has been advanced about two-thirds or three-fourths distance required to make smear with feathered edge, raise spreader slide directly upward. This produced smear with line of concentrated cells at its end instead of feathered edge.

stains, the evaluator can establish which times produce the preferred staining characteristics.

New Methylene Blue Stain: New methylene blue (NMB) stain is a useful adjunct to Romanowsky-type stains. It stains cytoplasm weakly, if at all, but gives excellent nuclear and nucleolar detail. Because NMB stains cytoplasm weakly, often the nuclear detail of cells in cell clumps can be visualized. Generally, RBCs do not stain but may develop a pale blue tint with NMB. As a result, marked RBC contamination does not obscure nucleated cells.

Papanicolaou Stains: The delicate Papanicolaou-type stains give excellent nuclear detail and delicate cytoplasmic detail. They allow the viewer to see through layers of cells in cell clumps and to evaluate nuclear and nucleolar changes very well. They do not stain cytoplasm as strongly as Romanowsky stains and, therefore, do not demonstrate cytoplasmic changes as well as Romanowsky stains. They also do not demonstrate bacteria and other organisms as well as Romanowsky stains.

Papanicolaou-type staining requires multiple steps and much time. Also, reagents often are difficult to locate, prepare, and maintain in practice. Papanicolaou stains and their derivatives require the specimen to be wet fixed, that is, the smear must be fixed before the cells have dried. Usually this is achieved by spraying the smear with a cytologic fixative or placing it in ethanol immediately after preparation. When the smear is to be placed in ethanol, it should be made on a protein-coated slide. This prevents the cells from falling off the slide when it is immersed.

Staining Problems

Poor stain quality often perplexes both the novice and the experienced cytologist. Most staining problems can be avoided if the following precautions are taken:

- Use new slides, fresh well-filtered (if periodic filtration is required) stain(s), and fresh buffer solution (if a buffer is required).
- Stain cytologic preparations immediately after air drying.
- Take care not to touch the surface of the slide or smear at any time.

Occasionally a sample may be contaminated with a foreign substance, such as K-Y Jelly and ultrasound gel, which alters the specimen's staining. Table 1-2 lists some of the problems that can occur with Romanowsky-type stains and some proposed solutions to these problems.

Microscopic Evaluation

After the smear has been stained and dried, it is scanned at low magnification (4× to 10× objective) to determine if all areas of the smear are stained adequately and if there are any localized areas of increased cellularity or areas

TABLE 1-2

Possible Solutions to Problems Seen with Common Romanowsky-type Stains

Problem	Solution
Excessive Blue Staining (RBC may be blue-green)	
Prolonged stain contact	Decrease staining time
Inadequate wash	Wash longer
Specimen too thick	Make thinner smears if possible
Stain, diluent, buffer, or wash water too alkaline	Check with pH paper and correct pH
Exposure to formalin vapors	Store and ship cytologic preparations separate from formalin containers
Wet fixation in ethanol or formalin	Air dry smears before fixation
Delayed fixation	Fix smears sooner if possible
Surface of slide alkaline	Use new slides
Excessive Pink Staining	
Insufficient staining time	Increase staining time
Prolonged washing	Decrease duration of wash
Stain or diluent too acidic	Check with pH paper and correct pH; may need fresh methanol
Excessive time in red stain solution	Decrease time in red stain solution
Inadequate time in blue stain solution	Increase time in blue stain solution
Mounting coverslip before preparation dry	Allow preparation to dry completely before mounting coverslip
Weak Staining	
Insufficient contact with stain solution(s)	Increase staining time
Fatigued (old) stains	Change stains
Another slide covered specimen during staining	Keep slides separate
Uneven Staining	
Variation of pH in different areas of slide surface (may result from slide surface being touched or slide being poorly cleaned)	Use new slides; avoid touching surface before and after preparation
Water allowed to stand on some areas of slide after staining and washing	Tilt slides close to vertical to drain water from surface or dry with fan
Inadequate mixing of stain and buffer	Mix stain and buffer thoroughly
Precipitate on Preparation	
Inadequate stain filtration	Filter or change stain(s)
Inadequate washing of slide after staining	Rinse slides well after staining
Dirty slides	Use clean new slides
Stain solution dries during staining	Use sufficient stain; do not leave stain on slide too long
Miscellaneous	
Overstained preparations	Destain with 95% methanol and restain; Diff-Quik–stained smears may have to be destained in red Diff-Quik stain solution to remove blue color, but this damages red stain solution
Refractile artifact on RBC with Diff-Quik stain (usually from moisture in fixative)	Change fixative

with unique features. If the smear is inadequately stained, it can be restained. However, not all areas of a slide need to be adequately stained. For example, only edges of thick smears may stain adequately, and yet the slides may be adequately evaluated. Any areas of increased and/or unique cellularity are mentally noted for future evaluation. Also, large objects, such as crystals, foreign bodies, parasites, and fungal hyphae, may be seen while scanning the slide at low magnification. When proper staining is assured and all areas of increased and/or unique cellularity are recognized, magnification is increased to the 10× or 20× objective. An impression of the cellularity and cellular composition (inflammatory cells, epithelial cells, spindle cells, etc) of the smear and of cell size usually is developed at this magnification. Areas of increased cellularity and/or unique cellularity are evaluated.

Next, the smear is viewed with the 40× objective. To improve resolution by decreasing light diffraction, a drop of oil can be placed on the smear; then a coverslip is placed over the drop of oil. This step is unnecessary if the microscope has a 50× (oil-immersion) objective instead of a 40× (dry) objective. At this magnification, individual cells are evaluated and compared to other cells in the smear. Usually, nucleoli and the chromatin pattern can be discerned. With experience, one can see most organisms visible microscopically with the 40× objective. However, it may be necessary to use the 100× (oil-immersion) objective to identify some organisms and inclusions and to confirm the identity of organisms seen with the 40× objective. Cell morphology (nuclear chromatin pattern, nucleoli, etc) is evaluated in detail with the 100× (oil-immersion) objective.

Interpretation

Cytologic examination can be a very useful tool for practicing veterinarians. While a definitive diagnosis is not always achieved, the general process (inflammation, etc) usually is recognized within a few minutes if a logical, methodical approach is used. Often definitive diagnosis is not necessary for practical management of the case. When a definitive diagnosis is necessary but cannot be achieved by cytologic examination, the cytologic results often help select the most rewarding procedure to perform next (eg, culture, biopsy, radiography). For example, a cytologic preparation containing only inflammatory cells, whether organisms are present or not, indicates that a culture might be helpful, whereas a preparation containing only tissue cells leads toward biopsy and away from culture.

Evaluation of a cytologic preparation should take only a few minutes once the evaluator has gained the basic skills of microscope operation. If cytologic changes are sufficient to establish a reliable diagnosis, they should be sufficiently plentiful and prominent for recognition within several minutes of serious viewing. When changes are not sufficiently plentiful or prominent for a reliable diagnosis, the preparation(s) should be sent to a veterinary clinical pathologist/cytologist for interpretation or an alternative diagnostic procedure should be employed. Occasionally, clinical and/or cytologic evidence of specific organism involvement is sufficient to merit a prolonged search for the organism suspected. For example, if a patient has clinical signs of coccidioidomycosis and macrophages and inflammatory giant cells are found in the cytologic preparation, a prolonged search for *Coccidioides immitis* might be rewarding. However, even in these cases, one should not spend so much time searching for the organism that it becomes frustrating. Instead, the cytologic preparation(s) should be sent to a veterinary clinical pathologist/cytologist or an alternative procedure used, such as biopsy or serologic testing.

Probably the most important judgment to be made when interpreting a cytologic sample is whether the lesion is inflammatory or neoplastic. If the lesion is strictly inflammatory, it can be treated with antiinflammatories, antibiotics, or other therapy. If the lesion is neoplastic in nature, however, it may need to be resected and/or treated by chemotherapy and/or radiation therapy. Often, the decision of whether the lesion is inflammatory or neoplastic is simple. Samples containing only inflammatory cells or inflammatory cells and a few nondysplastic tissue cells indicate an inflammatory lesion, whereas samples containing only tissue cells indicate a neoplastic or hyperplastic process. An admixture of inflammatory cells and tissue cells suggests either neoplasia with secondary inflammation or inflammation with secondary tissue cell dysplasia.

If there is confusion concerning whether the lesion is inflammatory or neoplastic, two approaches can be taken. First, the lesion can be treated with appropriate antibiotic therapy. If the lesion regresses, it was inflammatory. If the lesion does not regress, another aspirate can be taken to see if the inflammatory component has resolved, making the lesion recognizable as neoplastic. If the lesion does not regress and the decision of inflammation or neoplasia still cannot be made cytologically, the lesion can be removed or biopsied and submitted for histopathologic evaluation. Alternatively, without attempting treatment, the lesion can be removed and submitted for histopathologic examination.

Lesions determined to be inflammatory in nature can be classified into different categories of inflammation. Often, neoplastic lesions can be recognized as malignant or benign and as epithelial, mesenchymal (spindle-cell), or discrete round-cell tumors. Fig. 1-8 presents an algorithm to aid in general evaluation of cytologic preparations.

Inflammation

To determine the type of inflammatory lesion, the abundance and proportions of different inflammatory cells are evaluated. Types of inflammatory cells include

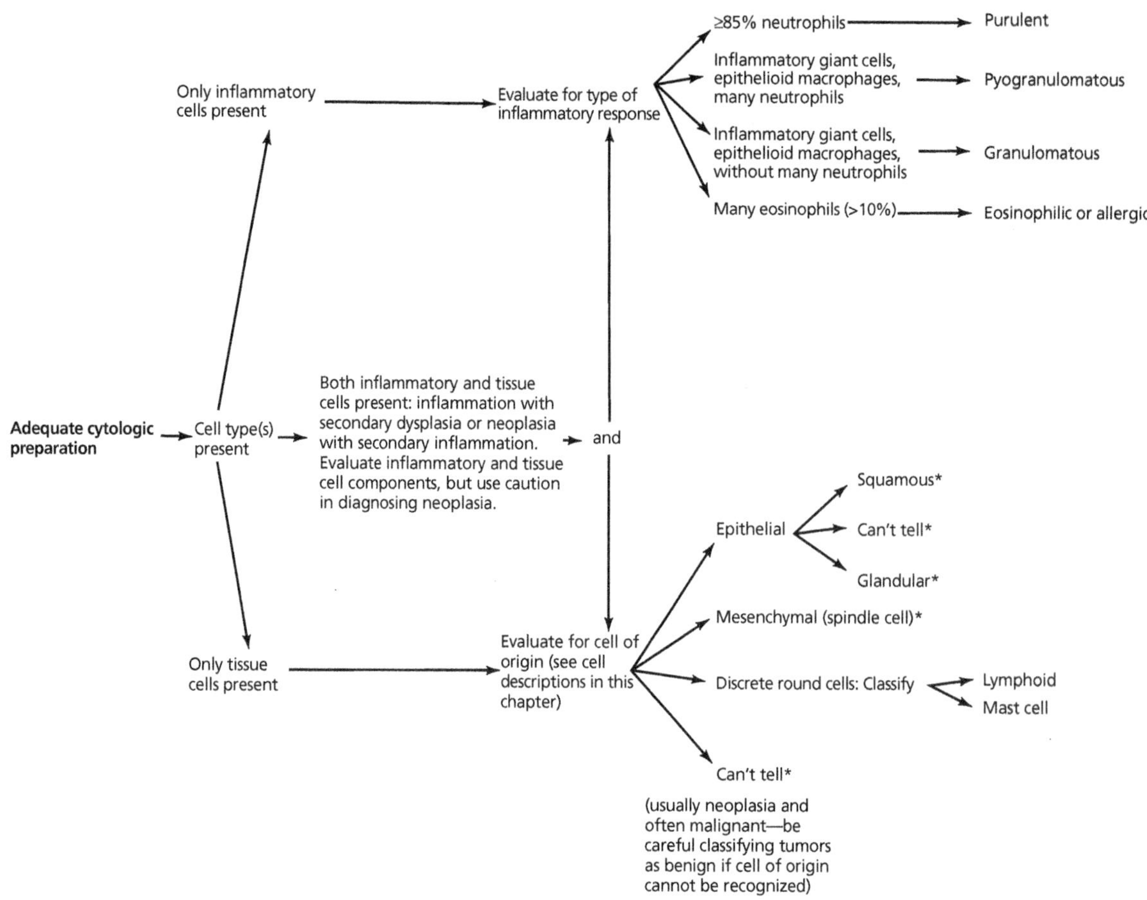

Fig. 1-8 Algorithm to aid evaluation of cytologic preparations.

neutrophils, eosinophils, tissue macrophages, epithelioid macrophages, and inflammatory giant cells. Also, a few mast cells may be present during some inflammatory responses, such as allergic inflammation.

Inflammation can be classified using terminology implying duration (acute, subacute, chronic-active, chronic) or by the type of inflammatory process (purulent, suppurative, granulomatous, eosinophilic). The qualifiers mild, moderate, and marked can be used to classify the severity of the inflammatory response.

The inflammatory process can be classified as acute when >70% of the inflammatory cells are neutrophils, as subacute or chronic-active when 50% to 70% of the inflammatory cells are neutrophils and 30% to 50% of the inflammatory cells are macrophages, and chronic when <50% of the inflammatory cells are macrophages.[9,10] The inflammatory response can be classified as purulent or suppurative if >85% of the inflammatory cells are neutrophils, granulomatous if inflammatory giant cells and/or numerous epithelioid macrophages are present, and eosinophilic or hypersensitivity reaction if eosinophils are numerous. The classifications of purulent/suppurative, granulomatous, and eosinophilic/allergic are not mutually exclusive. For example, purulent and granulomatous inflammation is termed "pyogranulomatous inflammation."

Neoplasia

When cellular components of a sample indicate the process is neoplastic, the neoplasm often can be recognized as an epithelial, mesenchymal (spindle-cell), or discrete round-cell tumor and/or benign or malignant.

Evaluation of Tumor Cell Types: Tumors are classified as epithelial, mesenchymal (spindle-cell), or discrete round-cell tumors based on their size, shape, and exfoliation characteristics (tendency to exfoliate individual cells or groups of cells and tendency to exfoliate numerous cells

TABLE 1-3

General Appearance of Basic Tumor Categories

Tumor Type	General Cell Size	General Cell Shape	Schematic Representation	Cellularity of Aspirates	Clumps or Clusters Common
Epithelial	Large	Round to caudate		Usually high	Yes
Mesenchymal (spindle cell)	Small to medium	Spindle to stellate		Usually low	No
Discrete round cell	Small to medium	Round	**Mast Cell** **Lymphosarcoma**	Usually high	No

or only a few cells) (Table 1-3). Some tumors do not demonstrate sufficient characteristics to be classified by cell types. Often, these tumors can be recognized as malignant. However, if they cannot be recognized as malignant, extreme caution should be used in classifying them as benign, since some types of malignant tumors show few cytologic criteria of malignancy. General characteristics of the different tumor cell types are described in the following discussion.

Epithelial neoplasms tend to exfoliate cells in sheets or clumps, though some individual cells usually are seen. Acinar or ductal arrangements may be identified with adenomas and adenocarcinomas. Cells from epithelial-cell tumors tend to be large to very large, with moderate to abundant cytoplasm and a round nucleus. The nucleus generally has a smooth to slightly coarse chromatin pattern that becomes more coarse and ropy as the tumor's malignant potential increases. The nucleus usually contains one or more prominent nucleoli that become larger and often irregular in shape as the tumor's malignant potential increases. Malignant epithelial-cell tumors often show marked variation in cellular, nuclear, and nucleolar size and shape. These variations are most significant when they occur within the same cell or same group of cells. Also, malignant epithelial-cell tumors often show a markedly increased nucleus to cytoplasm ratio and may show nuclear molding.

Benign epithelial-cell tumors not undergoing dysplasia subsequent to local inflammation or other irritation usually exfoliate cells indistinguishable from normal cells of the tissue of origin or cells that may be slightly more active than normal cells from the tissue of origin. The nucleolus may be a bit more prominent but still round and of reasonable size, the cytoplasm may be slightly more basophilic, and the nucleus to cytoplasm ratio may be mildly increased.

Local inflammation or other irritation can cause epithelial cells to become dysplastic. Epithelial cells undergoing dysplasia may show mild to moderate variation in cellular, nuclear, and nucleolar size and shape, increased nucleus to cytoplasm ratio, and coarse chromatin in a few cells. Dysplasia usually does not cause bizarre nuclear and nucleolar morphology. Again, when there is concern that the abnormal tissue cell morphology observed in a cytologic sample is caused by dysplasia, a biopsy from the lesion should be submitted for histopathologic evaluation or the cause of dysplasia should be treated and the lesion reevaluated cytologically.

Mesenchymal tumors are commonly referred to as spindle-cell tumors. These tumors tend to yield individual cells instead of groups, clumps, or sheets of cells, but a few groups of cells usually can be found. The term "spindle cell" arises from the fusiform or spindle shape of a few or many of the cells (depending on the specific cell of origin and malignant potential of the tumor). Spindle cells have a fusiform shape, with cytoplasmic tails trailing away from the nucleus in one or two directions. They usually are small to medium sized and have a moderate amount of light to medium blue cytoplasm. Nuclei are round to oval, stain with medium intensity, and have a smooth or fine lacy chromatin pattern. Usually nucleoli are not visible in nonneoplastic spindle cells. As malignant potential increases, nucleoli become prominent and the chromatin pattern becomes coarser. Also, the spindle shape of the cells becomes less prominent. Cytoplasmic basophilia and nucleus to cytoplasm ratio increase, and cellular, nuclear, and nucleolar size and shape vary markedly.

Spindle-cell tumors are often difficult or impossible to name cytologically. Also, granulation tissue produces plump, young fibroblasts that may have prominent criteria of malignancy. As a result, granulation tissue can be very difficult to differentiate from a spindle-cell neoplasm. In some cases, histopathologic examination may be necessary to definitively diagnose spindle-cell tumors.

Local inflammation or irritation can cause mesenchymal cells to become dysplastic. Cellular morphologic changes caused by dysplasia are very similar to changes caused by neoplasia but are usually mildly to moderately severe. Nuclear and nucleolar changes are less sensitive to dysplasia than cytoplasmic changes. If there is concern that cellular morphology is altered because of dysplasia instead of neoplasia, biopsy of the lesion should be submitted for histopathologic evaluation or, if possible, the stimulus for dysplasia (inflammation or irritation) can be treated and the lesion reevaluated cytologically.

Discrete round-cell tumors are also called cutaneous round-cell tumors and cutaneous discrete-cell tumors. These tumors tend to exfoliate small to medium-sized, single, round cells. The discrete round-cell tumors are mast-cell tumors and lymphosarcomas. Occasionally, malignant melanomas and basal-cell tumors also yield discrete round cells in cytologic smears.

Evaluation of Malignant Potential: The malignant potential of tumors is estimated by evaluating tumor cells for indications of anaplasia and asynchronous development (criteria of malignancy) (Table 1-4). Nuclear criteria of malignancy are more reliable than cytoplasmic criteria for estimating malignant potential. Cytoplasmic criteria of malignancy are more sensitive to cellular physiologic alterations caused by nonneoplastic processes, such as inflammation, than are nuclear criteria. As a result, cytoplasmic criteria of malignancy are encountered because of hyperplasia and/or dysplasia more commonly than nuclear criteria. Recognition of three or more nuclear criteria of malignancy in a high percentage of tumor cells is strong evidence that the tumor is malignant. When one to three criteria of malignancy are recognized in some tumor cells, the tumor may be

TABLE 1-4

Easily Recognized General and Nuclear Criteria of Malignancy

Criteria	Description	Schematic Representation
General Criteria		
Anisocytosis and macrocytosis	Variation in cell size, with some cell ≥1.5 time larger than normal	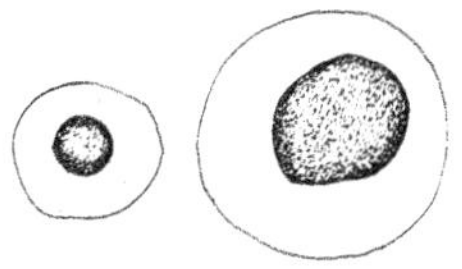
Hypercellularity	Increased cell exfoliation from decreased cell adherence	Not depicted
Pleomorphism (except in lymphoid tissue)	Variable size and shape in cells of same type	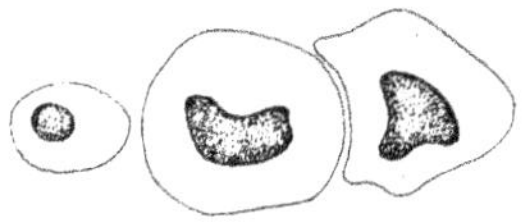
Nuclear Criteria		
Macrokaryosis	Increased nuclear size; cells with nuclei larger than 10μ in diameter suggest malignancy	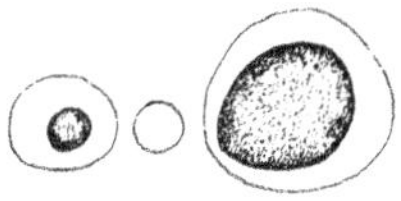 RBC
Increased nucleus to cytoplasm ratio (N:C)	Normal nonlymphoid cells usually have N:C of 1:3 to 1:8, depending on tissue; ratios ≥1:2 suggest malignancy	See Macrokaryosis
Anisokaryosis	Variation in nuclear size; especially important if nuclei of multinucleated cells vary in size	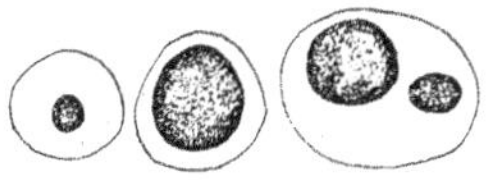
Multinucleation	Multiple nuclei in cell; especially important if nuclei vary in size	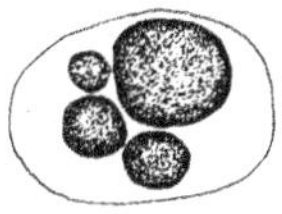
Increased mitotic figures	Mitosis rate in normal tissue	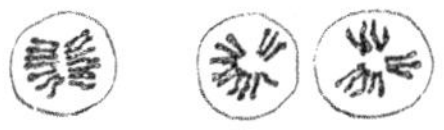 normal abnormal
Abnormal mitosis	Improper alignment of chromosomes	See Increased mitotic figures
Coarse chromatin pattern	Chromatin pattern coarser than normal; may appear ropy or cordlike	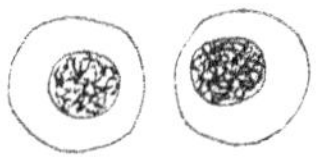
Nuclear molding	Deformation of nuclei by other nuclei within same or adjacent cell	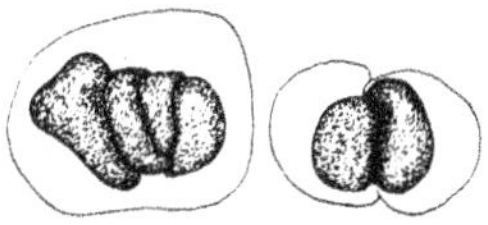
Macronucleoli	Nucleoli increased in size; nucleoli ≥5μ strongly suggest malignancy (for reference, RBCs are 5 to 6μ)	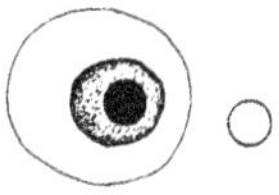 RBC
Angular nucleoli	Nucleoli fusiform or another angular shape instead of normal round to slightly oval shape	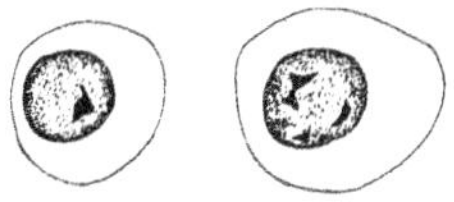
Anisonucleoliosis	Variation in nucleolar shape or size (especially important if variation occurs within same nucleus)	See Angular nucleoli

malignant or benign and histopathologic examination may be needed for definitive determination.

If malignant criteria are not recognized, the tumor is most likely benign. However, some tumors may be malignant but show few, if any, criteria of malignancy. Therefore, if the cell type of a tumor cannot be recognized or if the evaluator is not aware of which malignant tumor types are less likely to show criteria of malignancy, caution must be exercised in classifying the tumor as benign. Instead, the cytologic preparation can be sent to a veterinary clinical pathologist/cytologist for interpretation or a biopsy can be submitted for histopathologic examination.

Submission of Cytologic Preparations and Samples for Interpretation

When in-house evaluation of a cytologic preparation does not furnish sufficient reliable information for managing a case, the preparation can be submitted to a clinical pathologist/cytologist for interpretation or an alternative procedure, such as biopsy and histopathologic evaluation, can be performed. If possible, the person to whom the cytologic preparation is sent should be contacted and specifics concerning sample handling should be discussed, such as the number of smears to send, whether to fix or stain the smears before mailing, etc. The following discussion gives some general guidelines for submitting cytologic preparations for interpretation.

When possible, two or three air-dried unfixed smears and two or three air-dried Romanowsky-stained smears should be submitted. The air-dried unfixed smears can be stained by the pathologist with the Romanowsky-type or new methylene blue stains of his or her choice. The Romanowsky-stained smears are a safety factor. Some tissues stain poorly when they are air dried but not stained for several days. Also, slides occasionally are shattered during transport and cannot be stained upon receipt. Sometimes, microscopic examination of shards from the broken prestained smears allows diagnosis. If only a couple of smears can be prepared from the sample, one should be submitted air dried and unfixed and the other submitted air dried and stained. Smears should be well labeled with pencil, alcohol-resistant ink, or another permanent labeling method.

If a Papanicolaou-type stain is to be used, several wet-fixed smears should be submitted.

Fluid samples should have smears prepared from them immediately. Both direct smears and concentrated smears should be submitted. Also, an EDTA (lavender top) and serum tube (red top) fluid sample should be submitted. A total nucleated cell count and total protein concentration can be performed on the EDTA tube sample and, if necessary, chemical analyses can be performed on the serum tube sample.

Slides must be well protected when mailed. Simple cardboard mailers do not provide sufficient protection to prevent slide breakage if they are mailed in unpadded envelopes. Marking the envelope with such phrases as "Fragile," "Glass," "Breakable," and "Please Hand Cancel" have little success. Usually, placing a pad of bubble-paper or Styrofoam on each side of the slide holder prevents slide breakage. Also, slides can be mailed in plastic slide holders or innovative holders, such as small pill bottles. Slides should not be mailed with formalin-containing samples and should be protected against moisture. Formalin fumes alter the staining characteristics of smears and water causes cell lysis.

Submission of Samples for Culture

Culture results are strongly influenced by sample collection, preparation, and transport. Following are procedures suggested to optimize success in culturing lesions and fluids:

- Call the laboratory before collecting the sample.
- Collect the sample as aseptically as possible.
- Submit fresh samples for culture.
- Use proper equipment for collection and transport of the sample.
- Use a timely transportation service.

Call the Lab before Collecting the Sample

Techniques, media, days when cultures are read or subcultures are performed, and the like often vary from laboratory to laboratory. By contacting the laboratory to which the sample will be submitted, such things as optimum sample type, transport medium, and day of the week to submit the sample can be discussed. Also, some laboratories furnish culture supplies. Expensive and/or quickly outdated supplies, such as blood culture tubes, may be ordered from the laboratory as needed. Early communication with the laboratory also allows the laboratory to prepare for the sample and ensure that any special culture requirements are available.

Collect Samples as Aseptically as Possible

All samples should be collected as aseptically as possible. Even samples collected from lesions that naturally are exposed to secondary contamination, such as cutaneous ulcers, should be protected from further contamination. When samples are collected from more than one lesion, care should be taken not to cross-contaminate the samples. Finding the same organism in several different lesions is strong evidence that the organism is involved in development of the lesions. Therefore, cross-contamination of samples from different lesions can lead to misinterpretation of culture results. When fluids are collected, anticoagulant and serum tubes should not be assumed to be sterile.[8,22] Also, EDTA, through its effect on bacterial cell walls, can be bacteriostatic or bactericidal.

Submit Fresh Samples

Samples should be submitted as soon after collection as possible. Fluid aspiration, resection of lesions to be cultured, exploratory surgeries during which culture is anticipated, and other procedures that may produce samples to be cultured should be scheduled to allow immediate transportation of samples to the laboratory. During transport, samples should be kept cool but not frozen.

Tissue and fluid samples usually are more rewarding than swab samples for isolation of a causative agent. Individual tissue samples submitted for culture should be about 4 cm square or larger. Whirl-Pak bags (Nasco, Ft. Atkinson, WI), which are sterile and sealable, are excellent for submission of surgical biopsies in which the tissue surfaces need to be kept free of contaminants. Zipper-type or heat-sealable plastic bags, although not sterile, are fine for transport of tissue samples that have normal microbial flora or a contaminated surface. Tissues for anaerobic culture should be transported in self-contained atmosphere-generating anaerobic bags such as the Gas-Pak Pouch (Becton-Dickinson, Rutherford, NJ). Such samples as abscesses and skin, known to contain bacteria, must be packaged separately from other tissues. Culturette-type transport systems should be used to prevent small biopsies from drying during transport. Biopsies should not be shipped in sterile saline, since this may cause negative culture results.

Fluid samples (urine, milk, joint fluid, thoracic fluid, abdominal fluid, abscess aspirates) can be submitted in sterile Vacutainer tubes, small Whirl-Pak bags, or sterile disposable syringes. Fluids for anaerobic cultures should be collected in syringes, with air excluded, and then capped and transported immediately to the laboratory for culture. However, for optimal results or if a time delay is anticipated, the fluid should be placed in a transport system that supports both aerobic and anaerobic bacteria. These systems often can be obtained from the laboratory performing the culture. Containers such as Port-A-Cul Vials (BBL Microbiology Systems, Cockeysville, MD) are commercially available for fluid samples. These systems usually support a wide variety of anaerobic and aerobic organisms for up to 72 hours at 20° to 25° C.

When biopsies or aspirates are not obtainable or warranted, swabs are useful for sample collection, especially of mucosal surfaces and deep within soft tissue lesions. Culturette-type transport swabs such as Culture Collection and Transport Tube (Curtin Matheson Scientific, Burbank, CA) containing Amies medium with charcoal are suggested for aerobic cultures. These are excellent transport and holding media for fastidious bacteria. Anaerobic swab systems, such as the Marion Scientific Anaerobic Culturette (Kansas City, MO), have prereduced Cary-Blair transport medium and are necessary for transport of swabs for anaerobic culture. Swabs without medium can dry out in transport, resulting in false-negative results, whereas swabs submitted in broth medium often are overgrown by contaminants. Separate swabs should be submitted if additional cultures for fungi and/or viruses are desired.

In horses, elongated swabs often are needed to reach the sample site. Such swabs generally have an outer protective sleeve to prevent contamination when the swab must be passed through areas with normal bacterial flora or surface contaminants. Accu-CulShure swabs (Accu-Med, Pleasantville, NY) are guarded swabs with a self-contained transport medium and are available in various lengths. Other elongated, guarded swabs, such as Tiegland Swabs (Haver-Lockhart, Kansas City, KS) and Guarded Culture Instruments (Kalayjian Industries, Long Beach, CA), may be used to collect the sample. The swab then should be placed in an appropriate transport system by replacing the transport swab with the elongate swab, which is trimmed to an appropriate length to fit the transport tube.

In general, samples submitted for fungal culture, with the exception of dermatophyte suspects, should be collected and transported in the same manner as samples for bacterial culture. Again, tissues and body fluids are preferred to swabs. Suspect dermatophyte lesions should be cleaned gently with 70% alcohol to decrease bacterial contamination before plucking hair and scraping keratin scales from the periphery of the lesion. Dermatophyte samples need to be kept dry to inhibit growth of skin contaminants. Thus hair and scales should be transported in clean, dry, breathable containers such as envelopes or other paper containers. Tightly sealed glass or plastic tubes or containers often have condensate formation during transport and should not be used. Swab samples should never be submitted for dermatophyte cultures. If one is in doubt about proper sample submission or transport for fungal cultures, the rapid and easy solution is to contact the chosen laboratory.

REFERENCES

1. Allen and Prasse: Cytologic diagnosis of neoplasia and perioperative implementation. *Comp Cont Ed Pract Vet* 8:72-80, 1986.
2. Barton: Cytologic diagnosis of neoplastic diseases: an algorithm. *Texas Vet Med J* 45:11-13, 1983.
3. Boon et al: A cytologic comparison of Romanowsky stains and Papanicolaou-type stains. I. Introduction, methodology and cytology of normal tissues. *Vet Clin Pathol* 11:22-30, 1982.

4. DeNicola: Diagnostic cytology, collection techniques and sample handling. *Proc 4th Ann Mtg ACVIM*, 1987, pp 15-25.
5. Griffith and Lumsden: Fine needle aspiration cytology and histologic correlation in canine tumors. *Vet Clin Pathol* 13:13-17, 1984.
6. Meyers and Feldman: Diagnostic cytology in veterinary medicine. *Southwestern Vet* 25:277-282, 1972.
7. Meyers and Franks: Clinical cytology, management of tissue specimens. *Mod Vet Pract* 67:255-259, 1986.
8. O'Rourke: Cytology technics. *Mod Vet Pract* 64:185-189, 1983.
9. Rebar: Diagnostic cytology in veterinary practice. *Proc 54th Ann Mtg AAHA*, 1987, pp 498-504.
10. Rebar, in Kirk: *Current Veterinary Therapy VII*. Saunders, Philadelphia, 1980, pp 16-27.
11 Seybold et al: Exfoliative cytology. *VM/SAC* 77:1029-1033, 1982.
12. Bottles et al: Fine needle aspiration biopsy. *Am J Med* 81:525-529, 1986.
13. Cochland-Priolett et al: Comparison of cytologic examination of smears and histologic examination of tissue cores obtained by fine needle aspiration biopsy of the liver. *Acta Cytol* 31:476-480, 1987.
14. Kline and Neal: Needle aspiration biopsy: a critical appraisal. *JAMA* 239:36-39, 1978.
15. Kline et al: Needle aspiration biopsy: diagnosis of subcutaneous nodules and lymph nodes. *JAMA* 235:2848-2850, 1976.
16. Ljung et al: Fine needle aspiration biopsy of the prostate gland: a study of 103 cases with histological follow-up. *J Urol* 135:955-958, 1986.
17. Lundquist: Fine needle aspiration biopsy of the liver. *Acta Med Scand* (suppl) 520:1-28, 1971.
18. Mills and Griffiths: The accuracy of clinical diagnoses by fine-needle aspiration cytology. *Aust Vet* J 61:269-271, 1984.
19. Livraghi et al: Risk in fine needle abdominal biopsy. *J Clin Ultrasound* 11:77-81, 1983.
20. Zajicek: Aspiration biopsy cytology: 1. Cytology of supradiaphragmatic organs. *Monogr Clin Cytol* 4:1-211, 1974.
21. Menard and Papageorges: Fine-needle biopsies: how to increase diagnostic yield. *Comp Cont Ed Pract Vet* 19:738-740, 1997.
22. Meyer: The management of cytology specimens. *Comp Cont Ed Pract Vet* 9:10-16, 1987.

CHAPTER 2

Cutaneous and Subcutaneous Lesions

Masses, Cysts, and Fistulous Tracts

Ronald D. Tyler, James H. Meinkoth, Rick L. Cowell, Charles G. MacAllister, and Kimberly J. Caruso

Cytologic examination can be very useful when a cutaneous or subcutaneous lesion is not easily diagnosed by simple clinical evaluation, especially when such lesions are not responsive to therapy. Cutaneous and subcutaneous lesions are easily accessible, and there are no significant contraindications to collecting samples from them. Tranquilization and/or anesthesia is seldom needed for sample collection. Often the cytologic preparation can be collected, prepared, stained, and microscopically evaluated in minutes, providing a diagnosis, prognosis, indication of appropriate therapy, and/or indication of the next diagnostic procedure.

Collection Techniques

Lesions may be swabbed, imprinted, scraped, and/or aspirated, depending on the character of the lesion and the tractability of the patient. Ulcerated lesions should be imprinted, then cleaned, dried, and reimprinted. After imprints are made, scrapings should be obtained. Aspirates are then collected from deep within the lesion or mass. Obviously, lesions without an eroded or ulcerated surface must be aspirated.

Swabs

Generally, cytologic swab smears are collected only when imprints, scrapings, and aspirates cannot be made. Sterile cotton swabs moistened with sterile isotonic fluid, such as 0.9% NaCl, are used. Moistening the swab helps minimize cell damage during sample collection and smear preparation but is unnecessary if the lesion itself is very moist. After sample collection, gently roll the swab along the flat surface of a clean glass slide. Do not rub the swab across the slide surface, since this causes excessive cell damage. If a Romanowsky-type stain is used, air dry the smears before staining (see Chapter 1).

Imprints

Imprints are made by removing any scab covering the lesion and then touching the surface of a clean glass slide to the surface of the lesion. If *Dermatophilus congolensis* infection is suspected, the underside of the scab is imprinted also. The lesion is then cleaned with a nonirritating antiseptic, wiped dry with a sterile gauze sponge or other clean absorbent material, and reimprinted. High-quality cytologic smears can also be made by imprinting biopsy specimens (see Chapter 1).

Scrapings

Scrapings of cutaneous lesions are made by rubbing the edge of a blunt instrument, such as a glass slide or the back of a scalpel blade, across the lesion. This results in accumulation of cells along the edge of the blunt instrument. These cells are then spread onto a clean, dry glass slide by one of the techniques described in Chapter 1.

Aspirates of Solid Masses

Aspiration Technique: Aspirates are obtained by using a 20- to 25-gauge needle attached to a 3- to 20-ml syringe. If microbiologic evaluation is to be performed on a portion of the sample, the area of aspiration should be surgically prepared. Otherwise, skin preparation is essentially that required for vaccination or venipuncture. An alcohol swab can be used to clean the area.

Hold the mass to be aspirated firmly to aid penetration of the skin and mass and control the direction of the needle. Introduce the needle, attached to a syringe, into the center of the mass and apply strong negative pressure by withdrawing the plunger about one-half to three-fourths the volume of the syringe (see Fig. 1-1). Sample several areas of the mass, but avoid aspiration of the sample into the barrel of the syringe and contamination of the sample by aspiration of tissue surrounding the mass. To accomplish this, when the mass is large enough to allow the needle to be redirected and moved to several areas in the mass without danger of the needle's leaving the mass, maintain negative pressure during redirection and movement of the needle. However, when the mass is not large enough for the needle to be redirected and moved without danger of the needle leaving the mass, relieve the negative pressure during redirection and movement of the needle. In this situation, apply negative pressure only when the needle is static.

When aspiration is complete (often, high-quality collections do not have sample showing in the syringe and sometimes not even in the hub of the needle), release negative pressure from the syringe and remove the needle from the mass. If negative pressure is not released before the needle is removed from the mass, cells and blood from the subcutaneous tissues and skin may be aspirated into the sample and interfere with interpretation of the aspirate. If negative pressure remains on the syringe when the needle exits the skin, the portion of the sample in the barrel and hub of the needle will be aspirated into the syringe. Frequently, when only a small amount of sample has been collected and it is aspirated into the syringe, the sample cannot be recovered from the syringe and another sample must be collected. Once the negative pressure has been fully released, remove the needle from the mass and skin.

Then remove the needle from the syringe and aspirate air into the syringe. Next, replace the needle onto the syringe and expel some of the tissue in the barrel and hub of the needle onto the middle of a glass slide by rapidly depressing the plunger.

Nonaspiration Technique: Alternatively, a nonaspiration technique may be used. This has proved useful in some instances where adequate numbers of cells are difficult to retrieve without contaminating the sample with peripheral blood. With an aspiration technique, the tissue obtained will be the tissue of least resistance. Once small blood vessels are ruptured, peripheral blood will be the tissue of least resistance. The nonaspiration technique collects cells within the needle by capillary action after shearing cells loose from surrounding tissue with the point of the needle.

Use a needle and syringe of similar size as with the aspiration technique; however, fill the syringe with air before the aspiration procedure. Since aspiration is not required, hold either the distal end of the barrel of the syringe or the hub of the needle, gripping it like a pencil. This allows much greater control over directing the tip of the needle to the proper area. Firmly hold the mass to be aspirated with one hand, while using the other hand to guide the tip of the needle into the mass. Instead of aspirating, rapidly and repeatedly advance the needle through most of the thickness of the mass, using an action like a sewing machine. The repeated needle puncture of the tissue will dislodge some cells from the mass, creating a slurry of cells and tissue fluid. Some of this material will enter the needle. After 8 to 10 passages, withdraw the needle from the mass and expel the material onto a glass slide as usual. There is often enough material for just one slide in the needle. Repeated collections at various sites within the mass is recommended to get a representative sampling of the lesion.

Smears of Aspirates from Solid Masses

A combination of slide preparation techniques can be used to spread aspirates of solid masses (see Figs. 1-2 to 1-5). One combination procedure (see Fig. 1-2) is to spray the aspirate onto the middle of a slide (prep slide). Keeping the prep slide on a flat, solid, horizontal surface, pull another slide (spreader slide) backward at a 45-degree angle to the first slide until it contacts about one third of the aspirate. Then slide the spreader slide forward smoothly and rapidly as if making a blood smear. Next, place the spreader slide horizontally over the back third of the aspirate at a right angle to the prep slide. Use the weight of the top slide to spread the material, resisting the temptation to compress the slides manually. Keeping the top slide flat and horizontal, slide it quickly and smoothly across the prep slide. This makes a squash prep of the back third of the aspirate. The middle third of the aspirate is left untouched.

This procedure leaves the front third of the aspirate gently spread. If the aspirate is of fragile tissue, this area should contain sufficient unruptured cells to interpret. The back third of the aspirate has been spread with the shear forces of a squash prep. If the aspirate contains clumps of cells that are difficult to spread, there should be some clumps sufficiently spread in the back third of the preparation. If the aspirate is of very low cellularity, the middle third will be more concentrated and the most efficient area to study.

The squash prep (see Fig. 1-3) is commonly used to spread samples. In expert hands this procedure can yield excellent cytologic smears; however, in less experienced hands it often yields smears that cannot be evaluated because too many cells are ruptured or the sample is not sufficiently spread. Make a squash prep by expelling the aspirate onto the middle of a microscope slide (prep slide). Then place a second slide (spreader slide) over the aspirate at right angles to the first slide. Keeping the spreader slide horizontal with the prep slide, slide the spreader slide rapidly and smoothly across the prep slide. A modification of the squash preparation that has less tendency to rupture cells can be performed by placing the second slide (spreader slide) over the aspirate at right angles to the first slide (prep slide), then rotating the second slide 45 degrees and then lifting it upward (see Fig. 1-4).

Another technique for spreading aspirates (see Fig. 1-5) is to drag the aspirate peripherally in several directions with the point of a needle, producing a starfish-shaped preparation. This technique tends not to damage fragile cells but leaves a thick layer of tissue fluid around the cells. Sometimes the thick layer of fluid

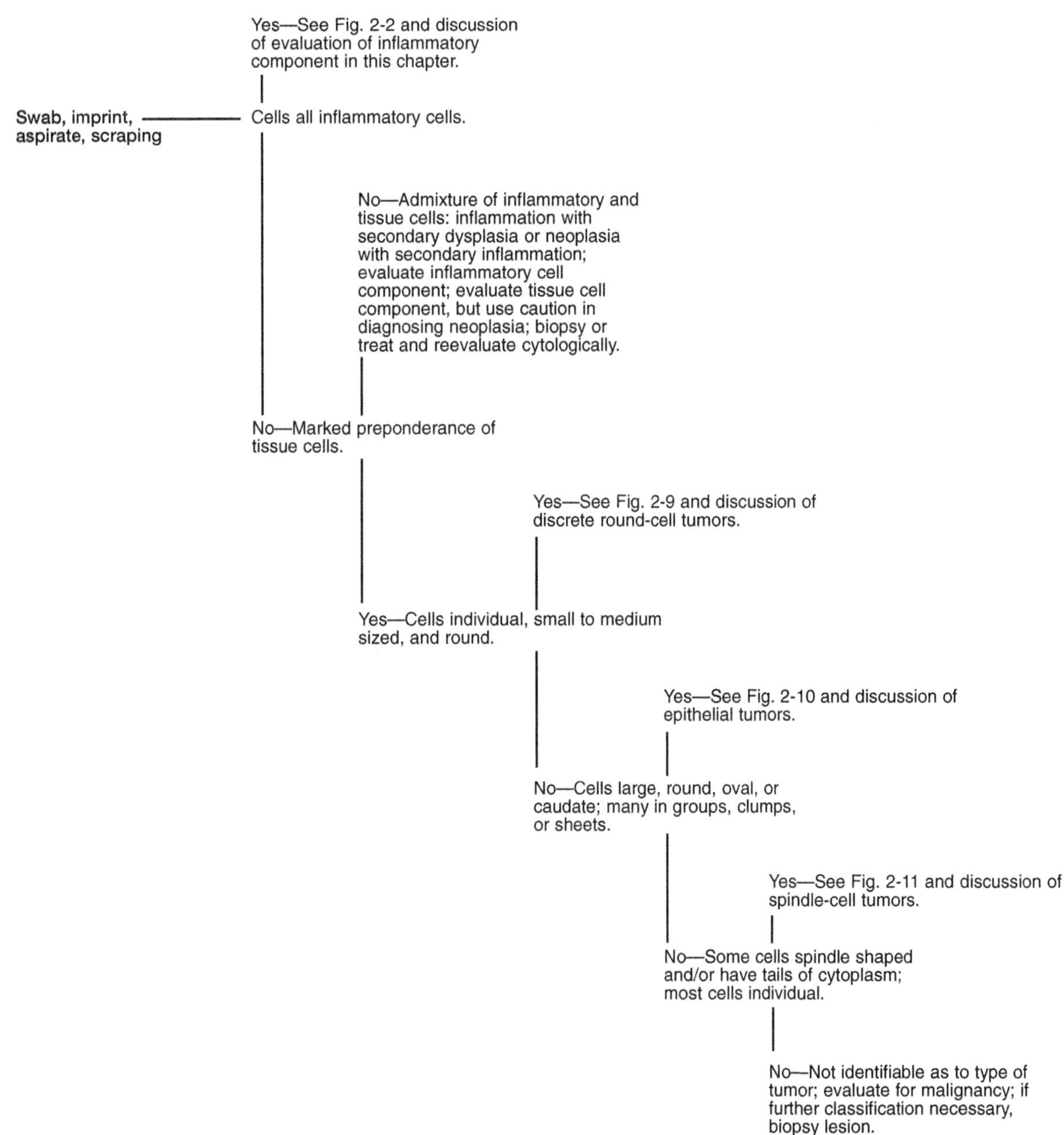

Fig. 2-1 Algorithm to aid classification of cellular components of cytologic preparations from solid lesions.

prevents individual cells from spreading well, causing them to appear contracted and interfering with evaluation of cell detail. Usually, however, some acceptable areas are present.

Aspirates of Fluid-Filled Masses and Cysts

Aspirates can be collected from fluid-filled masses and cysts with a 20- to 25-gauge needle attached to a 3-ml syringe. When possible, aspirate enough fluid to prepare several cytologic smears, perform a nucleated cell count and total protein analysis, and obtain a sample for culture. A sample of 1 to 3 ml usually is sufficient.

The lesion is prepared as described for solid masses. Smears can be prepared directly from the aspirated fluid or from the sediment of centrifuged fluid using the blood smear, line smear, and/or squash prep techniques as described in Chapter 1.

When lesions contain both solid and fluid areas, separate aspirates of each area should be collected if possible.

General Appearance of Lesion

The general physical appearance of the lesion is helpful in interpreting cytologic findings.

Fistulous Tracts

Fistulous tracts are usually caused by foreign bodies, bone sequestra, or infectious agents. They should be probed for foreign bodies and, if possible, radiographed for sequestra or osteomyelitis. Culture and cytologic swab samples should be collected from deep within the tracts. Cytologic preparations should be carefully perused for filamentous rods staining light blue with intermittent pink to purple dots with Romanowsky-type stains (Plate 3F). This morphology is characteristic of *Nocardia* spp. and *Actinomyces* spp., which can cause fistulous tracts, but occasionally occurs with some anaerobic bacteria also, such as *Fusobacterium* spp.

Ulcerated Lesions

Ulcerated lesions may be areas of skin that have been injured and/or infected and become ulcerated and indurated due to the subsequent inflammatory reaction or may be areas of ulcerated skin overlying a cutaneous or subcutaneous mass. Generally, physical examination of the lesion indicates whether there is an underlying mass. Ulcerated lesions can result from infectious, foreign body, allergic, parasitic, or neoplastic causes.

Nonulcerated Masses

Nonulcerated masses may be solid or fluid filled. Slowly developing, nonulcerated solid masses usually are neoplastic in origin. However, inflammatory conditions can produce rapidly developing, nonulcerated, solid masses. Fluid-filled nonulcerated masses usually are nonneoplastic in origin, but occasionally they represent cystic neoplasia.

General Evaluation of Cytologic Smears

The first step in cytologic evaluation of a smear is to determine whether sufficient numbers of intact cells are present and whether the sample is spread and stained adequately to allow evaluation of cell morphology. If repeated collection attempts fail to yield sufficient numbers of cells for cytologic evaluation, an alternative procedure, such as biopsy or culture (depending on the character of the lesion), may be necessary.

Once a suitable cytologic preparation has been produced, the smears are evaluated for evidence of inflammation and/or neoplasia (Fig. 2-1). If all the cells from a solid mass are tissue cells (ie, no inflammatory cells are present), either the lesion is caused by neoplasia or hyperplasia or the lesion was not sampled and surrounding tissues were sampled. If all the cells are inflammatory cells, an inflammatory process is most likely the primary cause of the lesion, but an inflamed neoplasm cannot be ruled out. An admixture of inflammatory cells and dysplastic tissue cells can be caused by inflammation with secondary tissue-cell dysplasia or neoplasia with secondary inflammation. Therefore, caution must be used in diagnosing neoplasia if evidence of inflammation is detected.

Evaluation of Inflammatory Cell Population

Fig. 2-2 provides an algorithm to aid evaluation of the inflammatory-cell component of cutaneous and subcutaneous lesions. Table 2-1 gives some general considerations for some inflammatory responses. If most of the inflammatory cells are neutrophils (Plates 1A-D, 3A) but no bacteria are found, a covert infection may be present or the neutrophilic inflammatory response may be due to one of the conditions listed under *Marked predominance of neutrophils* in Table 2-1. The lesion can be cultured to identify a covert infection. If culture results reveal an infectious agent, appropriate therapy can be instituted. If culture results do not reveal an infectious agent or if therapy for the infectious agent identified by culture is not effective, cytologic evaluation can be repeated or a biopsy can be submitted for histopathologic evaluation.

When >15% of the inflammatory cells are macrophages (Plates 2A-D, 3B) and/or giant inflammatory cells are present (Plate 3B), fungal infection or foreign body granuloma should be considered. The slide should be carefully perused for organisms or signs of foreign material, such as refractile debris (Fig. 2-3, *A*) or eosinophilic material typical of adjuvant (Fig. 2-3, *B*).

TABLE 2-1

Some Conditions Suggested by Certain Proportions of Inflammatory Cells

Inflammatory Cell Population	First Considerations	Second Considerations
Marked Predominance (85%) of Neutrophils		
Many neutrophils degenerate	Gram-negative bacteria Gram-positive bacteria	Abscess secondary to neoplasia, foreign bodies, etc
Few degenerate neutrophils	Gram-positive bacteria Gram-negative bacteria Higher bacteria (*Nocardia, Actinomyces,* etc)	Fungi Protozoa Foreign body Immune mediated Chemical or traumatic injury Abscess secondary to neoplasia
No degenerate neutrophils	Gram-positive bacteria Higher bacteria (*Nocardia, Actinomyces,* etc) Chemical or traumatic injury Panniculitis	Abscess secondary to neoplasia Fungi Foreign body Abscess secondary to neoplasia
Admixture of Inflammatory Cells		
15%-40% macrophages	Higher bacteria (*Nocardia, Actinomyces,* etc) Fungi Protozoa Neoplasia Foreign body Panniculitis Any resolving inflammatory lesions	Nonfilamentous gram-positive bacteria Parasites Chronic allergic inflammation
>40% macrophages	Fungi Foreign body Protozoa Neoplasia Panniculitis Any resolving inflammatory lesions	Parasites Chronic allergic inflammation
Giant inflammatory cells present	Fungi Foreign body Protozoa Collagen necrosis Panniculitis Parasites (if eosinophils are present)	
>10% eosinophils	Allergic inflammation Parasites Collagen necrosis Mast-cell tumor	Neoplasia Foreign body Hyphating fungi

Also, historical information concerning possible introduction of foreign material should be sought. If no organisms or foreign materials are found and there is no historical information indicating introduction of a foreign substance into the area, the tissue can be cultured or a biopsy can be submitted for histopathologic examination.

If the proportion of eosinophils exceeds 10% (Plate 3C), an allergic, parasitic, or foreign body reaction and certain hyphating fungi (eg, phycomycosis) should be considered. Again, the slide should be carefully searched for organisms or signs of foreign material. If none is found, the lesion can be cultured (including fungal cultures) or

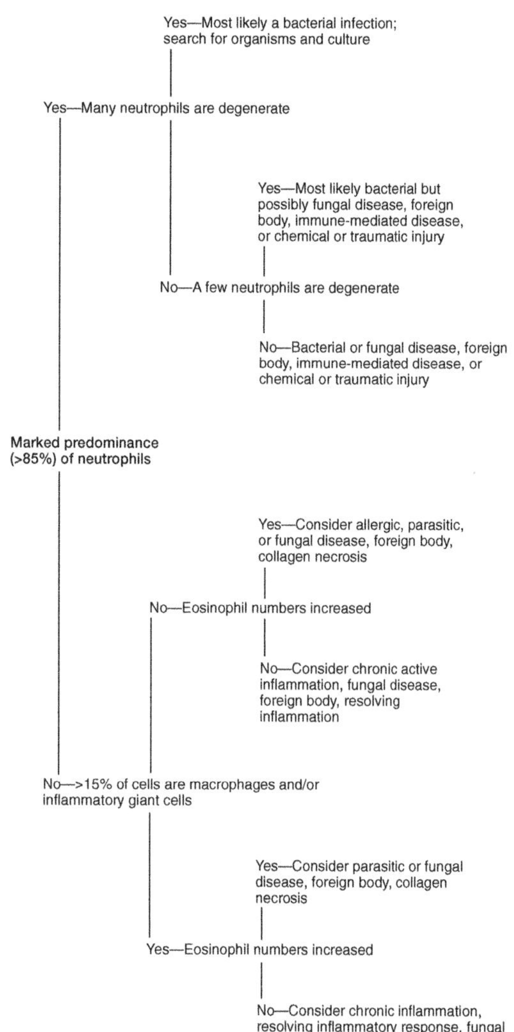

Fig. 2-2 Algorithm to aid in evaluation of aspirates containing preponderance of inflammatory cells.

a biopsy can be submitted for histopathologic evaluation.

When tissue cells showing criteria of malignancy are accompanied by inflammatory cells (Fig. 2-4), the sample should be interpreted cautiously. Dysplasia in tissue cells adjacent to inflammatory reactions can alter tissue cell morphology. As a result, cells undergoing dysplasia in response to a local inflammatory process can be erroneously classified as neoplastic cells. As the intensity of the inflammatory reaction increases, the assurance with which neoplasia can be diagnosed decreases.

Typical Cytologic Characteristics of Selected Infectious Agents

Infectious agents invariably cause lesions containing inflammatory cells. Bacteria usually produce lesions characterized by >85% neutrophils (Plates 1D, 3A) (many of which may be degenerate), a few macrophages, and a few lymphocytes and plasma cells. On the other hand, fungi tend to produce lesions containing more macrophages than in bacterial lesions, but neutrophils often predominate and occasionally eosinophils are plentiful with certain hyphating fungi. Mycotic lesions also often contain lymphocytes, plasma cells, and fibroblasts. The infectious agent, location of the lesion, chronicity of the lesion, and immune status of the animal influence the character of the lesion.

Bacterial Cocci

Most pathogenic bacterial cocci are gram positive and of the genus *Staphylococcus* or *Streptococcus* (Plate 3E). Staphylococci usually occur in clusters of 4 to 12 bacteria, while streptococci tend to occur in short or long chains of organisms. When cocci are identified in cytologic preparations and are considered as causing or contributing to the lesion, aerobic and anaerobic cultures and sensitivity tests should be performed to identify the organism and appropriate antibacterial therapy. Because most pathogenic cocci are gram positive, antibacterial therapy effective against gram-positive organisms should be used when it is necessary to initiate therapy before culture and sensitivity results are received.

Dermatophilus congolensis: *Dermatophilus congolensis* is an aerobic to facultatively anaerobic actinomycete that infects the superficial epidermis, causing exudative, crusty lesions. Removal of these crusty lesions reveals eroded to ulcerated skin lesions. Cytologic preparations from the undersurface of scabs from these crusty lesions are most rewarding in demonstrating organisms. These preparations usually contain mature epithelial cells, keratin bars, debris, and organisms. A few neutrophils may also be found. If the undersurface of scabs is dry and does not yield adequate cytologic preparations, crusts and scabs may be minced in saline and smears made for cytologic evaluation. *Dermatophilus congolensis* replicates by transverse and longitudinal division, producing chains of coccoid cells arranged in two to eight parallel rows. These chains resemble small, blue railroad tracks (Fig. 2-5). Also, many individual coccoid cells may be seen cytologically.

Small Bacterial Rods: Most small bacterial rods are gram negative; however, some, such as *Corynebacterium* spp, are gram positive. Some gram-negative rods can be recognized cytologically as bipolar (Plate 3D). All pathogenic bipolar bacterial rods are gram negative. Rod bacterial infections are usually associated with a marked neutrophilic inflammatory response. When small bacterial rods are recognized in cytologic preparations, the lesion should be cultured to identify the organism and sensitivity tests performed to determine appropriate antibacterial therapy. If it is necessary to institute antibacterial therapy before culture and sen-

A 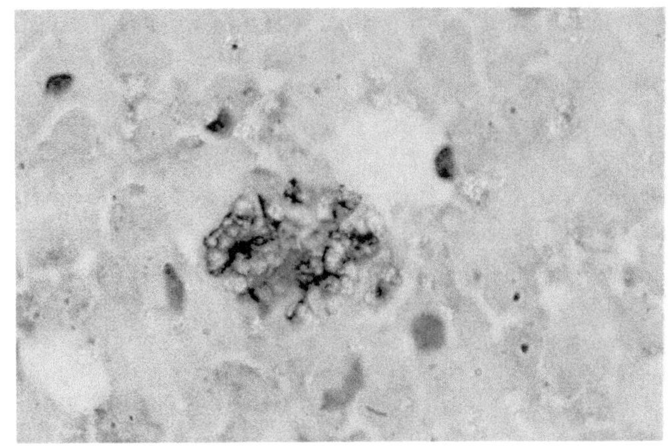

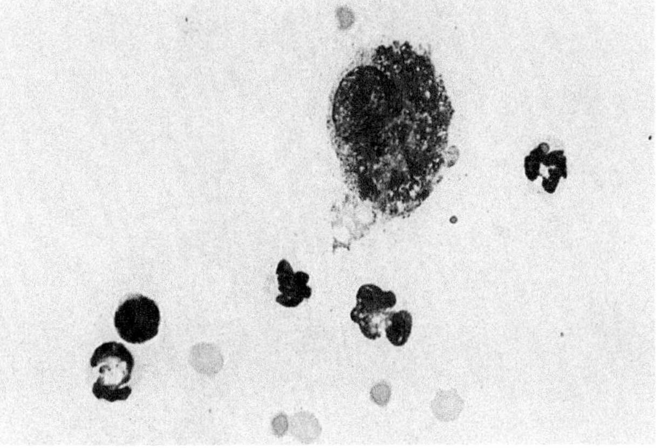 B

Fig. 2-3 Fine-needle aspirate.
A, Fine-needle aspirate from foreign body reaction. Refractile foreign material is scattered throughout micrograph. Large clump of cell debris and refractile foreign body is in center. (Wright's stain; original magnification 100X) **B,** Aspirate from injection site reaction in gelding. Large macrophage contains brightly eosinophilic noncellular material typical of adjuvant. Scattered neutrophils are also present. (Wright's stain; original magnification 125X)

sitivity results are received, therapy employed should be effective against gram-negative organisms, since most pathogenic small rods are gram negative.

Filamentous Rods: Filamentous rods that can cause cutaneous infections include *Nocardia* spp., *Actinomyces* spp., certain anaerobes (eg, *Fusobacterium* spp.), and *Mycobacterium* spp. Because these organisms are often refractory to common antibacterial therapy and reliable culture of these organisms has special requirements, cytologic evaluation is very useful in indicating that special cultures are needed.

Rarely, the pathogenic filamentous rods of *Nocardia* spp or *Actinomyces* spp. (Plate 3F) may cause cutaneous or subcutaneous lesions (abscesses, ulcers, draining tracts, lumps) in horses. These lesions are sometimes referred to as actinomycotic mycetomas. Infection with these agents is uncommon and usually occurs secondary to contamination of existing wounds.[1] Also, *Mycobacterium* spp. and some anaerobes, such as *Fusobacterium*, rarely may be filamentous. *Nocardia* and *Actinomyces* generally have a distinctive morphology in cytologic preparations stained with Romanowsky-type stains. They are characterized by long, slender (filamentous) strands that stain pale blue and have intermittent, small, pink to purple areas (dots). This morphology is characteristic of both *Nocardia* and *Actinomyces* spp. and the filamentous form of *Fusobacterium* spp. When these features are recognized cytologically, cultures should be performed specifically for *Nocardia*, *Actinomyces*, and anaerobes.

Mycobacterium spp. (atypical mycobacterial infections and cutaneous tuberculosis), on the other hand, often do not stain with Romanowsky-type stains. As a result, negative images (Plate 4A-B) may be observed in the cytoplasm of macrophages and/or inflammatory giant cells. When epithelioid macrophages and/or inflammatory giant cells are encountered in cytologic preparations not containing any obvious organisms, a careful search for negative images of *Mycobacterium* spp. should be made. *Mycobacterium* spp. stain with acid-fast stains. Therefore, when negative images are encountered or when the character of the lesion suggests *Mycobacterium* spp., an acid-fast stain can be performed to demonstrate the organism

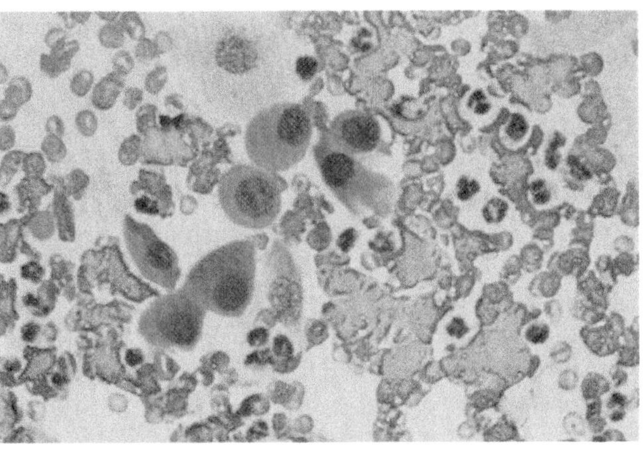

Fig. 2-4 Aspirate from nasal polyp caused by *Rhinosporidium seeberi.*
Note dysplastic epithelial cells (mild anisocytosis, anisokaryosis, prominent nucleoli, coarse chromatin, cytoplasmic basophilia) and numerous neutrophils. *Rhinosporidium* organisms were found in other areas of smear. (Wright's stain; original magnification 100X)

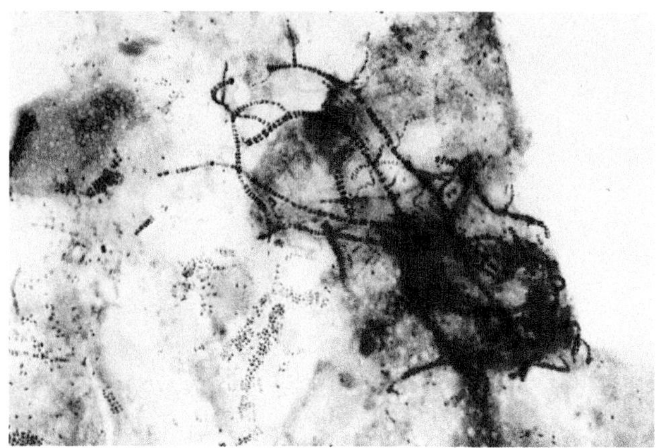

Fig. 2-5 Imprint from underside of scab caused by *Dermatophilus congolensis.*
There is a background of squamous debris and numerous chains of bacterial doublets. Scattered individual bacteria are also present. (Wright's stain; original magnification 250X)

and/or cultures for *Mycobacterium* spp. can be performed to identify the organism.

Large Bacterial Rods: Large bacterial rods found in cytologic preparations may be pathogenic or nonpathogenic. Those that are pathogenic and sometimes infect cutaneous and subcutaneous tissues include *Clostridium* spp. and, infrequently, *Bacillus* spp. When large bacterial rods are thought to be pathogenic, both aerobic and anaerobic cultures should be performed. Also, the smears should be inspected for large bacterial rods that contain spores.

Sporothrix schenckii: *Sporothrix schenckii* infection (sporotrichosis) (Plate 4D) most commonly occurs in a cutaneolymphatic form; however, a primary cutaneous form with no lymphatic involvement is seen occasionally. In the cutaneolymphatic form, hard subcutaneous nodules develop along lymphatics and the lymphatics may become *corded*. The nodules may ulcerate. In horses, the organisms are scarce and cytologic preparations must be perused carefully. If organisms are not found, the lesion should be cultured and a biopsy of the lesion should be submitted for histopathologic evaluation.

In cytologic preparations stained with Romanowsky stains, *Sporothrix schenckii* organisms are round to oval to fusiform (cigar shaped). They are 3 to 9 μ long and 1 to 3 μ wide and stain pale to medium blue with a slightly eccentric pink to purple nucleus (Plate 4D). They may be confused with *Histoplasma capsulatum* if only a few organisms are found and the classic fusiform (cigar shape) is not seen.

Histoplasma capsulatum, Blastomyces dermatitidis, Cryptococcus neoformans, and Coccidioides immitis: Cutaneous lesions secondary to infection with *Blastomyces, Cryptococcus, Coccidioides*, or *Histoplasma* organisms are rare. These organisms may on rare occasion produce a primary cutaneous lesion or disseminate from other sites and secondarily infect the skin.[2-4] Characteristics of these organisms in cytologic preparations stained with Romanowsky-type stains are as follows:

Histoplasma organisms (Plate 4C) are round to slightly oval but are not fusiform or cigar shaped. They are 2 to 4 μ in diameter (about half the size of a RBC), stain pale to medium blue, and contain an eccentric pink to purple nucleus. There is usually a thin, clear halo around the yeast.

Blastomyces dermatitidis organisms are blue, spherical, 8 to 20 μ in diameter, and thick walled (Plates 4E-G). Most organisms are single, but occasionally those showing broad-based budding are found. Imprints of these lesions usually have a cell composition characteristic of pyogranulomatous inflammation (Plate 3B) and few to many organisms.

Cryptococcus neoformans organisms are spherical and usually have a thick mucoid capsule; occasionally, nonencapsulated (rough) forms are found. The organism is 4 to 8 μ in diameter excluding the capsule and 8 to 40 μ in diameter including the capsule. The organism stains light pink to blue-purple and may be slightly granular (Plate 4H). The capsule usually is clear and homogeneous, but it may stain light to medium pink. Cryptococcosis usually evokes a minor granulomatous response of epithelioid macrophages and/or inflammatory giant cells. In some cytologic preparations, *Cryptococcus* organisms may outnumber inflammatory and tissue cells. Weakly encapsulated (rough) forms tend to elicit a greater inflammatory response than heavily encapsulated forms.

Coccidioides immitis organisms are large (10 to 100 μ in diameter), double-contoured, blue to blue-green spheres with finely granular protoplasm (Plate 5A). Round endospores 2 to 5 μ in diameter may be seen in larger organisms. Cytologic preparations usually have a cell composition characteristic of pyogranulomatous or granulomatous inflammation (Plate 3B). *Coccidioides* organisms usually are scarce. The tremendous variation in size, presence of endospores, and green tint to the organism differentiate *Coccidioides immitis* from nonbudding *Blastomyces dermatitidis*.

Dermatophytes: The dermatophytes *Trichophyton* spp. and *Microsporum* spp. cause cutaneous lesions that may have the typical ringworm-like appearance or appear as gray to yellow-brown crusty lesions or as follicular papules.[2] Scrapings from the edge of the lesion are most rewarding when searching for dermatophytes.

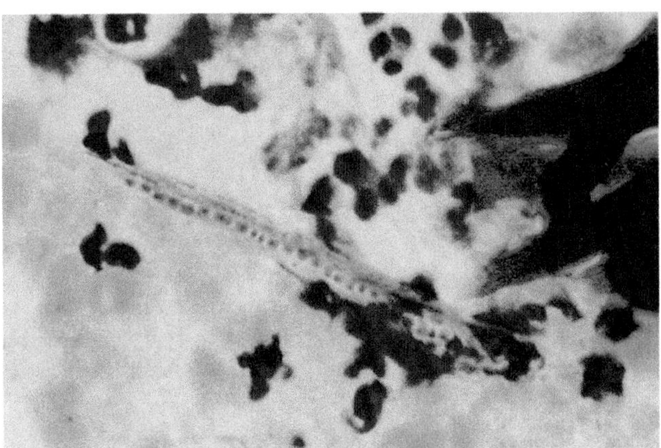

Fig. 2-6 Scraping from animal with ringworm. Several degenerating neutrophils are present, along with RBCs and a row of dermatophyte organisms attached to a hair shaft. (Wright's stain; original magnification 330X)

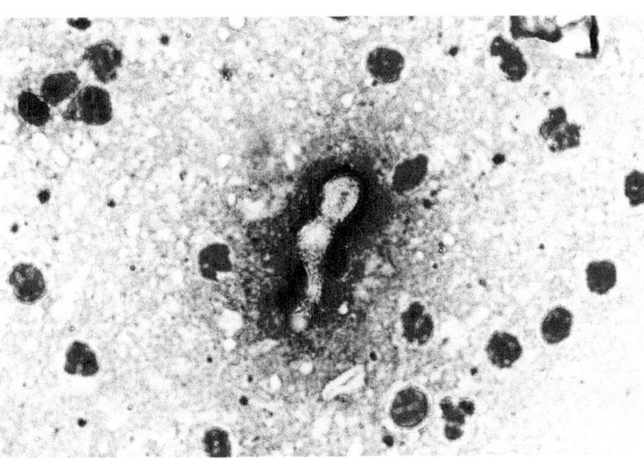

Fig. 2-7 Aspirate from cutaneous mass on horse. Negative image of poorly staining fungal hyphae is evident in center. (Wright's stain; original magnification 250X) (Courtesy Oklahoma State University.)

They can be identified in cytologic preparations using the standard 20% potassium hydroxide, in wet mount preparations stained with new methylene blue, or in air-dried preparations stained with Romanowsky-type stains. Cytologically, conidia are found free within the smears as well as within hair shafts (endothrix invasion) or on the hair shaft surface (ectothrix invasion). With Romanowsky-type stains, conidia stain medium to dark blue with a thin clear halo (Fig. 2-6). An inflammatory reaction composed of an admixture of neutrophils, macrophages, lymphocytes, eosinophils, and plasma cells may be seen in cytologic preparations from skin scrapings.

Fungi That Form Hyphae in Cutaneous and Subcutaneous Tissues: Many fungi can infect and form hyphae in cutaneous and subcutaneous tissues. They may cause single or multiple, small to very large lesions that range from nodules to ulcers to draining tracts. These fungi induce a granulomatous inflammatory response characterized by epithelioid macrophages and inflammatory giant cells (Plates 3B, 5B). Neutrophil, lymphocyte, plasma-cell, and eosinophil numbers are variable. Phaeohyphomycosis refers to infections by pigmented fungi. While most fungi stain well with Romanowsky-type stains, some do not and are recognized as negative images (Fig. 2-7 and Plate 5C).

Fungal culture or histopathologic examination with special immunohistochemical stains may be used to definitively classify the fungus.

Leishmania: *Leishmania donovani* can infect skin and subcutaneous tissues of horses, producing small to very large, thickened, nonhealing ulcerated areas with depressed granulating centers.[5] Imprints, scrapings, and aspirates yield numerous admixed neutrophils, macrophages, lymphocytes, and plasma cells. Either neutrophils or macrophages may predominate. Usually, numerous, small (2 to 4 μ), round to oval organisms with light blue cytoplasm, a red, oval, eccentric nucleus, and a small dark (red-purple) kinetoplast at right angles to the nucleus usually are found within macrophages and free in the preparation (Plate 5E).

Noninfectious Inflammatory Lesions

Some inflammatory lesions are not caused by infectious agents. Such conditions as immune-mediated diseases, allergic reactions, and sterile foreign body reactions elicit inflammatory lesions. Cytologic evaluation along with clinical evaluation may be helpful in diagnosing these lesions.

Allergic Inflammatory Reactions: Cytologically, allergic inflammatory reactions often are characterized by numerous eosinophils (Plate 3C). Neutrophil and mast-cell numbers are variable. Lymphocytes, plasma cells, and macrophages may also be present if the condition is chronic.

Parasite-Induced Inflammatory Reactions: Parasite-induced inflammatory reactions are characterized by numerous eosinophils and few to many neutrophils. Macrophages may be present in large numbers also. Variable numbers of lymphocytes and plasma cells may be present; occasionally, the parasitic organism is found.

Immune-Mediated Skin Lesions (Pemphigus): Cytologic preparations from immune-mediated skin lesions such as pemphigus usually contain many nondegenerative neutrophils. Acantholytic squamous epithelial cells may

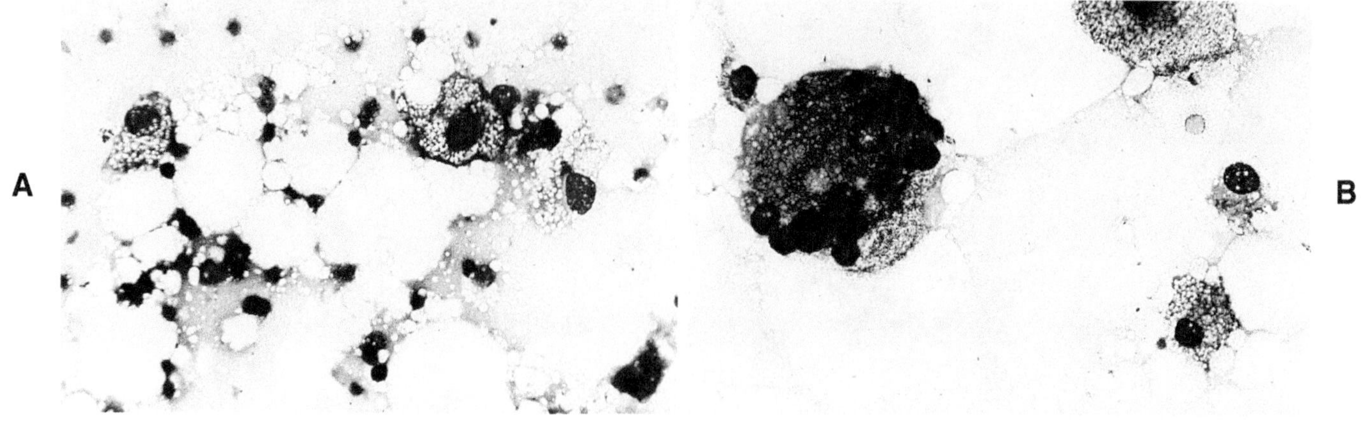

Fig. 2-8 Cytologic preparation from area of fat necrosis.
A, Numerous macrophages interspersed among normal fat droplets. Macrophages contain many fine clear vacuoles within their cytoplasm. (Wright's stain; original magnification 50X) **B,** Large multinucleated inflammatory giant cell and scattered macrophages. (Wright's stain; original magnification 125X)

be present and are highly suggestive of pemphigus foliaceus. Acantholytic epithelial cells are noncornified squamous cells that are rounded and intensely basophilic. They are often scattered individually (due to loss of cohesion) among the inflammatory cells. A few lymphocytes and plasma cells may be present. Open lesions may be secondarily infected. While cytologic findings may be suggestive of these lesions, definitive diagnosis requires histopathologic evaluation and immunofluorescent studies of properly collected and prepared biopsy specimens.

Traumatic Skin Lesions: Traumatic skin lesions may be caused by physical, thermal, or chemical injury. Cytologic preparations from these lesions usually contain numerous neutrophils and may contain abundant necrotic material and/or bacteria from secondary infection. History and physical examination usually help establish the suspicion of either physical, thermal, or chemical injury.

Sterile Foreign Body–Induced Inflammation: Cytologic preparations from inflammatory lesions induced by sterile foreign bodies usually contain an admixture of neutrophils and macrophages. Many of the macrophages in foreign body reactions may be epithelioid macrophages; inflammatory giant cells may be present also. Occasionally eosinophils are present. Lymphocytes and plasma cells may be present in variable numbers. Sometimes refractile material can be found (see Fig. 2-3, *A*). When a sterile foreign body is suspected, the smear can be viewed under polarized light. Some foreign material refracts polarized light, whereas endogenous breakdown products, such as hemosiderin, that might be mistaken as particulate foreign body material do not refract polarized light.

Injection Site Reactions: Sometimes, vaccinations or other injections can result in foreign body reactions. The cytologic reaction is similar to other forms of foreign body reactions, but the vaccine adjuvant or drug vehicle may be seen as an amorphous brightly eosinophilic material either extracellularly or within macrophages (see Fig. 2-3, *B*).

Fat Necrosis/Steatitis/Panniculitis: Necrosis and inflammation of adipose tissue (steatitis/panniculitis) rarely occurs in horses. It may present as single or multiple, nodule, and/or plaque-like lesions. Cytologic preparations from areas of fat necrosis/steatitis/panniculitis usually contain variable numbers of inflammatory cells intermixed with numerous lipid droplets (Fig. 2-8). The inflammatory cells are predominantly macrophages and a few to many large, multinucleated, inflammatory giant cells may be observed also (Fig. 2-8, *B*). Reactive spindle cells may be present. Often the spindle cells are dysplastic and, if caution is not used, can be misclassified as neoplastic.

Eosinophilic Granuloma with Collagen Degeneration: This condition, also termed nodular necrobiosis, nodular collagenolytic granuloma, collagenolytic granuloma, eosinophilic granuloma, or acute collagen necrosis, is characterized by single or multiple nodules that are generally well circumscribed and firm. Collagen degeneration elicits an inflammatory response characterized by marked infiltration of eosinophils and monocytes, with development of epithelioid macrophages and inflammatory giant

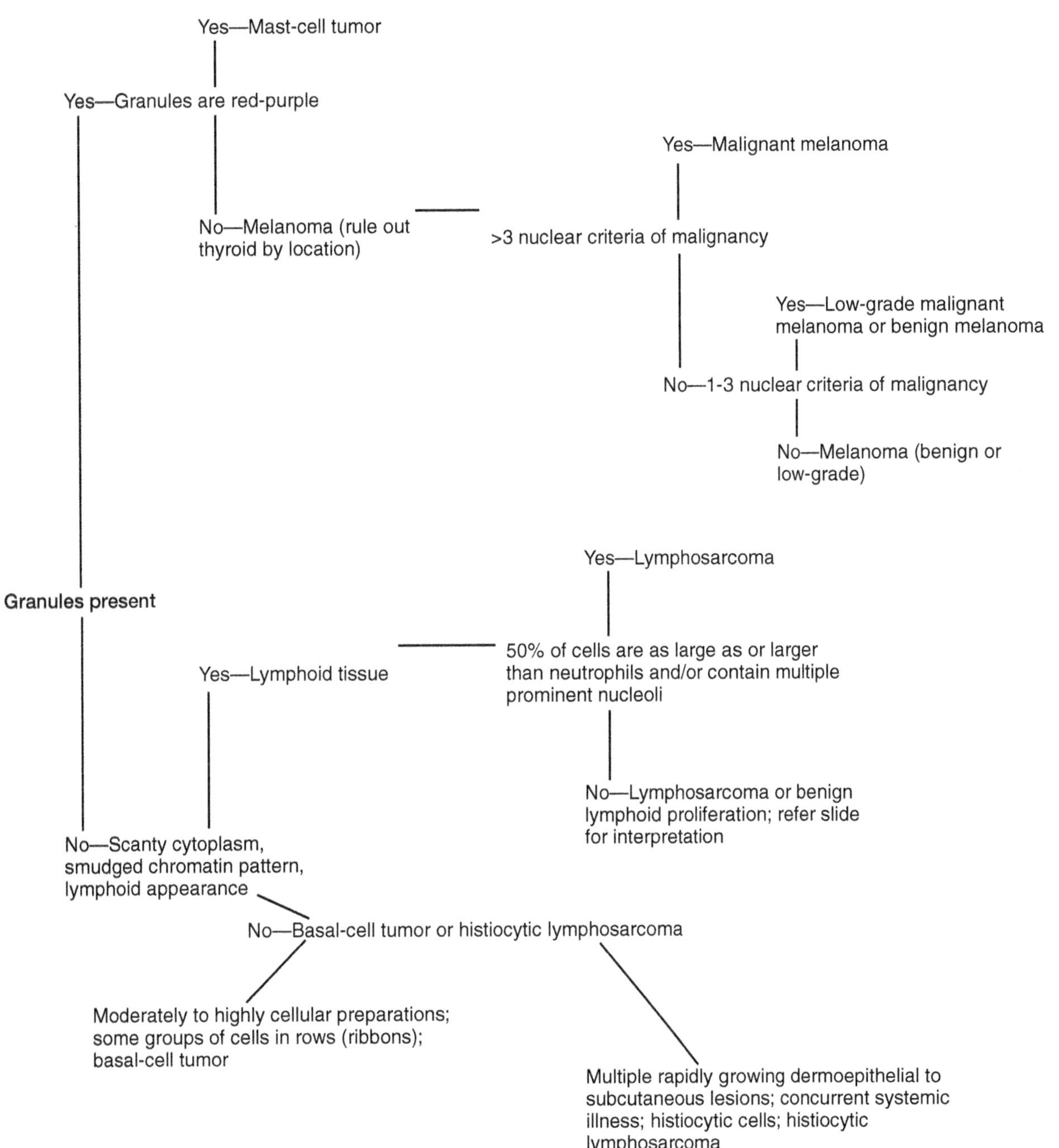

Fig. 2-9 Algorithm to aid in evaluation of aspirates containing discrete round cells from solid masses.

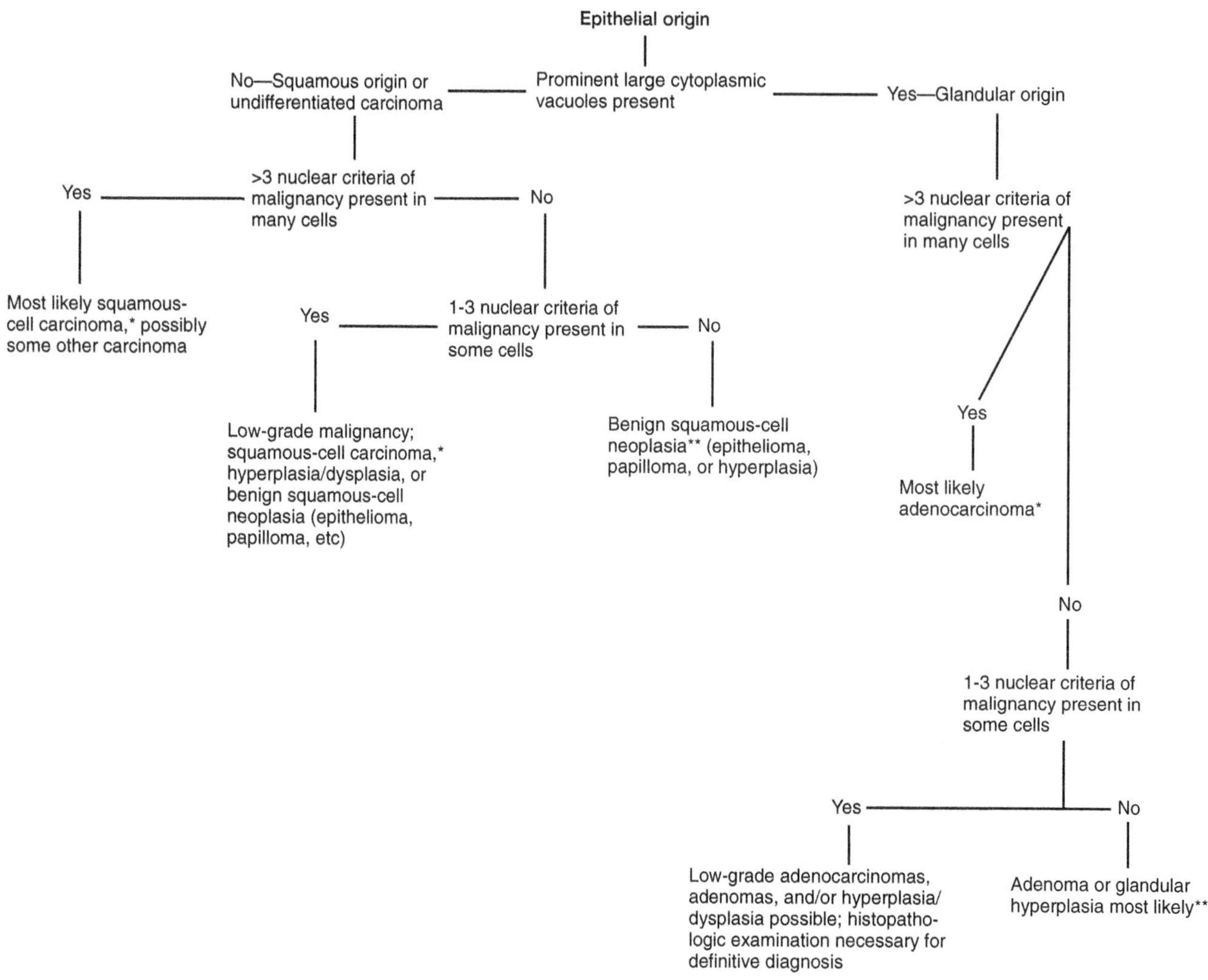

Fig. 2-10 Algorithm to aid in evaluation of cytologic smears containing epithelial cells from cutaneous or subcutaneous tissues.
Epithelial cells are large round to caudate cells with many cell clumps.

cells. As a result, cytologic preparations from areas of collagen degeneration contain numerous eosinophils and variable numbers of macrophages, epithelioid macrophages, and inflammatory giant cells. Eosinophilic amorphous debris representing the necrotic zone may be found. Lymphocytes and plasma cells are scarce and no microorganisms are seen. Histopathologic evaluation of a biopsy from the lesion usually is necessary for definitive diagnosis. The above findings support a clinical diagnosis of eosinophilic granuloma with collagen degeneration.

Insect Bites: Cytologic preparations from wheals caused by acute allergic reactions, such as bee stings, usually contain only a few local tissue cells and a few neutrophils and/or eosinophils. Older bumps caused by insect bites may contain a few neutrophils, eosinophils, macrophages, lymphocytes, and plasma cells, along with a few local tissue cells. Rarely, moderate to high numbers of basophils may be present due to cutaneous basophil hypersensitivity (Jones-Mote reaction).

Snake Bites: The muzzle, head, and legs are sites most commonly bitten by snakes. Cytologic preparations from recent snake bites tend to be of low cellularity. The cells present are local tissue cells and a few neutrophils. Neutrophil infiltration of the bitten area is very rapid. Within a few hours of the bite, neutrophil numbers begin to increase markedly. Within a couple of days they contain

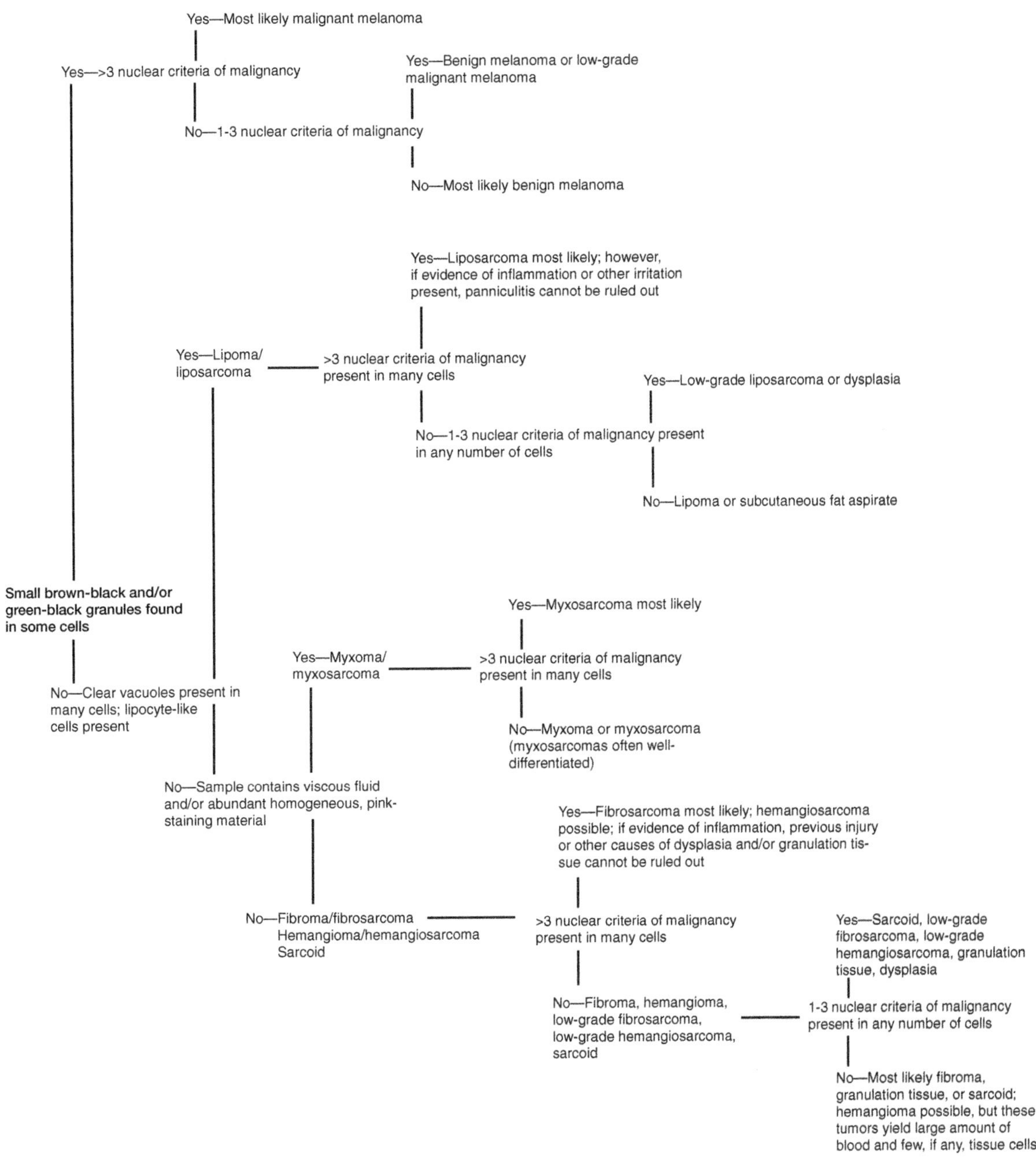

Fig. 2-11 Algorithm to aid in evaluation of aspirates containing spindle cells.

necrotic debris, numerous neutrophils, and variable numbers of macrophages.

Evaluation of Tumor Cells

Tissue cells found on cytologic smears may arise from normal tissue, hyperplastic and/or dysplastic tissue, or neoplastic tissue. The skin is the most common site for neoplasms in horses, with most skin tumors being benign and of mesenchymal origin. However, cutaneous and subcutaneous neoplasms may be of epithelial or mesenchymal (spindle-cell tumors) origin or may be discrete round-cell tumors. Cytologic evaluation often indicates the cell of origin and/or malignant potential of the tumor. In general, epithelial tumors yield medium to large, round to polygonal cells, with many clumps,

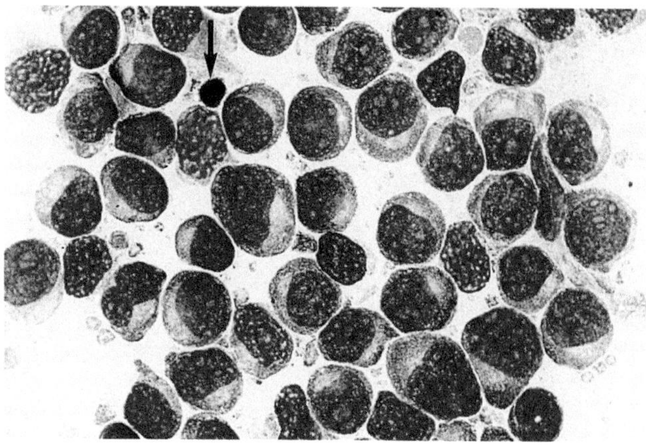

Fig. 2-12 Cutaneous lymphosarcoma.
Cutaneous lymphosarcoma is recognized by large number of lymphoblasts in aspirate. A single small lymphocyte (*arrow*) is also present. (Wright's stain; original magnification 250X) (Courtesy Oklahoma State University.)

groups, or sheets of cells. Mesenchymal tumors yield few to many cells, some of which are fusiform or stellate. Most mesenchymal cells exfoliate individually, but a few cell groups may be found. Discrete round-cell tumors yield small to medium, round, individual cells.

Cell morphology should be evaluated for criteria of malignancy (see Table 1-4). When no inflammatory cells are present, criteria of malignancy are more meaningful than when inflammatory cells are present. If many of the cells show three or fewer nuclear criteria of malignancy and no inflammatory cells are present, the lesion is most likely a malignant neoplasm. If fewer significant criteria of malignancy are present or only a few cells are affected, the cytologic preparation should be referred for interpretation or a biopsy of the lesion should be submitted for histopathologic examination. Sometimes tumors cannot be classified as spindle-cell tumors, epithelial-cell tumors, or discrete round-cell tumors cytologically. However, these tumors may demonstrate sufficient criteria of malignancy for classification as malignant.

Figs. 2-9 to 2-11 provide algorithms to aid evaluation of cytologic smears containing discrete round cells, epithelial cells, and spindle cells, respectively. The typical cytologic characteristics of selected tumors are discussed in the following paragraphs.

Discrete Round-Cell Tumors

Discrete round-cell tumors (Plate 7D-E) yield cytologic preparations containing individual, small to medium-sized, round cells. Lymphosarcoma and mast-cell tumor are the most common discrete round-cell tumors. Occasionally, melanomas and basal-cell tumors exfoliate as discrete round cells. Fig. 2-9 provides an algorithm to aid evaluation of aspirates containing discrete round cells.

Lymphosarcoma: Cutaneous lymphosarcoma is rare in horses and usually affects adult to old animals, though any age may be affected. They usually produce multiple lesions but occasionally produce solitary nodules.[6] Aspirates of these lesions usually yield highly cellular cytologic preparations.

Preparations from *lymphoblastic lymphosarcoma* (the most common cutaneous lymphoid neoplasm) contain numerous lymphoblasts (Fig. 2-12). Lymphoblasts are larger than neutrophils and have a small to moderate amount of light to medium blue-staining cytoplasm that is usually displaced to one side of the nucleus and not as abundant as in the other discrete round-cell tumors. They have indented to irregular nuclei, with smudged to stippled chromatin patterns and often several prominent nucleoli (Plate 7E).

Preparations from *lymphocytic lymphosarcoma* are composed of small lymphocytes that cannot be readily differentiated from normal lymphocytes. These tumors require histopathologic examination for definitive diagnosis.

Preparations from *histiocytic lymphosarcoma* lesions contain medium-sized, round cells. Some cells are multinucleated and other cells contain pleomorphic indented nuclei, similar to monocyte nuclei.

Mast-Cell Tumors: Cutaneous mastocytomas are uncommon in horses and usually occur as a solitary lesion on the head or legs; multiple lesions in foals have been reported.[6] Cutaneous mastocytomas (mast-cell tumors) are benign proliferative lesions that do not metastasize and seldom recur after excision.[7] They yield few to many cells with a moderate amount of cytoplasm, usually containing many small, red-purple granules. Often many extracellular mast-cell granules are scattered throughout the background of the smear due to rupturing of some mast cells during collection or smear preparation. The cells usually have round nuclei that often stain palely because of the intense staining of the highly granulated cytoplasm (Plate 7D). Diff-Quik sometimes fails to stain mast-cell granules.

Epithelial Tumors

Epithelial cells tend to adhere to each other; as a result, epithelial-cell tumors tend to exfoliate clumps of cells, but usually some individual cells are present also. Acinar or ductal arrangements may be identified with adenomas and adenocarcinomas. Cells from epithelial-cell tumors tend to be large to very large, with moderate to abundant cytoplasm and round nuclei. The nuclei generally have smooth to slightly coarse chromatin patterns that become more coarse and ropy as malignant potential increases. The nuclei usually contain one or more prominent nucleoli that become larger and more irregular in shape as malignant potential increases. Malignant epithelial-cell tumors often show marked variation in cellular, nuclear, and nucleolar size and shape. These variations are most significant when they occur within the same cell or same group of cells.

Malignant epithelial-cell tumors also often show a markedly increased nucleus to cytoplasm ratio and may show nuclear molding.

Local inflammation or other irritation can cause epithelial cells to become dysplastic. Epithelial cells undergoing dysplasia may show mild to moderate variation in cellular, nuclear, and nucleolar size and shape, increased nucleus to cytoplasm ratio, and coarse chromatin in a few cells. Dysplasia usually does not cause bizarre nuclear and nucleolar morphology. When there is concern that the abnormal cell morphology observed in a cytologic sample is caused by dysplasia instead of neoplasia, a biopsy from the lesion should be submitted for histopathologic evaluation, or the cause of dysplasia should be treated and the lesion reevaluated cytologically.

Neoplasms of epithelial origin are often ulcerated and may have a superficial secondary infection. Imprints of ulcerated areas on epithelial-cell tumors often yield only inflammatory cells with or without bacteria. When cells are collected by imprinting ulcerated areas, the changes in cellular morphology caused by neoplasia are difficult to distinguish from dysplastic changes caused by inflammation. It is more rewarding, therefore, to collect cytologic samples from ulcerated lesions by deep aspiration or deep scraping of the lesion after it has been cleaned and debrided. Scrapings have the advantage of collecting many tissue cells. A disadvantage is that the sample is collected from an area undergoing an inflammatory response that may have caused sufficient cellular dysplasia to impair cytologic interpretation. Aspirations from deep within the lesion have the advantage of being collected farther from the site of possible inflammation and the disadvantage of usually yielding fewer cells for evaluation.

Fig. 2-10 provides an algorithm to aid identification of epithelial-cell tumors. Some epithelial-cell tumors are discussed in the following paragraphs.

Normal Squamous Epithelium: Normal superficial squamous epithelial cells (Plate 6D) are very large, appear flattened, have abundant light blue to blue-green staining cytoplasm, and are anucleate or have a small, contracted, dark-staining nucleus without a discernible nucleolus. Normal squamous epithelial cells from the basal layer (Plate 6D) tend to be round, with a moderate amount of light to medium blue cytoplasm. They have a single medium to dark purple-staining nucleus with a smooth to slightly coarse chromatin pattern. Their nuclei may contain a single small, round, indistinct nucleolus. As maturation progresses, the morphology of squamous epithelial cells changes from that of basal squamous epithelial cells to that of larger, mature superficial squamous epithelial cells. As a result, cells with morphology varying from that of normal basal epithelial cells to that of normal mature squamous epithelial cells may be collected from cutaneous lesions, depending on the manner of collection and the erosion of the lesion.

Benign Tumors of Squamous Epithelium: Benign epithelial-cell tumors not undergoing dysplasia subsequent to local inflammation or other irritation usually exfoliate cells either indistinguishable from normal cells of the tissue of origin or showing mild neoplastic changes. The mild neoplastic changes often include nucleoli that are slightly more prominent but still round and of small size, cytoplasm that is slightly more basophilic, and nucleus to cytoplasm ratio that is slightly increased.

Papillomatosis: Papillomatosis (warts) is a common benign tumor of squamous epithelium. It usually occurs as multiple lesions, most commonly on the muzzle, distal legs, and genitalia and occasionally as aural plaques on the inner surface of the pinna.[6] Cytologic samples are composed predominantly of mature squamous epithelial cells. A few basal and intermediate stages of squamous maturation may also be present. If there is any concern that the lesion might be a well-differentiated squamous-cell carcinoma, a biopsy of the lesion should be submitted for histopathologic evaluation.

Epidermal Cysts: These are discussed under cysts.

Basal-Cell Tumors: These uncommon benign tumors occur most commonly on the neck, pectoral region, and trunk.[6] Basal-cell tumors yield some cells in groups and some individual cells. Sometimes a row or ribbon of several cells is found (Fig. 2-13). This pattern is caused by the tendency of basal cells to line up along basement membranes within the tumor. This gives the characteristic ribbon-like histologic pattern of the basal-cell tumor.

The individual cells of basal-cell tumors have morphology similar to that of normal basal cells (Plate 6D). They are medium-sized cells with a round to oval nucleus, stippled to finely clumped nuclear chromatin, and an indistinct or no visible nucleolus. The cytoplasm is moderately abundant and stains clear.

Squamous-Cell Carcinomas *(Plate 6E):* Squamous-cell carcinomas may occur anywhere in the skin of horses but most commonly occur as a solitary lesion on the head, mucocutaneous junction, or genitalia.[6] They may be ulcerated, with a secondary superficial bacterial infection. Imprints of ulcerated areas may yield only bacteria and inflammatory cells (Plate 3A). Scrapings of cleaned and debrided ulcerated areas may yield numerous tissue cells, but interpretation often is impaired by secondary inflammation. Deep aspirates from squamous-cell carcinomas usually do not yield as many cells as do scrapings, but aspirates usually are very helpful in diagnosis, since interpretation usually is not impaired by local inflammation.

A

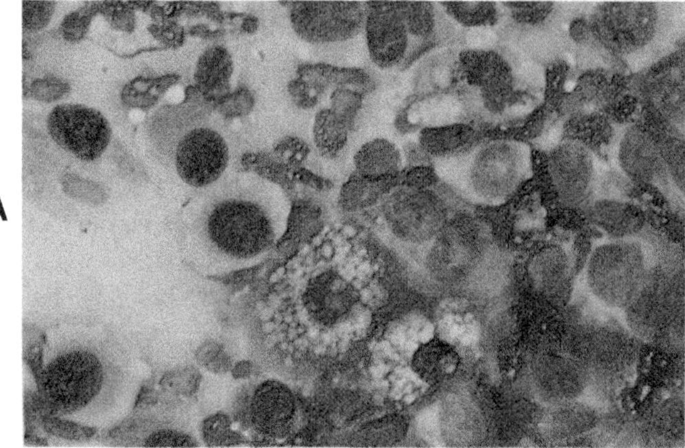

B

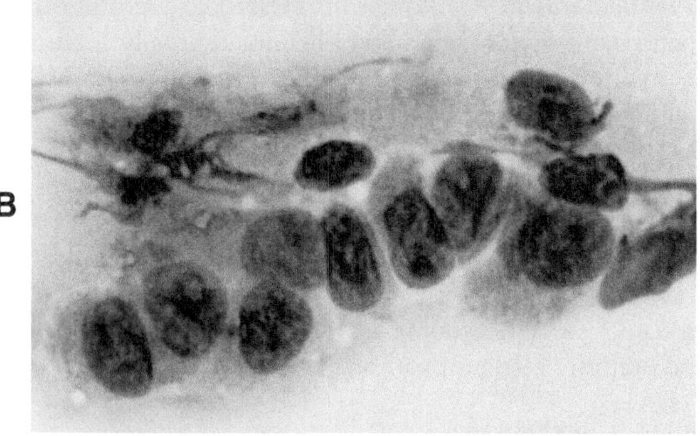

Fig. 2-13 Aspirate from basal-cell tumor.
A, The two cells containing numerous cytoplasmic vacuoles are probably sebaceous cells. (Wright's stain; original magnification 250X) **B,** Basal cells show row formation sometimes seen in cytologic preparations from basal-cell tumors. (Wright's stain; original magnification 400X)

Squamous-cell carcinomas tend to yield groups of cells and a few individual cells. Many groups of cells may be too thick to evaluate, but thinner groups and individual cells can be evaluated to determine the cell of origin and malignant potential. Often there is marked variation in cellular, nuclear, and nucleolar size, nucleolar number and shape, nucleus to cytoplasm ratio, and cytoplasmic basophilia. Some cells may contain small clear vacuoles. Occasionally the vacuoles may aggregate around the nucleus (perinuclear vacuolation) and appear to coalesce, forming a clear ring around the nucleus. These cells strongly suggest carcinoma. The cytoplasm of some cells may stain homogeneous blue-green. Occasionally an individual cell has its cytoplasm displaced to one side and a blunted cytoplasmic tail. These *tadpole cells* suggest squamous-cell carcinoma. Individual cellular morphology varies from normal large, mature squamous cells to small or medium-sized round cells, with a small amount of very basophilic cytoplasm and large, round nuclei that may have a very coarse, ropy chromatin pattern and contain multiple, prominent, irregularly shaped and sized nucleoli.

***Sebaceous-Cell Adenomas** (Plate 6B):* Sebaceous-cell adenomas usually appear as wartlike growths. They generally exfoliate cells in groups; however, a few individual cells may be present. Occasionally the cells of a group may be arranged in an acinar pattern. The morphology of sebaceous adenoma cells is very similar to that of normal sebaceous cells. They are large cells, with foamy cytoplasm and a small, central to slightly eccentric nucleus. The nucleus usually stains darkly and has a slightly coarse chromatin pattern. Usually the nucleolus is indistinct or indiscernible. In preparations from sebaceous-cell adenomas, some cells may have a slightly larger nucleus that stains with less intensity, a slightly coarse chromatin pattern, and a small to medium-sized, round, discernible nucleolus.

Basilar reserve cells may be found also. These cells are immature and contain little or no secretory material. They have basophilic cytoplasm and a nucleus to cytoplasm ratio of about 1:2. Tumors that consist primarily of normal-appearing reserve cells with lesser numbers of sebaceous cells are called sebaceous epitheliomas. Sebaceous cysts are described below in the section on cysts.

Sebaceous-Cell Adenocarcinomas: Sebaceous-cell adenocarcinomas are much less common than sebaceous-cell adenomas. The cytologic characteristics are similar to those of other adenocarcinomas (Plate 6C). Cytologic preparations usually consist of groups of extremely basophilic reserve cells showing numerous criteria of malignancy. Cells containing secretory material are scarce; however, signet-ring cells (cells containing large secretory vacuoles that press the nucleus against the cell membrane) occasionally may be found.

Sweat-Gland Adenomas/Adenocarcinomas: Sweat-gland tumors are usually solitary, firm to cystic tumors that occur most frequently on the pinna and vulva of adult to aged horses.[6] Adenomas occur more frequently than adenocarcinomas.

Sweat-gland adenomas usually yield cytologic preparations that are moderately cellular. Most cells are in clumps. The cells are of medium size and round to oval, with a slightly eccentric nucleus. They may contain one or more large droplets of secretory material.

Sweat-gland adenocarcinomas yield groups of basophilic round cells similar to those found with other adenocarcinomas (Plate 6C). These cells often show numerous criteria of malignancy (see Table 1-4).

Thyroid-Gland Lesions: Thyroid enlargement may occur with goiter, adenomas, and carcinomas. Thyroiditis, while uncommon in horses, may also cause thyroid enlargement. Thyroid aspirates are often very bloody and many of the nucleated cells may be ruptured. Aspirates of normal thyroid gland consist of a blue to gray amorphous colloid (Fig. 2-14) and thyroid epithelial cells occurring individually and in clusters. These epithelial cells have a moderate amount of basophilic cytoplasm and round to oval nuclei, with moderately clumped chromatin.

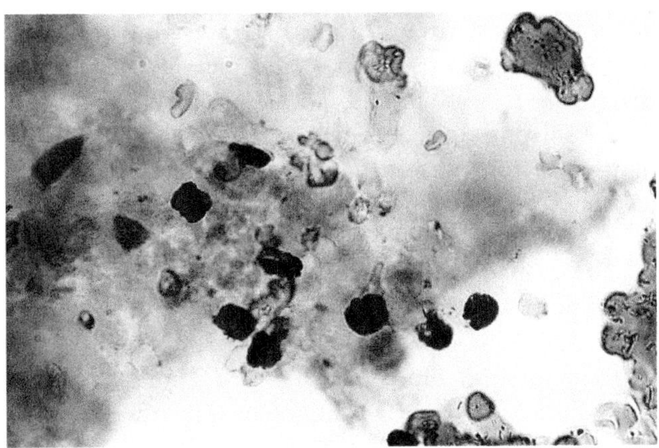

Fig. 2-14 Aspirate from thyroid gland.
Large amount of bluish amorphous colloid is present, along with some ruptured thyroid epithelial cells. (Wright's stain; original magnification 250X) (Courtesy Oklahoma State University.)

Intracytoplasmic blue-black tyrosine granules occasionally are present (Fig. 2-15, *A*).

Thyroid epithelial cells aspirated from thyroid adenomas and goitrous thyroid glands generally appear cytologically similar to epithelial cells aspirated from normal thyroid tissue. Thyroid carcinomas occur less commonly than thyroid adenomas in horses.[8] A well-differentiated thyroid carcinoma may be difficult to distinguish from a thyroid adenoma. Cytologically, thyroid carcinomas are identified by recognizing criteria of malignancy, such as variation in cell size, variation in nuclear size, and large prominent nucleoli (Fig. 2-15, *B*). Tyrosine granules are typically not observed in cells from a thyroid carcinoma, unless the tumor is functional.[9] Aspirates from cystic areas may contain macrophages, neutrophils, cholesterol crystals, and degenerating cells.

Undifferentiated Carcinoma: Undifferentiated carcinomas are malignant tumors that morphologically appear to be of epithelial origin, but the specific cell of origin (squamous epithelial cell or glandular epithelial cell) cannot be determined. Obviously, these tumors may vary greatly in cellular morphology. To classify them as carcinomas, characteristics of epithelial cells must be present without characteristics of spindle cells. Because of their undifferentiated (anaplastic) nature, numerous criteria of malignancy usually are present, and they are easily recognized as malignant.

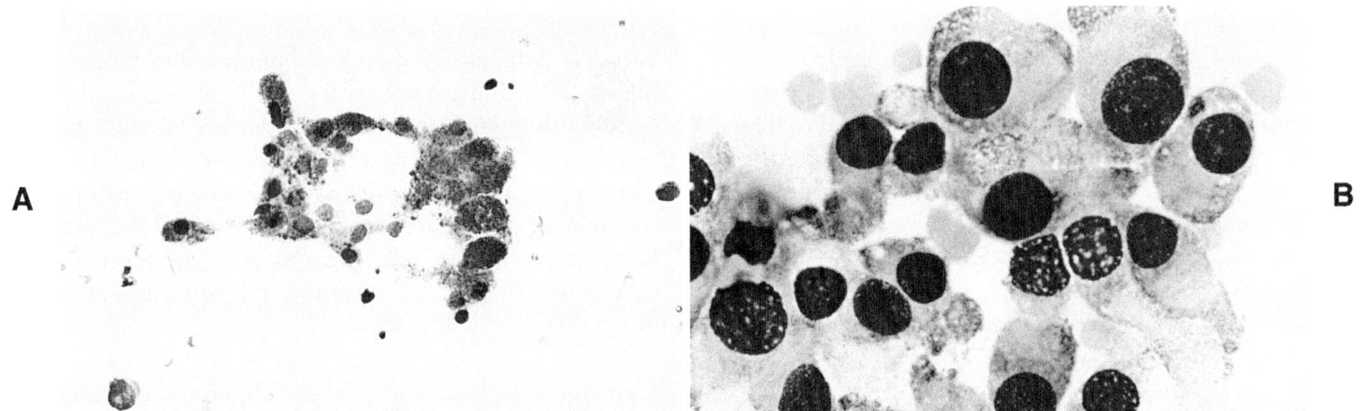

Fig. 2-15 Aspirate from thyroid gland.
A, Aspirate from thyroid gland shows small cluster of thyroid cells containing numerous blue-black tyrosine granules. (Wright's stain; original magnification 100X) **B,** Aspirate of thyroid adenocarcinoma from aged gelding. Epithelial cells are less cohesive than those in **A** and show anisocytosis, anisokaryosis, and a variable C:N ratio. No tyrosine granules were present in cells from this tumor. (Wright's stain; original magnification 250X) (**A** courtesy Oklahoma State University.)

Tumors of Mesenchymal Origin (Spindle-Cell Tumors)

Tumors of mesenchymal origin are commonly referred to as spindle-cell tumors. These tumors tend to yield individual cells instead of groups, clumps, or sheets of cells, but a few groups of cells usually can be found. The term "spindle cell" arises from the fusiform or spindle appearance that a few to many (depending on the specific cell of origin and malignant potential of the tumor) cells may show. Spindle cells have a fusiform shape with cytoplasmic tails trailing away from the nucleus in one or two directions. They usually are small to medium sized and have a moderate amount of light to medium blue cytoplasm. The round to oval nucleus stains with medium intensity and has a smooth to fine lacy chromatin pattern. Nucleoli usually are not visible in nonneoplastic spindle cells. As the malignant potential of spindle-cell tumors increases, nucleoli become prominent. The spindle shape becomes less prominent, and cellular, nuclear, and nucleolar size and shape vary markedly. The chromatin pattern becomes coarser, and cytoplasmic basophilia and the nucleus to cytoplasm ratio increase.

Spindle-cell tumors are often difficult or impossible to definitively classify as to type by cytologic examination. Also, granulation tissue produces plump, young fibroblasts that may have prominent criteria of malignancy. As a result, granulation tissue can be very difficult to differentiate from a spindle-cell neoplasm. In some cases, histopathologic examination is necessary to definitively diagnose spindle-cell tumors.

Local inflammation or other irritation can cause mesenchymal cells to become dysplastic. Cellular morphologic changes caused by dysplasia are very similar to the changes caused by neoplasia, but usually they are only mildly to moderately severe. Nuclear and nucleolar changes are less sensitive to dysplasia than cytoplasmic changes. If there is concern that cellular morphology is altered due to dysplasia instead of neoplasia, a biopsy of the lesion should be submitted for histopathologic evaluation. Alternatively, the stimulus for dysplasia (inflammation or other irritation) can be treated and the lesion reevaluated cytologically.

Fig. 2-11 provides an algorithm to aid identification of spindle-cell tumors. Some spindle-cell tumors are discussed below.

Fibromas: Fibromas are uncommon benign tumors that occur most commonly as solitary masses in adult to aged horses. They may be firm (fibroma durum) or soft (fibroma molle) and seldom ulcerate. Aspirates and imprints yield very few cells. Scrapings from excised fibromas yield more cells, but even scrapings do not yield many cells. The cells collected usually are individuals, but an occasional group of two to several cells may be found.

Cells from fibromas are uniform in size and shape (Plate 7A). They tend to have very elongated spindle shapes, with a moderate amount of light blue cytoplasm streaming away from the nucleus in two opposing directions. Their nuclei are round to oval and stain with medium to marked intensity, have a smooth to lacy chromatin pattern, and may contain one or two small, round, indistinct nucleoli.

Fibrosarcomas: Fibrosarcomas can arise from cutaneous or subcutaneous tissues. They may ulcerate and become secondarily infected. Aspirates, imprints, and scrapings from fibrosarcomas tend to collect more cells than those from fibromas.

Cells from fibrosarcomas are less spindle-shaped than cells from fibromas (Plate 7C). Many cells may be plump and/or oval shaped. Others may be stellate or have only a single, indistinct tail of cytoplasm. Occasionally multinucleated fibroblasts may be found. Mild to marked variation in cellular, nuclear, and nucleolar size and shape, cytoplasmic basophilia, increased nucleus to cytoplasm ratio, and enlarged and/or angular nucleoli develop as malignant potential increases.

Granulation Tissue: Excessive formation of granulation tissue (proud flesh) in wounds, especially on the distal extremities, is a well-recognized problem in horses. Granulation tissue is composed of proliferating fibroblasts and small blood vessels. Because fibroblasts are young, plump spindle cells with anaplastic characteristics, granulation tissue cannot be reliably differentiated from fibrous-tissue neoplasia cytologically. If granulation tissue is suspected, a biopsy of the lesion should be submitted for histopathologic evaluation to definitively differentiate granulation tissue from fibrous-tissue neoplasia.

Sarcoids: Sarcoids are the most common skin tumor in horses. Sarcoids may be solitary or multiple. Though most common in young horses, they may affect horses of any age. Sarcoids are locally aggressive, fibroblastic skin tumors that cytologically consist of spindle cells, with mild to moderately coarse nuclear chromatin and small nucleoli. Sarcoids cannot be differentiated from other fibrous tumors (eg, fibroma, fibrosarcoma) and granulation tissue by cytologic evaluation alone.

Lipomas: Lipomas are uncommon benign tumors that most frequently occur in the subcutaneous tissue of the trunk and proximal limbs.[6] They seldom ulcerate. Aspirates of lipomas usually yield abundant free fat and a few lipocytes. As a result, cytologic smears have an oily appearance and do not dry. Fat does not stain with Romanowsky-type stains and is dissolved by alcohol in stains containing alcohol. Therefore, microscopic evaluation of the smear reveals clear areas and a variable number

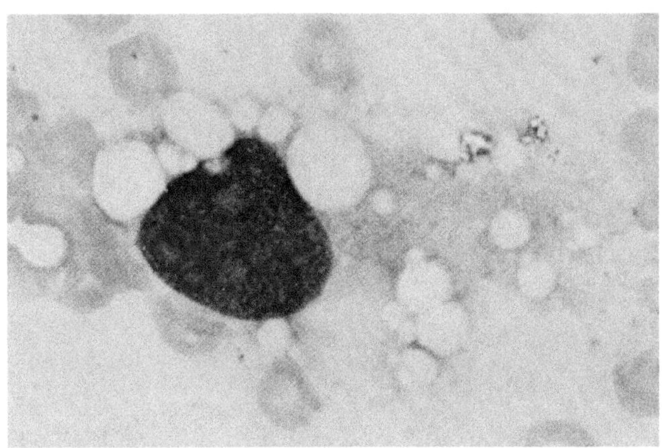

Fig. 2-16 Aspirate from liposarcoma. Note vacuolated cytoplasm with indistinct borders, large nucleus, ropy chromatin pattern, and multiple prominent nucleoli. (Wright's stain; original magnification 400X) (Courtesy University of Georgia.)

of lipocytes. Lipocytes have small dark nuclei that are pressed against the side of the cell membrane by huge fat globules (Plate 6H). Fat stains, such as Sudan IV and oil red O, may be used on fresh smears before alcohol fixation to establish the presence of lipids.

Lipomas usually do not become secondarily infected. Therefore, when inflammatory cells are found concurrently with lipid and lipocytes, inflammation of fat tissue (fat necrosis/steatitis/panniculitis) should be suspected.

Liposarcomas: Liposarcomas are rare in horses. Aspirates, imprints, and scrapings from liposarcomas may contain free fat and some mature lipocytes and lipoblasts and appear greasy. Or they may contain very little free fat and few mature lipocytes, along with many lipoblasts, and not appear greasy.

Cells from liposarcomas often have very light cytoplasm with indistinct cell borders (Fig. 2-16). Within the same tumor, cells may vary in morphology from that of lipocytes to that of bizarre blastic cells similar to those found in fibrosarcomas. Large to small lipid globules may be found in any of the cells. However, in general, the more immature and anaplastic cells have fewer and smaller fat globules. Smears that have not been exposed to alcohol or other lipid solvents can be stained with fat stains, such as Sudan IV and oil red O, to establish the presence of lipid.

Inflammation can cause fat cells to become dysplastic. The cellular morphology of fat cells undergoing dysplasia can be similar to that of cells from liposarcomas. Because liposarcomas do not usually become secondarily infected or inflamed, evidence of inflammation concurrent with cellular changes suggestive of dysplasia or neoplasia indicates inflammation or necrosis of fat tissue (fat necrosis/steatitis, panniculitis) (see Fig. 2-8), but secondary inflammation of neoplastic fat tissue cannot be totally ruled out. To definitively differentiate neoplasia from dysplasia, a biopsy of the lesion can be submitted for histopathologic evaluation.

Hemangiomas: Hemangiomas are uncommon benign tumors of blood vessel endothelium and are contiguous with the blood vascular system. They may occur at any age and may be congenital. Cutaneous hemangiomas are usually solitary, bluish to blackish lesions that occur most commonly on the distal limbs.[6] Aspirates of hemangiomas usually yield a large amount of blood that may contain a few endothelial cells. Because of the tendency for neutrophils to marginate, neutrophil numbers may be higher in blood aspirated from hemangiomas and hemangiosarcomas than in peripheral blood. Even when a few tumor cells are collected, they are difficult to differentiate from non-neoplastic reactive endothelial cells. They tend to be oval, spindle or stellate, have a moderate to abundant amount of light to medium blue cytoplasm, and contain a medium-sized round to slightly oval nucleus (Plate 7B). The nucleus usually has a smooth to fine lacy chromatin pattern and may have one or two small, round, indistinct nucleoli. Because hemangiosarcomas may be well differentiated, tumors thought to be hemangiomas or hemangiosarcomas that do not yield sufficient cytologic evidence for classification as hemangiosarcomas should not be classified as hemangiomas by cytologic examination alone. Instead, they should be excised and submitted for histopathologic evaluation.

Cytologic evaluation can be used to help differentiate hemangiomas and hemangiosarcomas from hematomas. Blood collected from hemangiomas and hemangiosarcomas contains platelets, whereas aspirates collected from hematomas do not, unless blood has hemorrhaged into the hematoma within a few hours of sample collection or blood contamination has occurred during sample collection. Also, aspirates from hematomas usually contain macrophages with phagocytized RBCs (Plate 2B) and/or RBC breakdown products, whereas blood from hemangiomas and hemangiosarcomas does not. Hemorrhage/hematoma may develop within or around any tumor, including hemangioma/hemangiosarcoma. Thus evidence of hemorrhage/hematomas by cytologic evaluation does not totally rule out hemangioma/hemangiosarcoma.

Hemangiosarcomas: Hemangiosarcomas are rare tumors that are usually solitary, rapidly growing lesions of adult to aged horses.[6] They are malignant tumors of the vascular endothelium and are contiguous with the vascular system. Aspirates from hemangiosarcomas usually yield abundant blood, with a few endothelial cells. Occasionally,

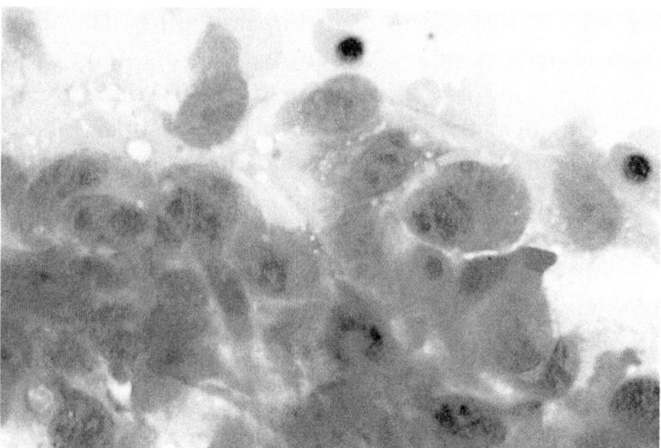

Fig. 2-17 Impression smear from hemangiosarcoma. Cells are very pleomorphic, with distinct cell margins and variable amounts of blue cytoplasm. Variation in nuclear size and shape is marked. Nucleoli are prominent and vary in size, shape, and number. (Wright's stain; original magnification 480X) (Courtesy Dr. P.S. MacWilliams, University of Wisconsin.)

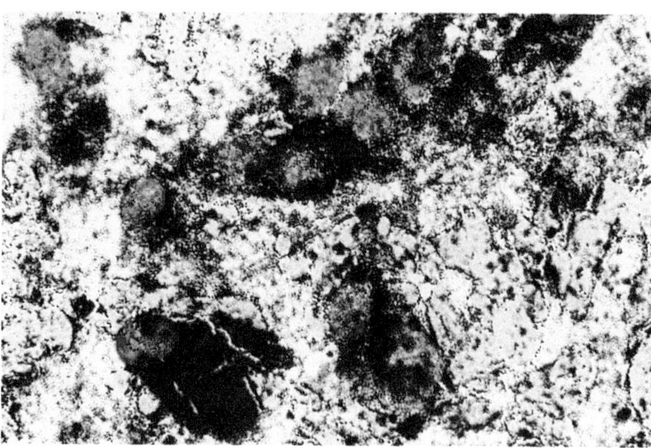

Fig. 2-18 Aspirate from melanoma. Melanoma cells contain abundant amount of green-black pigment. Background contains abundant pigment released from cells ruptured during aspiration and slide preparation. (Wright's stain; original magnification 250X) (Courtesy Oklahoma State University.)

a moderate number of endothelial cells may be collected. Because of the tendency of neutrophils to marginate, neutrophil numbers in blood collected from hemangiosarcomas may exceed neutrophil numbers in the peripheral blood. Neoplastic endothelial cells collected from hemangiosarcomas range in morphology from normal-appearing endothelial cells to medium or large cells with marked variation in cellular, nuclear, and nucleolar size and increased nucleus to cytoplasm ratio, nucleolar prominence, nucleolar angularity, and cytoplasmic basophilia (Fig. 2-17).

When ≥3 nuclear criteria of malignancy (see Table 1-4) are prominent in many of the cells collected and there is no evidence of inflammation or granulation tissue, the tumor can be classified as malignant. However, often sufficient numbers of cells are not collected or the criteria of malignancy are not sufficiently prominent to allow the tumor to be classified as malignant. Tumors thought to be hemangiomas or hemangiosarcomas and not yielding sufficient cytologic evidence to be recognized as hemangiosarcomas should not be classified as hemangiomas based on cytologic examination alone. Instead, they should be excised and submitted for histopathologic evaluation.

Melanomas: Melanomas may be benign or malignant and occur as solitary or multiple nodules. They occur at any age, but most occur in adult to aged horses. Melanomas are common in gray horses; about 80% of gray horses over 15 years of age have clinical melanomas.[6,10]

Cytologic preparations from melanomas usually are moderately cellular and contain a small to moderate amount of blood, but occasionally they are of low cellularity and contain a large amount of blood. Most of the cells are found as individual cells, but a few small groups of cells may be found. The cells may be round, oval, stellate, or spindle shaped. Amelanotic melanomas composed predominantly of round to oval cells may be confused with round-cell tumors. Generally, however, a few spindle-shaped cells can be found. The cells have a moderate to abundant amount of cytoplasm. Even cells from malignant melanomas often contain a large amount of cytoplasm and, therefore, have a low nucleus to cytoplasm ratio. The cytoplasm usually contains granules of brown-black to green-black pigment (Plate 6F). These granules may be densely packed and obscure the nucleus in some cells or may be absent from other cells. Often the background of the smear contains abundant black pigment from ruptured cells (Fig. 2-18). Amelanotic melanomas, which are often malignant, contain only a small amount of pigment that is often not discernible by histopathologic examination. However, a careful search of cytologic preparations invariably identifies a few cells containing a few small pigment granules interspersed throughout their cytoplasm. Some malignant melanomas demonstrate numerous cytologic criteria of malignancy, but others are well differentiated and do not demonstrate significant criteria of malignancy. Therefore, caution should be used in classifying melanomas as benign by cytologic evaluation alone.

Melanocytes must be differentiated from melanophages (macrophages containing phagocytized melanin), hemosiderophages (macrophages containing hemosiderin), and mast cells. Melanophages usually contain a few clear vacuoles, along with few to many large phagocytic vacuoles packed with melanin pigment. These

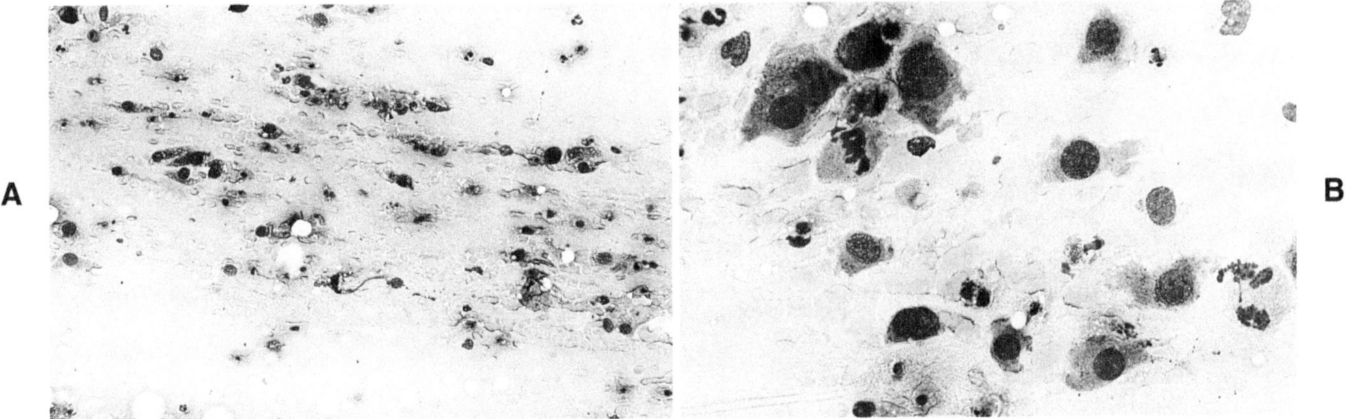

Fig. 2-19 Aspirate from myxosarcoma.
A, Low magnification shows mesenchymal cells and erythrocytes present in rows, suggesting a viscous nature to material being spread. Note lightly eosinophilic nature to background. (Wright's stain; original magnification 50X) **B,** Higher magnification shows pleomorphic population of spindle-shaped mesenchymal cells. Granules of eosinophilic secretory material are visible in cell in lower right. (Wright's stain; original magnification 125X)

melanin-packed vacuoles are much larger than the small granules in melanocytes and melanoblasts. Hemosiderophages have few to many phagocytic vacuoles stuffed with hemosiderin. The hemosiderin-laden vacuoles are blue-black to brown-black and usually are much larger than the small granules of melanocytes and melanoblasts. Mast cells (Plate 7D) are round to oval and contain a few to many red purple granules. Usually these granules are larger than the small green-black to brown-black granules of melanocytes and melanoblasts but are smaller than the melanin-laden phagocytic vacuoles of melanophages and the hemosiderin-laden phagocytic vacuoles of hemosiderophages.

Myxomas/Myxosarcomas: Myxomas and myxosarcomas are rare tumors of the subcutaneous tissues. They are usually solitary masses that can occur anywhere on the body. On aspiration, a small to large amount of viscid material usually is obtained. Cytologic preparations of myxomas and myxosarcomas contain a few to many individual cells in a background of pink homogeneous material. The cells vary in morphology from oval to stellate or spindle shaped and have a small to abundant amount of cytoplasm that sometimes contains small vacuoles of pink secretory material (Fig. 2-19). The oval cells often have eccentric nuclei and medium to dark blue cytoplasm, giving them an appearance similar to plasma cells. Myxosarcomas exhibit variable degrees of criteria of malignancy.

Neurofibromas/Neurofibrosarcomas: Neurofibromas and neurofibrosarcomas are rare tumors of the nerve cell sheath. They occur most commonly around the eyelids in young (3- to 6-year-old) horses.[6] Cytologically, they

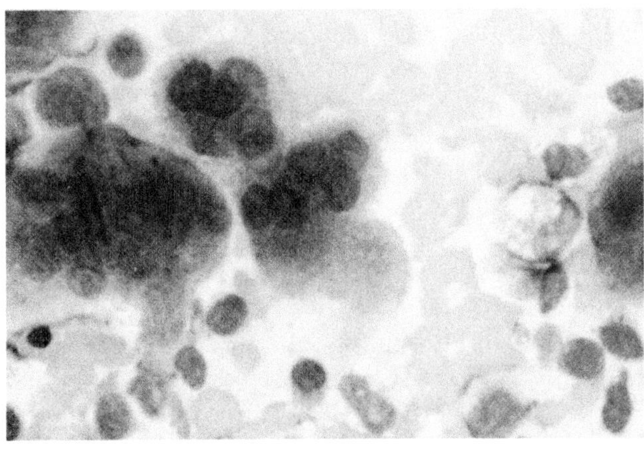

Fig. 2-20 Aspirate from malignant fibrous histiocytoma (giant-cell tumor).
Several multinucleated cells and a few histiocytic cells are present. One cell has tail of cytoplasm trailing away from it. (Wright's stain; original magnification 200X)

cannot be reliably differentiated from other spindle-cell tumors, such as fibromas and fibrosarcomas. Histologic demonstration of tumor involvement with a nerve sheath is necessary for a definitive diagnosis.

Malignant Fibrous Histiocytomas (Giant-Cell Tumors of Soft Parts): These tumors are rare in horses and generally occur as solitary lesions. They occur most frequently on the neck and proximal limbs.[6] These tumors seldom metastasize but are locally invasive; recurrence following incomplete surgical removal is common.

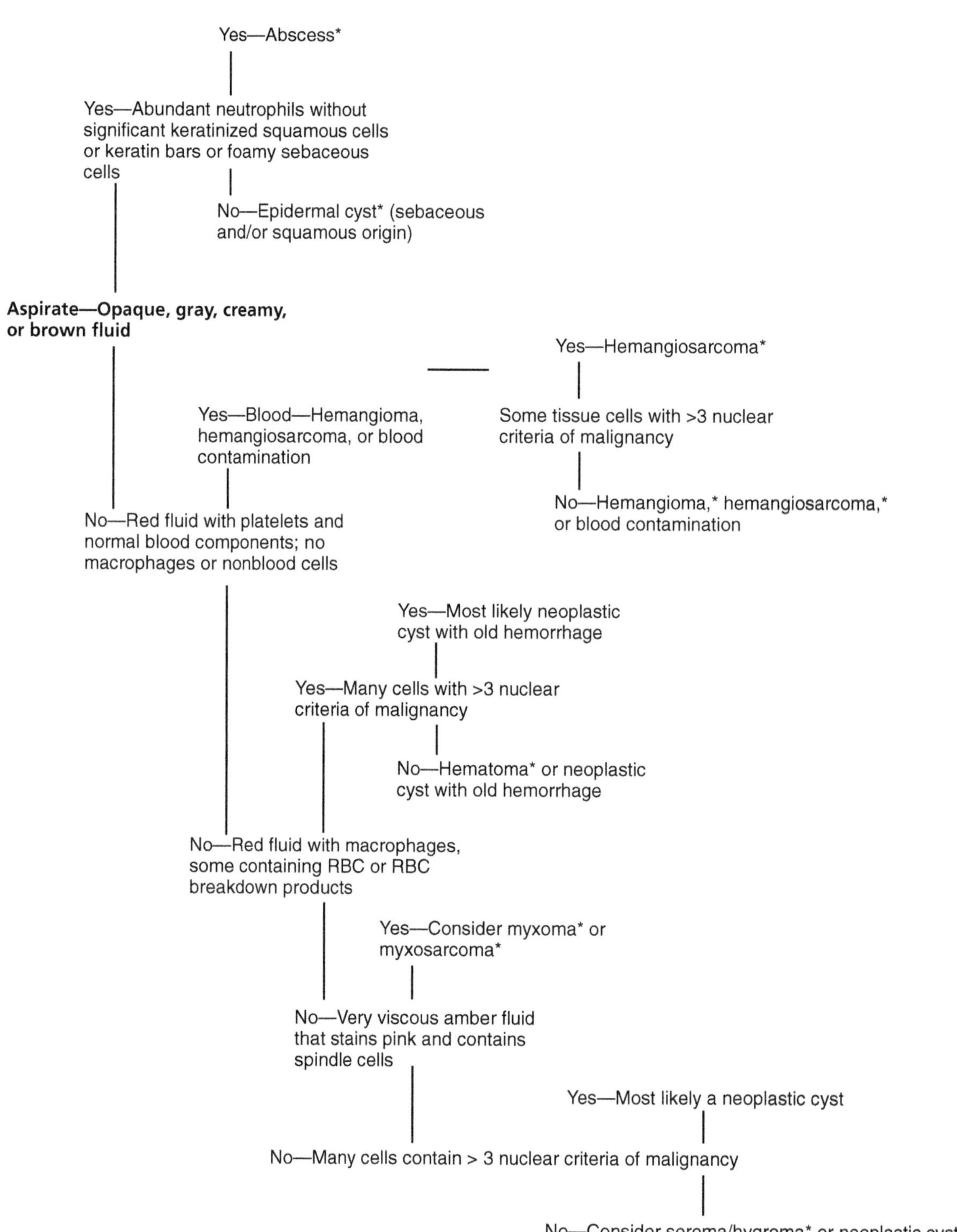

Fig. 2-21 Algorithm to aid in evaluation of cytologic preparations from fluid-filled lesions.

Fig. 2-22 Aspirate from epidermal cyst.
Note abundant blue amorphous debris. (Wright's stain; original magnification 50X)

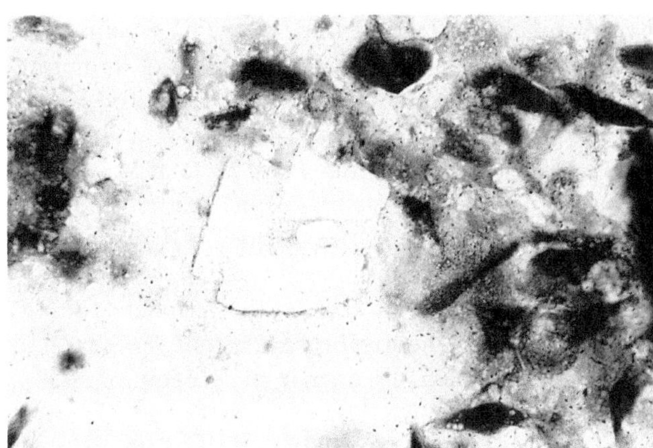

Fig. 2-23 Aspirate from epidermal cyst.
Cholesterol crystal is present in a background of degenerating squamous cells and basophilic cell debris. (Wright's stain; original magnification 50X)

Cytologic preparations are best collected by aspiration, which generally yields sufficient cells for a diagnosis. The preparations generally consist of multinucleated giant cells (Fig. 2-20), fibroblastic cells (see description of fibrosarcomas above), and smaller round cells that resemble histiocytes.

Undifferentiated Sarcomas: Undifferentiated sarcomas are malignant tumors that morphologically appear to be of mesenchymal origin, but the specific cell of origin (fibroblasts, endothelial cell, etc) cannot be determined. Obviously, these tumors may vary greatly in cellular morphology. To classify them as sarcomas, some spindling must be recognized. Because of their undifferentiated and anaplastic nature, they usually are easily recognized as malignant. Their cellular characteristics are those described above in the general description of spindle-cell tumors.

Carcinosarcomas: Carcinosarcomas are malignant tumors that do not show sufficient cellular differentiation to be classified as carcinomas or sarcomas. Because of the anaplastic nature of these tumors, they usually are easily classified as malignant. Their cellular characteristics are a variable admixture of the characteristics for carcinomas and sarcomas.

Evaluation of Fluid-Filled Lesions

Fluid-filled lesions may be neoplastic or nonneoplastic in origin. Neoplastic fluid-filled lesions of the cutaneous and subcutaneous tissues include hemangiomas/hemangiosarcomas, adenomas/adenocarcinomas, neurofibromas/neurofibrosarcomas, and myxomas/myxosarcomas. Nonneoplastic fluid-filled lesions of the cutaneous and subcutaneous tissues include hematomas, seromas, hygromas, abscesses, and epidermoid cysts. Cytologic evaluation of fluid from these lesions can be very helpful in their differentiation. Fig. 2-21 provides an algorithm to aid evaluation of fluid-filled lesions. Some common fluid-filled lesions are discussed below.

Epidermoid Cysts

Epidermoid cysts arise from tissues of squamous cell differentiation. Fluid from epidermoid cysts is usually creamy white to brown to gray. With previous hemorrhage or peripheral blood contamination during collection, the fluid may appear pink to red.

Smears prepared from these cysts contain abundant amorphous blue to gray-staining material and a few to many squamous epithelial cells (Fig. 2-22). Neutrophils and macrophages may be present if the cyst has ruptured. Blood components (RBCs, neutrophils, etc) are present if hemorrhage or blood contamination has occurred. Sometimes, cholesterol clefts and/or cholesterol crystals are seen (Fig. 2-23). Cholesterol crystals form from cholesterol that accumulates from degradation of cells exfoliating into the cyst. Cholesterol clefts are the negative images left after cholesterol crystals have been dissolved by the alcohol in Romanowsky-type stains. When cholesterol crystals are abundant, some may remain undissolved in Romanowsky-stained smears.

Hematomas

Fluid from hematomas is red to red-brown. Supernatant from centrifuged samples usually has a total protein content between 2.5 g/dl and that of peripheral blood. Cytologically, the fluid contains nondegenerate neutrophils, macrophages, and numerous RBCs. A few lymphocytes may be present also. Usually the macrophages are activated and often contain intact RBCs (Plate 2B), hematoidin (Plate 2A), and other RBC breakdown products. Platelets are not found in fluid from hematomas unless there has been hemorrhage into the hematoma within a few hours of sample collection or the sample is contaminated with peripheral blood. Differentiation of hematomas from hemangiomas and hemangiosarcomas is discussed in the hemangiomas section of this chapter.

Seromas/Hygromas

Fluid from seromas/hygromas is typically clear to amber and usually has a total protein concentration >2.5 g/dl. The fluid usually is of low cellularity. The cell population is composed predominantly of mononuclear cells with characteristics of macrophages or cyst lining cells. These cells are medium to large and round and have moderate to abundant cytoplasm that is often highly vacuolated. Their nuclei may be central but are often eccentric. Usually the nucleus is round, has a smooth to fine lacy chromatin pattern, and may contain one or two indistinct nucleoli. A few nondegenerate neutrophils may also be found. A few cyst-lining cells may be spindle shaped. Occasionally, some cells may be very dysplastic and exhibit criteria of malignancy.

With hemorrhage into the seroma/hygroma or if the sample is contaminated with peripheral blood, a combination of the cytologic characteristics of hematomas and/or peripheral blood and the cytologic characteristics of seromas/hygromas is observed.

Abscesses

Fluid from abscesses usually is creamy and yellow, pink, or brown. The total protein concentration usually cannot be determined because of the turbidity of the fluid. Even the supernatant of centrifuged samples often is too turbid for accurate total protein measurement. When the total protein concentration can be determined, it usually is >4.0 g/dl.

Smears prepared from abscesses are highly cellular. The cell composition usually is over 90% neutrophils, with a few macrophages. Scattered lymphocytes and plasma cells may be present also. Abscesses caused by gram-negative bacteria usually contain numerous degenerate neutrophils (Plate 1D). Abscesses caused by gram-positive bacteria often contain a few to many degenerate neutrophils. In other abscesses, usually only a few or no neutrophils are degenerate. Occasionally, macrophages may compose greater than 50% of the nucleated cells, especially with sterile foreign body abscesses. Sterile foreign body abscesses, such as those caused by oil-based injections, may contain refractile material as well as the inflammatory cells (see Fig. 2-3).

REFERENCES

1. Ackerman: *Practical Equine Dermatology*. 2nd ed. Goleta, CA, 1989, American Veterinary Publications, pp 62-63.
2. Scott: *Large Animal Dermatology*. Philadelphia, 1988, Saunders, pp 168-196.
3. Crane: Equine coccidioidomycosis. *Vet Med* 57:1073-1078, 1962.
4. Weidman: Cutaneous torulosis. *Arch Dermatol Syphilol* 31:58-61, 1935.
5. Bennett: Equine leishmaniasis: treatment with berberine sulphate *J Comp Pathol* 48:241-243, 1935.
6. Scott: *Large Animal Dermatology*. Philadelphia, 1988, Saunders, pp 419-458.
7. McEntee: Equine cutaneous mastocytoma: morphology, biological behavior and evolution of the lesion. *J Comp Pathol* 104:171-178, 1991.
8. Held et al: Work intolerance in a horse with thyroid carcinoma. *JAVMA* 10:1044-1045, 1985.
9. Ramirez et al: Hyperthyroidism associated with a thyroid adenocarcinoma in a 21-year-old gelding. *J Vet Int Med* 12(6):475-477, 1998.
10. McFadyean: Equine melanomatosis. *J Comp Pathol* 38:186-204, 1933.

CHAPTER 3

Eyes and Ocular Adnexa

Elizabeth A. Giuliano and Cecil P. Moore

Cytologic evaluation of cellular material collected from the equine eye and ocular adnexa is a valuable tool in the diagnosis and treatment of many ophthalmic diseases affecting the horse. Cytologic collection and examination are simple to perform, are inexpensive, and hold minimal risk for the patient. Also, cytologic results can be obtained more expeditiously than by histopathology. Although an important procedure used by both the general practitioner and the specialist in ophthalmology, cytology should not be considered a replacement for other diagnostic tools, including culture and biopsy. Microbial culture and histopathology have been shown to maximize the positive identification of infectious organisms and improve the interpretation of cytology alone.[1,2] Cytology evaluates individual cells without regard to the architectural structure of the tissue, so histologic examination is more appropriate for the classification and prognosis of neoplastic disease.[3]

Collection of cytologic specimens from the eye and ocular adnexa generally adheres to the same principles as for collection of any cytologic specimen and has been reviewed elsewhere in this text (see Chapter 1). This chapter will first highlight some special considerations in the preparation of cytologic specimens from ocular tissues and then review normal ocular cytologic findings. Following these considerations, a more detailed description of the more common infectious, inflammatory, and neoplastic diseases affecting the equine globe and associated structures is given.

Cytologic Collection of Ocular Tissues

Proper sample collection is essential for accurate diagnosis. Examination or manipulation of the equine eye may be difficult due to severe ocular pain associated with the disease process. Adequate restraint—in the form of an ear or nose twitch, auriculopalpebral motor and supraorbital sensory nerve blocks, topical anesthetics, and intravenous sedation—is often required to allow proper examination and initial diagnostic testing of the affected globe.[4] Diagnostic procedures performed on the eye and associated adnexa should proceed in an organized, sequential fashion to prevent initial procedures from adversely affecting subsequent test results. It is recommended that samples for aerobic and fungal culture be obtained prior to the application of fluorescein stain or topical anesthetic.[5] For routine culture of samples from the eyelids, cornea, or conjunctiva, recommended media include blood agar, the basic culture medium for most aerobic bacteria, and Sabouraud's agar for suspected fungal infection. Chocolate agar should be used in addition to blood agar if more fastidious bacteria, such as nutritionally variant streptococci, are suspected.[6] Agar inoculation followed by immediate incubation is preferred to use of transport media.

Cytology may be indicated in acute conditions as well as refractory or recurrent cases of external ocular disease that manifest as exudative, purulent, or proliferative processes affecting the eyelid, membrana nictitans, conjunctiva, and/or cornea. Cytology is an essential tool used to help characterize the cellular response (neutrophilic, lymphocytic, eosinophilic, granulomatous) and to identify parasites, bacteria, or fungi. In humans, scrapings are most helpful when done in the early, active phases of disease before secondary ocular changes ensue.[7]

Before cytologic samples are collected, exudate should be gently cleaned from the ocular surfaces using a cotton swab or by flushing with a sterile, nonbacteriostatic, commercial eyewash. Exudate containing mucus, neutrophils, and pleomorphic bacteria occurs as a nonspecific reaction in many ophthalmic diseases, regardless of the underlying etiology. A preliminary cleaning of the eye and associated structures helps ensure proper sampling of the affected tissue rather than collections of nonrepresentative, and sometimes misleading, cellular debris.

The preferred site for scraping is the specific area involved in the disease. For example, if neoplasia is suspected, scrapings should be taken from the surface of the abnormal tissue. In corneal disease, the margin of the corneal lesion is scraped. If a diffuse conjunctival lesion is present, the lower palpebral conjunctiva is everted and scraped, avoiding the lower lid margin with its keratinized epithelium.

Cytologic harvesting methods include impression, fine-needle aspiration, swabbing, and brushing techniques. In ophthalmology, impression cytology has been most frequently used in the study of goblet cells and corneal and conjunctival epithelial cells.[8-11] Swabbing the conjunctiva and cornea using cotton-tipped applicators does not yield a high enough cell count and therefore is not a recommended cytologic technique for the eye.[12] Scraping is a common cytologic technique used for collection of ocular surface cells. Various instruments have been used in this technique, including Kimura spatulas, iris repositioning spatulas, butt of scalpel blade handles, and chemistry measuring spatulas (Fig. 3-1).[3, 13-14] More recently, exfoliative cytology of the conjunctiva and cornea using a brush technique has been reported.[15-16] This method has been shown to yield sufficient number of cells for cytologic interpretation, and a consistent epithelial cell monolayer can be produced.

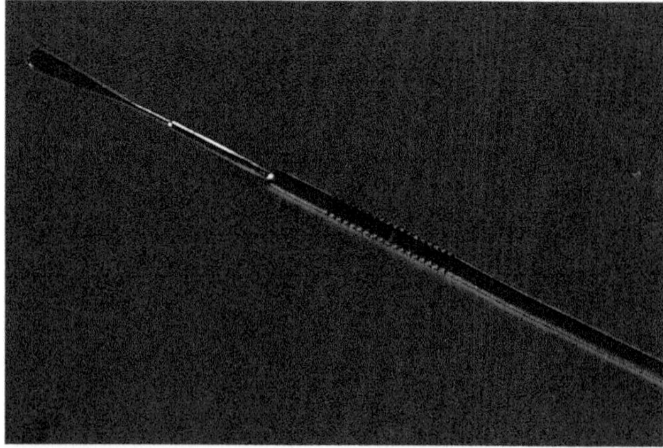

Fig. 3-1
Kimura platinum spatula, designed for collection of ocular cytologic samples.

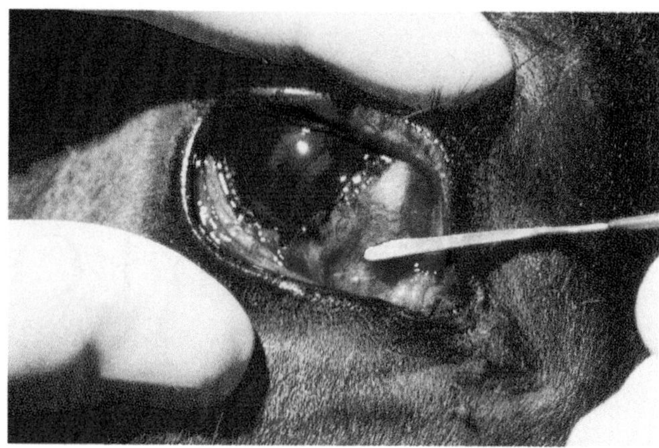

Fig. 3-2
Sterilized Kimura spatula is scraped along the surface or margins of the lesion several times in the same direction until a small droplet of material is collected on the top of the spatula.

If a spatula is used for the collection of ophthalmic cytologic specimens, repeatedly flame sterilize the tip of the instrument and allow it to cool prior to touching the ocular surface. The platinum tip of the Kimura spatula permits rapid heating and cooling of this instrument, making it ideal for cytologic sampling. After cleaning mucopurulent exudate from the ocular surfaces and anesthetizing the cornea and conjunctiva with a topical ophthalmic anesthetic, scrape the sterilized spatula along the surface or margins of the lesion several times in the same direction (not back and forth) until a small droplet of material is collected on the edge or tip of the spatula (Fig. 3-2). Use gentle pressure so that the sample does not become contaminated by blood. Immediately transfer the collected material to a glass slide and gently spread or smear it as described in Chapter 1. If the material is sticky and thick, add a drop of sterile saline before spreading the sample. Ideally, spread the cells thinly so the smear is only one cell layer thick.

Corneal Scrapings

In cases of ulcerative keratitis, the corneal ulcer margin is sampled directly for both cytologic preparations and cultures. Cytologic examination of conjunctival scrapings or

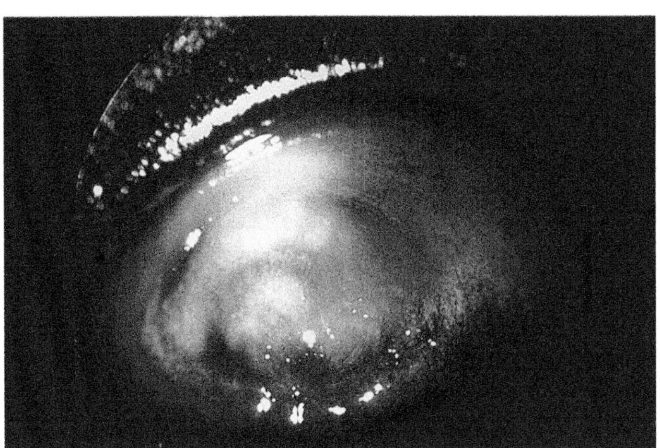

Fig. 3-3 Mycotic keratitis.
Satellite lesions are frequently present in cases of mycotic keratitis. Fungal hyphae may be found in these areas if the epithelium is first scraped off the cornea.

exudate smears alone in cases of ulcerative keratitis may be misleading because the number and types of organisms in the exudate may be different from those present in the corneal stroma. Although it is generally recommended to collect corneal samples for culture prior to application of topical anesthetic, 2 drops of 0.5% proparacaine HCl does not significantly affect the numbers and types of organisms cultured from ocular surfaces.[5,17] Moistening the swab with thioglycolate broth before collecting the culture specimen increases the chance of recovering organisms from the ocular surface.[18] Because various species of bacteria and fungi can be isolated from the eyelid margins and conjunctival fornices in normal horses, it is important to obtain samples from the corneal lesion and not the eyelids, conjunctiva, or ocular discharges when bacterial or mycotic keratitis is suspected.[19,20]

Corneal scrapings may require vigorous but careful debridement of the involved area to obtain sufficient cellular material for diagnosis. A topical anesthetic, such as 0.5% proparacaine HCl, should be applied to the cornea before a corneal scraping is collected. However, with deep ulcers or descemetocele formation, excessive pressure on the eye or eyelids must be avoided to prevent iatrogenic globe rupture. In cases of equine keratomycosis, fungi most commonly inhabit the deeper corneal layers, with an apparent affinity for Descemet's membrane.[21,22] If a corneal lesion infected with fungal hyphae has epithelialized prior to any diagnostic procedures being performed, it may be necessary to remove the superficial epithelium to obtain meaningful culture and cytology samples. Multiple, deep corneal scrapings may be required to establish the diagnosis, especially in cases with satellite lesions (Fig. 3-3).[23,24] Finally, a partial keratectomy or corneal biopsy may be necessary to demonstrate fungal elements if corneal scrapings are negative.[25] Impression imprints of the biopsied portion of cornea can be made for cytologic examination before the tissue is fixed in formalin for histopathologic examination. Special stains may help detect fungal elements (see discussion of special stains later in this chapter).

Conjunctival and Corneal Excision Biopsy

Conjunctival or corneal biopsy is a useful diagnostic technique, especially for detecting neoplasia, parasites, or fungi. At least two instillations of topical anesthetic several minutes apart are required to sufficiently anesthetize the conjunctival or corneal tissue for biopsy. For larger lesions, local anesthesia may be better achieved by gently holding a premoistened cotton-tipped applicator, soaked in topical anesthetic, directly on the area to be biopsied for 1 or 2 minutes prior to tissue collection. Additional injectable regional anesthesia and systemic sedation may be necessary to obtain an adequate sample.

Grasp the tissue directly adjacent to the affected area with fine forceps, and use scissors or scalpel with trephine to excise a biopsy sample (Fig. 3-4). Make imprints for cytologic evaluation of the excised tissue before fixing the specimen in formalin for histologic processing. Examine wet preparations of the excised tissue for microfilariae. To make wet preparations, mince the tissue with a drop of warm physiologic saline and place it on a glass slide. Keep the specimen warm and examine it periodically over 5 to 60 minutes for microfilariae. Microfilariae may be observed under low-power magnification.[26]

Aqueous, Vitreous, and Subretinal Paracentesis

Severe anterior uveitis is sometimes associated with an inflammatory cell egress into the anterior chamber that may settle ventrally, resulting in hypopyon (Figs. 3-5 and 3-6). Aqueous paracentesis may be indicated in severe, nonresponsive anterior uveitis when the aqueous humor is cloudy or opaque, as in cases of infectious anterior

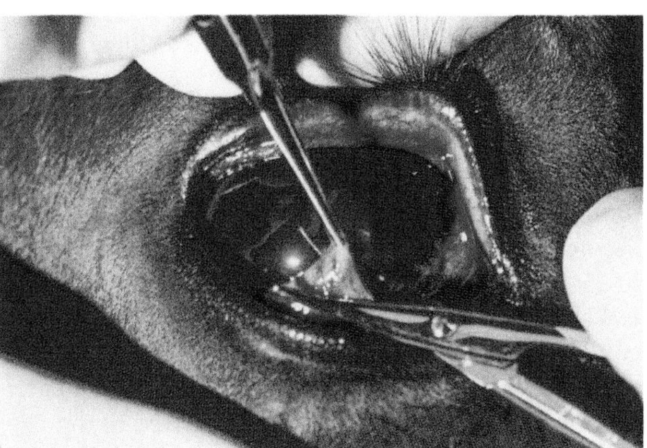

Fig. 3-4 Conjunctival biopsy.
Small scissors are used to snip off a portion of conjunctiva.

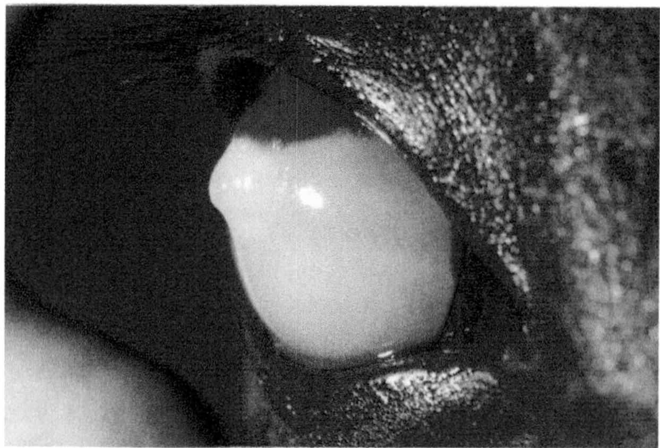

Fig. 3-5 Hypopyon.
Severe anterior uveitis resulting in hypopyon in the anterior chamber.

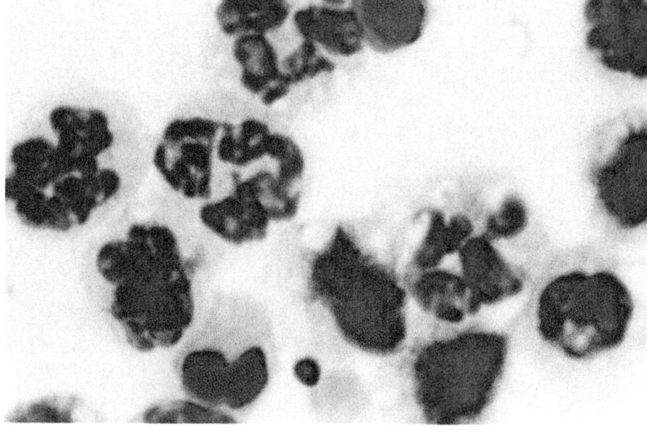

Fig. 3-6 Smear of hypopyon aspirate.
Smear from the horse shown in Fig. 3-5. The cellular response is primarily neutrophilic, though fibrin and small numbers of erythrocytes, plasma cells, lymphocytes, and pigment-containing cells may be present.

uveitis or intraocular neoplasia. Vitreous or subretinal paracentesis should be considered in horses with marked vitreous opacification, exudative retinal separations, or suspected bacterial or fungal endophthalmitis. Blood cultures may aid diagnosis of bacterial endophthalmitis; therefore, intraocular paracentesis may not be needed in cases of *Rhodococcus equi* infection.[27]

Aqueous, vitreous, or subretinal paracentesis in the horse requires general anesthesia and must be undertaken with caution. When performing ocular paracentesis, the clinician must be aware of possible complications, including exacerbation of existing uveitis, intraocular hemorrhage, lens perforation with secondary phacoclastic uveitis, endothelial damage, and corneal edema, or introduction of microorganisms into the globe. Therefore, this procedure should be reserved for eyes where other diagnostic methods have failed to yield sufficient information to allow rational case management.

Tap the anterior chamber through a simple limbal approach (Fig. 3-7). Initially, clean the conjunctiva and cornea with a dilute (5%) aqueous povidone-iodine solution and rinse with sterile 0.9% saline. Use an eyelid speculum to retract the eyelids from the anterior surface of the eye during this procedure. Using a delicate thumb forceps, grasp the bulbar conjunctiva and stabilize near the point of entry into the globe. Attach a 22- or 25-gauge needle to a 1-ml syringe (with the plunger seal already broken) and then insert it under the bulbar conjunctiva, 3 to 4 mm from the limbus. Thread the needle under the conjunctiva toward the limbus, and enter the anterior chamber parallel to the surface of the iris. Collect a 0.5- to 1.0-ml sample of aqueous humor with slow, gentle aspiration. The region of bulbar conjunctiva that is threaded by the needle prior to insertion into the anterior chamber helps to create a small "tunnel" that will act as a seal once the needle is slowly withdrawn. Gentle pressure over the exit wound using a thumb forceps or sterile cotton-tipped applicator will also help control further aqueous egress. An alternative method of performing aqueocentesis has been described using an aqueous paracentesis pipette.[28]

Vitreous and subretinal paracenteses are performed through a pars plana approach, taking care not to puncture the lens (Fig. 3-8). General anesthesia and ocular surface preparation are similar to those described for aqueocentesis. In addition, pharmacologically dilate the pupil to provide better visualization of the posterior segment

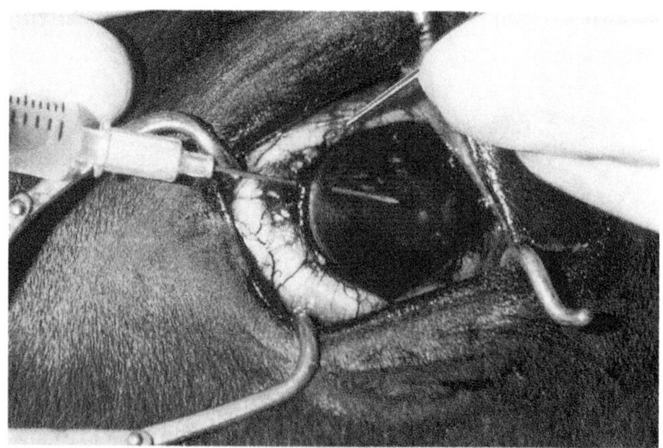

Fig. 3-7 Anterior chamber paracentesis.
A 25- or 22-gauge needle attached to a sterile 1-ml syringe is inserted into the bulbar conjunctiva, 3 to 4 mm from the limbus. The needle is threaded deep to the conjunctiva toward the limbus and enters the anterior chamber parallel to the surface of the iris.

during the sampling procedure. In vitreal and subretinal paracenteses, attach a 22- or 23-gauge hypodermic needle to a 1-ml syringe (with the plunger seal already broken) and insert approximately 7 mm behind the limbus in the dorsolateral quadrant, avoiding the inferior and medial quadrant, where the retina extends more anteriorly in most species.[29] The vitreous is usually liquefied in disease, so only a small amount of negative pressure on the syringe attached to the needle is required. However, neoplastic or granulomatous cellular material may require a larger needle or greater suction. The amount of fluid aspirated from the vitreous or subretinal space usually does not exceed 0.2 ml. After sample collection, withdraw the needle and hold the conjunctival site with a forceps for a few seconds to seal the wound.

Samples collected via paracentesis can be submitted for cytology, culture, antibody titers, and other more specialized diagnostic techniques. When preparing the sample for cytology, deposit a few drops of the collected fluid onto a glass slide, spread, fix, and stain as described in Chapter 1. In poorly cellular samples, centrifugation of the sample may help concentrate the cells and give a higher yield for interpretation. Make cytologic preparations from aqueous humor as soon as possible after collection to avoid disintegration of cells in the low-protein aqueous humor.[30] If special diagnostic techniques are desired, it is prudent to contact the laboratory to which the sample will be sent prior to paracentesis to ensure that the material collected is handled promptly and correctly after being obtained from the equine globe.

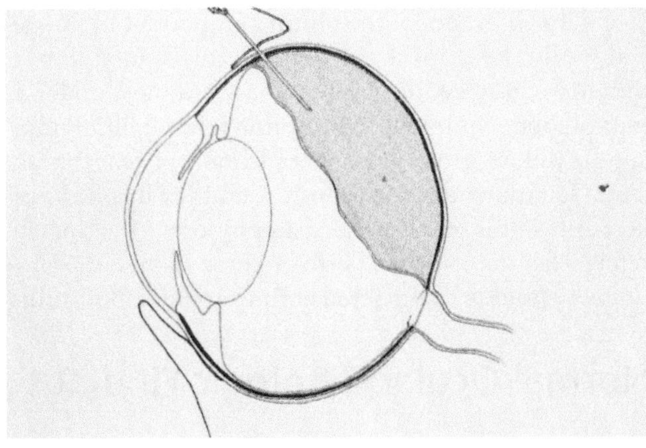

Fig. 3-8
Vitreous or subretinal paracentesis is performed through a pars plana approach, taking care not to puncture the lens. (Courtesy Don Connor, University of Missouri–Columbia.)

Orbital Aspiration

Retrobulbar fine-needle aspiration may be the least invasive way to acquire diagnostic specimens from space-occupying orbital lesions. The globe and the optic nerve must be avoided. In humans, fine-needle aspirates of the orbit have been useful for diagnosis of unresectable malignant orbital neoplasms, possibly eliminating a need for further surgical intervention.[31] Despite being more efficient and economical in some cases, cytologic diagnosis obtained by orbital aspiration is not as accurate when compared to surgical biopsy.[32,33]

Staining Ocular Specimens

Romanowsky-type stains (Wright's, Giemsa, modified Wright's-Giemsa stain) are useful for identifying inflammatory and neoplastic cells, bacteria, fungi, or cytoplasmic inclusions. With Romanowsky stains, it is possible to recognize and differentiate bacterial cocci *(Staphylococci, Streptococci)*, large rods *(Bacillus)*, and small (some bipolar) rods *(Pseudomonas*, coliforms). Most fungi readily stain with Romanowsky stains. Gram stain may be used to characterize bacteria as gram positive or negative. It may be difficult to identify gram-negative organisms in the red background of exudates, including ocular discharges, stained with Gram stain. Identification of the organism from culture and antimicrobial sensitivity

TABLE 3-1
Gram-Staining Reactions in Conjunctivitis and Keratitis

Staining Characteristics	*Most Probable Causative Organism*
Gram-Positive	
Cocci, singly or in clusters	*Staphylococcus* spp.
Cocci in chains	*Streptococcus* spp., nutritionally variant *Streptococcus* spp.
Rods	*Bacillus* spp.
Filaments	Fungi, especially *Aspergillus* spp., *Fusarium* spp., *Penicillium*, Phycomycetes
Gram-Negative	
Diplobacilli	*Moraxella* spp.
Rods	*Pseudomonas aeruginosa*, coliforms
Filaments	Fungi

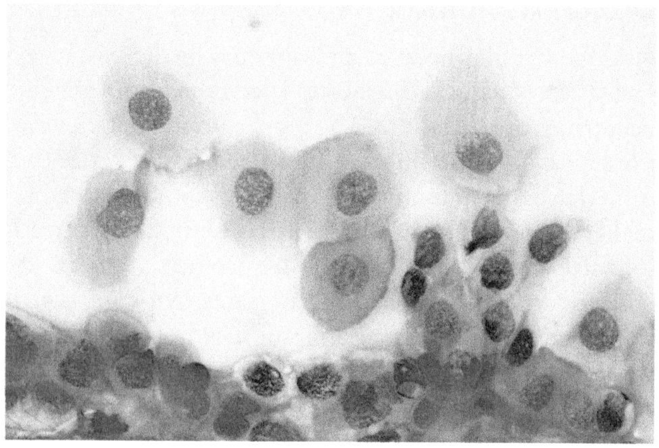

Fig. 3-9 Conjunctival smear.
Epithelial cells have pale blue cytoplasm and round to oval, central, basophilic nuclei.

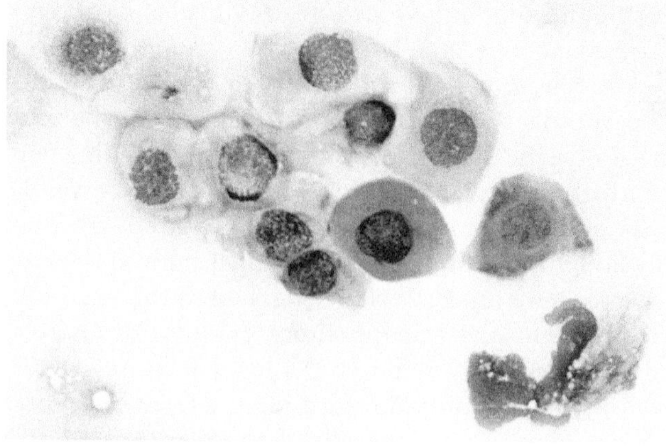

Fig. 3-10 Conjunctival smear.
Cells from the deeper (basal or parabasal cells) are round to cylindric, with less but darker-staining cytoplasm than more superficial cells.

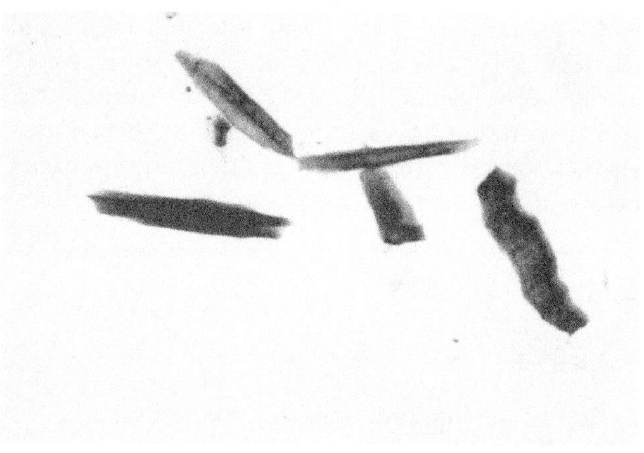

Fig. 3-11 Conjunctival smear.
Keratinaceous debris appears spike-like and results from "scrolling" of flattened epithelial cells.

testing directs definitive therapy; however, immediate treatment may be instituted based on the staining properties and morphologic features of the offending organism and knowledge of common equine ocular pathogens (Table 3-1).

Special stains, such as periodic acid–Schiff (PAS), Gomori methenamine silver (GMS), or Cellufluor (see next section), may be used to detect fungi. However, special stains are not readily available to most practitioners evaluating their own preparations. Special stains are available at most referral laboratories if requested or if the pathologist evaluating the samples decides they are indicated. When collecting specimens, prepare several smears, leaving some unstained so they are available for additional special staining procedures later if deemed necessary.

Special Stains

Immunofluorescent antibody (IFA) testing is not commonly used in diagnosis of equine ocular diseases. The IFA test has been used for conjunctival antigen detection in chlamydial and rabies virus infections.[34,35] *Borrelia burgdorferi* spirochetes have been detected in the anterior chamber of a pony using IFA techniques.[36] Confirmation of equine herpesvirus, serotype 2, has been reported using fluorescent antibody staining.[37] The Calcofluor white–potassium hydroxide technique is a much more sensitive test for microscopic detection of fungi than PAS or GMS staining.[38] Calcofluor white (Cellufluor) is a fluorescent stain that is readily absorbed by the chitin component in fungal cell walls. Diagnostic specimens are stained for 1 minute, counterstained, and then examined under a microscope equipped with ultraviolet light. Fungi appear yellow-green against a red-orange background. The Cellufluor examination is useful for diagnosis of keratomycoses and for dermatophytoses.[39-41] Not all referral laboratories can perform these tests, so the laboratory should be contacted before sample submission.

Normal Ocular Cytologic Findings

Conjunctival and Corneal Epithelial Cells

Morphologic features of normal corneal and conjunctival cells of horses are similar to those described for dogs and cats.[13,14] Scrapings from healthy cornea or conjunctiva characteristically yield sheets of epithelial cells containing

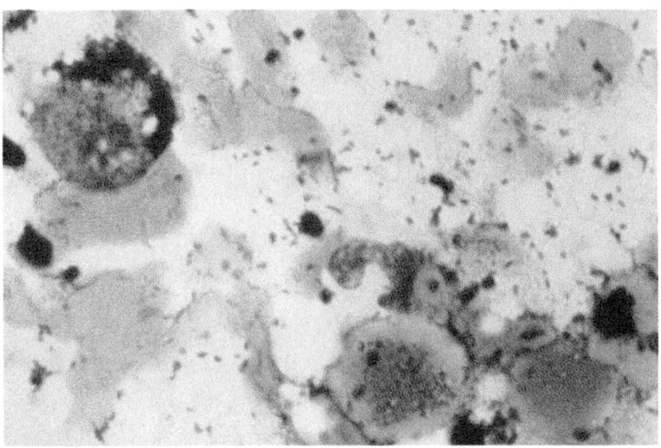

Fig. 3-12 Conjunctival smear.
Melanocytes and melanin granules appear dark green to brown or black. Numerous melanin granules are dusted throughout the background.

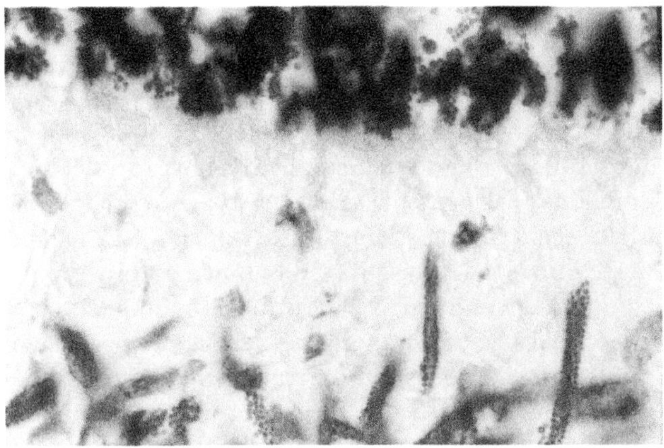

Fig. 3-13 Iris melanin granules.
Melanin granules from the iris (shown here) or ciliary body are oval or round, in contrast to the more lanceolate melanin granules present in retinal pigment epithelial cells.

cells from one or more of their representative layers. Superficial epithelial cells are flattened with large amounts of pale blue cytoplasm and round to oval, central, basophilic nuclei (Fig. 3-9). Cells from the intermediate zone are more polyhedral in appearance when compared to superficial epithelial cells. Basal or parabasal cells, originating from the deepest layers of the cornea and conjunctiva, are round or cylindrical, with less abundant but darker-staining cytoplasm (Fig. 3-10). Keratinized corneal or conjunctival epithelial cells are abnormal, except for conjunctival cells adjacent to the eyelid margin, which are normally keratinized. Epithelial cells that are keratinized have dark blue to blue-green cytoplasm, with a degenerate, pyknotic, or absent nucleus. Many of these cells "scroll" when smeared, resulting in a jagged or sharply pointed and long rectangular appearance (Fig. 3-11). This artifact should not be mistaken for foreign material.

Melanin Granules

Intracytoplasmic melanin granules are common in epithelial cells collected from pigmented areas, such as the limbus, or pigmented ocular lesions. Pigment granules are not found in normal corneal epithelial cells. Melanin granules appear dark green to brown or black (Fig. 3-12) and may demonstrate slightly different shapes, depending on their location. Melanin granules in iridal cells are generally oval to round versus more lanceolate shaped in retinal pigmented epithelial cells (Fig. 3-13).[29] Small amounts of free melanin granules and a few melanin-containing cells (melanocytes, melanophages) may be seen in aqueous paracentesis samples.[42]

Microorganisms

Populations of bacterial flora normally inhabit the ocular mucosal surface and can be found on routine cytologic specimens from healthy horses. Gram-positive isolates predominate, with some gram-negative organisms found less commonly.[19,43] Long-term use of topical ophthalmic antibacterials may lead to the overgrowth of pathogenic bacteria, yeast, or fungi.[44]

Goblet Cells and Mucus

Goblet cells are large, distended cells with a peripheral nucleus. The round to oval nucleus may be molded into a crescent shape when the goblet-cell cytoplasm becomes laden with mucus. Intracellular mucus may appear as a clear area or may stain red to blue (depending on the quantity present) with Romanowsky stains (Fig. 3-14). With periodic acid–Schiff (PAS) stain, mucus stains a dark pink (Fig. 3-15). Goblet cells tend to occur in clusters and are found in greatest concentration in the lower nasal fornix in some species.[45]

Erythrocytes and Inflammatory Cells

Occasional erythrocytes, lymphocytes, monocytes, plasma cells, and neutrophils are usually present in conjunctival scrapings from normal horses. If scraping has been overzealous, the number and type of these cells may be increased due to peripheral blood contamination. Inflammatory diseases usually result in much higher numbers of neutrophils, lymphocytes, monocytes, or plasma cells than occur with peripheral blood contamination alone. Therefore, if these cells are present in large numbers without accompanying erythrocytes, an inflammatory response is most likely present. The bulbar surface of the membrana nictitans normally contains some lymphoid follicles. Scrapings from this area may contain

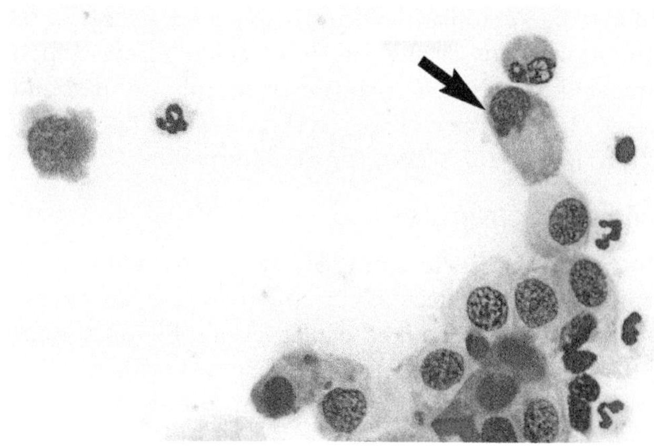

Fig. 3-14 Conjunctival smear.
A goblet cell, featured near the top of this image, has an eccentric nucleus and a clear, pale blue cytoplasm.

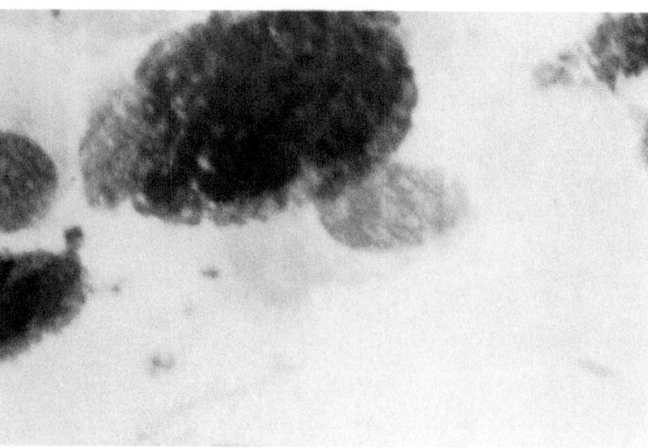

Fig. 3-15
Goblet cell with eccentric nucleus and granular intracellular mucin that stains dark pink with PAS stain.

numerous, variably sized lymphocytes, similar to those found in normal lymph nodes. Therefore, correct interpretation of a cytologic specimen where inflammatory cells are present should be made with consideration to the presence or absence of clinical signs of ocular inflammation and the number and type of inflammatory cells seen. Eosinophils and basophils are not normally present in conjunctival or corneal scrapings from horses.

Pseudoinclusions

Improper spreading of cells on the glass slide may result in rupture of the nuclear membrane and subsequent herniation of nuclear material into the cytoplasm. This artifact may give the appearance of an inclusion body and is referred to as a pseudoinclusion.

Aqueous Humor

Anterior chamber aspirates from normal eyes are virtually acellular.[30] A few erythrocytes, mature lymphocytes, histiocytes, free pigment granules, and pigment-containing cells are occasionally present. Because the protein content of normal aqueous humor is very low, in vitro disintegration of cells may be rapid.[30]

Eyelids

Bacterial Lesions

Primary bacterial blepharitis is rare in horses. Eyelid abscesses are usually secondary to a foreign body reaction.[46] High numbers of degenerate and nondegenerate neutrophils, with or without bacteria, are seen cytologically. Chronic blepharitis with draining tract formation secondary to a bone sequestrum of the zygomatic arch was reported in one horse.[47] *Moraxella* sp. may cause ulcerative dermatitis with erosions of the mucocutaneous junction of the eyelids and medial canthus.[48,49]

Fungal Lesions

The eyelids of horses may become infected by cutaneous and systemic fungi. Dermatophytosis due to infection with *Trichophyton* sp. or *Microsporum* sp. may result in eyelid alopecia, crusting, scaling, and dermatitis (see Chapter 2). Definitive diagnosis is based on microscopic examination of hairs and surface debris, fungal culture, and skin biopsy. Because most domestic animal dermatophyte infections are of the ectothrix type, it is not usually necessary to use hair shaft–clearing techniques involving potassium hydroxide to visualize the fungi.[50] Hair and keratin can be examined for fungal hyphae and conidia simply by suspending the specimens in mineral oil or saline. Arthroconidia may be seen on the hair shaft, with hyphae invading and penetrating the hair shaft. Cutaneous scrapings may also be stained with Wright's stain. Arthroconidia appear as small (2 to 4 μ), dark blue, round to oval spores (see Chapter 2).

Phycomycosis (mycetomas) are subcutaneous infections occurring in tropical climates that may be caused by several different species.[51] The eyelids may be involved when lesions occur on the head and are characterized by pruritus, granulation tissue, and necrotic draining tracts.

Histoplasma farciminosum is enzootic in Africa, Asia, and Eastern Europe. Epizootic lymphangitis, caused by *H. farciminosum*, may be characterized by a localized granuloma along the free margin of the eyelid.[52] Conjunctival and lacrimal involvement may also occur. Diagnosis is made by seeing the double-contoured, thin-walled, budding, oval yeast cells, 2 to 3 μ in diameter (Plate 4C) on smears or aspirates from the affected

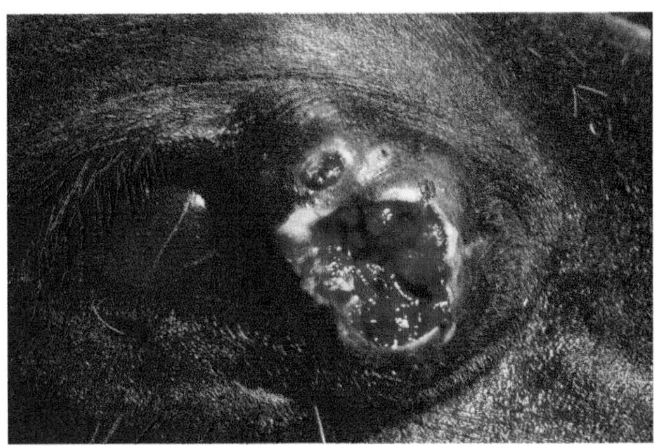

Fig. 3-16 Habronemiasis.
Habronemiasis is characterized by nonhealing, raised, ulcerated lesions containing yellow, caseous, gritty nodules.

tissue. *Histoplasma* infections are associated with a mononuclear-cell response, with monocytes and macrophages predominating. Neutrophils are generally found in fewer numbers than mononuclear cells and are nondegenerate. Reactive lymphocytes may be present. *Cryptococcus mirandi* may also cause ulcerative eyelid lesions (Plate 4H).[46]

Viral Lesions

Viral causes of equine eyelid disease include facial papillomas and horsepox virus.[46] Equine papillomas (warts) resulting from a papova virus can be commonly found on the face of young horses. These warts may regress spontaneously in several months or can be treated via surgical removal, cryotherapy, or autogenous vaccination.[53]

Horsepox is a rare, benign disease of horses in Europe caused by an unclassified poxvirus. Horsepox has been reported once in North America in a donkey.[54] The buccal form of horsepox (contagious pustular dermatitis) is characterized by multiple vesicles, umbilicated pustules, and crusts on the lips and buccal mucosa. In severe cases, the eyelids and conjunctiva may be affected. It may be possible to find large, eosinophilic, intracytoplasmic poxvirus inclusions in vacuolated keratinocytes in cutaneous scrapings and conjunctival scrapings.

Parasitic Lesions

Eyelid disease may result from ectoparasitism or migrating helminth larvae. Habronemiasis is a common cause of eyelid, conjunctival, caruncular, and membrana nictitans granulomas.[55,56] House flies and stable flies (*Habronema muscae, H. microstoma*, or *Draschia megastoma*) act as the biologic vectors of habronemiasis, so ocular lesions are seasonal in occurrence, predominating in warm months.[46] Larvae deposited on moist ocular tissues migrate into the skin, conjunctiva, and nasolacrimal system and cause an intense inflammatory reaction. The ocular lesions are characterized by pruritic, nonhealing, raised, ulcerative, granulomatous lesions, sometimes associated with fistulous tracts (Fig. 3-16). Other clinical signs are discussed in later sections.

Cytologic examination of eyelid habronemiasis is characterized by numerous eosinophils, mast cells, neutrophils, and plasma cells, often without positive larvae identification (Fig. 3-17).[46] Larvae may be better identified in minced tissue preparations from a nodule. Without observation of the definitive cytologic presence of larvae, it may be difficult to distinguish eyelid habronemiasis from a mast-cell tumor, eosinophilic granuloma with collagen degeneration (nodular necrobiosis), or phycomycosis.[57] *Habronema* and *Draschia* larvae may also invade other ulcerative dermatoses, such as sarcoid or squamous-cell carcinoma, which may complicate the cytologic findings, making definitive diagnosis more difficult. Therefore, histopathologic examination of any granuloma, in addition to cytologic examination, is recommended for definitive diagnosis.

Though naturally occurring demodectic mange is rare in horses, two species of demodecid mites, *Demodex equi* and *D. folliculorum* var *equi*, may cause meibomitis, eyelid alopecia, papulopustular dermatitis, and mild blepharitis secondary to their presence in the meibomian glands or modified sebaceous glands of the eyelids.[58-60] Diagnosis is made by gently expressing meibomian-gland secretions from the eyelid margin and microscopic examination of the material for the cigar-shaped mites.

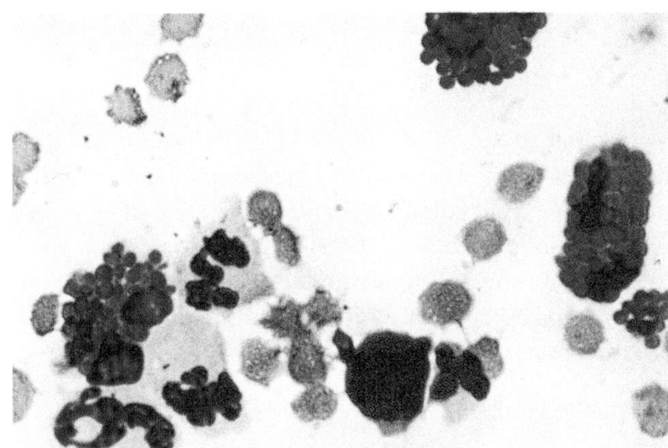

Fig. 3-17 Habronemiasis.
Cytologic preparation from horse with habronemiasis. Numerous eosinophils, mast cells, neutrophils, and plasma cells are usually present.

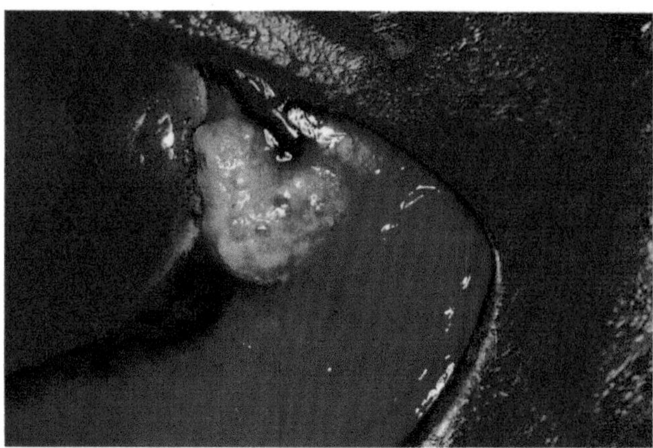

Fig. 3-18 Squamous-cell carcinoma.
Squamous-cell carcinoma involving the temporal limbus and adjacent cornea.

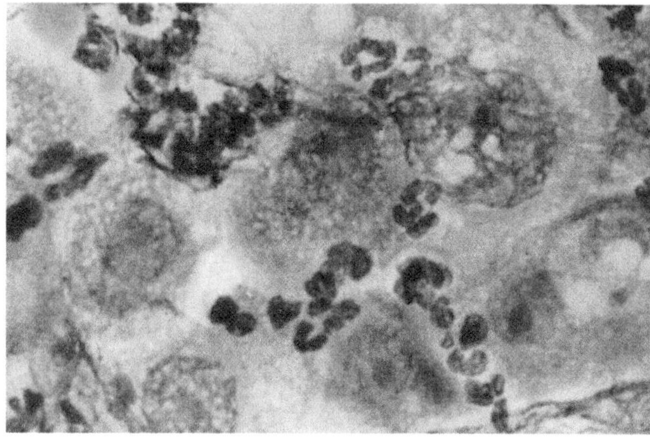

Fig. 3-19 Squamous-cell carcinoma.
Squamous-cell carcinoma is characterized by pleomorphic basophilic epithelial cells with a variable nucleus-to-cytoplasm ratio and prominent, often multiple, nuclei.

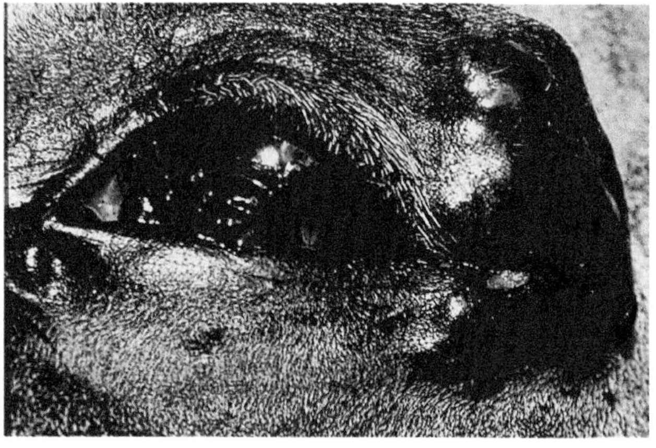

Fig. 3-20 Equine sarcoid.
This benign fibrovascular tumor presented as a darkly pigmented, lobulated mass involving the temporal aspect of the upper and lower eyelids.

Edematous eyelids, epiphora, jaundiced ocular mucous membranes, conjunctival hemorrhage, distention of the supraorbital fossa, and blood-stained tears are ocular manifestations of *Babesia caballi* or *Babesia equi* infections.[61] The characteristic *Babesia* organisms may be seen in erythrocytes in conjunctival scrapings or nasolacrimal secretions (Plate 5G).

Neoplastic Lesions

The most common equine eyelid tumors are squamous-cell carcinoma, sarcoid, and melanoma.[62] Various other neoplasms have been less frequently reported, including fibroma, fibrosarcoma, neurofibroma, schwannoma, papilloma, lymphosarcoma, plasmacytoma, mastocytoma, adenoma, adenocarcinoma, basal-cell carcinoma, and angiosarcoma.[46]

Squamous-cell carcinoma (SCC) usually arises in a zone of epithelial transition, such as the limbus or mucocutaneous eyelid junctions. However, SCC can arise from any epithelial surface and may affect the eyelid, conjunctiva, membrana nictitans, caruncle, and/or cornea (Fig. 3-18). Environmental (ie, solar radiation) as well as host factors such as breed, age, and amount of adnexal pigmentation are factors that may increase a horse's risk of developing this neoplasm.[63,64] Clinically, the tumor can range from small, white, elevated, hyperplastic plaques or papilloma-like structures with verrucous surfaces to irregular, nodular, pink, erosive, necrotic lesions. Squamous-cell carcinoma is characterized by pleomorphic basophilic epithelial cells with a variable nucleus to cytoplasmic ratio and prominent, often multiple, nucleoli (Fig. 3-19). Numerous mitotic figures may be seen. Obtaining a biopsy specimen is the cornerstone for diagnosis and may incorporate treatment with diagnosis in one step if the lesion is small.[65]

Equine sarcoids are benign fibroblastic tumors that present as single or multiple masses of the eyelids and periocular area (Fig. 3-20).[66] Grossly, sarcoids may be smooth, ulcerated, or verrucous in nature, with the overlying skin usually alopecic or secondarily infected.[67] Histologically, sarcoids are composed mainly of fibrous tissue and generally yield few cells by aspiration, scrapings, or touch impressions. While cytologic samples containing scattered spindle cells support the clinical diagnosis of sarcoid, histologic examination of tissue from these lesions is needed to confirm the diagnosis. Sarcoids must be differentiated from fibromas and schwannomas.

Melanomas of the equine eyelid arise as localized, slowly growing, pigmented tumors with minimal risk

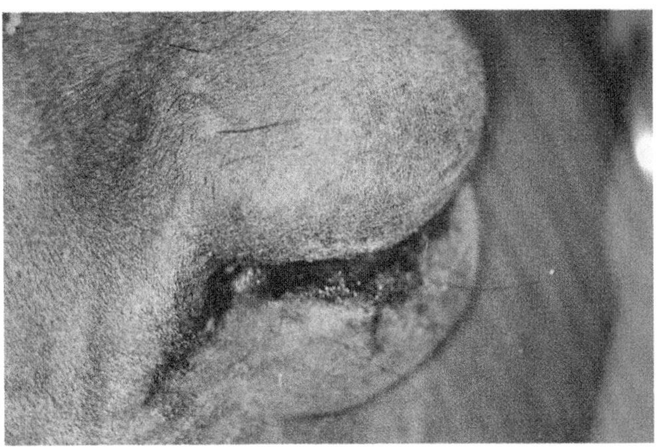

Fig. 3-21 Lymphosarcoma.
Eyelid swelling attributable to lymphosarcoma. (Courtesy Dr. Christopher Murphy, University of Wisconsin–Madison.)

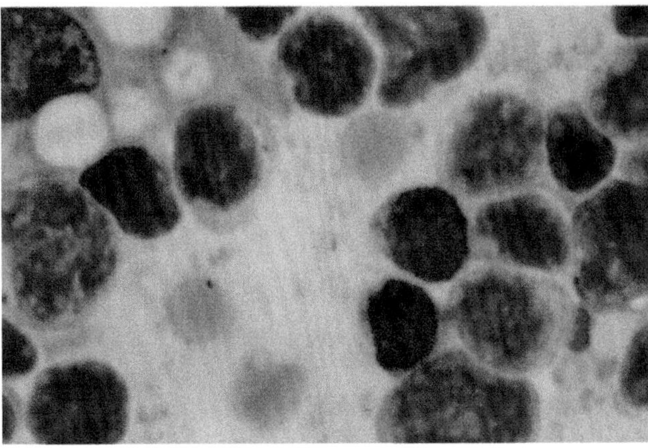

Fig. 3-22 Aspirate from eyelid lymphosarcoma.
These pleomorphic lymphoblasts have prominent, large nucleoli and vacuolated basophilic cytoplasm.

of distant metastasis. Arabian, Percheron, and gray horses appear more at risk than other horses to develop this neoplasm.[62] Cytologically melanocytes may appear as round, spindle, or epithelial cells. They generally contain abundant greenish-black pigment that may obscure the nucleus. The absence of malignant criteria, especially if the nucleus cannot be adequately evaluated due to heavy granulation, does not rule out malignancy. Diagnosis should be confirmed by biopsy and histopathologic examination.

Although lymphosarcoma is not a common ocular disease in horses, one review demonstrated that the most common equine ocular manifestation was infiltration of the eyelids and palpebral conjunctiva (Fig. 3-21).[68] Additional reports of horses affected with ocular adnexal lymphosarcoma have been sporadic.[69,70] Lymphosarcoma should be suspected when a monomorphic population of atypical or large immature lymphocytes is observed in smears (Fig. 3-22). The immaturity of these cells may be realized by comparing erythrocyte size to lymphoid cell size. The equine red blood cell is about 5 μ in diameter, while benign lymphoid cells are usually no larger than 15 μ in diameter. Typically, a mixture of predominantly small cells with a few medium-sized or occasionally large lymphocytes may be found in any lymphoid reaction. In contrast, neoplastic lymphocytes have larger amounts of basophilic, sometimes vacuolated cytoplasm; homogeneous or irregularly clumped, pale-staining, lace-like nucleochromatin; and prominent, irregular, and sometimes multiple nucleoli.[71] Difficulty in finding a heterogeneous population of lymphocytes predominated by small cells with condensed dark nuclei or, alternatively, an abundance of immature blast-like cells should increase the index of suspicion for lymphoid neoplasia.

Other Lesions

Chalazia (meibomian cysts) are not common in horses and must be differentiated from parasitic granulomas and other granulomas. The upper or lower eyelid may be affected with single or multiple chalazia. The affected site appears white to yellow and may be abscessed. The mass may contain a hard concretion or a caseous substance. Fine-needle aspirates from a chalazion contain numerous foamy macrophages. Sebaceous-gland epithelial cells, lymphocytes, giant cells, and amorphous debris may also be present (Fig. 3-23). Meibomianitis, in which the meibomian glands become abscessed, is unusual in horses. Lesions may appear similar to chalazia, except numerous glands in one or more eyelids are affected. The abscesses may open and drain. One horse with meibomianitis had a chronic granulomatous reaction characterized by numerous eosinophils.[57]

Pemphigus foliaceus may affect the equine eyelid, as well as other parts of the body. Microscopic examination of aspirates from intact vesicles or pustules may contain acanthocytes and nondegenerate neutrophils or eosinophils. Occasional acanthocytes may be seen in any suppurative condition; however, when these cells are present in clusters or large numbers, pemphigus is strongly suspected.[50] Acanthocytes are difficult to reliably identify in cytologic preparations; histopathologic examination of excised tissue from these lesions is required to confirm a diagnosis of pemphigus foliaceus.

Eosinophilic granulomas with collagen degeneration may occasionally occur on the eyelid. The nodules are usually firm, rounded, well circumscribed, nonalopecic, and nonulcerated. Aspirates of the nodules contain eosinophils, mast cells, histiocytes, lymphocytes, and no microorganisms.[50] Differential diagnoses include mast-cell tumors and parasitic granulomas.

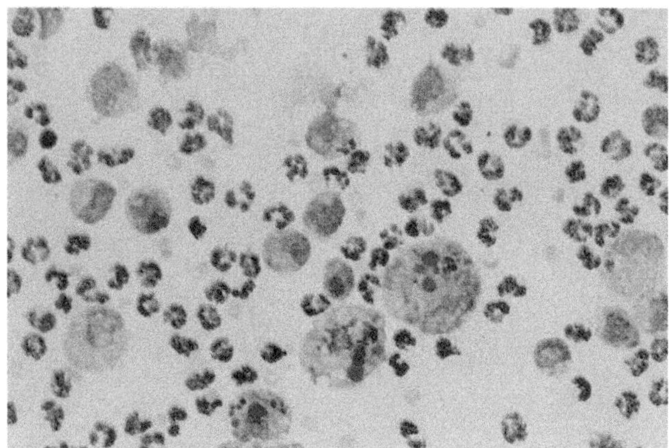

Fig. 3-23 Fine-needle aspirate of chalazion. Note the vacuolated and foamy macrophages among nondegenerate neutrophils.

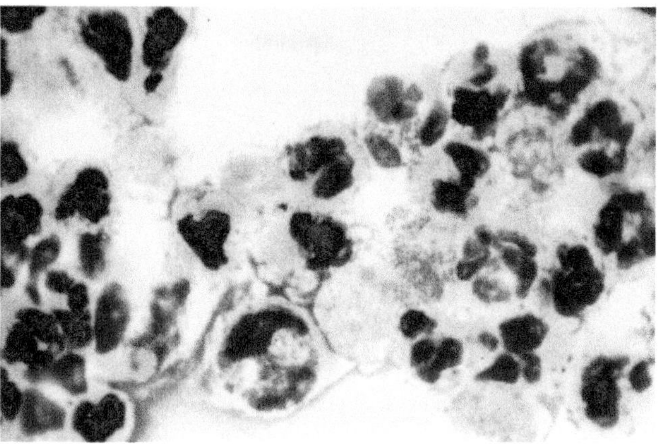

Fig. 3-24 Streptococcal conjunctivitis. Numerous cocci and degenerate and nondegenerate neutrophils are seen.

Subpalpebral lavage systems are commonly used as a means of providing frequent topical administration to the equine eye.[72] Complications such as tube slippage can occur, allowing medication to enter the subcutaneous tissue and resulting in severe palpebral cellulitis or mechanical abrasion of the cornea.[73,74] Acute and chronic allergic blepharitis, solar blepharitis of nonpigmented skin, and St. John's wort photosensitization of the lids have also been reported.[46]

Conjunctiva, Membrana Nictitans, and Caruncle

Bacterial Lesions

Primary bacterial conjunctivitis is uncommon in horses. Secondary conjunctivitis often accompanies other primary equine ocular problems such as trauma, toxic insult, allergic stimuli, lid abnormalities, decreased tear production, dacryocystitis, keratitis, or uveitis.[62]

Moraxella equi has been isolated from horses with primary bacterial conjunctivitis.[75,76] Clinical findings in affected horses include bacterial conjunctivitis with mucocutaneous eyelid erosions. Cytologically, short, round-ended, gram-negative coccobacillus organisms occurring in pairs and short chains can be found.[75-77] Conjunctival cultures are necessary to definitively diagnose the causative organism.

Systemic bacterial infectious agents that often manifest with conjunctivitis as part of the disease syndrome include chlamydial, pseudomonal, and streptococcal infections. Foals with chlamydial polyarthritis may have an associated conjunctivitis.[78] *Chlamydia* was the reported cause of an outbreak of keratoconjunctivitis in a stable of horses.[79] Chlamydial organisms appear as basophilic intracytoplasmic inclusion bodies within conjunctival cells.

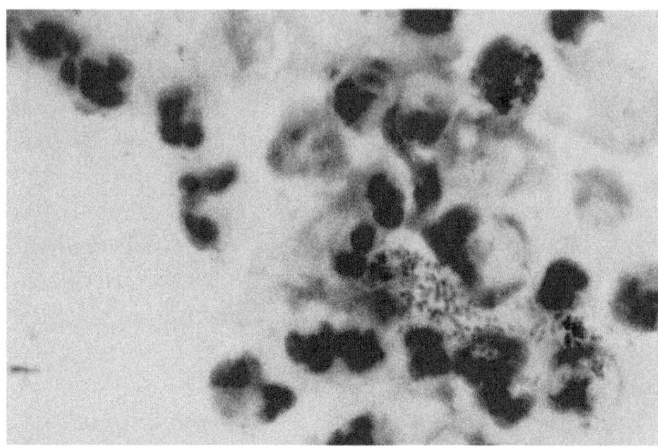

Fig. 3-25 Streptococcal conjunctivitis (Gram stain).

Bacterial conjunctivitis has been associated with *Streptococcus equi* infection (Figs. 3-24 and 3-25). Large numbers of neutrophils with intracellular or extracellular cocci are present. Cytologically, secondary bacterial infection is identical to primary bacterial infection, characterized by a marked inflammatory response containing neutrophils and intracellular as well as extracellular bacteria.

Horses with "glanders" (*Pseudomonas mallei* infection) may develop raised gray to purple nodules (5 to 12 mm) at the limbus.[57] The disease is restricted to Eastern Europe, Asia, and North Africa. Causative bacteria are gram-negative, short rods with rounded ends.

Fungal Lesions

Mycotic conjunctivitis, as a primary condition in North America, occurs infrequently in horses and when present is most commonly associated with keratomycosis (see Cornea). In tropical climates, *Blastomyces* may infect the conjunctiva and nasolacrimal system. Pyogranulomatous lesions containing the organism can be found adjacent to the nasolacrimal puncta.

Histoplasma farciminosum causes epizootic lymphangitis, which may be manifested as mild self-limiting conjunctivitis, severe wound infection of the eyelid and conjunctiva, or nasolacrimal infection.[80] The disease probably no longer occurs in North America but is still common in some countries, notably China, India, Egypt, and Sudan.[81] *Cryptococcus mirandi* may cause eyelid ulcerations that involve the conjunctiva.[46] Phycomycosis may appear similar to habronemiasis. Phycomycosis caused by *Hyphomyces destruens* can be diagnosed by finding hyphae in aspirates or conjunctival scrapings and by culture.[82]

Viral Lesions

Conjunctivitis in horses may be due to a variety of viral etiologies, including equine adenovirus, equine herpes virus, equine viral arteritis, influenza virus, and African horse sickness.[53] Intracellular inclusion bodies in conjunctival epithelial cells may not always be found in these diseases in cytologic preparations. A lymphocytic cellular response usually predominates in the acute phase of ocular viral infections, while neutrophils predominate in the more chronic phases.

Adenoviral conjunctivitis in immunodeficient Arabian foals is accompanied by mucopurulent nasal and ocular discharge.[83] Characteristic intranuclear inclusion bodies may be found in conjunctival epithelial cells. With Giemsa stain, the inclusions are deep red-purple and centrally located in the nucleus, with marginated chromatin surrounding the inclusion bodies. The cellular response includes macrophages, neutrophils, swollen epithelial cells, and large amounts of mucus.[83]

Parasitic Lesions

Eyelid, membrana nictitans, and caruncular conjunctival granulomas are most commonly caused by habronemiasis. Clinical signs associated with habronemiasis include pruritic, yellow, raised, plaque-like, gritty, conjunctival nodules. The nodules, sometimes referred to as "sulfur granules," are approximately 1 to 2 mm in diameter and are considered pathognomonic when seen.[55] These gritty conjunctival nodules are made up of calcified concretions embedded in necrotic tissue. The medial canthus may be affected with raised, painful, ulcerative granulomas with fistulous tracts. Proliferative, papillomatous, reddened lesions that later turn yellow can develop on the third eyelid.[55] Cytologic features have been discussed (see Eyelids).

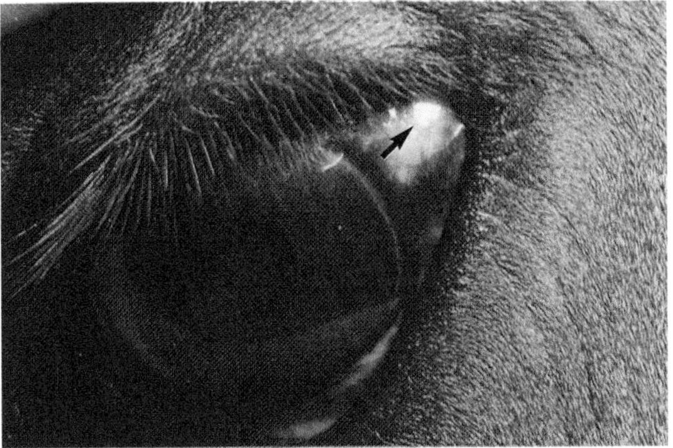

Fig. 3-26 Onchocercal hypersensitivity reaction. Perilimbal bulbar conjunctival nodules, follicles, and vitiligo (*arrow*) suggest onchocercal hypersensitivity reaction.

Onchocerciasis, caused by *Onchocerca cervicalis* and its vector the *Culicoides* sp. midge, can cause several forms of ocular disease, including conjunctivitis, keratitis, and uveitis.[84] Small firm perilimbal nodules and follicles with associated bulbar conjunctival vitiligo at the temporal limbus are particularly characteristic (Fig. 3-26). Some horses also have chronic corneal vascularization and edema.[55]

Corneal and conjunctival cytology of affected regions reveal a pleocellular reaction consisting of eosinophils, neutrophils, lymphocytes, plasma cells, and macrophages. The presence of eosinophils in horses with characteristic clinical findings is highly suggestive, though not definitive, of onchocerciasis. Fragments of dead microfilariae, as well as live ones, may occasionally be seen cytologically. Onchocercal microfilariae are approximately 200 to 240 μ long and 4 to 5 μ in diameter, with a short, unsheathed tail.[85,86] Microfilariae may be more easily seen with a wet-mount preparation of conjunctival tissue from the affected region. A portion of excised conjunctiva is moistened with warm saline and minced with a razor blade for direct observation of microfilariae (Fig. 3-27). The remainder is fixed in formalin for histologic examination. Microfilariae may also be observed in conjunctival tissues from clinically normal horses. Superficial keratectomy and histologic examination of the perilimbal corneal tissue adjacent to the affected conjunctival region may reveal onchocercal microfilariae when the conjunctival biopsy is negative.[57] Histologically, *Onchocerca* microfilariae have been found in the subepithelial layer of the cornea.[87,88]

Thelazia lacrimalis, a spiruroid nematode, is a commensal parasite that inhabits the conjunctiva and nasolacrimal duct of the horse.[46] Most horses are asymptomatic, but chronic conjunctivitis with nodule formation, dacryocystitis, blepharedema, superficial keratitis, and seromucoid exudates can occur when *Thelazia* burrow into the ocular tissues and incite an inflammatory response.[53,55] The cellular reaction is predominantly lymphoplasmacytic with moderate numbers of eosinophils.[89] *Thelazia* are 8 to 18 mm long and milky white, with prominent annular cuticular striations.[90] A variety of other infectious ocular parasitic diseases manifesting with

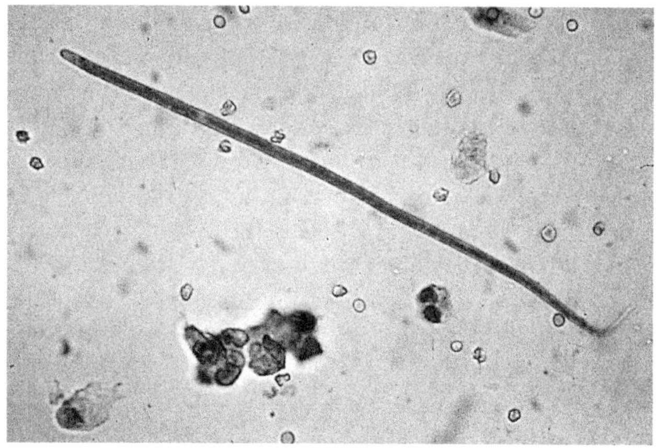

Fig. 3-27 ***Onchocerca*** **microfilariae in minced conjunctival specimen.**

ocular signs have been reported, including cestodiasis, myiasis, and systemic parasites. The reader is referred to a review article, which discusses these rarer conditions in more detail.[55]

Neoplastic Lesions

Tumors involving the conjunctiva of the horse include squamous cell carcinoma, lymphosarcoma, papilloma, and hemangiosarcoma, among others.[62] Cytologic specimens from conjunctival neoplasia may be difficult to interpret due to concurrent bacterial, parasitic, or mycotic infections that may secondarily infiltrate the neoplastic area. While aspirates or scrapings of a conjunctival neoplastic mass may be diagnostic, biopsy with histopathologic examination remains the gold standard for proper identification of any ocular neoplastic process.

While various neoplasms affect the conjunctiva of the eyelid, membrana nictitans, and caruncle, squamous-cell carcinoma is the most common (see Eyelid). A review of 21 equine cases with ocular lymphosarcoma found that neoplastic infiltration of the palpebral conjunctiva and eyelids was the most common ocular lesion.[68] Sebaceous adenocarcinoma and basal-cell tumor of the membrana nictitans have been reported.[91,92] See Chapter 2 for cytologic details of these tumor types.

Aspirates or scrapings of vascular neoplasms usually yield a large amount of blood that may contain few endothelial cells. A moderate number of endothelial cells occasionally may be collected. These tend to be oval, spindle, or stellate, with a moderate to abundant amount of light to dark blue cytoplasm and a round to oval nucleus. Criteria of malignancy may be minimal to marked. Hemangiomas should not be separated from hemangiosarcomas by cytologic examination alone. They should be excised and submitted for histopathologic examination.

One report of a conjunctival hemangioma described a raised red lesion at the lateral limbus, attached to the conjunctiva and underlying sclera.[93] Histopathologically, the mass consisted of irregular blood-filled spaces. Angiosarcomas originating from the equine conjunctiva are considered highly malignant neoplasms. An intense lymphocytic/plasmacytic inflammatory infiltrate may be present within and surrounding an ocular angiosarcoma and may lead to misdiagnosis as cellulitis.[94,95]

Equine conjunctival melanoma has been described.[96,97] In the first case report, a darkly pigmented, raised, pedunculated mass was found arising from the limbal bulbar conjunctiva with corneal involvement.[96] Cytologic examination contained numerous anisokaryotic, karyorrhectic melanocytes containing large amounts of melanin. A presumptive diagnosis of conjunctival melanoma was later confirmed by histologic examination. A second case report of equine conjunctival melanoma has recently been published.[97] In this more recent report, the conjunctival melanoma demonstrated locally aggressive behavior and recurred following two separate treatment episodes, eventually necessitating orbital exenteration.

Other Lesions

Allergic conjunctivitis is characterized by hyperemic and edematous conjunctiva and is usually bilateral. The eyelids may be edematous, and a serous discharge may be present.[57] Pruritus and self-trauma are typical of allergic conjunctivitis. Conjunctival cytologic preparations may reveal a mixed inflammatory cellular response with variable numbers of eosinophils and/or mast cells.

Follicular conjunctivitis may develop when chronic ocular disease induces lymphoid follicle formation on the bulbar and/or palpebral conjunctiva and/or on the palpebral surface of the third eyelid. Conjunctival follicles are most often associated with environmental irritants but have also been reported with ocular parasites.[55]

Raised, red conjunctival masses may develop following trauma due to exuberant growth of granulation tissue. The slowly growing mass must be differentiated from neoplasia or a granuloma. Cytologically, granulation tissue yields low to high numbers of fibroblasts. Fibroblasts are spindle cells that have an oval nucleus with ropy nuclear chromatin and often visible nucleoli (Plate 7A, *right*). Fibroblasts from granulation tissue may show marked variation in cell and nuclear size and are easily confused with spindle cell tumors cytologically. Biopsy and histopathology are needed to definitively differentiate granulation tissue from fibrous tissue (spindle-cell) neoplasia.

Orbital fat, or fat surrounding the base of the membrana nictitans, may herniate beneath the conjunctiva.[62] Herniated fat appears as a beige or yellow, smooth to slightly lobulated subconjunctival mass (Fig. 3-28). The conjunctiva may become stretched by the mass and appear to be quite thin. Aspiration and cytologic evaluation confirm the presence of adipose cells.[98] Grossly, the smears appear greasy. Cytologically, adipose cells are large (30 to 40 μ) cells with a clear vacuolated central area and a small peripheral nucleus (4 to 6 μ) found within a thin rim of cytoplasm and are often found in clusters or rafts (Plate 6H). The commonly used Romanowsky stains are alcohol based and dissolve free lipid. Therefore, if the aspirated adipocytes are ruptured and only free fat is present on the smear, it will dissolve during the staining procedure and not be visible on stained smears.

Nasolacrimal System

Material is collected from the nasolacrimal system by flushing the nasolacrimal canaliculi or ducts with sterile saline from the upper eyelid punctum or through the nasolacrimal meatus at the rostral end of the nose. Cytologic examination is performed on sediments of washings or exudate collected.[46]

Dacryocystitis may develop secondary to a foreign body in the nasolacrimal system, parasites, bacterial or mycotic infections, or neoplastic lesions. Inflammatory exudates may contain variable numbers of neutrophils, macrophages, and bacteria as well as mucus. Exudates should be examined carefully for fungi, plant material, and neoplastic cells.

The nasolacrimal system and paranasal sinuses may become infected with streptococcal species. Streptococcal infections are characterized by a neutrophilic response, with phagocytized bacterial cocci. *Streptococcus equi* may produce abscessation of the lacrimal gland.[57] "Necrotic granulomatous lesions" in the lacrimal sac and nasolacrimal ducts in donkeys from Egypt have been described.[80] The etiologic agent was *Histoplasma farciminosum*.

Severe bilateral eosinophilic granulomatous dacryoadenitis of the lacrimal and membrana nictitans gland was possibly caused by parasites in one horse.[99] Findings of conjunctival cytologic preparations were consistent only with abnormally low tear production, including epithelial hyperplasia and dysplasia, and lymphoid hyperplasia. Lacrimal-gland aspirates were not examined.

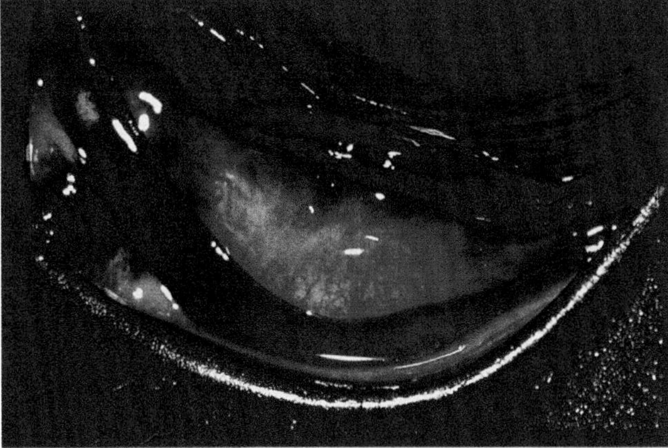

Fig. 3-28 Orbital fat prolapse in horse.
Note the smooth protruding subconjunctival mass behind the nictitating membrane. (Courtesy Dr. David Maggs, University of California–Davis.)

Cornea and Sclera

The equine cornea is constantly exposed to a wide variety of bacterial and fungal agents, both from the environment and from normal conjunctival flora.[43] Corneal abrasion or epithelial defects with subsequent infectious keratitis can develop secondary to traumatic abrasion, corneal edema, exposure keratitis, keratoconjunctivitis sicca, neurotrophic keratitis from equine protozoal myeloencephalitis, and neuroparalytic keratitis.[53,100] Equine infectious keratitis may be classified as ulcerative or nonulcerative (stromal abscess).[101] Cytology and culture with sensitivity are essential diagnostic tests to be performed in any case of equine keratitis that has a history of poor response to previous therapy or evidence of infection with or without stromal melting.[102]

Bacterial Lesions

Common gram-positive pathogens known to infect the equine cornea include *Staphylococcus* and *Streptococcus* spp.[20,103,104] *Pseudomonas* sp. and assorted coliform bacteria such as *E. coli* are gram-negative organisms that may also colonize the damaged equine cornea.[105]

Corneal stromal abscesses occur when microorganisms infect the cornea and the epithelium subsequently regrows and seals bacteria within the corneal stroma.[106] Stromal abscesses may occur as single, multifocal, or diffuse areas of yellow-white stromal infiltrates (Fig. 3-29). In cases of nonulcerated stromal abscesses, cytologic examination of scrapings of the corneal epithelium may be insufficient for diagnosis because the organisms are embedded deep within the stroma. Therefore, scrapings of both the corneal epithelium and the deeper stroma should be examined. Neutrophils are the predominant inflammatory cell present.[105] Cocci are seen most frequently, but bacilli or a mixed bacterial and fungal population may also be seen.[107] Bacteria cultured from stromal abscesses include *Streptococcus* and *Staphylococcus* spp., *E. coli*, and *Corynebacterium*, among others.[6,105,108] Stromal abscesses occasionally are sterile.

Pseudomonas keratitis may be strongly suspected when corneal cytology reveals large numbers of gram-negative rods (Fig. 3-30).[109,110] *Pseudomonas* infections can provoke liquefaction of corneal stromal proteoglycans with rapid

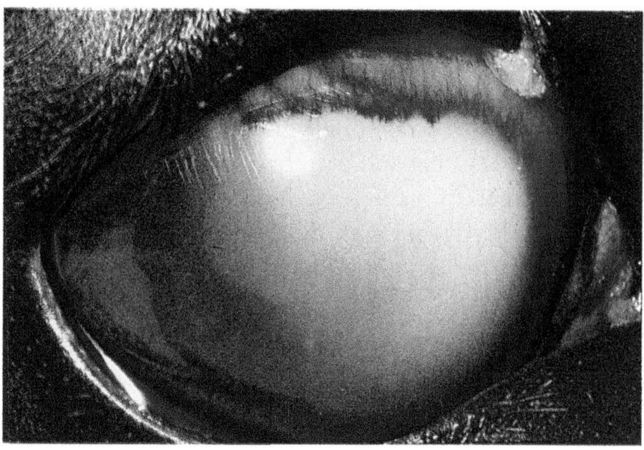

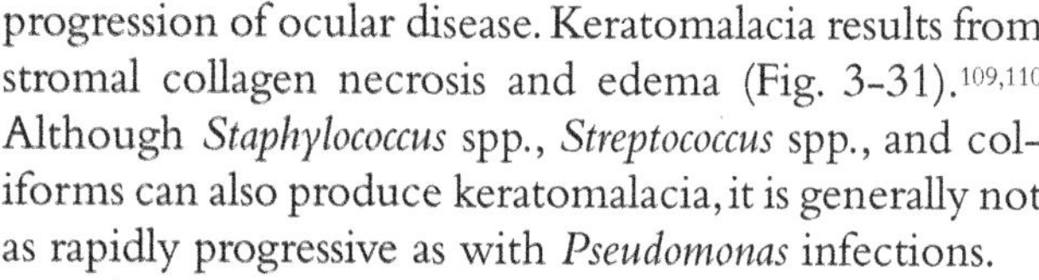

Fig. 3-29 Diffuse stromal abscess.
Stromal abscesses occur as single, multifocal, or diffuse (shown here) areas of yellow-white corneal stromal infiltrates. (Courtesy Dr. David Maggs, University of California–Davis.)

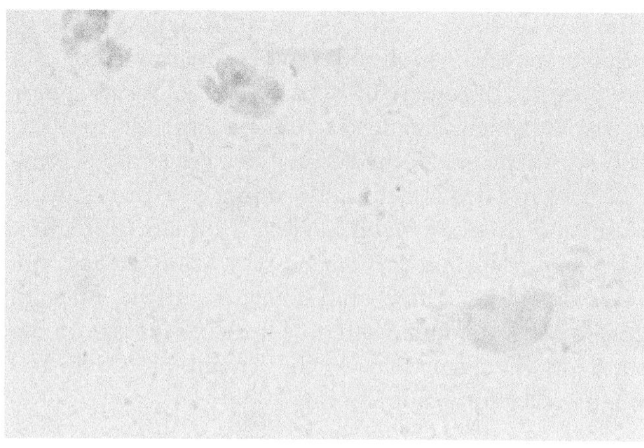

Fig. 3-30 *Pseudomonas* keratitis.
In *Pseudomonas* keratitis, corneal scrapings contain large numbers of gram-negative rods.

progression of ocular disease. Keratomalacia results from stromal collagen necrosis and edema (Fig. 3-31).[109,110] Although *Staphylococcus* spp., *Streptococcus* spp., and coliforms can also produce keratomalacia, it is generally not as rapidly progressive as with *Pseudomonas* infections.

Other less common causes of equine ulcerative keratitis include *Salmonella arizonae* and *Clostridium perfringens* infections.[111,112] Cytologic examination of the latter revealed neutrophils and large gram-positive rods suggestive of a *Clostridium* species (Plate 3H) that was later confirmed by culture.[112]

Fungal Lesions

Keratomycosis is a well-recognized problem that affects horses worldwide. Fungal organisms are ubiquitous in the environment and can also be present as part of the normal equine conjunctival flora.[19,25,43,113-115] Clinical presentations of equine keratomycosis include ulcerative keratitis, stromal abscessation, and iris prolapse.[53,116] Mycotic keratitis may be difficult to diagnose due to the propensity of fungal organisms to inhabit the deeper corneal tissues.[117]

Several different species of fungi have been reported to infect the equine cornea, with *Aspergillus* spp. and *Fusarium* spp. being the most commonly cultured.[20,105,118,119] *Penicillium* spp., *Phycomyces* spp., *Pseudallescheria boydii, Papulospora* spp., *Cylindrocarpon* spp., *Torulopsis* spp., *Cladorrhinum bulbillosum*, and yeast keratomycosis have also been reported.[120-125]

Special considerations for collecting appropriate samples for diagnosis of keratomycosis have already been discussed (see Collection of Corneal Scrapings). Cytologic preparations of mycotic keratitis are moderately to markedly cellular. Predominant cells include epithelial cells and nondegenerated neutrophils. Fungal organisms are often numerous but may not stain well. These organisms are essentially identified by "negative staining" areas, that is, poorly or nonstaining regions admixed among unidentifiable debris that stain well. Septate filamentous fungi are more commonly involved in keratomycosis (Fig. 3-32). Cytologically, these fungi (eg, *Aspergillus* sp.) will demonstrate short, slender, dichotomously branching hyphae with multiple crosswalls that divide the hyphae into distinct cells containing one or more nuclei. Fungal cultures should be a part of every workup for cases of suspected equine keratomycosis.

Viral Lesions

Equine herpesvirus-2 (EHV-2) has been incriminated in ocular disease. Clinically, this infection is characterized by multiple, superficial, white, punctate or linear opacities with or without fluorescein stain retention.[37,126,127] Unique

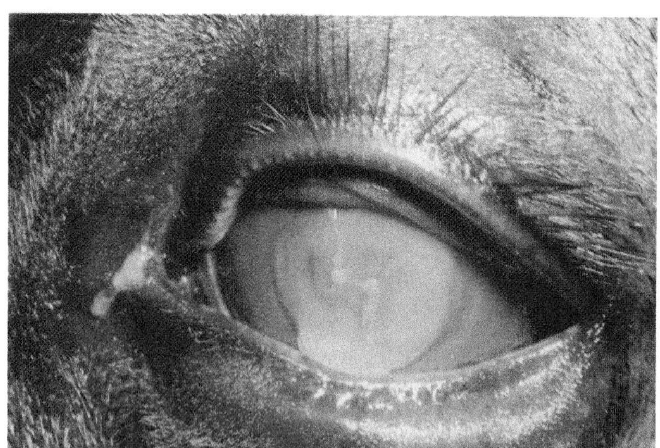

Fig. 3-31 Keratomalacia secondary to *Pseudomonas* keratitis.

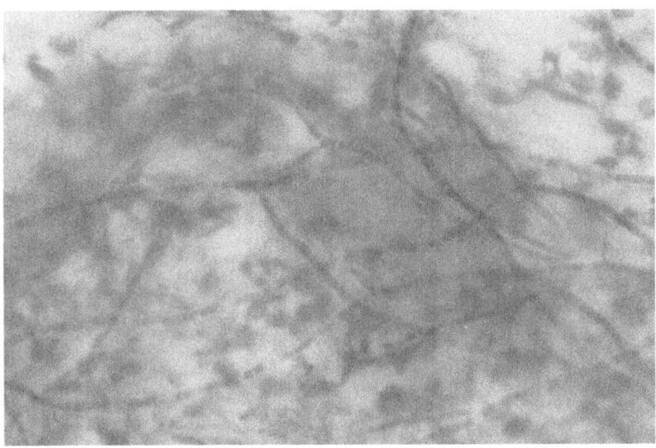

Fig. 3-32 Mycotic keratitis.
Corneal swab from a horse with mycotic keratitis shows numerous fungal hyphae.

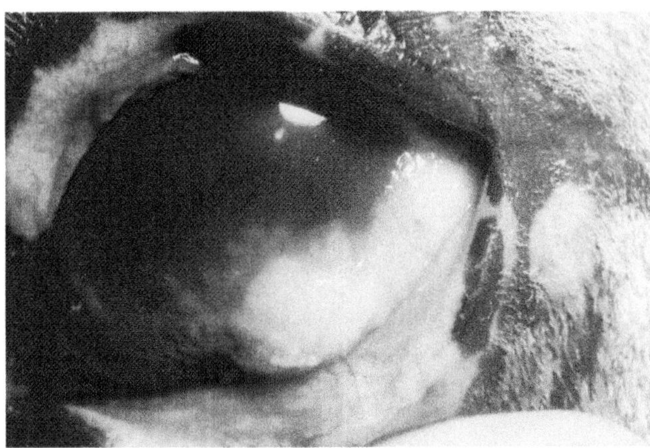

Fig. 3-33 Corneal squamous-cell carcinoma.

cytologic characteristics of this infection that might lead to a definitive diagnosis, such as intracellular inclusions, have not been reported. Virus isolation, polymerizing chain reaction, DNA fingerprinting, and fluorescent antibody testing have been used as diagnostic methods for EHV-2; however, not all of these tests are commercially available at this time.[37,126-129]

Parasitic Lesions

Primary corneal onchocerciasis and thelaziasis, as well as secondary corneal pathology due to habronemiasis, have been reported.[19,87,89] Clinical signs reported are variable, depending on the nature of the disease process involved, and include stromal opacities, corneal edema, subepithelial "fluffy" white opacities, corneal erosions with superficial or deep neovascularization, pigmentary keratitis, granulation tissue, and radial corneal streaks. In humans, punctate keratitis is the most commonly reported lesion of ocular onchocerciasis.[130] Corneal scrapings or a wet-mount preparation of a superficial keratectomy sample may be examined for onchocercal microfilariae (see Conjunctiva).

Neoplastic Lesions

Primary tumors of the cornea, other than squamous-cell carcinoma, are extremely rare. Squamous-cell carcinomas arise at the limbus and grow across the adjacent cornea (Fig. 3-33). The clinical and cytologic appearance of corneal squamous-cell carcinoma is similar to conjunctival or eyelid squamous-cell carcinoma (see previous sections). Differential diagnoses for corneal neoplasia include dermoid and granulation tissue.

Melanocytic neoplasia involving the cornea and epibulbar region of the equine globe has been reported.[96,97,131] Melanomas are moderately cellular and contain variable amounts of blood. Melanoma cells are found in a variety of shapes and sizes (mostly round but also oval and spindle shaped), and may be arranged singly or in groups, rafts, and clusters. These cells contain variable amounts of cytoplasm, but the nucleus-to-cytoplasm ratio may not be increased.

All melanomas, including amelanotic melanomas, have varying degrees of pigment. Often the pigment is "dusted" throughout the cytoplasm. Macrophages containing melanin are often present. Melanin granules may be clustered in macrophage cytoplasmic vacuoles. Melanin can be differentiated from other intracytoplasmic contents by the black-green cast achieved by changing the focus of the microscope objective. By contrast, mast cells contain red- to blue-staining granules with routine stains.

Ocular mastocytosis involving the equine cornea has been reported.[132,133] Mast cells and eosinophils predominated in cytologic preparations (Fig. 3-34). In a recent review of horses with ocular lymphosarcoma, two horses had corneoscleral presentations of this neoplastic process.[68] (See previous sections for cytologic descriptions.) The cornea may become involved in neoplastic processes that originate from the conjunctiva or eyelids (see previous sections for further details). Biopsy and histopathologic examination are recommended for definitive diagnosis of any suspected corneal neoplasm.

Other Lesions

Equine eosinophilic keratitis is an idiopathic unilateral or bilateral disease that has recently been recognized.[134,135] Clinically affected horses present with raised, white, subepithelial, necrotic plaques involving the cornea and associated conjunctiva (Fig. 3-35). Cytologically, the disease is characterized by numerous

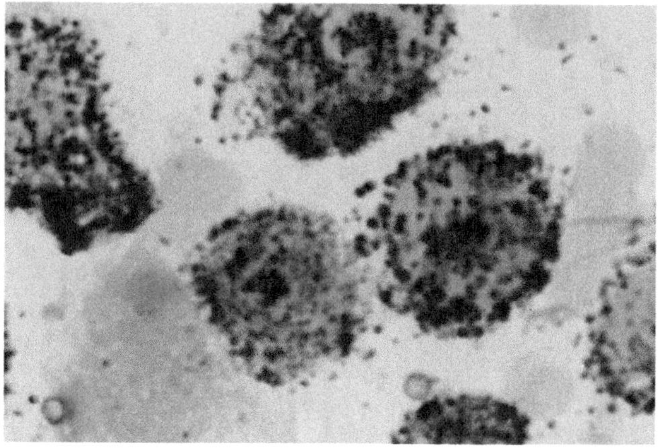

Fig. 3-34 Mastocytoma.
Aspirate of eyelid mass shows numerous mast cells indicative of mastocytoma. (Courtesy Dr. Donald Schmidt, University of Missouri–Columbia.)

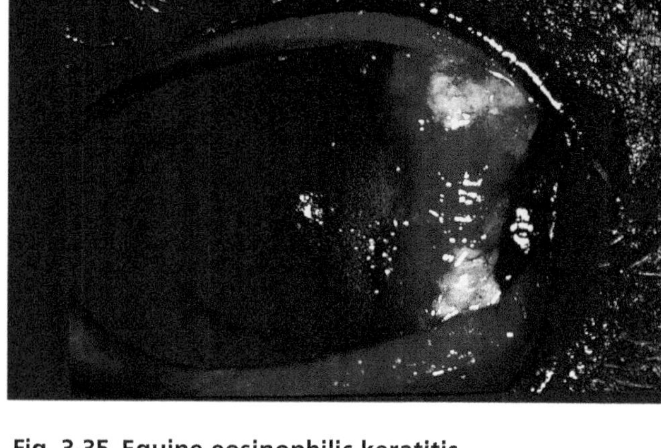

Fig. 3-35 Equine eosinophilic keratitis.
Equine eosinophilic keratitis at the temporal limbus with characteristic white surface plaques. Corneal fibrovascular proliferation is often a feature of this condition.

eosinophils and neutrophils, with occasional mast cells, plasma cells, and lymphocytes (Fig. 3-36). This condition is diagnosed on the basis of supportive clinical and cytologic findings and concurrent absence of all other possible causes of keratitis, including fungal, bacterial, allergic, and parasitic etiologies.

Calcific band keratopathy may occur on the equine cornea secondary to inflammatory disease.[136] Clinically, dense, white, dystrophic bands are present in the interpalpebral region of the central cornea. Calcium, in the form of hydroxyapatite, is deposited at the level of the epithelial basement membrane. Progressive accumulation of calcium may cause vascularizing keratitis with or without ulceration. Cytologic findings have not been described except during the scraping procedure to give audible and tactile evidence of mineralization. Histologic examination of von Kossa and Alizarin red–stained keratectomy specimens confirms the presence of calcium. Dystrophic calcium deposition occurs in response to a variety of stromal keratopathies, especially in older horses, in which the calcium deposition coincides with the site of previous insult or inflammatory process.[137] By contrast, calcific band keratopathy is unique in that calcium deposition is more restricted to the subepithelial, interpalpebral corneal zones and can occur in horses of any age.[136]

Keratoconjunctivitis sicca (KCS) has been rarely documented in horses.[99,138-142] In those reports, causes of equine KCS were of traumatic, poisonous, parasitic, immune-mediated, or idiopathic origins. Corneal and conjunctival scrapings most commonly reveal nonspecific changes secondary to decreased tear production. Cytologic findings may include keratinized epithelial cells admixed with neutrophils, lymphocytes, plasma cells, occasional eosinophils, and any infectious organisms that may have secondarily infected the cornea and conjunctiva.

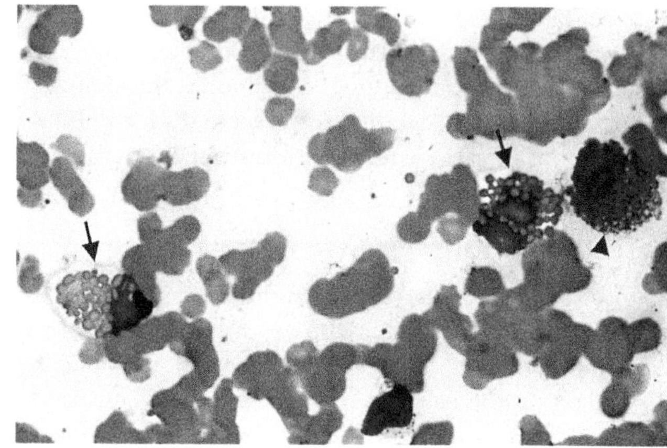

Fig. 3-36 Equine eosinophilic keratitis.
Cytologic specimen taken from the horse in Fig. 3-35. Note prominent eosinophils (*arrows*) and a mast cell (*arrowhead*).

Uvea

Infectious Agents

Equine uveitis is a multifactorial condition with a number of different bacterial, viral, and parasitic agents implicated in the disease process.[143] A detailed discussion of the individual infectious agents is beyond the scope of this text; the reader is encouraged to consult other, more detailed references.[53,143] Cytologic diagnostic techniques for this intraocular region of the globe are limited to aqueous, vitreal, or subretinal paracentesis. Paracentesis techniques (described in an earlier section of this chapter) require general anesthesia and may further aggravate the uveal inflammation already present.

Neoplastic Lesions

Intraocular tumors in which cytologic examination might be helpful include medulloepithelioma, melanoma, and metastatic tumors.[144,145] Intraocular tumors are difficult to aspirate, since fine-needle aspiration of space-occupying uveal masses must be performed under general anesthesia and aspiration may cause severe complications.[32,145] Lymphosarcoma is one of the few intraocular tumors that may readily exfoliate into the vitreous or aqueous humor.[146] In cases of hypopyon due to ocular lymphosarcoma, numerous atypical or immature lymphocytes can be found on cytologic examination of aqueous humor aspirates. If an intraocular tumor is strongly suspected, enucleation and histopathology are recommended to establish a definitive diagnosis.

Orbit

The globe and optic nerve must be avoided during retrobulbar aspiration. The needle may be directed through the conjunctiva or through the eyelid to reach the retrobulbar area. Considerations when performing fine-needle aspiration of orbital lesions have been discussed in an earlier section of this chapter.

Bacterial Lesions

Bacterial orbital cellulitis is uncommon in horses. Bacterial inflammation involving the nose, mouth, teeth, guttural pouch, orbital bones, or frontal, sphenopalatine, or maxillary sinuses may spread to the orbit. Orbital foreign bodies may result in cellulitis. Clinical signs of orbital cellulitis include edema of the eyelids and supraorbital fossa, pain, serous or mucopurulent ocular discharge, conjunctival hyperemia, fever, protrusion of the membrana nictitans, and occasionally exophthalmos. Bacteria and inflammatory cells (variable numbers of neutrophils, lymphocytes, eosinophils, mast cells, mononuclear cells) may be observed in orbital aspirates.

Fungal Lesions

Exophthalmos may be caused by retrobulbar fungal granulomas. Orbital maduromycosis (infection by Ascomycetes, Deuteromycetes, Actinomycetes) and cryptococcosis (*Cryptococcus neoformans*) have been described in horses.[147,148] Definitive diagnosis is based on finding fungal organisms in orbital aspirates. Fungal organisms are often accompanied by large numbers of neutrophils and macrophages, and a pyogranulomatous response is usually found on cytologic examination. Commonly isolated fungal species, their morphologic features found on cytology, and special stains used to aid in the diagnosis of fungal organisms have been discussed previously in this chapter.

Neoplastic Lesions

Tumors affecting the equine orbit include adenocarcinoma, lymphosarcoma, melanoma, sarcoid, squamous-cell carcinoma, nerve-cell tumors (schwannoma, malignant schwannoma, neurofibroma, neurofibrosarcoma), mast-cell tumor, angiosarcoma, hemangioma, hemangiosarcoma, multilobular osteosarcoma, optic nerve neuroepithelioma, lipoma, and paraganglioma.[149-151] Concurrent orbital cellulitis may make tumor recognition difficult. As with all ocular and adnexal neoplasia, histopathology is recommended over cytologic examination alone for diagnosis.

Parasitic Lesions

Hydatid cyst formation from larval forms of *Echinococcus granulosa* or *Echinococcus multilocularis* can occur within the equine orbit.[57] Retrobulbar tissues of one affected horse contained an inflammatory infiltrate of eosinophils, lymphocytes, and macrophages.[152]

Other Lesions

Orbital hematoma resulting from trauma can result in exophthalmos. Aspirates collected from hematomas usually contain macrophages with phagocytosed red blood cells and/or red blood cell breakdown products. These findings support a diagnosis of hematoma.

Seromas or orbital abscesses may form after enucleation and/or implantation of an intraorbital silicon or methylmethacrylate prosthesis. In these cases, cytologic examination of orbital aspirates can distinguish septic from nonseptic processes. A septic process is diagnosed by finding infectious organisms in conjunction with a neutrophilic cellular response. Cytology performed on aspirates from a septic orbit may reveal bacteria within phagosomes of neutrophils or mononuclear cells. Free bacteria suggest contamination in the collection process, especially in the absence of inflammation. Neutrophils displaying age-related change only (pyknotic nucleus) do not indicate sepsis. However, neutrophils displaying karyolysis (pale, swollen, or shapeless nucleus) may indicate an underlying septic process. These cellular changes may also be seen in sterile but toxic processes. Stain debris may mimic bacteria but is more variable in size and shape than most microorganisms.

Acknowledgments: The authors would like to acknowledge the co-authors of the first edition, J.M.A. da Silva Curiel, J.A. Taylor, and B.F. Feldman, for their contributions to this chapter, and Howard Wilson for technical assistance.

REFERENCES

1. Massa et al: Usefulness of aerobic microbial culture and cytologic evaluation of corneal specimens in the diagnosis of infectious ulcerative keratitis in animals. *J Am Vet Med Assoc* 215:1671-1674, 1999.
2. Hamilton et al: Histological findings in corneal stromal abscesses of eleven horses: correlation with cultures and cytology. *Equine Vet J* 26:448-453, 1994.
3. Severin and Thrall: Ocular exfoliative cytology. *Proc 5th Ann Kal Kan Symp*, 1981, pp 11-15.
4. Lavach: *Large Animal Ophthalmology*, St. Louis, 1990, Mosby, pp 3-28.
5. Helper: Diagnostic techniques in conjunctivitis and keratitis. *Vet Clin North Am* 3:357-365, 1973.
6. da Silva Curiel et al: Nutritionally variant *Streptococci* associated with corneal ulcers in horses: 35 cases. *J Am Vet Med Assoc* 197:624-626, 1990.
7. Fedukowicz and Stenson: *External Infections of the Eye*, Norwalk, CT, 1985, Appleton-Century-Crofts.
8. Adams et al: Monitoring ocular disease by impression cytology. *Eye* 2:506-516, 1988.
9. de Rojas et al: Impression cytology in patients with keratoconjunctivitis sicca. *Cytopathology* 4:347-355, 1993.
10. Maskin: Diagnostic impression cytology for external eye disease. *Cornea* 8:270-273, 1989.
11. Nelson: Impression cytology. *Cornea* 7:71-81, 1988.
12. Cordozo et al: Exfoliative cytology in the diagnosis of conjunctival tumors. *Ophthalmologica* 182:157-164, 1981.
13. Lavach et al: Cytology of normal and inflamed conjunctivas in dogs and cats. *J Am Vet Med Assoc* 170:722-727, 1977.
14. Murphy: Exfoliative cytologic examination as an aid in diagnosing ocular diseases in the dog and cat. *Sem Vet Med Surg* 3:10-14, 1988.
15. Bauer: Exfoliative cytology of conjunctiva and cornea in domestic animals: a comparison of four collecting techniques. *Vet Comp Ophthalmol* 6:181-186, 1996.
16. Willis et al: Conjunctival brush cytology: evaluation of a new cytological collection technique in dogs and cats with a comparison to conjunctival scraping. *Vet Comp Ophthalmol* 7:74-81, 1997.
17. Champagne and Pickett: The effect of topical 0.5% proparacaine HCL on corneal and conjunctival culture results. *Proc 26th Ann Mtg ACVO*, 1995, p 144.
18. Hacker et al: A comparison of conjunctival culture techniques in the dog. *J Am Anim Hosp Assoc* 15:223-225, 1979.
19. Whitley and Moore: Microbiology of the equine eye in health and disease. *Vet Clin North Am Food Anim Pract* 6:451-465, 1984.
20. Moore et al: Bacterial and fungal isolates from equidae with ulcerative keratitis. *J Am Vet Med Assoc* 182:600-603, 1983.
21. Ishibashi and Kauffman: Corneal biopsy in the diagnosis of keratomycosis. *Am J Ophthalmol* 101:288-293, 1986.
22. Peiffer et al: in Gelatt: *Veterinary Ophthalmology*, 3rd ed, Philadelphia, 1999, Lippincott Williams & Wilkins, pp 355-425.
23. Beech and Sweeney: Keratomycoses in 11 horses. *Equine Vet J* (Suppl) 2:39-44, 1983.
24. Kern et al: Equine keratomycosis: current concepts of diagnosis and therapy. *Equine Vet J* (Suppl) 2:33-38, 1983.
25. Andrew et al: Equine ulcerative keratomycosis: visual outcome and ocular survival in 39 cases (1987-1996). *Equine Vet J* 30:109-116, 1998.
26. Cello: Ocular onchocerciasis in the horse. *Equine Vet J* 3:148-154, 1971.
27. Blogg et al: Blindness caused by Rhodococcus equi infection in a foal. *Equine Vet J* (Suppl) 2:25-26, 1983.
28. O'Rourke et al: An aqueous paracentesis pipette. *Ophthalmic Surg* 22:166-167, 1991.
29. Samuelson: in Gelatt: *Veterinary Ophthalmology*, 3rd ed, Philadelphia, 1999, Lippincott Williams & Wilkins, pp 31-150.
30. Hazel et al: Laboratory evaluation of aqueous humor in the healthy dog, cat, horse and cow. *Am J Vet Res* 46:657-659, 1985.
31. Kennerdell et al: Fine-needle aspiration biopsy: its use in orbital tumors. *Arch Ophthalmol* 97:1315-1317, 1979.
32. Midena et al: Fine-needle aspiration biopsy in ophthalmology. *Surv Ophthalmol* 20:410-422, 1985.
33. Krohel et al: Inaccuracy of fine needle aspiration biopsy. *Ophthalmology* 92:666-670, 1985.
34. Burrell et al: Isolation of *Chlamydia psittaci* from the respiratory tract and conjunctivae of thoroughbred horses. *Vet Record* 119:302-303, 1986.
35. Rajan and Padmanaban: Clinical diagnosis of rabies in herbivores. Examination of corneal impression smears by fluorescent antibody technique. *Indian Vet J* 63:882-885, 1986.
36. Burgess et al: Arthritis and panuveitis as manifestations of *Borrelia burgdorferi* infection in a Wisconsin pony. *J Am Vet Med Assoc* 189:1340-1342, 1986.
37. Miller et al: Herpetic keratitis in a horse. *Equine Vet J* (Suppl) 10:15-17, 1990.
38. Sutphin et al: Improved detection of oculomycoses using induced fluorescence with Cellufluor. *Ophthalmology* 93:416-417, 1986.
39. Arffa et al: Calcofluor and ink-potassium hydroxide preparations for identifying fungi. *Am J Ophthalmol* 100:719-723, 1985.
40. Hageage and Harrington: Use of Calcofluor white in clinical mycology. *Lab Med* 15:1984.
41. Robin et al: Rapid visualization of three common fungi using fluorescein-conjugated lectins. *Invest Ophthalmol Vis Sci* 27:500-506, 1986.
42. Olin: Examination of the aqueous humor as a diagnostic aid in anterior uveitis. *J Am Vet Med Assoc* 171:557-559, 1977.
43. Moore et al: Prevalence of ocular microorganisms in hospitalized and stabled horses. *Am J Vet Res* 49:773-777, 1988.
44. Eichenbaum et al: Immunology of the ocular surface. *Comp Cont Ed Pract Vet* 9:1101-1115, 1987.
45. Moore et al: Density and distribution of canine conjunctival goblet cells. *Invest Ophthalmol Vis Sci* 28:1925-1932, 1987.
46. Moore: Eyelid and nasolacrimal disease. *Vet Clin North Am (Equine Pract)* 8:499-519, 1992.
47. Boulton and Campbell: Orbital bone sequestration as a cause of equine recurrent blepharitis and ulcerative keratitis. *Vet Med Small Anim Clin* 77:1057-1058, 1982.
48. Hughes and Pugh: Isolation and description of a *Moraxella* from horses with conjunctivitis. *J Am Vet Med Assoc* 31:457-462, 1970.
49. Huntington et al: Isolation of a *Moraxella* sp. from horses with conjunctivitis. *Aust Vet J* 64:118-119, 1987.
50. Scott: *Large Animal Dermatology*, Philadelphia, 1988, WB Saunders, pp 169, 308.
51. Blackford: Superficial and deep mycosis in horses. *Vet Clin North Am Food Anim Pract* 6:47-58, 1984.
52. Singh: Studies on epizootic lymphangitis. *Indian J Vet Sci* 36:45-49, 1966.
53. Brooks: in Gelatt: *Veterinary Ophthalmology*, 3rd ed, Philadelphia, 1999, Lippincott Williams & Wilkins, pp 1053-1116.
54. Jayo et al: Poxvirus infection in a donkey. *Vet Pathol* 23:635-637, 1986.
55. Moore et al: Equine ocular parasites: a review. *Equine Vet J* (Suppl) 2:76-85, 1983.
56. Rebhun et al: Habronemic blepharoconjunctivitis in horses. *J Am Vet Med Assoc* 179:469-472, 1981.
57. Lavach: *Handbook of Equine Ophthalmology*, Fort Collins, CO, 1987, Giddings Studio Publishing.
58. Bennison: Demodicidosis of horses with particular reference to members of the genus *Demodex*. *J Royal Army Vet Corps* 14(2):34-73, 1943.
59. Besch and Griffiths: Demonstration of *Demodex equi* from a horse in Minnesota. *J Am Vet Med Assoc* 128:82-83, 1956.
60. Scott and White: Demodicidosis associated with systemic glucocorticoid therapy in 2 horses. *Equine Pract* 5:31-35, 1983.
61. Knowles et al: Equine piroplasmosis. *J Am Vet Med Assoc* 148:407-410, 1966.
62. Barnett et al: *Color Atlas and Text of Equine Ophthalmology*. London, 1995, Mosby-Wolfe, Times Mirror International Publishers Limited, pp 49-97.
63. Dugan et al: Epidemiologic studies on ocular/adnexal squamous cell carcinoma in horses. *J Am Vet Med Assoc* 198:251-256, 1991.
64. Dugan et al: Prognostic factors and survival of horses with ocular/adnexal squamous cell carcinoma: 147 cases (1978-1988). *J Am Vet Med Assoc* 198:298-303, 1991.
65. Garma-Avina: The cytology of squamous cell carcinomas in domestic animals. *J Vet Diagn Invest* 6:238-246, 1994.
66. Martis et al: Report of the first international workshop on equine sarcoid. *Equine Vet J* 25:397-407, 1993.
67. Bertone and McClure: Therapy for sarcoids. *Comp Cont Ed Pract Vet* 12:262-265, 1990.

68. Rebhun and Del Piero: Ocular lesions in horses with lymphosarcoma: 21 cases (1977-1997). *J Am Vet Med Assoc* 212:852-854, 1998.
69. Murphy et al: Bilateral eyelid swelling attributable to lymphosarcoma in a horse. *J Am Vet Med Assoc* 194:939-942, 1989.
70. Glaze et al: A case of equine adnexal lymphosarcoma. *Equine Vet J* (Suppl) 10:83-84, 1990.
71. Scott: *Large Animal Dermatology*, Philadelphia, 1988, WB Saunders, pp 419-458.
72. Giuliano et al: Inferomedial placement of a single-entry subpalpebral lavage tube for treatment of equine eye disease. *Vet Ophthalmol* 3:153-156, 2000.
73. Miller: Principles of therapeutics. *Vet Clin North Am (Equine Pract)* 8:479-497, 1992.
74. Sweeney and Russell: Complications associated with use of a one-hole subpalpebral lavage system in horses: 150 cases (1977-1996). *J Am Vet Med Assoc* 211:1271-1274, 1997.
75. Huntington et al: Isolation of a *Moraxella* sp from horses with conjunctivitis. *Aust Vet J* 64:118-119, 1987.
76. Hughes and Pugh: Isolation and description of a *Moraxella* from horses with conjunctivitis. *Am J Vet Res* 31:457-462, 1970.
77. Inzana: in Carter and Cole: *Diagnostic Procedures in Veterinary Bacteriology and Mycology*, 5th ed, San Diego, 1990, Academic Press, pp 165-176.
78. McChesney et al: Chlamydial polyarthritis in a foal. *J Am Vet Med Assoc* 165:259-261, 1974.
79. Pienaar and Schutte: The occurrence and pathology of chlamydiosis in domestic and laboratory animals: a review. *Onderstepoort J Vet Res* 42:77-90, 1975.
80. Fouad et al: Studies on the lacrymal histoplasmosis in donkeys in Egypt. *Zentralbl Veterinarmed* 20B:584-593, 1973.
81. Jones and Hunt: *Veterinary Pathology*. 5th ed, Philadelphia, 1983, Lea & Febiger, p 688.
82. da Silva Curiel et al: in Cowell and Tyler: *Cytology and Hematology of the Horse*. Goleta, 1992, American Veterinary Publications, Inc., pp 47-68.
83. McChesney et al: Adenoviral infection in foals. *J Am Vet Med Assoc* 162:545-549, 1973.
84. Klei et al: Prevalence of *Onchocerca cervicalis* in equids in the gulf coast region. *Am J Vet Res* 45:1646-1648, 1984.
85. Soulsby: *Textbook of Veterinary Clinical Parasitology*. Philadelphia, 1965, FA Davis, p 884.
86. Cummings and James: Prevalence of equine onchocerciasis in southeastern and midwestern United States. *J Am Vet Med Assoc* 186: 1202-1203, 1985.
87. Schmidt et al: Equine ocular onchocerciasis: histopathologic study. *Am J Vet Res* 43:1371-1375, 1982.
88. Hammond et al: Equine ocular onchocerciasis: a case report. *Equine Vet J* (Suppl) 2:74-75, 1983.
89. Patton and McCracken: The occurrence and effect of Thelazia in horses. *Equine Pract* 2:53-57, 1981.
90. Barker: *Thelazia* lacrymalis from the eyes of an Ontario horse. *Can Vet J* 11:186-189, 1970.
91. Kunze et al: Sebaceous adenocarcinoma of the third eyelid of a horse. *J Equine Med Surg* 3:452-455, 1979.
92. Baril: Basal cell tumor of the third eyelid in a horse. *Can Vet J* 14:66-67, 1973.
93. Vestre: Conjunctival hemangioma in a horse. *J Am Vet Med Assoc* 180:1481-1482, 1982.
94. Hacker et al: Ocular angiosarcoma in four horses. *J Am Vet Med Assoc* 189:200-203, 1986.
95. Moore et al: Ocular angiosarcoma in the horse: morphological and immunohistochemical studies. *Vet Pathol* 23:240-244, 1986.
96. Hamor et al: Melanoma of the conjunctiva and cornea in a horse. *Vet Comp Ophthalmol* 7:52-55, 1997.
97. Moore et al: Conjunctival malignant melanoma in a horse. *Vet Ophthalmol* 3:201-206, 2000.
98. Vestre and Steckel: Episcleral prolapse of orbital fat in the horse. *Equine Pract* 5(8):34-37, 1983.
99. Spiess et al: Eosinophilic granulomatous dacryoadenitis causing bilateral keratoconjunctivitis sicca in a horse. *Equine Vet J* 21:226-228, 1989.
100. van der Woerdt et al: Ulcerative keratitis secondary to single layer repair of a traumatic eyelid laceration in a horse. *Equine Pract* 18:33-38, 1996.
101. McLaughlin et al: Infectious keratitis in horses: evaluation and management. *Comp Cont Ed Pract Vet* 14:372-379, 1992.
102. Bistner: Clinical diagnosis and treatment of infectious keratitis. *Comp Cont Ed Pract Vet* 3:1056-1066, 1981.
103. Moore et al: Antimicrobial agents for treatment of infectious keratitis in horses. *J Am Vet Med Assoc* 207:855-862, 1995.
104. Moore et al: Antibacterial susceptibility patterns for microbial isolates associated with infectious keratitis in horses: 63 cases (1986-1994). *J Am Vet Med Assoc* 207:928-933, 1995.
105. McLaughlin et al: Pathogenic bacteria and fungi associated with extraocular disease in the horse. *J Am Vet Med Assoc* 182:241-242, 1983.
106. Rebhun: Corneal stromal abscesses in horses. *J Am Vet Med Assoc* 181:677-679, 1982.
107. Rebhun: Corneal stromal infections in horses. *Comp Cont Ed Pract Vet* 14:363-371, 1992.
108. Hendrix et al: Corneal stromal abscesses in the horse: a review of 24 cases. *Equine Vet J* 27:440-447, 1995.
109. Divers and George: Hypopyon and descemetocele formation associated with *Pseudomonas* ulcerative keratitis in a horse: a case report and review. *J Equine Vet Sci* 2:104-107, 1982.
110. Sweeney and Irby: Topical treatment of Pseudomonas sp-infected corneal ulcers in horses: 70 cases (1977-1994). *J Am Vet Med Assoc* 209:954-957, 1996.
111. Adamson and Jang: Ulcerative keratitis associated with Salmonella arizonae infection in a horse. *J Am Vet Med Assoc* 186:1219-1220, 1985.
112. Rebhun et al: Presumed clostridial and aerobic bacterial infections of the cornea in horses. *J Am Vet Med Assoc* 214:1519-1522, 1999.
113. Samuelson: Conjunctival fungal flora in horses, cattle, dogs, and cats. *J Am Vet Med Assoc* 184:1240-1242, 1984.
114. Ball: Equine fungal keratitis. *Comp Cont Ed Pract Vet* 22(2):182-186, 2000.
115. Whitley et al: Microbial isolates of the normal equine eye. *Equine Vet J* (Suppl) 2:138-140, 1983.
116. Gaarder et al: Clinical appearances, healing patterns, risk factors, and outcomes of horses with fungal keratitis: 53 cases (1978-1996). *J Am Vet Med Assoc* 213:105-112, 1998.
117. Whittaker et al: Therapeutic penetrating keratoplasty for deep corneal stromal abscesses in 8 horses. *Vet Comp Ophthalmol* 7:19-28, 1997.
118. Grahn et al: Equine keratomycosis: clinical and laboratory findings in 23 cases. *Prog Vet Comp Ophthalmol* 3:2-7, 1993.
119. Coad et al: Antifungal sensitivity testing for equine keratomycosis. *Am J Vet Res* 46:676-678, 1985.
120. Friedman et al: *Pseudallescheria boydii* keratomycosis in a horse. *J Am Vet Med Assoc* 195:616-618, 1989.
121. Shadomy and Dixon: A new *Papulospora* species from the infected eye of a horse: *Papulospora equi*. *Mycopathologica* 106:35-39, 1989.
122. Hendrix et al: Keratomycosis in 4 horses caused by *Cylindrocarpon destructans*. *Vet Comp Ophthalmol* 6:252-257, 1996.
123. Brooks et al: Antimicrobial susceptibility patterns of fungi isolated from horses with ulcerative keratomycosis. *Am J Vet Res* 59:138-142, 1998.
124. Ball et al. Evaluation of itraconazole-dimethyl sulfoxide ointment for treatment of keratomycosis in nine horses. *J Am Vet Med Assoc* 211:199-203, 1997.
125. Chopin et al: Keratotomy costs in a percheron cross horse caused by *Cladorrhinum bulbillosum*. *J Med Vet Mycol* 35:53-55, 1997.
126. Borchers et al: Virological and molecular biological investigations into equine herpes virus type 2 (EHV-2) experimental infections. *Virus Res* 55:101-106, 1998.
127. Collinson et al: Isolation of equine herpesvirus type 2 (equine gammaherpesvirus 2) from foals with keratoconjunctivitis. *J Am Vet Med Assoc* 205:329-331, 1994.
128. Mathews and Handscombe: Superficial keratitis in a horse: treatment with the antiviral drug idoxuridine. *Equine Vet J* (Suppl) 2:29-31, 1983.
129. Thein: in Bryans and Gerber: *Equine Infectious Diseases IV: The association of EHV-2 infection with keratitis and research on the occurrence of equine exanthema (EHV-3) in horses in Germany*. Princeton, 1978, Veterinary Publications, pp 33-41.
130. Gunders and Neumann: Parasitology and diagnosis of onchocerciasis with special reference to the outer eye. *Isr J Med Sci* 8:1139-1142, 1972.
131. Hirst et al: Benign epibulbar melanocytoma in a horse. *J Am Vet Med Assoc* 183:333-334, 1983.

132. Martin and Leipold: Mastocytoma of the globe in a horse. *J Am Anim Hosp Assoc* 8:32-34, 1972.
133. Hum and Bowers: Ocular mastocytosis in a horse. *Aust Vet J* 66:32, 1989.
134. Ramsey: Eosinophilic keratoconjunctivitis in a horse. *J Am Vet Med Assoc* 205:1308-1311, 1994.
135. Yamagata et al: Eosinophilic keratoconjunctivitis in seven horses. *J Am Vet Med Assoc* 209:1283-1286, 1996.
136. Rebhun et al: Calcific band keratopathy in horses. *Comp Cont Ed Pract Vet* 15:1402-1409, 1993.
137. Wouters and De Moor: Band-shaped opacities and corneal edema in two horses. *Vlaams Diergeneesk Tijdschr* 48:107-114, 1979.
138. Collins et al: Immune-mediated keratoconjunctivitis sicca in a horse. *Vet Comp Ophthalmol* 4:61-65, 1994.
139. Joyce and Bratton: Keratoconjunctivitis sicca secondary to fracture of the mandible. *Vet Clin North Am Small Anim Pract* 6:619-620, 1973.
140. Spurlock et al: Keratoconjunctivitis sicca associated with fracture of the stylohyoid bone in a horse. *J Am Vet Med Assoc* 194:258-259, 1989.
141. Van Kampen and James: Ophthalmic lesions in locoweed poisoning of cattle, sheep, and horses. *Am J Vet Res* 32:1293-1295, 1971.
142. Wolf and Merideth: Parotid duct transposition in the horse. *J Equine Vet Sci* 1:143-145, 1981.
143. Schwink: Equine uveitis. *Vet Clin North Am (Equine Pract)* 8:557-574, 1992.
144. Ramadan: Primary ocular melanoma in a young horse. *Equine Vet J* 7:49-50, 1975.
145. Augsburger et al: Fine-needle aspiration biopsy in the diagnosis of intraocular cancer. *Ophthalmology* 92:39-49, 1985.
146. Prasse and Winston: in Cowell et al: *Diagnostic Cytology and Hematology of the Dog and Cat.* 2nd ed., St. Louis, 1999, Mosby, pp 68-82.
147. Johnson et al: Maduromycosis in a horse in Western *Canada. Can Vet J* 16:341-344, 1975.
148. Scott et al: Cryptococcosis involving the post orbital area and frontal sinus in a horse. *J Am Vet Med Assoc* 165:626-627, 1974.
149. Sweeney and Beech: Retrobulbar melanoma in a horse. *Equine Vet J* (Suppl) 2:123-124, 1983.
150. Dugan: Ocular neoplasia. *Vet Clin North Am (Equine Pract)* 8:609-626, 1992.
151. Goodhead et al: Retrobulbar extra-adrenal paraganglioma in a horse and its surgical removal by orbitotomy. *Vet Comp Ophthalmol* 7:96-100, 1997.
152. Barnett: Retrobulbar hydatid cyst in the horse. *Equine Vet J* 20:136-138, 1988.

CHAPTER 4

Oral and Nasal Cavities, Pharynx, Guttural Pouches, and Paranasal Sinuses

Kenneth D. Clinkenbeard, Charles G. MacAllister, Rick L. Cowell, Ronald D. Tyler, and Sylvie Beaudin

Indications for Cytologic Examination

Oral Cavity

Clinical signs associated with pathologic conditions of the oral cavity include ptyalism, quidding, foul odor, dysphagia, and depression. Conditions of the nasal passages may result in nasal discharge, epistaxis, dyspnea, inspiratory stridor, and foul breath. Involvement of the nasopharynx can be associated with dysphagia, dyspnea, abnormal respiratory noise, and exercise intolerance.[1]

Horses have four pairs of paranasal sinuses: frontal, maxillary, sphenopalatine, and ethmoidal. Pathologic conditions of the paranasal sinuses may result in unilateral purulent nasal discharge, facial distortion, foul breath, dullness on percussion of the involved sinus, and formation of a chronic fistula.

Guttural Pouches

Clinical signs associated with guttural pouch disease include nasal discharge (usually unilateral), unilateral epistaxis, and swelling and/or pain in the area of the parotid salivary gland. The amount of nasal discharge often increases when the head is lowered. Because cranial nerves IX (glossopharyngeal), X (vagus), XI (spinal accessory), and XII (hypoglossal), the sympathetic trunk, and the cranial cervical ganglion are associated with the wall of the guttural pouch, neurologic disease caused by inflammation of the guttural pouch wall (Horner's syndrome, etc) also may be present.

Examination

If disease of the oral cavity is suspected, a thorough examination can usually be conducted in the standing animal. Sedation is often necessary. Food material in the oral cavity may conceal the lesion and should be removed by flushing with water before examination. A mouth speculum also may facilitate visualization. Lesions near the base of the tongue are often difficult to visualize, and careful digital palpation may be necessary. Radiographic evaluation is sometimes helpful, especially if teeth or bony structures are involved.

Diseases of the nasal passages and nasopharynx often require endoscopic examination for adequate visualization.[1] Sedation may distort the nasopharynx by relaxation of the soft tissues. Therefore, initial endoscopic examination of this area should be conducted without the aid of sedation if possible. Radiography may also help define the extent of lesions in this area.

The paranasal sinuses on each side communicate and drain into the middle meatus via the nasomaxillary opening. The nasomaxillary opening is not visible endoscopically. However, if nasal discharge is observed endoscopically to originate at the caudal portion of the middle meatus, paranasal sinus disease should be suspected. Confirmation of paranasal sinus involvement requires percussion and often radiography. Once primary sinus involvement is confirmed, the involved sinus can be aspirated for culture and cytologic evaluation.

The guttural pouches can be evaluated by palpation, endoscopy, and radiography. Two different methods may be used to insert a flexible endoscope into the guttural pouch. In the first method, place a biopsy instrument or cleaning brush in the biopsy channel of the endoscope and extend it 2 or 3 cm past the end of the endoscope. Then insert the biopsy instrument or cleaning brush into the guttural pouch opening and rotate the endoscope to open the guttural pouch flap. Then advance the endoscope into the guttural pouch. With the second method, place a Chambers mare catheter into the guttural pouch and rotate to open the flap (Fig. 4-1). Pass the flexible endoscope dorsal or ventral to the catheter and into the pouch as the Chambers catheter is withdrawn.

Sample Collection

Lesions in the oral cavity, nasal passages, nasopharynx, paranasal sinuses, and guttural pouches may be defined by cytologic evaluation, histopathologic examination, and culture (bacterial, fungal). Cytologic samples from the oral cavity are usually limited to fine-needle aspirates of masses or imprints for cytologic examination from excised tissues (see Chapter 1 for a discussion of slide preparation techniques). Cytologic preparations from ulcerative lesions may be collected by imprinting, swabbing, or scraping.

Nasal Passages and Nasopharynx

Cytologic samples from nasal passages and nasopharynx are collected directly via the external nares or with a flexible endoscope. Atheromas are accessible for percutaneous aspiration, and fungal polyps often are close enough to the external nares to make direct imprints, biopsy, and/or fine-needle aspiration possible. Samples of exudates in nasal passages can be collected via polyethylene tubing passed through the biopsy port of a flexible endoscope. Masses and fungal plaques can be sampled with the endoscopic biopsy instrument.

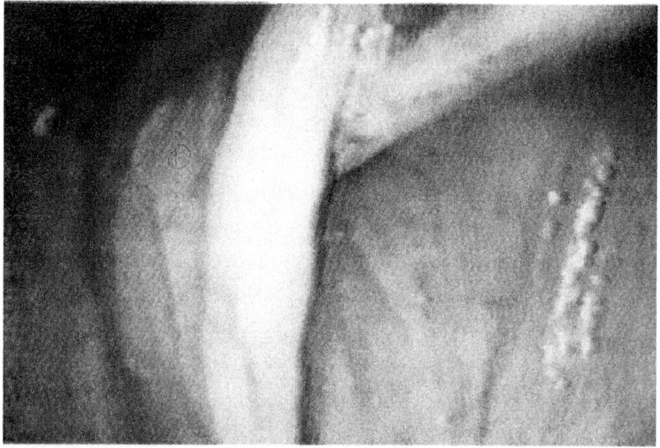

Fig. 4-1
Endoscopic view of openings to guttural pouch, with a Chambers mare catheter in place. Note the yellowish exudate draining from the guttural pouch opening. (Courtesy Dr. C.G. MacAllister, Oklahoma State University, Stillwater.)

Paranasal Sinuses

Though exudate from paranasal sinuses can sometimes be detected endoscopically in the middle meatus, samples for cytologic evaluation and culture should be taken directly from the involved sinus. Sinus aspiration is usually possible in a standing horse using sedation and local anesthesia. The landmarks for frontal sinus aspiration are 2.5 cm caudal to the point at which the nasal bones start to diverge and 2.5 cm lateral to the midline. For superior maxillary sinus aspiration, the landmarks are dorsal to the facial crest and about 2 cm rostral to the bony orbit. To avoid the lacrimal canal, the practitioner must not perform trephining more dorsally than a line drawn from the medial canthus to the infraorbital foramen.[2]

After surgical preparation and local anesthetic infiltration, make a stab incision in the skin and use a small Steinmann pin to drill into the sinus. Anatomic landmarks and the technique for trephination of paranasal sinuses are described in detail elsewhere.[1] Retrieve exudate by aspiration with a male canine urinary catheter or intravenous catheter. If exudate is not easily obtained, infuse and aspirate 30 to 40 ml of physiologic saline. If sinus contents are too thick for aspiration, use the eyed end of a large suture needle for sample collection.

Guttural Pouches

The technique for endoscopic entrance into the guttural pouches is described above. To collect cytologic samples from the guttural pouch, pass polyethylene tubing through the biopsy port of the endoscope and into the guttural pouch. In most instances, exudate is present on the floor of the pouch and is easily aspirated into the tubing. If exudate is not present, infuse 20 to 30 ml of physiologic saline through the tubing and onto the lesion. The saline pools on the floor of the guttural pouch and is easily aspirated.

Sample Preparation

To make smears from swabbed samples, the practitioner gently rolls the swab across a clean glass microscope slide and allows it to air dry. Rolling the swab avoids the rupturing of cells that often occurs if the swab is rubbed or dragged across the slide. Samples collected by brushing can be impressed on the slide. Rubbing or dragging the brush across the slide surface should be avoided to prevent excessive damage to cells.

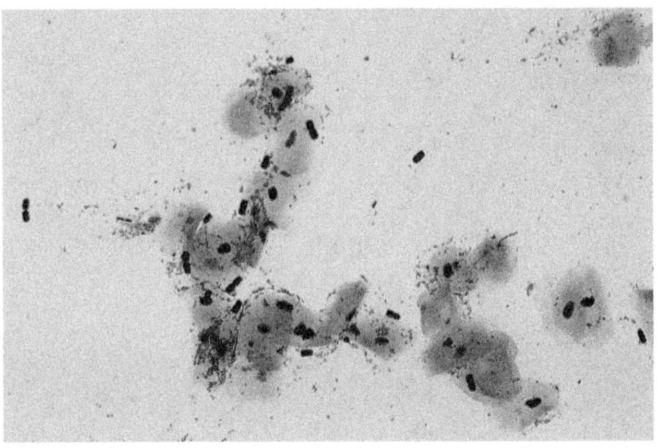

Fig. 4-2 Swab smear from oral cavity of normal horse. Squamous epithelial cells and a multimorphic bacterial population, including *Simonsiella*, are evident. (Original magnification 100X) (Courtesy Oklahoma Veterinary Diagnostics.)

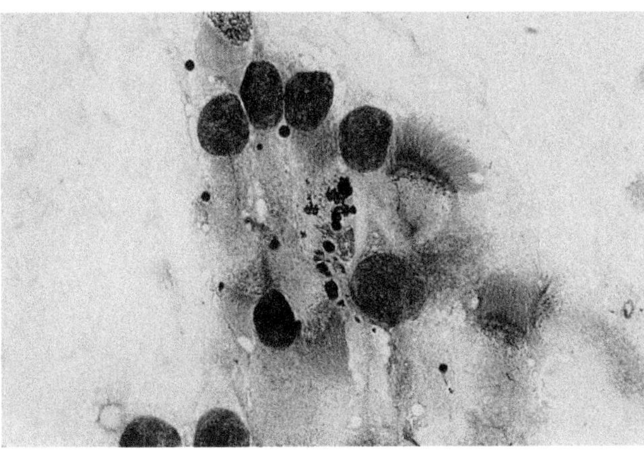

Fig. 4-3 Swab smear from nasal cavity of normal horse. Ciliated columnar epithelial cells and goblet cells are evident. (Original magnification 250X) (Courtesy Oklahoma Veterinary Diagnostics.)

Cells collected by washes can be harvested by centrifugation in a clinical centrifuge using the same speed as is used for urine sedimentation. The supernatant is poured off, the pelleted material is gently resuspended, and a drop of the suspension applied to a clean glass microscope slide with an applicator or pipet. The sediment is then spread using a blood smear technique (see Chapter 1) and allowed to air dry.

Preparation of fine-needle aspirate smears and impressions of biopsied samples is covered in Chapter 1. Staining with hematologic stains is satisfactory for cytologic examination of samples from the oral cavity and upper respiratory tract. A more complete discussion on sample collection, slide preparation, and staining is given in Chapter 1.

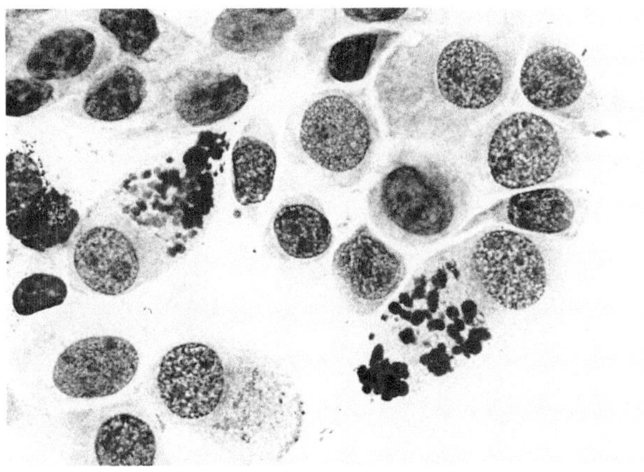

Fig. 4-4 Goblet cells.
Two goblet cells appear as columnar to cuboid epithelial cells, with numerous rose-colored cytoplasmic granules. (Original magnification 330X) (Courtesy Dr. R.L. Cowell, Oklahoma State University, Stillwater.)

Normal Cytologic Features

The oral cavity and upper respiratory tract are composed of several mucous membrane–lined, communicating passages and cavities: the oral and nasal cavities, pharynx, guttural pouches, and paranasal sinuses. Cytologic samples of the normal oral cavity or upper respiratory tract, collected by washing, swabbing, or brushing, consist of the exfoliated epithelial cells characteristic of the area sampled.

Oral Cavity and Nasal Passages

The epithelium of the mucous membranes lining the oral cavity and rostral portion of the nasal passages consists of keratinized and nonkeratinized stratified squamous epithelium; therefore, these surfaces exfoliate squamous epithelial cells (Fig. 4-2). Squamous epithelial cells appear cytologically as large flattened cells with angular borders and abundant, pale-staining cytoplasm and a condensed to pyknotic central nucleus.

The nasal epithelium caudal to the vestibule progresses from stratified squamous epithelium to pseudostratified ciliated and nonciliated columnar epithelium containing numerous goblet cells and exfoliates these various epithelial cells and goblet cells (Fig. 4-3). Columnar epithelial cells appear cytologically as medium-sized, elongated cells with basophilic cytoplasm and central to basal nuclei. Ciliated cells have pink-staining, hair-like cilia extending

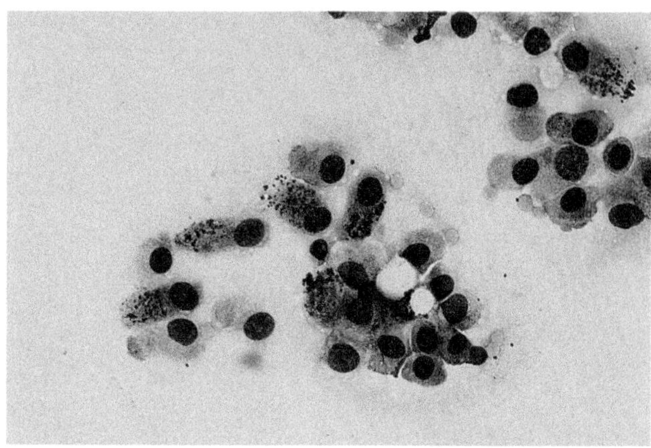

Fig. 4-5 Swab smear of normal pharyngeal recess. Note cuboidal and columnar epithelial cells and goblet cells. (Original magnification 100X) (Courtesy Oklahoma Veterinary Diagnostics.)

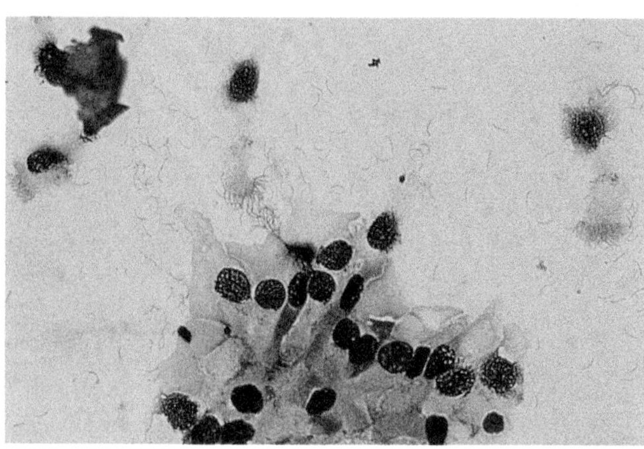

Fig. 4-6 Wash sediment from normal guttural pouch. Note cuboidal and columnar epithelial cells and free cilia. (Original magnification 100X) (Courtesy Oklahoma Veterinary Diagnostics.)

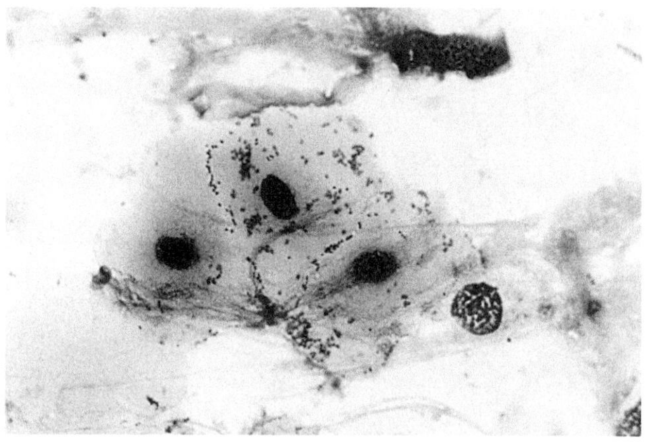

Fig. 4-7
Oral swab smear shows superficial squamous epithelial cells coated with commensal bacteria. (Original magnification 200X) (Courtesy Dr. R.L. Cowell, Oklahoma State University, Stillwater.)

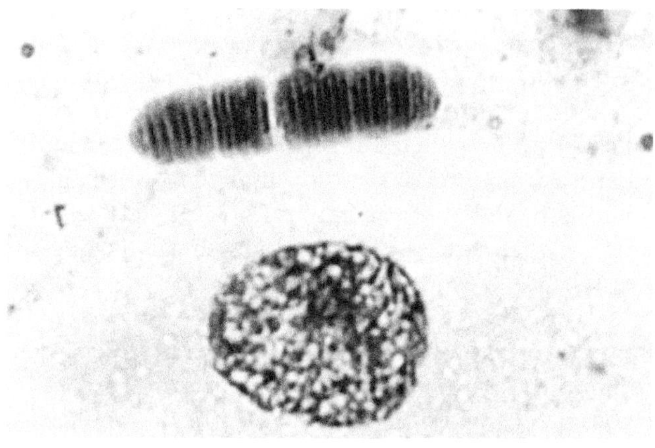

Fig. 4-8
In this oral swab, the striated structure at the top consists of *Simonsiella* spp. bacterial, alongside a squamous epithelial cell (*bottom*). (Original magnification 250X) (Courtesy Dr. R.L. Cowell, Oklahoma State University, Stillwater.)

as a fringe from one end of the cell (Fig. 4-3). Goblet cells contain numerous, red-staining cytoplasmic mucin granules (Fig. 4-4). The cytologic appearance of cells from the oral cavity and upper respiratory tract can be complicated by the presence of cells from specialized structures of the mucosa, such as papillae of various types, and taste and olfactory cells.

Pharynx, Guttural Pouches, and Paranasal Sinuses

The type of cells exfoliated from the pharyngeal mucosa depends on the area sampled. The pharynx is lined primarily by pseudostratified ciliated columnar epithelium, but it also has areas of stratified squamous epithelium (Fig. 4-5). The mucosa of the guttural pouches and paranasal sinuses consists of transitional epithelium and simple ciliated columnar or cuboidal epithelium containing goblet cells (Fig. 4-6). Cytologically, cuboidal epithelial cells of transitional epithelium appear as medium-sized, cuboidal cells with rounded borders, basophilic cytoplasm, and large central nuclei composed of finely stippled chromatin with areas of condensed chromatin.

Microorganisms

Bacteria from numerous commensal species normally inhabit the oral cavity and upper respiratory tract, and

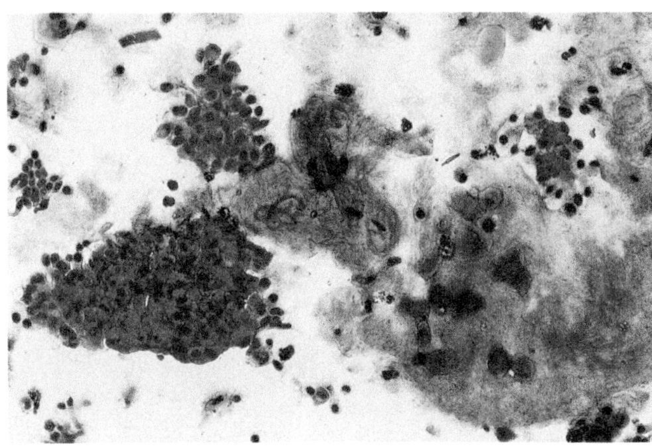

Fig. 4-9 Wash sediment from horse with guttural pouch irritation.
Large amounts of amorphous pink-staining mucin are evident, with clusters of columnar epithelial cells. (Original magnification 50X) (Courtesy Oklahoma Veterinary Diagnostics.)

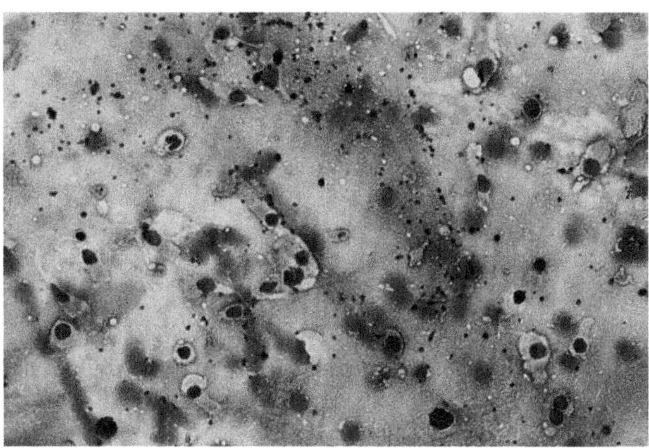

Fig. 4-10 Wash sediment from horse with guttural pouch irritation.
Large amounts of mucin and free mucin granules are evident, with cuboidal and columnar epithelial cells. (Original magnification 100X) (Courtesy Oklahoma Veterinary Diagnostics.)

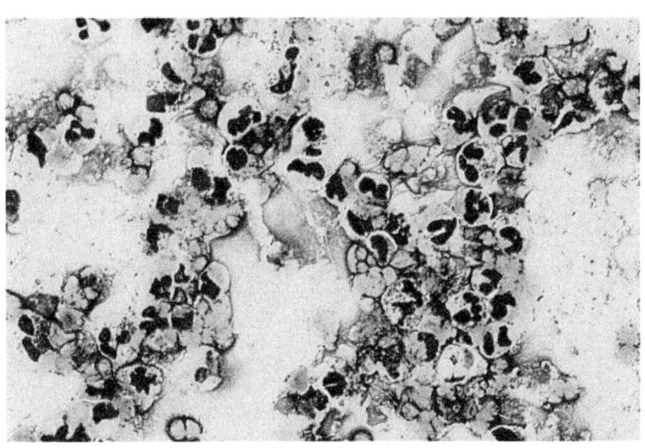

Fig. 4-11 Smear of exudate from paranasal sinus.
Smear contains large numbers of neutrophils and extracellular and intracellular bacteria. (Original magnification 100X). (Courtesy Oklahoma Veterinary Diagnostics.)

the bacterial population can be quite heavy in the oral cavity (see Fig. 4-2). This normal bacterial flora do not elicit a significant inflammatory response (*ie*, neutrophil exudation) (Fig. 4-7). Perhaps the most striking of the normal bacterial flora of the oral cavity are *Simonsiella* spp., which appear as giant rod-like structures (Fig. 4-2). These apparent giant rods are composed of multiple *Simonsiella* rods apposed side-to-side (Fig. 4-8 and Plate 3G).

Cytologic samples of the oral cavity and upper respiratory tract of horses also often contain "barn mold," that is, mycelial and fruiting bodies of saprophytic fungi commonly encountered in barn air and feed. Cytologically, these are typically large (>1-2 RBC diameters in size), green- to turquoise-staining, round to elliptical structures.

Underlying Structures

In addition to the mucosal epithelium, numerous and varied structures underlie the mucosa of the oral and upper respiratory tracts (cartilage, bone, adipose tissue, salivary glands, lymphoid tissue). Core biopsies, surgical biopsies, or fine-needle aspirates can be used to obtain cells characteristic of these structures.

Abnormal Cytologic Features

Irritation

Conditions that irritate the mucosal lining of the upper respiratory tract can result in increased goblet cells and production of increased amounts of mucin, which appears cytologically as mats of homogeneous, pink- to red-staining material or as a finely mottled pink background (Fig. 4-9). Goblet cells are rarely seen in washes of normal oronasopharyngeal structures.[3] Free mucin granules may also be seen in smears from irritated mucosa. These appear as small, round, rose-colored structures ($\frac{1}{2}$ RBC diameter) (Fig. 4-10).

Inflammation and Infection

The cytologic hallmark of inflammation is increased numbers of inflammatory cells (neutrophils, macrophages, etc)

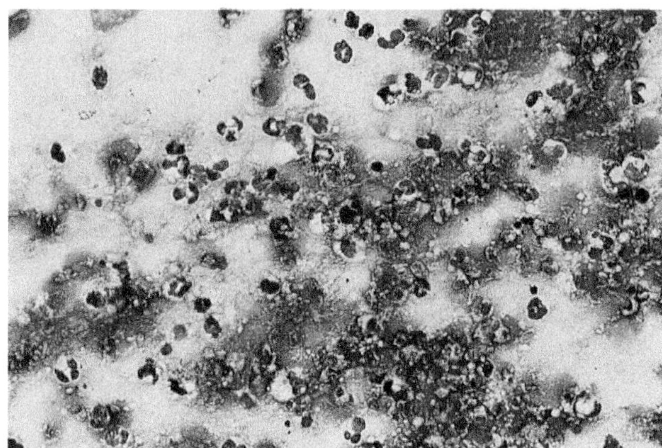

Fig. 4-12 Smear of exudate from paranasal sinus. Note large numbers of degenerate neutrophils, debris from lysed neutrophils, and small numbers of small rods in short chains. (Original magnification 100X) (Courtesy Oklahoma Veterinary Diagnostics.)

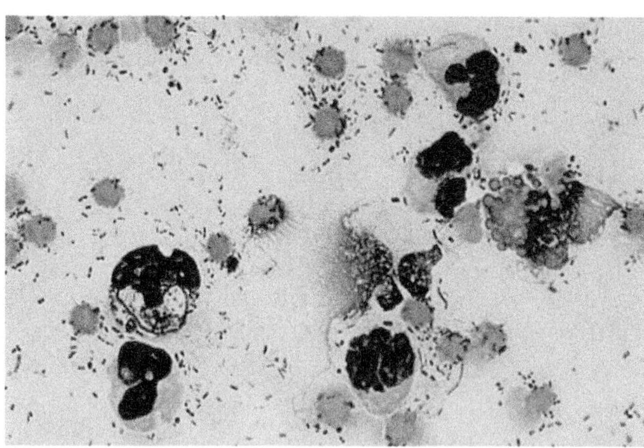

Fig. 4-13 Smear of exudate from paranasal sinus. Note large multimorphic bacterial population seen extracellularly and within neutrophils. (Original magnification 250X) (Courtesy Oklahoma Veterinary Diagnostics.)

(Fig. 4-11). Normally, only small numbers (<5%) of inflammatory cells are associated with the mucosa, submucosa, and associated structures of the oral cavity and upper respiratory tract.[3] Noxious stimuli, such as foreign bodies, trauma causing tissue necrosis, or infectious organisms, can provoke an inflammatory response resulting in increased inflammatory cells (>25%) in smears.[3]

Bacterial Infection: Bacterial infections are readily detected by cytologic examination. Typically, bacterial infection is associated with intense infiltration of neutrophils into tissues and exudation of neutrophils through the mucosa (Fig. 4-11). Because many bacteria produce toxins, neutrophils migrating into infected sites often become degenerate. In cytologic preparations, degenerate neutrophils appear swollen, lose their nuclear segmentation, and have lighter, pink-staining chromatin that gives them a monocytoid appearance (Fig. 4-12). The presence of degenerate neutrophils in a neutrophilic cytologic smear suggests bacterial infection, even if bacteria are not directly observed.

Cytologically, bacteria appear as collections of uniform rod-like to coccoid structures that typically stain dark blue with hematologic stains (see Fig. 4-11). Bacteria can be located extracellularly or intracellularly (Figs. 4-13 and 4-14). If bacteria are located only extracellularly and only small numbers of neutrophils are seen, one must exercise caution in differentiating bacterial infection from normal flora or contamination of the sample. In contrast, the presence of phagocytized bacteria indicates bacterial infection (primary or secondary).

Free mucin granules (Fig. 4-10), free cilia (Fig. 4-6), stain precipitate, or necrotic debris on cytologic smears

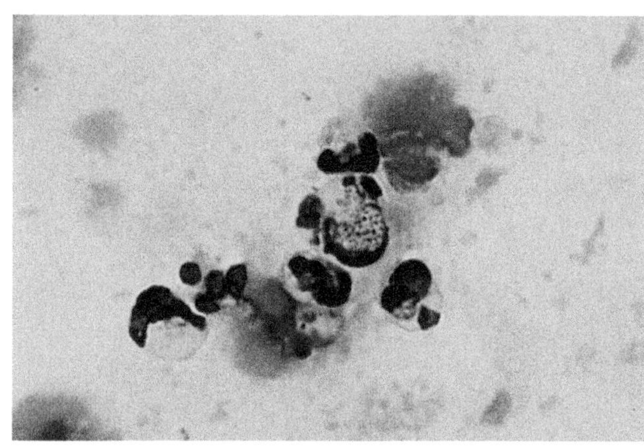

Fig. 4-14 Smear of exudate from paranasal sinus. Note ruptured cells and degenerate neutrophils containing phagocytized coccobacilli. (Original magnification 250X) (Courtesy Oklahoma Veterinary Diagnostics.)

can be mistaken for bacteria. As discussed before, bacterial infection is almost always associated with neutrophilic infiltration and phagocytized bacteria. Caution should be exercised in interpreting structures like bacteria if neutrophilic infiltration and phagocytized bacteria are not seen.

Bacterial infections of oral and upper respiratory mucosae can involve numerous bacterial species. Identification of particular bacterial pathogens based on their cytologic appearance is not reliable; therefore,

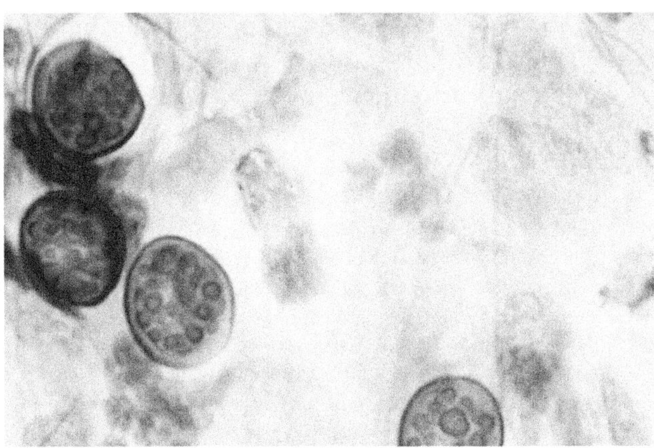

Fig. 4-15 Rhinitis caused by *Rhinosporidium seeberi*.
This smear shows several spherical rhinosporidia about the size of a neutrophils, with enclosed endospores. Inflammatory cells are present in the background. (Original magnification 100X) (Courtesy Oklahoma Veterinary Diagnostics.)

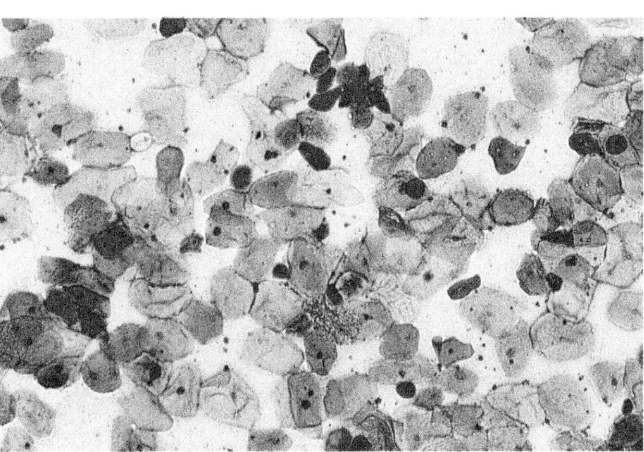

Fig. 4-16 Epidermal cyst.
This fine-needle aspirate contains large numbers of squamous epithelial cells, many with pyknotic nuclei or no nucleus and some that are keratinized. (Original magnification 25X) (Courtesy Oklahoma Veterinary Diagnostics.)

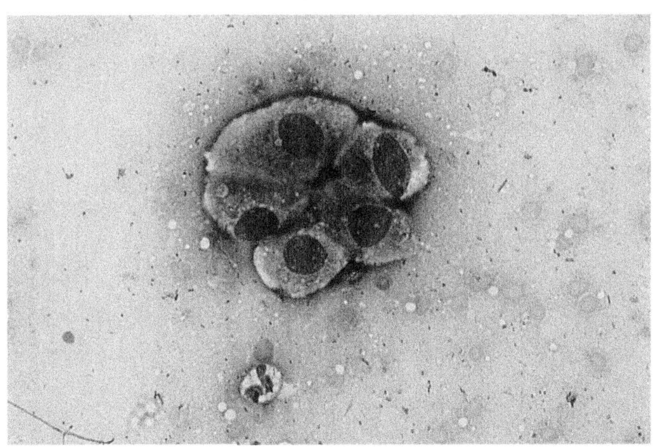

Fig. 4-17 Oral squamous-cell carcinoma.
This smear of a scraping shows a cluster of anaplastic epithelial cells that exhibit pleomorphism (anisocytosis, anisokaryosis), macrokaryosis, and multiple nucleoli. (Original magnification 100X) (Courtesy Oklahoma Veterinary Diagnostics.)

culture (and antimicrobial sensitivity testing) should be used to identify the organisms involved. Neutrophilic exudates are consistently observed in samples from oronasopharyngeal structures infected with *Streptococcus equi* but not with nonpathogenic streptococcal species or other commensals.[3]

Fungal Infection: Samples from horses with mycotic rhinitis, sinusitis, or guttural pouch infection typically contain large numbers of neutrophils and macrophages.[4] Multinucleated inflammatory giant cells, lymphocytes, and reactive stromal cells may also be seen. *Mycelium*-producing fungi are readily recognized as filamentous structures with a width greater than $\frac{1}{2}$ RBC diameter (wider than filamentous bacteria); some have septal divisions (Plate 5B). Determining the species of *mycelium*-producing fungi using cytologic features is not reliable. Mycotic rhinitis is occasionally associated with infection by *Rhinosporidium seeberi* (Fig. 4-15) or *Cryptococcus neoformans* (Plate 4H).

Hypersensitivity Reactions: Inflammatory processes involving hypersensitivity reactions can result in increased numbers of eosinophils, basophils, or mast cells in cytologic smears. Antigenic stimulation is associated with increased numbers of small lymphocytes and plasma cells. Pharyngeal lymphoid hyperplasia, like other forms of benign lymphoid hyperplasia, has no cytologic features that distinguish it from the normal cytologic appearance of lymphoid tissue; the cell population consists of ≥80% small lymphocytes.

Cysts and Hematomas

Cytologic examination of samples from fluid-filled structures of the dermis, mucosa, glands, or associated ducts often helps identify the process involved. *Atheromas* are epidermoid or sebaceous cysts of the nasal diverticulum. They consist of large numbers of squamous epithelial cells (Fig. 4-16) and a variable amount of sebum or cholesterol crystals.[5] *Cysts* involving the mucosa contain cells characteristic of their linings and may also contain mucins. *Hematomas* (eg, ethmoid hematomas) contain RBCs,

WBCs, and platelets, fresh or in various stages of RBC catabolism (erythrophagocytosis, bilirubin or biliverdin crystals, hemosiderin).[6] Mild or chronic cellular inflammatory processes are often associated with cystic structures such that increased neutrophils are often seen in the cytologic preparations of cystic fluid.[7]

Neoplasia

Neoplasms involving the oral cavity or upper respiratory tract consist of carcinomas arising from the mucosa and/or its associated glands or tumors of structures underlying the mucosa, such as osteosarcomas or lymphosarcomas. *Squamous-cell carcinomas* exfoliate moderate numbers of single- or multiple-cell clusters of medium-sized to large, pleomorphic epithelial cells.[8] These cells are polygonal and rounded, with distinct cell margins, abundant slightly granular blue to smooth turquoise cytoplasm, large round to oval single or double nuclei, reticulate to ropy chromatin pattern, and one or multiple nucleoli (Fig. 4-17). Other carcinomas have a similar anaplastic epithelial cytologic appearance (Plates 6A, 6C).

Nasal polyps are usually secondary to chronic inflammation and not of neoplastic origin. They consist of a mucosal lining, surrounding fibrous tissue.[9]

REFERENCES

1. Traub-Dargatz: Field examination of the equine patient with nasal discharge. *Vet Clin North Am (Equine Pract)* 13:561-588, 1997.
2. Schnieder: in Oehme and Prier: *Textbook of Large Animal Surgery*. Baltimore, 1974, Williams & Wilkins, pp 340-359.
3. Chiesa et al: Cytological and microbiological results from equine guttural pouch lavages obtained percutaneously: correlation with histopathological findings. *Vet Rec* 144:618-621, 1999.
4. Brearley et al: Nasal granuloma caused by *Pseudoallescheria boydii*. *Equine Vet J* 18:151-153, 1986.
5. Boles: Abnormalities of the upper respiratory tract. *Vet Clin North Am (Equine Pract)* 1:89-111, 1979.
6. Cook and Littlewort: Progressive haematoma of the ethmoid region in the horse. *Equine Vet J* 6:101-108, 1974.
7. Tremaine et al: Histopathological findings in equine sinonasal disorders. *Equine Vet J* 31:296-303, 1999.
8. Tuckey et al: Squamous cell carcinoma of the pharyngeal wall in a horse. *Aust Vet J* 72:227, 1995.
9. Hilbert et al: Tumours of the paranasal sinuses in 16 horses. *Aust Vet J* 65:86-88, 1988.

CHAPTER 5

Lower Respiratory Tract

Joseph G. Zinkl

Signs of lower respiratory tract disease include dyspnea, tachypnea, coughing, and stridor. A patient may expel mucus, exudate, or blood while coughing. If the respiratory disease is caused by an infectious agent, the horse may have a fever. Auscultation may reveal rales of various types, including crackles, wheezes, rhonchi, and pleural friction rubs. After the initial clinical examination of a patient with respiratory disease, a clinician may examine the patient in a variety of ways. With small animals the next phase is usually radiographic examination, but with larger animals radiographic examination may be difficult because of the relative lack of powerful radiographic equipment necessary for quality radiographic examination. However, quality radiographic examination should be conducted on horses with respiratory disease when possible.[1]

Pleural effusion may accompany conditions, especially infectious diseases, affecting the lower respiratory tract. Therefore signs referable to pleural effusion may also be found, and cytologic evaluation of pleural fluid may be indicated (see Chapter 8). Other general health examinations, such as hematologic and serum biochemical examinations, are also indicated in horses with respiratory disease. Specific examinations of the lower respiratory tract include bronchoscopy and laboratory evaluation of material from the lower respiratory tract. Laboratory examinations of this material include culture and microscopic examination. Material from the lower respiratory tract is usually obtained by transtracheal wash (TTW), bronchoalveolar lavage (BAL), and occasionally transthoracic aspiration.[1,2]

Sample Collection

Bronchoalveolar Lavage

Bronchoalveolar lavage (BAL) is usually performed during bronchoscopic examination of the lower respiratory tract. Fiberoptic endoscopy allows detailed examination and sampling of specific locations. The endoscope or catheter is passed into a major bronchus. Usually it is necessary to sedate the patient with xylazine (0.5 mg/kg body weight). Lidocaine (up to 60 ml of 0.5% lidocaine) is often infused through the endoscope to desensitize the airways.[3] After the endoscope is gently wedged in a small bronchus, 30 to 250 ml of sterile saline (without bacteriostatic preservative) is infused and as much as possible is immediately retrieved by aspiration with syringes or a suction pump.[3,4] In people, multiple infusions and aspirations have been used to obtain samples from the bronchioli and alveoli. The initial washing contains material primarily from the small airways, while subsequent washings contain material primarily from the alveoli.[5] Greater detail of BAL technique is described elsewhere.[3]

Tracheal Wash

Tracheal wash or lavage may be performed during endoscopic examination. Tracheal wash, however, is more frequently performed by the transtracheal method. With the transtracheal wash (TTW) technique, a catheter is passed through the skin, between tracheal rings, and into the tracheal lumen. The TTW technique is performed by first clipping approximately a 10-cm2 area in the region of the upper trachea, performing a surgical scrub, and anesthetizing the skin with a local anesthetic, such as 2% lidocaine. When the area is sufficiently anesthetized, a small stab incision is made through the skin. An intravenous cannula (eg, Medicut, Sherwood Medical, St. Louis, MO) or a large-bore hypodermic needle is inserted between two tracheal rings into the tracheal lumen. While the cannula is directed caudally, a sterile polypropylene catheter is passed approximately to the area of the tracheal bifurcation. Immediately after 30 to 60 ml of sterile saline (without bacteriostatic preservative) is infused, as much as possible is rapidly aspirated. Alternatively, the saline may be aspirated intermittently while withdrawing the catheter. It has been suggested that either gentle exercising or provoking a cough in a patient before sample collection helps obtain a representative sample.[3,6,7]

After the sample is collected, the catheter should be withdrawn and part of the sample readied for culture if culture is indicated by clinical signs or the gross appearance of the aspirated material (see Chapter 1). The remainder of the sample is retained for subsequent analysis. A small amount of antiseptic solution should be applied to the skin incision after the catheter and cannula are withdrawn.[3,6-9]

Complications: Complications of TTW are rare, but occasionally subcutaneous, peritracheal, and mediastinal emphysema may occur. Subcutaneous infection from leakage of exudate or from external contamination has been reported.[8] Rarely the cannula can sever the catheter when the catheter is withdrawn. This can be prevented by withdrawing the cannula or needle from the trachea before retrieving the catheter.[3] It is reported that horses quickly expel the severed end of the catheter by cough.[3,9]

Other Methods

Techniques for obtaining specimens with endoscopes and guarded brushes or protected aspiration catheters have been described. Such sample are uncontaminated by bacteria from the mouth or nasal passages of the upper airways.[10-12] The use of these methods for obtaining material for cytology evaluation has not been evaluated but potentially could provide cellular material from very localized lesions detected during bronchoscopic evaluation.

Percutaneous transthoracic biopsy is occasionally used to obtain biopsies of lungs and potentially could be used for fine-needle aspirates. A survey of large animal diplomates of the American College of Veterinary Internal Medicine indicated that sampling lung tissue in this way is useful for diagnosis of a variety of conditions, including those that produce a miliary pattern, suspicion for pulmonary infiltrative disease, pulmonary neoplasia, and pulmonary abscessation.[2]

Slide Preparation

Because TTW and BAL samples are collected in saline, they usually contain little protein, except for small amounts of mucus. Material obtained from inflamed lungs also contains plasma proteins. These proteins are markedly diluted by the saline used to obtain the sample. Therefore, total protein determination is of little or no value. Because of the dilution, cell numbers are usually low in BAL and TTW samples. The combination of low protein concentration and low cellularity decreases the quality of direct smears. Because of the low protein concentration, cells often disintegrate if smears are made by methods routinely used for blood and fluids with higher protein concentrations. Similarly, on smears made from material concentrated by centrifugation, many of the cells are often disrupted. Occasionally, TTW or BAL material contains sufficient mucus, other proteins, and well-preserved cells so direct smears can be examined. However, it is generally necessary to use methods that increase the cellularity of the smear and preserve the cells.

Cellularity can be improved by centrifuging a sample, pouring off the supernatant, and making smears from the sedimented pellet, provided that the cell pellet is first suspended in 1 or 2 drops of serum or commercial bovine serum albumin. A more direct method is to concentrate the wash material directly on a slide with a high-speed centrifuge (eg, Cytospin, Shandon Southern). Slides prepared by a high-speed centrifuge are usually very cellular, and the cells are well preserved.

Total and Differential Cell Counts

There is moderate to marked variation in the amount of fluid recovered after BAL or TTW procedures. The variation is less in BAL, however. Some investigators have suggested that total and differential cell counts may be of particular value for evaluating BAL fluid, but this is not commonly done in routine evaluation of BAL fluid.[4,8,13-15] Probably because different amounts of fluid have been infused in studies evaluating BAL cellularity, marked differences in total cell count have been reported.[16-19] When cell counts are determined, a hemacytometer technique is used. The sample dilution should be varied based on the estimated cellularity or the gross appearance of the fluid. One group suggested a 1:2 dilution for clear samples and up to 1:21 dilution for more turbid samples.[8] Differential cell counts may be of greater value than total cell counts. Cells are classified as epithelial cells, macrophages, neutrophils, lymphocytes, eosinophils, mast cells, and other cells (eg,

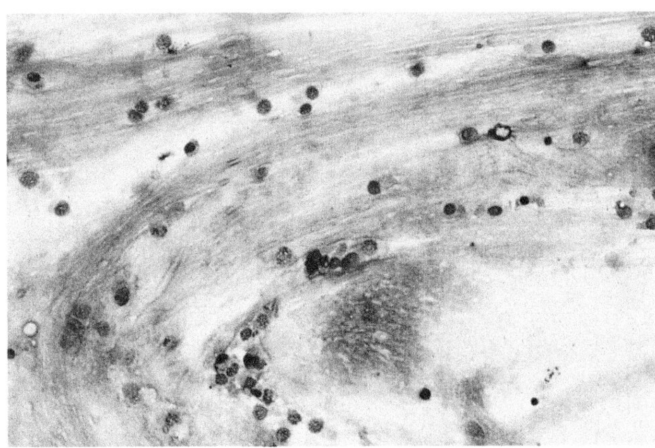

Fig. 5-1
Mucous strands, neutrophils, macrophages, and epithelial cells in TTW from horse with subacute, nonseptic pneumonia. (Wright's stain; original magnification 100X)

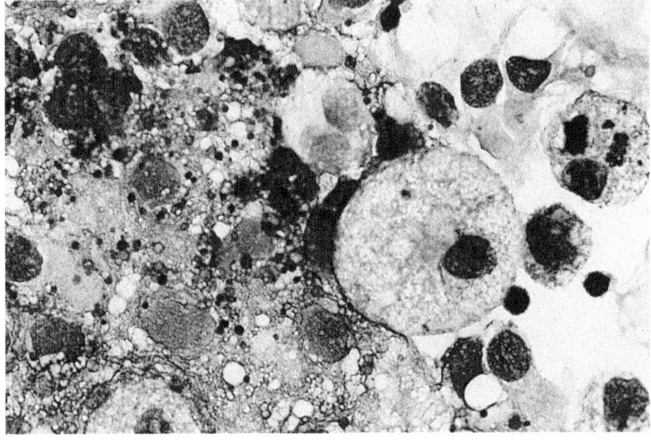

Fig. 5-2
Granules of mucus, mucus and cell debris, macrophages, and ciliated columnar epithelial cells in TTW from horse with chronic pneumonia and excessive mucous production. One macrophage has phagocytized a dark crystalline structure, suggesting impaired mucociliary clearance. (Wright's stain; original magnification 400X)

squamous cells). Epithelial cells may be further divided into columnar, cuboidal, and goblet cells.[16-19]

Staining Smears

Air-dried smears are usually stained by Romanowsky methods (Wright's, Giemsa, May-Grünwald Giemsa, etc). Hematoxylin and eosin, Sano's trichrome, and Papanicolaou stains also have been used.[8,17,20,21] Other stains, such as Gram stain to identify bacteria (especially gram-positive bacteria), PAS stain to define fungi, and Perl's Prussian blue or Gomori's stains for iron, are also useful.[17]

Microscopic Features

Elements in BAL and TTW Fluid

Mucus: Material obtained from the lower respiratory tract always contains some mucus.[17] In the collected fluid, mucus appears as strands of flocculent material. In Wright's-stained slides, mucus appears as pink to light blue amorphous strands (Fig. 5-1). Also, granular structures of similar staining quality sometimes are seen. These are mucus particles that have recently been released from goblet cells (Fig. 5-2). Mucus may also appear as dark-staining tight spirals (Curschmann's spirals), which are inspissated mucous casts of small bronchioli (Fig. 5-3). Curschmann's spirals are usually found in samples from animals with prolonged and excessive production of mucus.

Cells: Cells from the lower respiratory tract include epithelial cells, resident macrophages, and inflammatory cells.[17] Epithelial cells are of various types, depending on their origin. They consist of ciliated columnar epithelial cells, nonciliated epithelial cells of various types, and goblet cells (Figs. 5-4 and 5-5). Ciliated columnar epithelial cells are elongated and may have distinct, fine cilia at the end of the cell opposite the nucleus. Goblet cells are similar in shape to columnar epithelial cells, but they do not have cilia, and with some stains they may contain numerous azurophilic granules of mucus. Frequently, groups of basophilic epithelial cells are found in material from the lower respiratory tract. Usually these are adhered clusters of hyperplastic epithelial cells that have been stimulated by local irritation, especially with

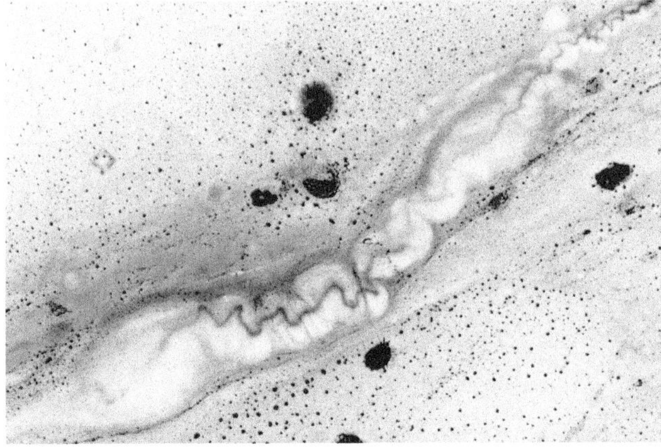

Fig. 5-3
Curschmann's spiral and several macrophages in background of mucus in TTW from horse with chronic lower respiratory disease. (Wright's stain; original magnification 200X)

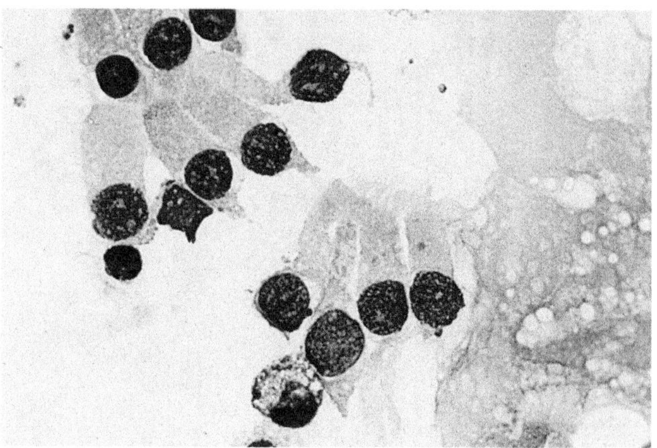

Fig. 5-4
Several ciliated epithelial cells, one alveolar macrophage, and lymphocyte in TTW from normal horse. (Wright's stain; original magnification 400X)

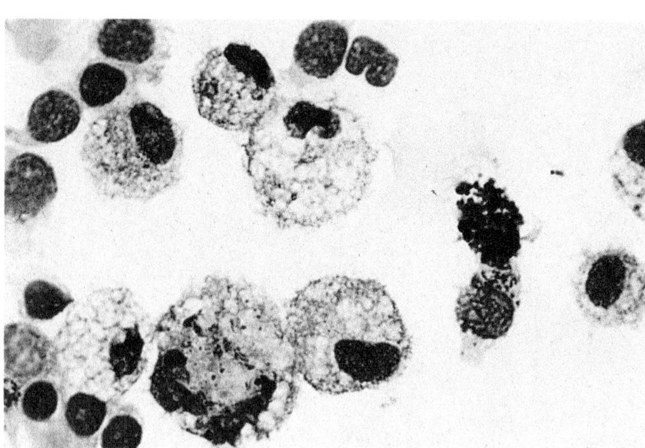

Fig. 5-5
Goblet cell and several alveolar macrophages in TTW from horse with chronic inflammation of lower respiratory tract. (Wright's stain; original magnification 400X)

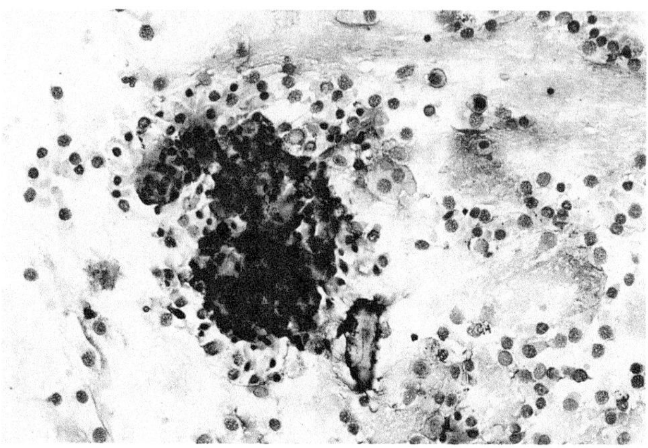

Fig. 5-6
Cluster of hyperplastic epithelial cells and individual epithelial cells in TTW from horse with long history of coughing and poor performance. A few alveolar macrophages are scattered among normal epithelial cells. (Wright's stain; original magnification 100X)

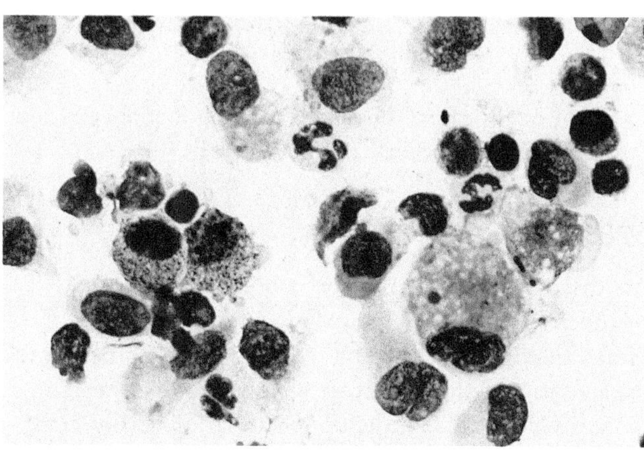

Fig. 5-7
Alveolar macrophages, lymphocytes, neutrophils, and mast cells in BAL from apparently normal horse. (Wright's stain; original magnification 400X)

conditions that cause chronic inflammation (Fig. 5-6).

Macrophages are resident cells of alveoli. They may transform into reactive inflammatory cells. Inflammatory cells include neutrophils, reactive macrophages, and eosinophils. Lymphocytes and mast cells are also found in lower respiratory samples from horses (Fig. 5-7). Erythrocytes are usually present, most frequently because of minor trauma of the epithelium that occurs during TTW or BAL, but they may also accompany inflammatory conditions or conditions that cause hemorrhage, such as exercise-induced pulmonary hemorrhage (EIPH).[17]

Substances from outside the lower respiratory tract also may be found. Usually these are the result of contamination during the TTW or BAL procedure, but they may be inhaled material that has not been expelled by the mucociliary action of the respiratory epithelium. Frequently, squamous epithelial cells or squamous-cell particles from the mouth or pharynx contaminate the sample (Figs. 5-8 and 5-9). Squamous cells are large cells with a distinctly flattened appearance. They may appear folded or rolled up. Usually they stain moderately basophilic, but occasionally they are slightly acidophilic. Their nuclei are often pyknotic or fragmented. Bacteria may be adhered to their surfaces. These organisms are contaminants from the mouth, pharynx, or nasal passages (Fig. 5-9).

Various other contaminants may be found in material obtained from the lower respiratory tract. These include some bacteria, plant material (pollen), fungal

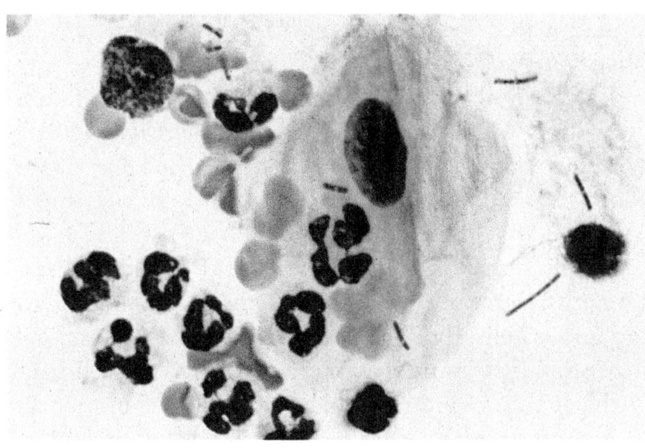

Fig. 5-8
Squamous epithelial cell, several large bacilli, and neutrophils in TTW sample contaminated with oral/pharyngeal material. (Wright's stain; original magnification 400X)

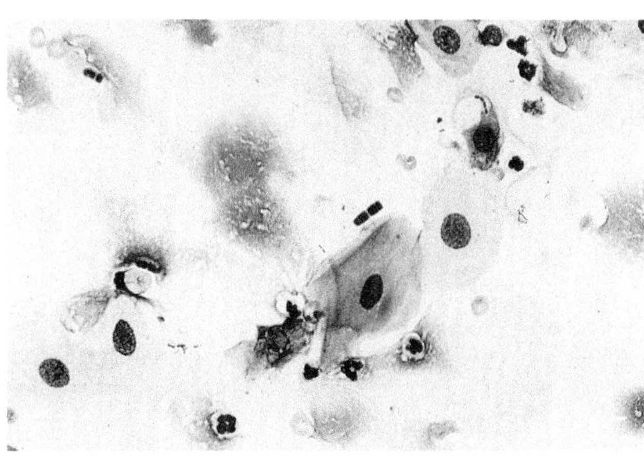

Fig. 5-9
Basophilic and eosinophilic squamous cell, *Simonsiella* organisms, several smaller bacteria, neutrophils, a granule of glove powder, and degenerated cell debris in TTW contaminated with oral/pharyngeal material. (Wright's stain; original magnification 200X)

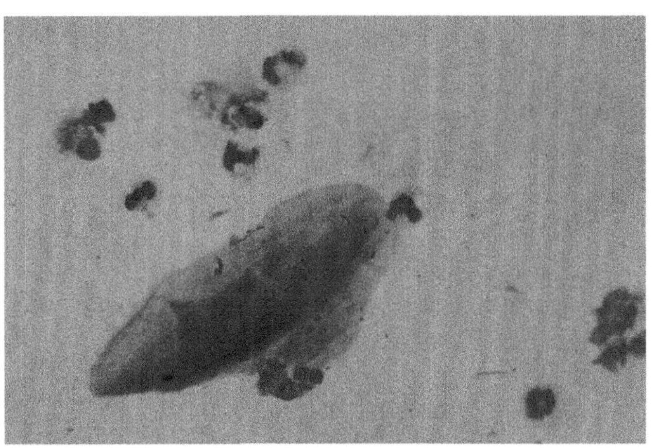

Fig. 5-10
Squamous cell with bacteria adhered to surface in TTW from foal with aspiration-induced pneumonia. A small *Simonsiella* sp. organism and degenerated neutrophils are also present. (Wright's stain; original magnification 400X)

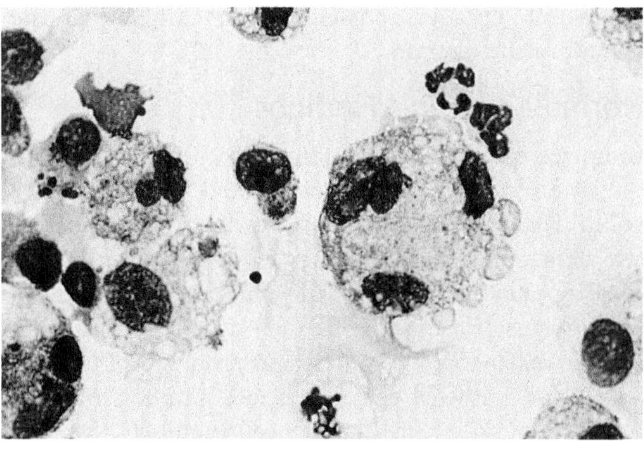

Fig. 5-11
Several alveolar macrophages in BAL from horse with chronic respiratory disease. Macrophage at right contains pollen particle. (Wright's stain; original magnification 400X)

elements, and crystals (Figs. 5-8 to 5-12). Most of these substances are usually contaminants. Bacteria may be either pathogens or contaminants obtained from the upper airways, the mouth, or the environment. Cytologic evaluation and the associated clinical signs are used to determine the significance of bacteria or the other elements. Granules of surgical glove powder (starch granules) (Fig. 5-9) are also found. Starch granules are light to moderate blue and round or imperfectly hexagonal. They have a refractile zone in their center. Microscopically, starch granules have a three-dimensional character. The depth dimension can be appreciated by observing the granules coming into focus in a different plane from the flattened cells on a slide. Other crystalline structures are also found occasionally. These crystals may be free or within macrophages. Generally they are clear and slightly refractile with straight borders and distinctly angular corners.

Superficial squamous-cell fragments are dark-staining, rolled scrolls that do not contain a nucleus. These structures usually come from superficial skin on the horse's neck, where the catheter was inserted, or from the hands of the person performing the TTW or BAL. Careful attention to technique, especially the use of a

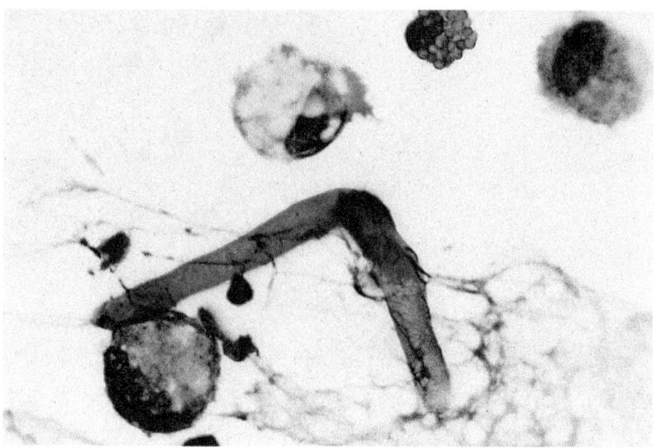

Fig. 5-12
Mucus, two macrophages, eosinophil, and plant fiber in BAL from horse with chronic respiratory disease. (Wright's stain; original magnification 400X)

cannula for inserting the catheter and only touching the cannula and catheter with gloved hands, helps avoid contamination by squamous-cell debris from either the patient or the operator.

Normal Cytologic Findings

In horses without lesions of the lower respiratory tract, the major cells in a TTW are ciliated and nonciliated columnar epithelial cells and alveolar macrophages. A few neutrophils and lymphocytes are usually found. A small amount of mucus is usually present.[13-15,17] BAL fluid from normal horses is significantly different from TTW fluid, in that it contains more macrophages (60% to 80%) and fewer epithelial cells. Moderate numbers of lymphocytes (20% to 35%), a few neutrophils (<5%), and rare mast cells (<2%) are also found in BAL fluid.[13,15,17] Total cell counts vary significantly depending on the technique used. In one study total cell counts of almost 4000/µl were reported,[19] but in most other studies counts of less than 1000 cells/µl have been found.[16,18,20,22]

Contamination by Oral/Pharyngeal Material

Occasionally, TTW and BAL samples are contaminated with oral or pharyngeal material. Cytologic features of oral/pharyngeal contamination include squamous epithelial cells and bacteria of various types, including *Simonsiella* spp. (see Figs. 5-8 and 5-9). Squamous cells are large, flat cells that usually stain lightly basophilic, but they may also stain lightly acidophilic. They appear flattened and often have straight borders with distinct corners. Squamous cells may have bacteria adhered to their surfaces. Contaminating organisms may be of many shapes and sizes. The presence of a large variety of organisms suggests that the sample has been contaminated from the mouth, nasal passages, or pharynx (see Fig. 5-10).

Extremely strong (nearly absolute) evidence of such contamination is provided when *Simonsiella* bacteria are found in TTW or BAL material (see Fig. 5-9). *Simonsiella* spp. divide lengthwise, and so line up in parallel rows, giving the impression of a single large organism with parallel light and dark stripes. Organisms may be free in the smear or adhered to squamous cells. Evidence of oral/pharyngeal contamination is also found in samples obtained from horses with aspiration-induced pneumonia. If inflammation is accompanied by cytologic evidence of oral/pharyngeal contamination, aspiration-induced inflammation of the respiratory tract must be considered (see following sections).

In some geographic areas, saprophytic "barn fungus" contaminants of hyphae, spores, and macroconidia are commonly found in horses housed indoors. A common contaminant is the saprophyte fungus, *Alternaria* sp. (Fig. 5-13). *Alternaria* is differentiated from other fungi, especially *Aspergillus*, by its large macroconidia that are divided transversely and vertically and the enlarged area at the joints of the hyphae.

Conditions Causing Abnormal Cytologic Findings

Septic and Nonseptic Inflammation: One of the most common lesions detected by examination of material from the lower respiratory tract is purulent (acute) inflammation.[8,14,17-20,23] Neutrophils are the primary cells in purulent inflammation (Fig. 5-14). Neutrophils collected from the respiratory tract often appear degenerated by displaying karyolysis and cytoplasmic vacuolization (Figs. 5-15 and 5-16). With fluids from other sites, neutrophils with these features are strong indications of sepsis. In TTW and

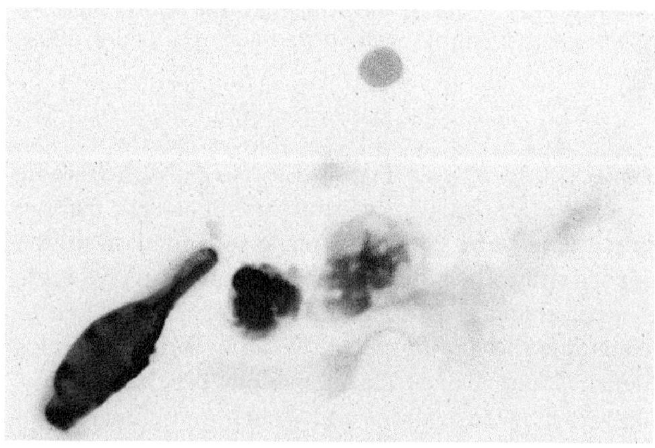

Fig. 5-13
Macroconidium of *Alternaria* in contaminated TTW. (Wright's stain; original magnification 200X)

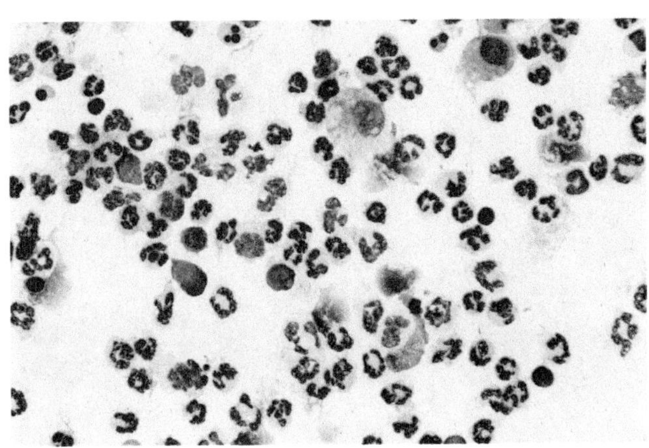

Fig. 5-14
Neutrophils (some degenerated) and macrophages in TTW from horse with purulent pneumonia. (Wright's stain; original magnification 200X)

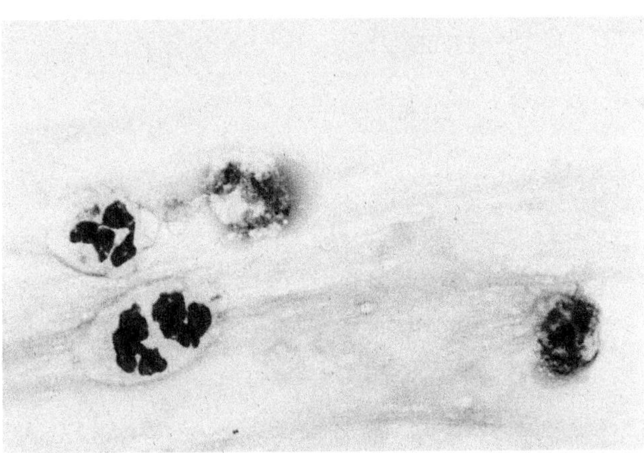

Fig. 5-15
Neutrophils and pair of small extracellular cocci in TTW from foal with *Streptococcus zooepidemicus* pneumonia. (Wright's stain; original magnification 400X)

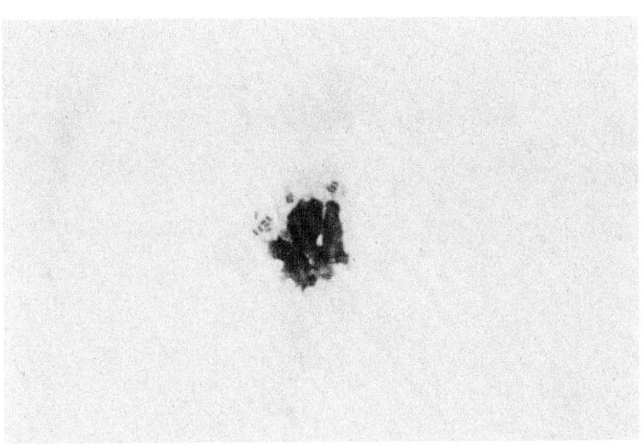

Fig. 5-16
Extremely degenerated neutrophil (note karyolysis) containing several small bacilli in TTW from foal with *Rhodococcus equi* pneumonia. (Wright's stain; original magnification 400X)

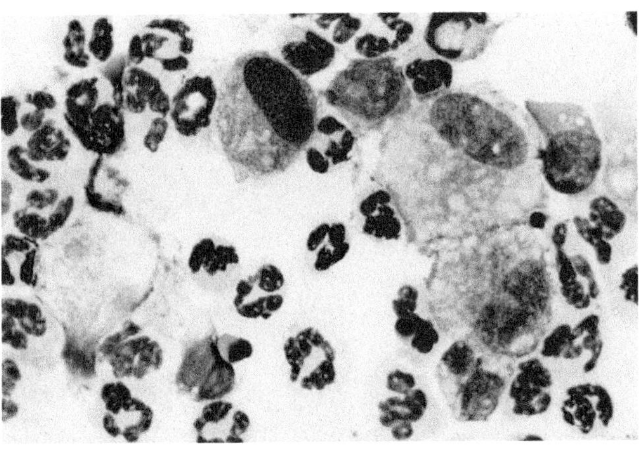

Fig. 5-17
Neutrophils and alveolar macrophages in TTW from horse with acute, nonseptic inflammation. Note occasional cell with darkly stained nucleus. These are neutrophils undergoing slow degeneration from aging, rather than toxicity. (Wright's stain; original magnification 400X)

BAL samples, however, the features of neutrophil degeneration may be found in nonseptic, purulent inflammation because the collection and handling of samples often impart features of degeneration to neutrophils. Lavage samples, particularly those left in the collection fluid for some time, often contain vacuolated, karyolytic neutrophils. Occasionally neutrophils may not display features of degeneration, especially when bacteria are present in low numbers and smears have been made soon after the sample was collected. Similarly, neutrophils from nonseptic inflammation on smears made soon after collection may be hypersegmented or show karyorrhexis (Fig. 5-17). When neutrophils are the dominant cell types and the horse has clinical features compatible with infection, the BAL or TTW fluid should be cultured for bacteria even if organisms are not identified by microscopic examination.

Alveolar macrophages (Figs. 5-14 and 5-17) are usually present with purulent inflammation, and columnar epithelial cells are often found in TTW fluid (but not from properly collected BAL fluid) from patients with acute purulent inflammation of the lower airways. Alveolar macrophages are large cells with abundant, foamy, basophilic to clear cytoplasm. They usually contain a single nucleus, but binucleate cells are common and multinucleated macrophages are found occasionally (Fig. 5-18). Columnar epithelial cells usually appear normal, but small clusters of hyperplastic epithe-

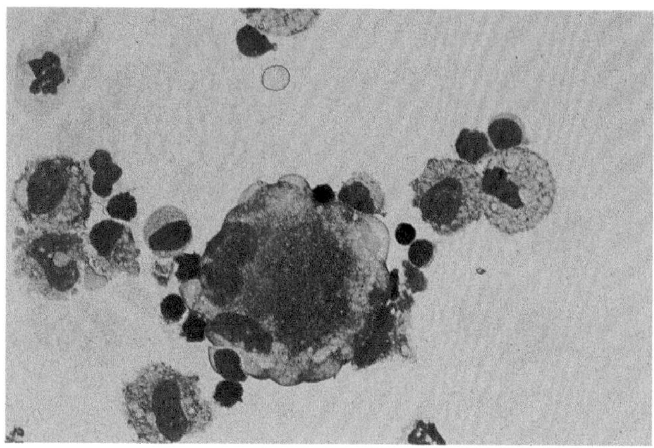

Fig. 5-18
Multinucleated macrophage, other macrophages, lymphocytes, and neutrophils in BAL from horse with silicosis (pneumoconiosis). Macrophage at upper right contains several pink crystals of cristobalite. (Wright's stain; original magnification 400X)

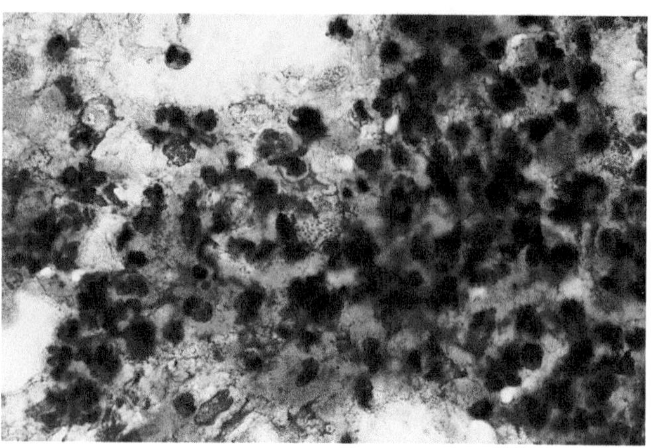

Fig. 5-19
Degenerated neutrophils embedded in cell debris and mucus in TTW from foal with pneumonia. Numerous small coccobacilli in center have "watermelon seed" appearance. *Rhodococcus equi* was cultured from fluid. (Wright's stain; original magnification 400X)

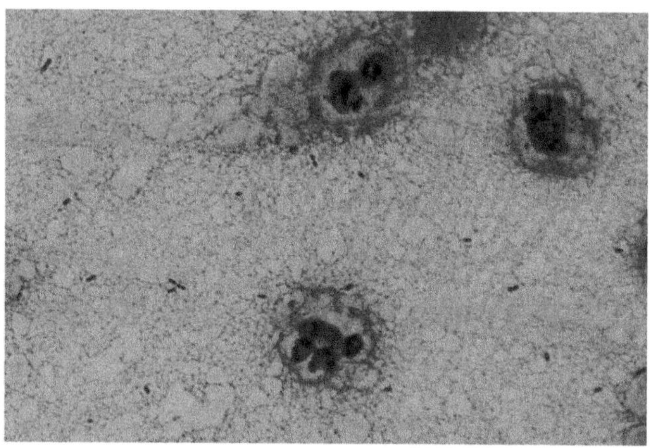

Fig. 5-20
Extracellular and intracellular bacteria scattered in thin layer of mucus and cell debris. Cocci and bacilli (rods) indicate mixed infection. *Streptococcus zooepidemicus* and *Actinobacillus suis*–like organisms were cultured from fluid. (Wright's stain; original magnification 400X)

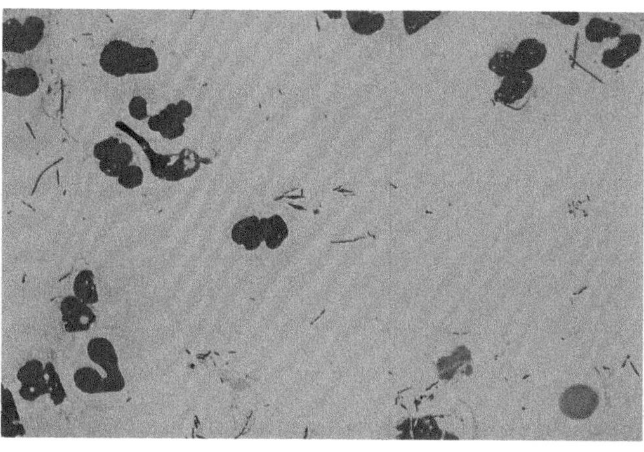

Fig. 5-21
Degenerated neutrophils and bizarre-shaped bacteria in TTW from adult horse with pneumonia. *Escherichia coli* and mixed anaerobic bacteria including *Fusobacterium necrophorus*, *Veillonella* sp., and *Peptostreptococcus* sp. were cultured from fluid. (Wright's stain; original magnification 600X)

lial cells occasionally are found in purulent inflammation.

When an inflammatory lesion persists, the ratio of neutrophils to alveolar macrophages decreases in favor of increased macrophages.[14,15,17,19,21] The relative numbers of macrophages and neutrophils determine the classification of the lesion, which varies from mixed, neutrophilic/mononuclear, to mononuclear. Terms indicating age of a lesion (ie, acute, subacute, and chronic) may be misleading because an alveolar macrophage response can be rather rapid and purulent inflammation can persist for a long time. There is a rough correlation between duration of the lesion and the type of cellular response, however.

All inflammatory lesions should be examined for etiologic agents. Bacteria may be found intracellularly and extracellularly (see Figs. 5-15 and 5-16). There are many bacterial pathogens, and frequently more than one species is found by culture or suggested by the organisms' morphology. Several organisms can cause pneumonia in adult and neonatal horses. It has been suggested that

TABLE 5-1

Microscopic and Other Features of Bacteria Found in Material Obtained from Horses with Pneumonia

Morphology	Gram reaction	Group	Classification*	Other Features
Cocci	Positive	Beta-hemolytic *Streptococcus*	*Streptococcus zooepidemicus,* **other *Streptococcus* spp.**	Single, pairs, and short chains (usually not more than four); most common *Streptococcus* in pneumonia of horses; *Streptococcus equi* may be long chains
		Anaerobic organisms	***Peptostreptococcus***	Single, pairs, or short chains
Coccobacilli	Positive	*Coryneform* organisms	*Rhodococcus equi*	*R. equi* are usually single, "watermelon seed"–like (may be difficult to differentiate from cocci), often intracellular; far more frequent in foals (<6 months) than in older horses
Bacilli (rods)	Negative	Enteric organisms	***Escherichia coli,*** *Klebsiella pneumoniae*, other enteric species.	*E. coli* is the most common enteric rod in pneumonia of horses
		Nonenteric organisms	***Actinobacillus suis*–like,** other *Actinobacillus, Pasteurella,* and *Bordetella* spp.	*A. suis*–like is most common nonenteric rod in pneumonia of horses
		Anaerobic organisms	*Bacteroides, Porphyomonas, Prevotella,* and *Fusobacterium* spp.	In addition to rod shape, may have bizarre shapes (pointed, bulge in the middle or at the end, bent, or curved)
	Positive	Anaerobic organisms	*Clostridium, Eubacterium, Bifidobacterium,* and *Propionibacterium* spp.	*Clostridium* spp. usually larger than other rod-shaped organisms

*Organisms in **bold** are the most common pathogens in pneumonia of horses.

approximately one third of the positive samples from infected horses will contain one species of microorganisms, one third will contain two, and the remaining one third will contain three or more.[24] Most bacteria stain dark with Romanowsky methods. Finding bacteria intracellularly is a strong indicator of sepsis. Although bacteria species cannot be determined by cytologic examination, the organisms can be classified according to their shape (Table 5-1). Further information can be obtained from their Gram reaction. The most common lung pathogens of horses, *Streptococcus zooepidemicus*, are gram-positive cocci that are usually found as single organisms or short chains of two to four organisms. *Rhodococcus equi*, an organism that is nearly exclusively a respiratory pathogen of young foals, is distinguished by gram-positive coccobacilli that are often intracellular and have the appearance of "watermelon seeds" (Fig. 5-19). Many rod-shaped organisms are lung pathogens in horses, and most are gram negative. These include *Actinobacillus suis*–like (Fig. 5-20)[25], *Pasteurella* spp., members of the Enterobacteriaceae family (*Escherichia coli, Klebsiella pneumoniae*, and *Enterobacter* spp.), and many anaerobes including *Fusobacterium necrophorum*, *Bacteroides* spp., and *Clostridium* spp.[24-29] Frequently anaerobic bacteria also have unusual or bizarre shapes such as sharply pointed ends, central or terminal bulges, bends, or curves (Fig. 5-21). It is necessary to distinguish bacteria from other small, round or elongated structures, including mucous granules, mast-cell granules, and precipitated stain. When evidence of oral/pharyngeal contamination is present along with severe purulent inflammation, aspiration-induced pneumonia must be considered a possible cause of the pneumonia. As discussed before, features of oral/pharyngeal contamination include squamous cells, mixed bacteria that may be adhered to squamous cells, and *Simonsiella* sp.

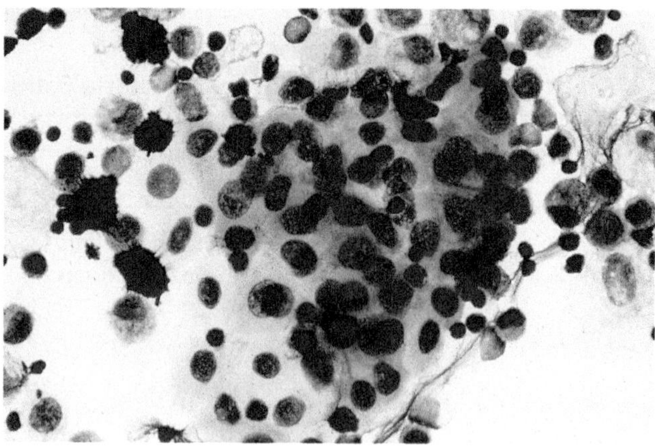

Fig. 5-22
Squamous metaplasia of epithelium in TTW from horse with chronic respiratory disease. Numerous macrophages and lymphocytes and a few darkly stained mast cells are scattered around the slide. (Wright's stain; original magnification 200X)

Fungal Infection: Probably most respiratory fungal infections are secondary to immunosuppression, other severe disease of the lungs, or other diseases such as enterocolitis, peritonitis, endotoxemia, or septicemia.[30] Infrequently, fungal elements may be found in or cultured from lavage fluid.[30-32] Quite often the inflammatory reaction is purulent, but occasionally the dominant cells are macrophages. The most frequently identified pathogenic fungus from the lower respiratory tract of horses is *Aspergillus* spp. (Plate 5B). However, other fungi may be identified, including *Coccidioides immitis* (Plate 5A), *Histoplasma capsulatum* (Plate 4C), and *Cryptococcus neoformans* (Plate 4H). Contaminating fungi, especially *Alternaria* spp., must be distinguished from true pathogens, especially *Aspergillus* spp.

Protozoal Infection: The protozoan *Pneumocystis carinii* can cause pneumonia in immunosuppressed foals or secondary to bacterial infection.[33-34] Mixed inflammatory reactions consisting of neutrophils and macrophages were noted in BALs from two foals with *P. carinii* infection.[34] The cyst stage of the organism can be identified cytologically in TTW or BAL samples, but free trophozoites are difficult to differentiate from debris. Intact cysts are distinctive, being 5 to 10 μ in diameter and containing four to eight dark-staining intracystic bodies that are 2 to 3 μ in diameter (Plate 5F).

Chronic Obstructive Pulmonary Disease (COPD): COPD occurs because of hypersensitivity and hyperirritability of the lungs to inhaled irritants or allergens.[4,35,36] A series of mechanisms mediated through the production of chemokines by macrophages results in purulent inflammation of bronchi and bronchioli.[37] Signs vary with severity of the condition and include exercise intolerance, coughing and wheezing, crackles on auscultation, and dyspnea characterized by accentuated effort at end respiration. Cytologic features are an increased amount of mucus accompanied by a mixed neutrophil and macrophage exudate.[4] Because of chronic increased mucus production and the relationship to hypersensitivity, Curschmann's spirals (Fig. 5-3) and/or increased numbers of eosinophils may be observed occasionally. In some horses, eosinophilic inflammation may be an early event in the natural progression of COPD.[38] In addition, there may be clusters of hyperplastic ciliated epithelial cells (Fig. 5-6) and increased numbers of goblet cells (see Fig. 5-5). Infrequently, squamous metaplasia of epithelium is found (Fig. 5-22). Cytologic findings are not specific, yet the findings reveal that inflammation is an important component of COPD.

Viruses: Horses may be affected by a variety of respiratory viruses. It has been suggested that epithelial atypias—including margination of chromatin, ciliocytophthoria (a particular type of degeneration resulting in ciliated tufts and basal cell fragments containing pyknotic nuclei and red cytoplasmic inclusion), and/or multinucleation—may indicate viral infection.[39] These changes are rarely recognized and may be nonspecific. Very frequently, severe viral infections are accompanied by secondary bacterial infection. TTW and BAL findings are not significantly different in secondary bacterial pneumonia from those of primary bacterial pneumonia, which consists of increased numbers of neutrophils.[40]

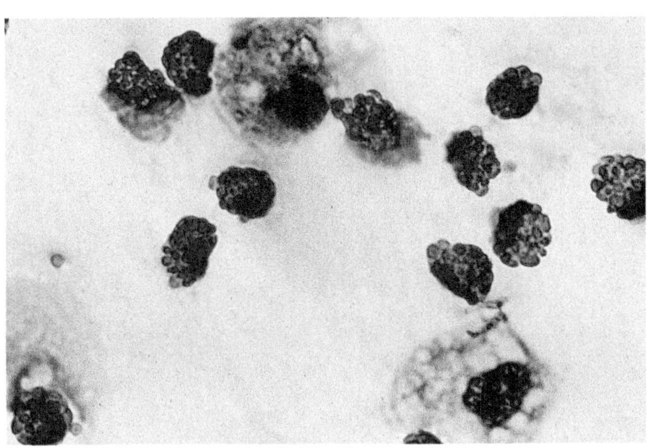

Fig. 5-23
Eosinophils and alveolar macrophages in TTW from mare infected with *Dictyocaulus arnfieldi* after grazing in pasture previously used by a donkey. (Wright's stain; original magnification 400X)

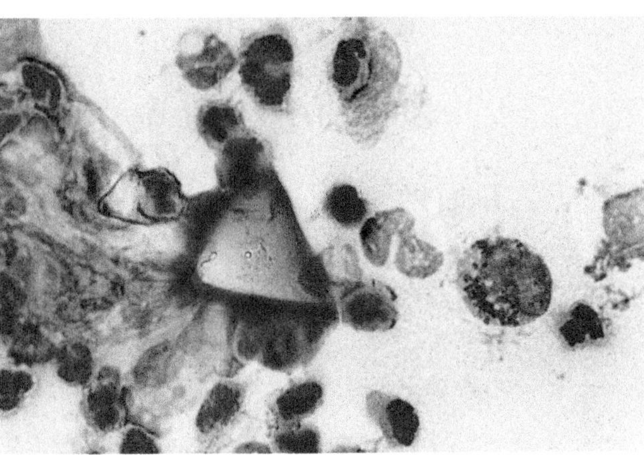

Fig. 5-24
Alveolar macrophage containing carbonaceous material in TTW from horse that survived a barn fire. There are also many neutrophils and a large crystal. (Wright's stain; original magnification 400X)

Increased numbers of lymphocytes are occasionally found in people with viral pneumonia.[5]

Eosinophilic Inflammation: Eosinophilic inflammation suggests hypersensitivity. Increased numbers of eosinophils are seen in allergic bronchitis and lungworm migration. Eosinophilic inflammation usually is accompanied by marked alveolar macrophage proliferation. Horses infected with the donkey lungworm, *Dictyocaulus arnfieldi*, may have severe respiratory signs.[41,42] Large numbers of eosinophils and alveolar macrophages are observed on cytologic preparations (Fig. 5-23). Larvae may occasionally be found in feces using the Baermann technique.[8,41,43] Eosinophilic inflammation is not specific for lungworm infection because eosinophilic infiltration is frequently part of an allergic reaction.[38] Eosinophilic inflammation of the respiratory tract in horses indicates a reaction to inhaled allergens or to migrating parasite larvae.

Smoke Inhalation: Smoke inhalation, such as may occur during a barn fire, causes severe damage to the respiratory tract. Although the upper respiratory tract is more vulnerable to the effects of heat, the lower respiratory tract is also affected by the noxious gases and particles generated by a fire.[44] The epithelium of the trachea, bronchi, and bronchioli may be destroyed or severely damaged, resulting in extreme edema and bleeding into the airways. Alveolar macrophages are laden with erythrocytes and black, carbonaceous particles (Fig. 5-24). Because of the extreme damage to the mucociliary clearance mechanism of the lungs, secondary bacterial and/or fungal infection may occur, and the TTW or BAL preparation may contain large numbers of neutrophils. Carbonaceous material may also be found in lower respiratory tract macrophages from horses living in highly polluted environments. A variety of other inhaled substances—such as crystalline structures (Fig. 5-24), pollen (Fig. 5-11), plant fibers (Fig. 5-12), and fungal elements (Fig. 5-13)—may also be found after smoke inhalation or from other conditions, such as viral infections or after septic purulent inflammation, that cause mucociliary dysfunction.

Exercise-Induced Pulmonary Hemorrhage (EIPH): EIPH occurs as a consequence of strenuous exercise.[45] Though some horses with EIPH have epistaxis, most horses bleed solely into the lower respiratory tract.[46] Examination ofTTW and BAL material can support the diagnosis of EIPH and may help determine whether a horse previously had EIPH.The presence of erythrocytes in the fluid, even with a history of recent strenuous exercise and obvious clinical signs, does not establish the diagnosis. Detection of blood in the airways by endoscopic examination is required to diagnose EIPH.There must be evidence that the erythrocytes are not a consequence of hemorrhage due to trauma during examination or sample collection.With preexisting hemorrhage, alveolar macrophages show erythrophagocytosis (Fig. 5-25), or they contain erythrocyte breakdown products, such as hematoidin (Plate 2A) or hemosiderin (Fig. 5-26).[47] Perl's Prussian blue and Gomori's stains are useful for determining whether material in macrophages contains iron. Hemosiderin-laden macrophages may

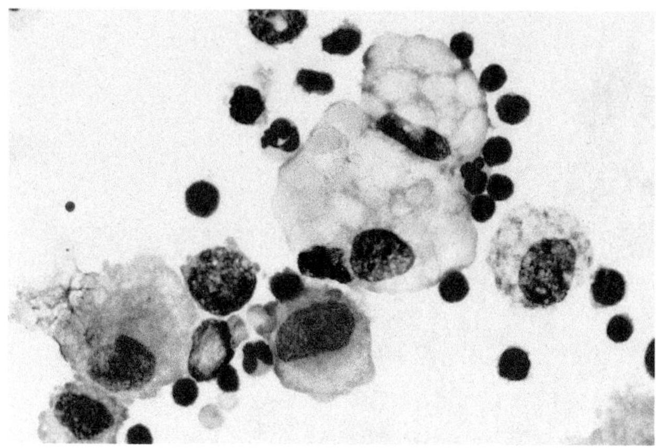

Fig. 5-25
Erythrophagocytosis by two macrophages in BAL from horse with exercise-induced pulmonary hemorrhage. There are also several other macrophages, numerous lymphocytes, and a few neutrophils. (Wright's stain; original magnification 400X)

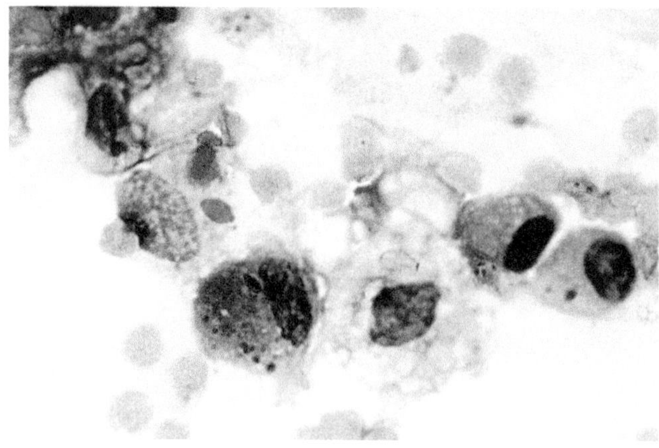

Fig. 5-26
Pigment (probably hemosiderin) in macrophage in TTW from horse with recurrent epistaxis. Several other macrophages and erythrocytes are also present. (Wright's stain; original magnification 400X)

present for at least 3 weeks after an episode of EIPH.[48] Many hemosiderophages were present for 21 days after inoculation of autologous blood into the lungs.[19] Hemosiderophages have also been found in horses after episodes of epistaxis because of inhalation of blood.[20]

Silicosis: Silicosis or pneumoconiosis has been best documented in horses in the Monterey area and Carmel Peninsula of California[49] and in some other coastal regions of California. The primary features are exercise intolerance and occasional respiratory distress. Affected horses often have restrictive breathing patterns, and auscultation reveals harsh respiratory sounds and some wheezing. TTW material contains large numbers of macrophages. Within some macrophages, irregular pink crystalline inclusions are found. These differ from many other crystalline inclusions found in alveolar macrophages by their distinctive pinkish color (Figs. 5-10 and 5-27). In addition to the macrophages, excessive mucus, including Curschmann's spirals, and increased numbers of neutrophils and hyperplastic epithelial cells can be found.

Neoplasia: Primary and metastatic lung tumors are very rare in horses.[50-53] I am unaware of any reports in which BAL/TTW has facilitated diagnosis of primary lung neoplasia in horses. In my experience, BAL/TTW has not been helpful in diagnosing tumors that have metastasized to the lungs of horses or other species. However, some metastatic lung tumors in people, such as melanomas, sarcomas, carcinomas, and leukemias, have been accurately identified by examination of BAL.[5]

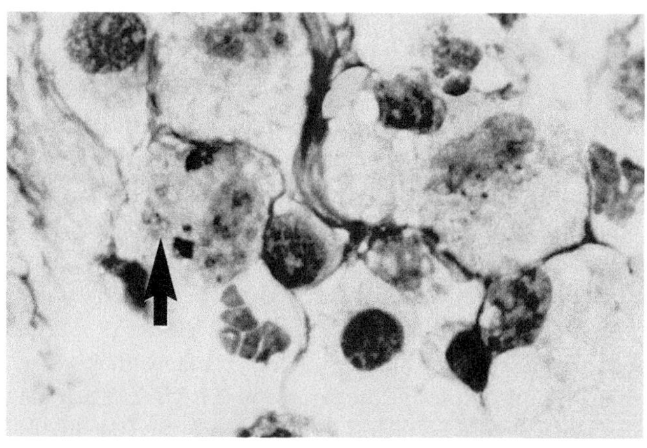

Fig. 5-27
Several macrophages, a neutrophil, and some mucus in TTW from horse with silicosis (pneumoconiosis). One macrophage contains several small pinkish crystals of cristobalite (*arrow*). (Wright's stain; original magnification 400X)

Diagnosis of neoplasia in BAL fluids from people was greatly facilitated by examining Papanicolaou-stained slides. However, Papanicolaou staining is not a common procedure in veterinary medicine. For neoplastic cells to be retrievable by BAL/TTW, the tumor must have invaded the bronchi or bronchioli and the bronchi or bronchioli must not be too peripherally located or blocked by mucus. A more reliable technique for obtaining material from suspected tumors of the lungs may be percutaneous lung biopsy or aspirates.[2,51] Primary tumors of lungs of horses include pulmonary

A 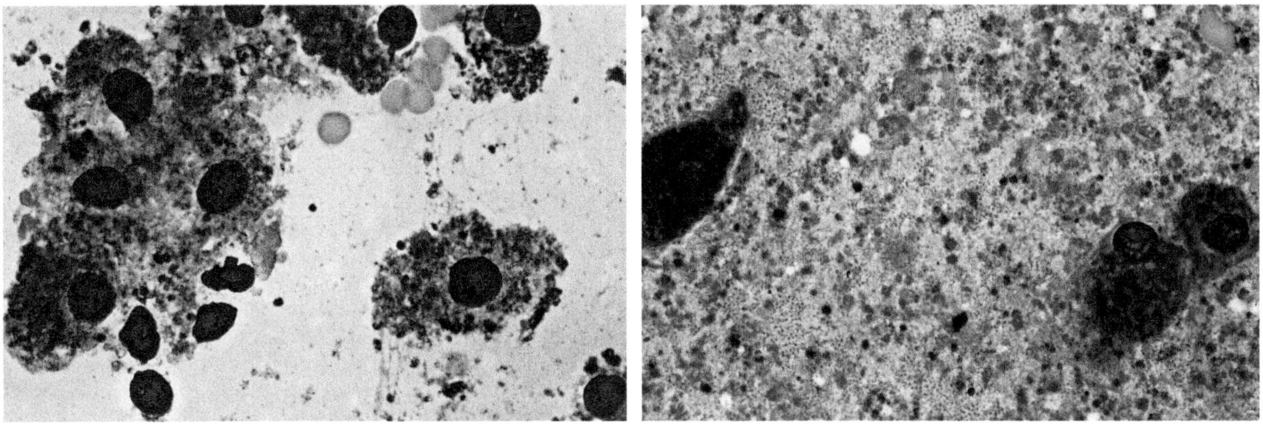 B

Fig. 5-28
Impression smear from ultrasound-guided Tru-Cut biopsy of lung mass (granular cell tumor) in horse. **A,** Large epithelial cells with eosinophilic cytoplasmic granules. (Wright's stain; original magnification 250X) **B,** Three epithelial cells and numerous eosinophilic granules from ruptured cells scattered in background of smear. (Wright's stain; original magnification 250X)

granular-cell tumor, pulmonary adenocarcinoma, bronchogenic carcinoma, pulmonary carcinoma, bronchogenic squamous-cell carcinoma, pulmonary chondrosarcoma, and bronchial myxoma.[50-53] Metastatic tumors of the lung or thorax include hemangiosarcoma, squamous-cell carcinoma, adenocarcinoma, renal carcinoma, rhabdomyosarcoma, malignant melanoma, fibrosarcoma, hepatoblastoma, chondrosarcoma, neuroendocrine tumor, undifferentiated sarcoma, and undifferentiated carcinoma.[51] Among the most frequent tumors that can metastasize to the lungs in horses are malignant melanomas.[53] Cytologic features of epithelial neoplasia were found in an ultrasound-guided aspirate of a lung mass in a horse, which was determined on histologic examination to be a bronchoalveolar carcinoma.[54] Granulosa-cell tumor was diagnosed in a mare by cytologic evaluation of impression smears of a biopsy (Fig. 5-28).[55] Lung aspirates from some other horses with pulmonary tumors failed to reveal neoplastic cells.[56,57]

REFERENCES

1. Wagner: in Smith: *Large Animal Internal Medicine*. St. Louis, 1996, Mosby, pp 550-565.
2. Savage et al: Survey of the large animal diplomates of the American College ofVeterinary Internal Medicine regarding percutaneous lung biopsy in the horse. *J Vet Internal Med* 12:456-464, 1998.
3. Hoffman and Viel: Techniques for sampling the respiratory tract of horses. *Vet Clin North Am* 13:463-475, 1997.
4. Derksen et al: Bronchoalveolar lavage in ponies with recurrent airway obstruction (heaves). *Am Rev Respir Dis* 132:1066-1070, 1985.
5. Linder and Rennard: *Bronchoalveolar Lavage*. Chicago, 1988, ASCP Press.
6. Mansmann and Knight: Transtracheal aspiration in the horse. *JAVMA* 160:1527-1529, 1972.
7. Beech: Technique of tracheobronchial aspiration in the horse. *Equine Vet J* 13:136-137, 1981.
8. Whitwell and Greet: Collection and evaluation of tracheobronchial washes in the horse. *Equine Vet J* 16:499-508, 1984.
9. Mansmann and Strouss: Evaluation of transtracheal aspiration in the horse. *JAVMA* 169:631-633, 1976.
10. Sweeney et al: Comparison of bacteria isolated from specimens obtained by use of endoscopic guarded tracheal swabbing and percutaneous tracheal aspiration in horses. *JAVMA* 195:1225-1229, 1989.
11. Darien et al: A tracheoscopic technique for obtaining uncontaminated lower airway secretions for bacterial culture in the horse. *Equine Vet J* 22:170-173, 1990.
12. Hoffman et al: Sensitivity and specificity of bronchoalveolar lavage and protected catheter brush methods for isolating bacteria from foals with experimentally induced pneumonia caused by *Klebsiella pneumoniae*. *Am J Vet Res* 54:1803-1807, 1993.
13. Mair et al: Cellular content of secretions obtained by lavage from different levels of the equine respiratory tract. *Equine Vet J* 19:458-462, 1987.
14. Larson and Busch: Equine tracheobronchial lavage: comparison of lavage cytology and pulmonary histopathologic findings. *Am J Vet Res* 46:144-146, 1985.
15. Derksen et al: Comparison of transtracheal aspirate and bronchoalveolar lavage in 50 horses with chronic lung disease. *Equine Vet J* 21:23-26, 1989.
16. McKane et al: Equine bronchoalveolar lavage cytology: survey of Thoroughbred racehorses in training. *Aust Vet J* 70:401-404, 1993.
17. Bain: Cytology of the respiratory tract. *Vet Clin North Am (Equine Pract)* 13:477-486, 1997.
18. Couetil and Denicola: Blood gas, plasma lactate and bronchoalveolar lavage cytology analyses in racehorses with respiratory disease. *Equine Vet J Suppl* 30:77-82, 1999.
19. McKane and Slocombe: Sequential changes in bronchoalveolar cytology after autologous blood inoculation. *Equine Vet J Suppl* 30:126-130, 1999.
20. Beech: Cytology of tracheobronchial aspirates in horses. *Vet Pathol* 12:157-164, 1975.
21. Bursh and Jensen: The use of cytology in the diagnosis and treatment of equine respiratory infections. *Equine Pract* 6(10):18-23, 1984.

22. Moore et al: Cytologic evaluation of bronchoalveolar lavage fluid obtained from Standard bred racehorses with inflammatory airway disease. *Am J Vet Res* 56:562-567, 1995.
23. Bursh and Jensen: The use of cytology in the diagnosis of equine respiratory infections. *Equine Pract* 9(2):7-10, 1987.
24. Hirsh and Jang: Antimicrobic susceptibility of bacterial pathogens from horses. *Vet Clin North Am (Equine Pract)* 3:181-190, 1987.
25. Jang et al: *Actinobacillus suis*-like organisms in horses. *Am J Vet Res* 48:1036-1038, 1987.
26. Traub-Dargatz: Bacterial pneumonia. *Vet Clin North Am (Equine Pract)* 7:53-61, 1991.
27. Hoffman et al: Association of microbiologic flora with clinical, endoscopic, and pulmonary cytologic findings in foals with distal respiratory tract infection. *Am J Vet Res* 54:1615-1622, 1993.
28. Warner: in Smith: *Large Animal Internal Medicine*. St Louis, 1996, Mosby, pp 566-575.
29. Carlson and O'Brien: Anaerobic bacterial pneumonia with septicemia in two racehorses. *JAVMA* 196:941-943, 1990.
30. Sweeney: in Smith: *Large Animal Internal Medicine*. St Louis, 1996, Mosby, pp 576-577.
31. Sweeney and Habecker: *JAVMA* 214:808-811, 1999.
32. Riley et al: Cryptococcosis in seven horses. *Aust Vet J* 69:135-139, 1992.
33. Ainsworth et al: Recognition of *Pneumocystis carinii* in foals with respiratory distress. *Equine Vet J* 25:103-108, 1993.
34. Ewing et al: *Pneumocystis carinii* pneumonia in foals. *JAVMA* 204:929-933, 1994.
35. Nuytten et al: Cytology, bacteriology, and phagocytic capacity of tracheobronchial aspirates in healthy horses and horses with chronic obstructive pulmonary disease (COPD). *Zbl Vet Med A* 30:114-120, 1983.
36. Beech: in Smith: *Large Animal Internal Medicine*. St Louis, 1996, Mosby, pp 594-597.
37. Franchini et al: The role of neutrophil chemotactic cytokines in the pathogenesis of equine chronic obstructive pulmonary disease (COPD). *Vet Immunol Immunopathol* 66:53-65, 1998.
38. Hare and Viel: Pulmonary eosinophilia associated with increased airway responsiveness in young racing horses. *J Vet Intern Med* 12:163-170, 1998.
39. Freeman et al: A review of cytological specimens from horses with and without clinical signs of respiratory disease. *Equine Vet J* 25:523-526, 1993.
40. Gross et al: Effect of moderate exercise on the severity of clinical signs associated with influenza virus infection in horses. *Equine Vet J* 30:489-497, 1998.
41. MacKay and Urquhart: An outbreak of eosinophilic bronchitis in horses possibly associated with *Dictyocaulus arnfieldi* infection. *Equine Vet J* 11:110-112, 1979.
42. Dixon et al: Equine pulmonary disease: a case control study of 300 referred cases. Part 3: Ancillary diagnostic findings. *Equine Vet J* 27:428-435, 1995.
43. Mair: Value of tracheal aspirates in the diagnosis of chronic pulmonary disease in the horse. *Equine Vet J* 19:463-465, 1987.
44. Beech: in Smith: *Large Animal Internal Medicine*. St Louis, 1996, Mosby, pp 595-596.
45. Roberts and Erickson: Exercise-induced pulmonary haemorrhage workshop. *Equine Vet J Suppl* 30:642-644, 1999.
46. Pasco et al: Exercise-induced pulmonary hemorrhage in racing thoroughbreds: a preliminary study. *Am J Vet Res* 42:703-707, 1981.
47. O'Callaghan et al: Exercise-induced pulmonary hemorrhage in the horse: results of a detailed clinical, postmortem and imaging study. I. Clinical profile of horses. *Equine Vet J* 19:384-388, 1987.
48. Meyer et al: Quantification of exercise-induced pulmonary haemorrhage with bronchoalveolar lavage. *Equine Vet J* 30:284-286, 1998.
49. Schwartz et al: Silicate pneumoconiosis and pulmonary fibrosis in horses from the Monterey-Carmel Peninsula. *Chest* 80:82S-85S, 1981.
50. Moulton: *Tumors of Domestic Animals*. 3rd ed. Berkeley, 1990, University of California Press, pp 308-346.
51. Scarratt and Crisman: Neoplasia of the respiratory tract. *Vet Clin North Am (Equine Pract)* 14:451-473, 1998.
52. Mair and Brown: Clinical and pathological features of thoracic neoplasia in the horse. *Equine Vet J* 25:220-223, 1993.
53. Dungworth: in Jubb et al: *Pathology of Domestic Animals*, 4th ed. New York, 1993, Academic Press, pp 688-696.
54. Anderson et al: Primary neoplasm in a horse. *JAVMA* 201:1399-1401, 1992.
55. Walker et al: What is your diagnosis. *Vet Clin Pathol* 22:35, 58-59, 1993.
56. Schultze et al: Primary malignant pulmonary neoplasia in two horses. *JAVMA* 193:477-480, 1998.
57. Van Rensburg et al: Bronchoalveolar adenocarcinoma in a horse. *Tydskr S Afr Vet Ver* 60:212-214, 1989.

CHAPTER 6

Gastrointestinal Tract

Carol B. Grindem and Heather L. DeHeer

Gastrointestinal disorders account for approximately half of all equine medical problems.[1] Cytology can be an invaluable quick, inexpensive aid in the diagnosis of these disorders. Sample procurement has previously limited gastrointestinal cytology to the evaluation of thoracic and abdominal fluid (Chapters 8 and 9), necropsy specimens, and fecal material. Endoscopy, laparoscopy, and ultrasonography have made visualization and biopsying of gastrointestinal lesions physically and economically possible.[2-6] Therefore, antemortem sampling of the gastrointestinal tract has become not only feasible but also an integral part of complete diagnostic workups.

Definitive cytologic diagnoses can often be made for mass lesions that are neoplastic or inflammatory/infectious. Cytologic patterns such as hemorrhage, chronic inflammation, or necrosis, although not specific diagnoses, may provide helpful prognostic information or presumptive diagnoses. A negative cytologic examination, however, cannot rule out a neoplastic or inflammatory disease. Sample size, quality of specimen, effect of therapy on tissue reactions, representativeness of sample, propensity of biopsied cells to exfoliate, and cytologic differentiation of reactive cells versus neoplastic disorders are concerns with cytologic diagnoses. Cytologic interpretations must always be correlated to clinical, endoscopic, and ultrasonographic findings.

Sampling

Investigation of gastrointestinal disorders usually begins with rectal palpation after collection of a minimum database. If an abnormality such as abnormal masses, enlarged lymph nodes, thickened loops of bowel, or excessive abdominal fluid is found, ancillary diagnostic tools such as endoscopy, ultrasonography, radiography, or abdominocentesis can more specifically define the disorder. Endoscopic biopsies are usually small (1.8 to 2.3 mm) but sufficient for diagnostic purposes. Collection of excellent quality biopsies is challenging, especially with endoscopy and laparoscopy. Experience and teamwork are essential for the collection of good endoscopic or laparoscopic biopsies. Biopsy instrument slippage, incorrect angle placement, hemorrhage, risks of full-thickness biopsying, and iatrogenic perforation of the diseased gut with the endoscope are serious problems to manage. Bacterial contamination is also a real problem with endoscopic samples. Culture results must be compared to cytologic findings to reduce the risk of misinterpretation.

Endoscopy, laparoscopy, and ultrasonography have become the new standards to visualize and biopsy the equine gastrointestinal tract. Gastrointestinal biopsy, brushings, and lavage samples can be collected by endoscopy. Additionally, tissue biopsies can be obtained by laparoscopy, exploratory surgery, or percutaneous ultrasound guidance.

There are authoritative texts describing endoscopic and ultrasonographic techniques.[2-7] Briefly, with endoscopes that are 3 meters in length, the esophagus, stomach, and proximal duodenum of most adult horses can be examined. Restraint may be minimal (twitch or light sedation), depending on the horse. Fasting is not required for esophagoscopy if anesthesia is not used.

Esophagoscopy is commonly performed by nasopharyngeal placement. Advance the scope smoothly and observe the characteristic whitish esophageal mucosa of a collapsed esophagus. If esophageal placement is uncertain or tracheal rings observed, withdraw the scope and make another attempt. Never force the endoscope without knowing its course. Pharyngo-oral retroflexion is a serious risk to equipment, and esophageal perforation is a serious risk to the horse. Examine the stomach along with the esophagus because gastric lesions frequently accompany esophageal lesions. For adequate visualization of the stomach in the adult horse, withhold food for at least 12 hours and water for 6 hours if the horse can tolerate water deprivation.[6] To examine the duodenum, pass the endoscope along the greater curvature of the stomach and through the pylorus. This takes patience and experience. For colonic and rectal endoscopy, remove the feces either manually or, in small horses, using an enema. Pass a well-lubricated endoscope into the rectum. Air insufflation distends the esophagus or gastrointestinal tract for better mucosal visualization, especially for ulcers. Transrectal (5 MHz) and transabdominal (2.5 to 3.5 MHz) ultrasonography can be used to visualize and take a transcutaneous aspiration or punch biopsy of a mass.[8]

Once collected, biopsy specimens can be gently rolled on glass slides or imprinted for cytology before placing in 10% buffered formalin for histopathologic examination. Additionally, firm or particulate material can be scraped or squashed and aspirated material can be smeared like a blood smear. Suspected infectious lesions should be cultured and cytology can be valuable in selecting the appropriate culture media.

Collection of gastric fluid is relatively easily accomplished by passing the appropriate-sized polyethylene tubing through the biopsy channel of an endoscope and aspirating fluid from the area of the lesion or flushing the lesion with physiologic saline and then reaspirating the fluid. Direct, concentrated direct, and cytospin smears are recommended on all fluid specimens in addition to squash preparation of any particulate material. Rectal scraping is performed with a blunt instrument such as a chemical spatula after feces are removed from the rectum. Gentle but firm pressure is used to scrape the rectal mucosa deep enough to sample the lamina propria but not perforate the rectum.

Cytologic Features of Normal Tissues

Esophagus and Stomach

The esophagus and nonglandular anterior region of the stomach are lined by stratified squamous epithelium (Fig. 6-1). A keratinized thick outer stratum corneum overlies the deeper stratum granularis (flattened cells with shrunken nuclei and large basophilic staining cytoplasmic keratohyaline granules), stratum spinosum (flattened cuboid cells), and stratum basale (columnar cells).[1] Superficial epithelial cells are large cells with abundant pale blue homogeneous cytoplasm, angular cytoplasmic borders, and sometimes small, dense, round to oval nuclei. Bacteria can adhere to the surfaces of these epithelial cells, but inflammatory cells are lacking. Deeper samples may contain some basal epithelial cells, which are round with darker blue, slightly granular cytoplasm, larger ovoid, nuclei, and a higher nucleus to cytoplasm (N:C) ratio.

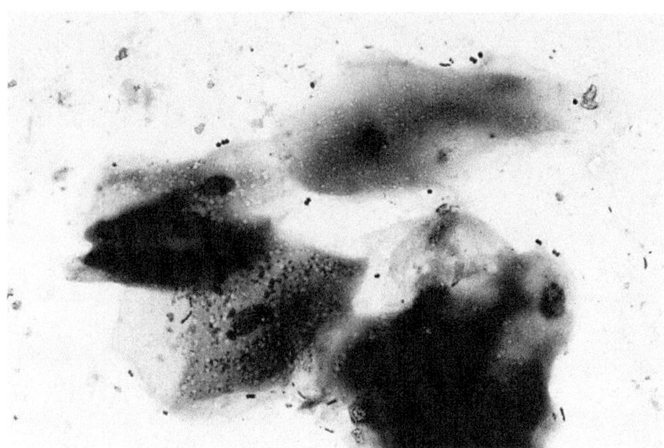

Fig. 6-1 Squamous epithelial cells scraped from stomach of horse.
Bacterial flora are seen on surfaces of some cells. (Wright-Giemsa stain)

Grossly, the margo plicatus forms a distinct boundary between the white-pink squamous region and the reddish glandular region of the equine stomach. The equine glandular stomach is lined by tall, periodic acid–Schiff–positive columnar epithelial cells that overlie deeper chief cells, parietal cells, mucous neck cells, and rare enteric endocrine cells.[1] Cytologic preparations from the glandular region of the stomach contain clusters and sheets of a uniform population of columnar epithelial cells. On low magnification the cells may have a honeycomb appearance (Fig. 6-2). Individualized cells exhibit a columnar shape with basal, round to oval nuclei, stippled chromatin pattern, and pale blue granular cytoplasm. Surface microvilli may give the apical margin a feathery appearance (Fig. 6-3).

Gastric fluid pH in the horse is variable. The horse appears to be a continuous, variable gastric hydrochloric acid secretor with intermittent periods of spontaneous alkalization.[9] Duodenogastric reflux, which is common in the horse, can contribute to this alkalization. Gastric fluid pH values are typically less than 2.0 during feed deprivation but can be greater than 6.0 after free access to timothy grass hay.[9] Cytologic examination

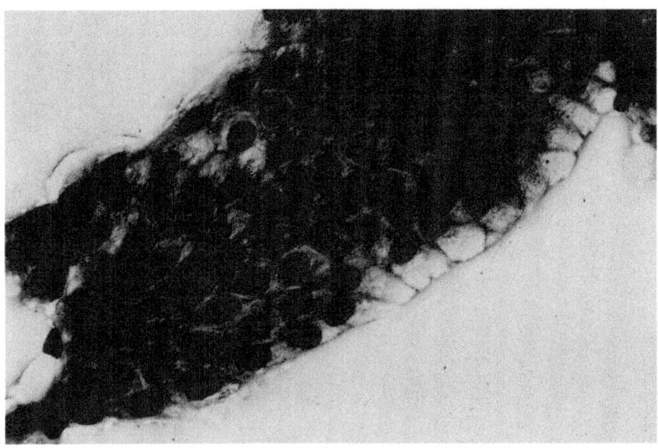

Fig. 6-2 Sheet of columnar epithelial cells from pyloric portion of stomach.
The uniform size and shape of the cells give this cluster a honeycomb appearance. (Wright's stain)

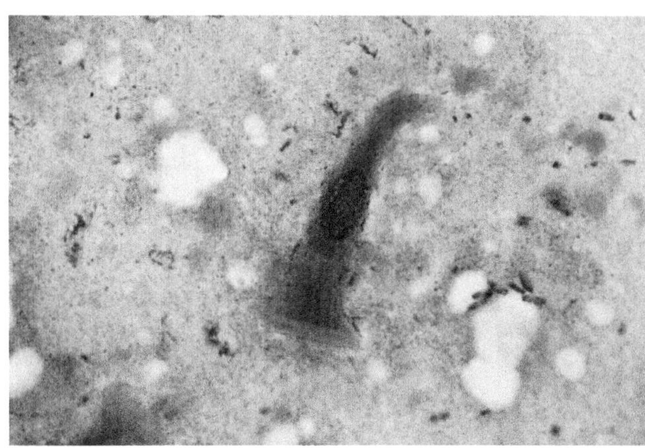

Fig. 6-3 Columnar epithelial cell imprinted from glandular region of stomach.
Cell has oval, basal nucleus and pale-staining microvillus apical border. (Wright-Giemsa stain)

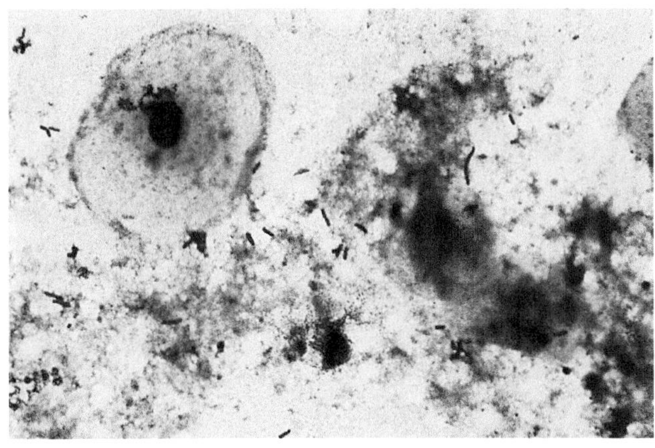

Fig. 6-4
Smear of gastric fluid from horse containing sloughed squamous epithelial cells, mixed population of bacteria, debris. (Wright-Giemsa stain)

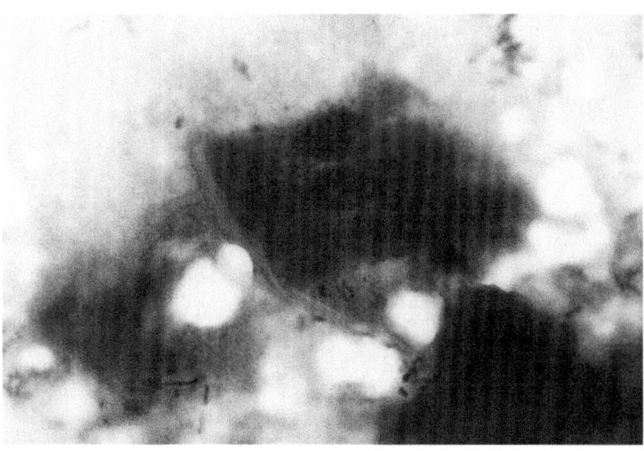

Fig. 6-5
Row of duodenal columnar epithelial cells with oval, basal nuclei and pale-staining microvillus apical "brush border" similar to gastric columnar epithelial cells. (Wright-Giemsa stain)

of gastric fluid contains exfoliated and degenerating squamous and columnar epithelial cells, mixed population of bacteria, and possibly plant material (Fig. 6-4).

Small and Large Intestine

Both small and large intestinal mucosal cells resemble stomach glandular epithelium (Fig. 6-5). Cells are columnar with pale blue, slightly granular cytoplasm, basal oval nuclei, and striated border composed of apical microvilli. Goblet cells, which have a vacuolated pale staining appearance and eosinophilic staining mucus, are more common in the colon and rectum (Fig. 6-6). Squamous epithelial cells are associated with the terminal rectum and anus. Endocrine cells, Paneth cells (pyramidal-shaped cells with prominent apical, spherical, acidophilic granules), and Brunner's gland cells (Alcian blue–positive submucosal serous-type intestinal glands) are present in the small intestine and granular cells are present in the colon, but these cells are infrequent and have not been cytologically described (Figs. 6-7 and 6-8).[1] A few lymphocytes are often seen in intestinal specimens from horses because of Peyer's patches and submucosal lymphoid tissue. Hemosiderin-laden macrophages have also been reported in the lamina propria of clinically normal horses.[10] Although neutrophils were not present in the

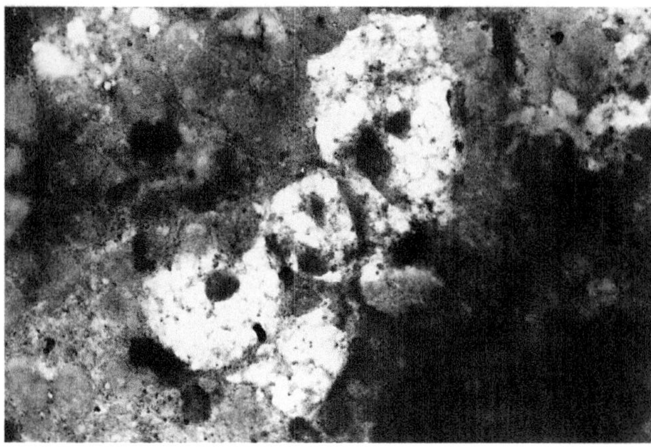

Fig. 6-6 Cluster of pale-staining goblet cells from colon of horse.
Note small central to eccentric nuclei and abundant clear to vacuolated cytoplasm. These cells are most prominent in the large intestine. (Wright-Giemsa stain)

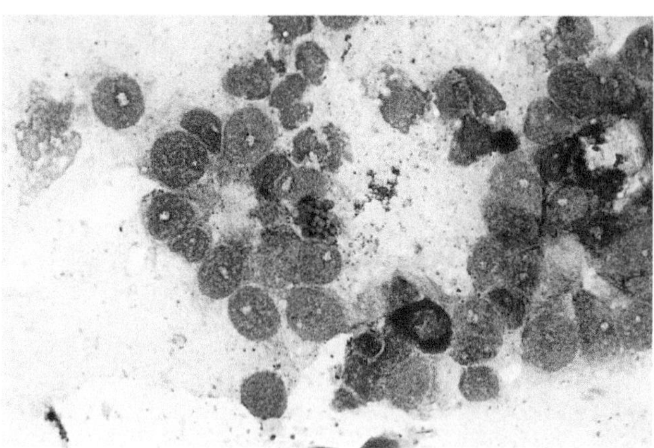

Fig. 6-7
Colonic scraping from healthy horse containing numerous clusters of epithelial cells in sheets or forming acinar-like structures. Mast cells are occasionally observed. (Wright-Giemsa stain)

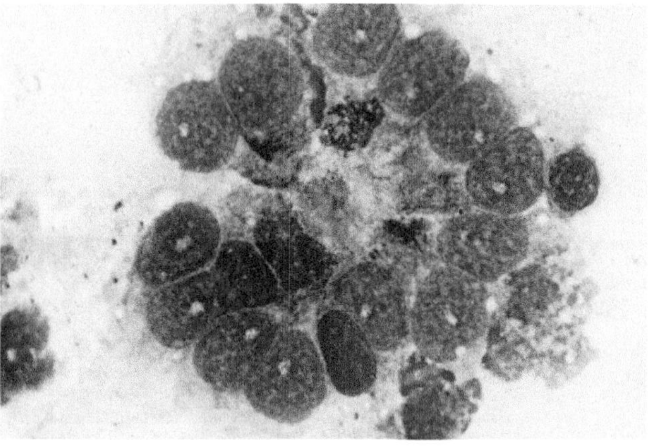

Fig. 6-8 Higher magnification of colonic epithelium.
A small granular cell with fine azurophilic granules is seen toward center of cell cluster. (Wright-Giemsa stain)

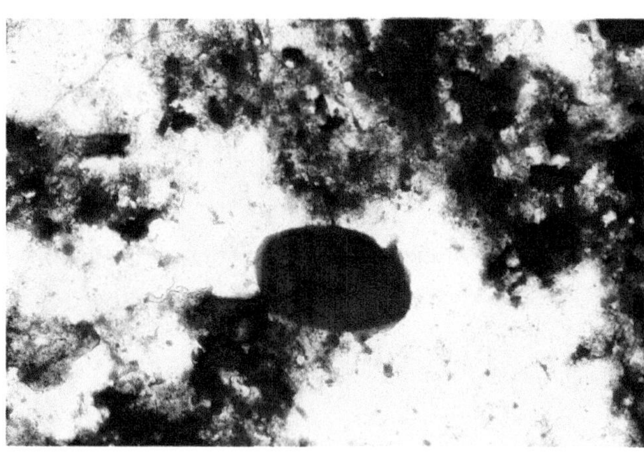

Fig. 6-9
Fluid from large intestine containing a large, dark-staining protozoa in center of field surrounded by plant material, a mixed population of bacteria, and cellular debris. (Wright-Giemsa stain)

surface epithelium of the equine rectum, scattered neutrophils and eosinophils have been reported in the rectal lamina propria of healthy horses.[11]

Intestinal fluid contains low numbers of squamous epithelial cells from the esophagus and stomach, a few columnar epithelial cells from the intestinal mucosa, a mixed population of bacteria, protozoa, fungal elements, food material, and rare to no inflammatory cells (Figs. 6-9 to 6-11). Minimal information is available on the microbial population inhabiting the gastrointestinal tract of the healthy horse. Proteolytic bacteria comprise a high proportion of culturable bacteria in the equine gastrointestinal tract.[12] Mean pH values reported for the equine duodenum, jejunum, ileum, and hindgut are 6.32, 7.10, 7.47, and 6.7, respectively.[12]

Cytologic Features of Abnormal Tissues

Neoplasia

Neoplasia of the gastrointestinal tract of horses is uncommon and usually occurs in older horses, except for lymphoma, which often occurs in younger horses (Table 6-1). General clinical signs associated with equine gastrointestinal neoplasia include weight loss, anorexia,

TABLE 6-1

Tumors of the Equine Gastrointestinal Tract

Esophagus Squamous cell carcinoma	**Cecum** Adenocarcinoma with/without osseous metaplasia Myxosarcoma
Stomach Squamous cell carcinoma Adenocarcinoma Leiomyosarcoma Leiomyoma Gastric polyp	**Colon** Adenocarcinoma with/without osseous metaplasia Lymphoma Lipoma Lipomatosis
Small intestine Lymphoma Adenocarcinoma Leiomyoma Leiomyosarcoma Adenomatous polyposis Lipoma Carcinoid	**Rectum** Lymphoma Lipoma Leiomyosarcoma Polyps

Data from Barker et al: in Jubb et al: *Pathology of Domestic Animals,* ed 4, Vol 2. San Diego, 1993, Academic Press, pp 33-317; East and Savage: Abdominal neoplasia (excluding urogenital tract). *Vet Clin North Am (Equine Pract)* 14:475-493, 1998; Orsini et al: Intestinal carcinoid in a mare: an etiologic consideration for chronic colic in horses. *JAVMA* 193:87-88, 1988; Patterson-Kane et al: Small intestinal adenomatous polyposis resulting in protein-losing enteropathy in a horse. *Vet Pathol* 37:82-85, 2000.

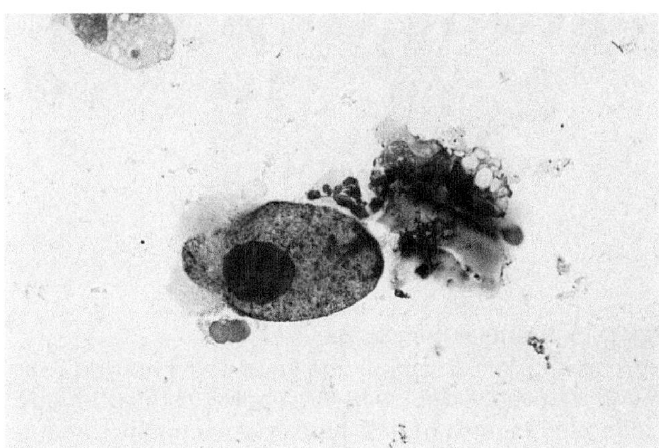

Fig. 6-10 Normal equine protozoa.
Large intestinal fluid illustrating the pleomorphic appearance of normal equine protozoa. Note large size of protozoa compared to red cells. Some plant material and cellular debris are adjacent to protozoa. (Wright-Giemsa stain)

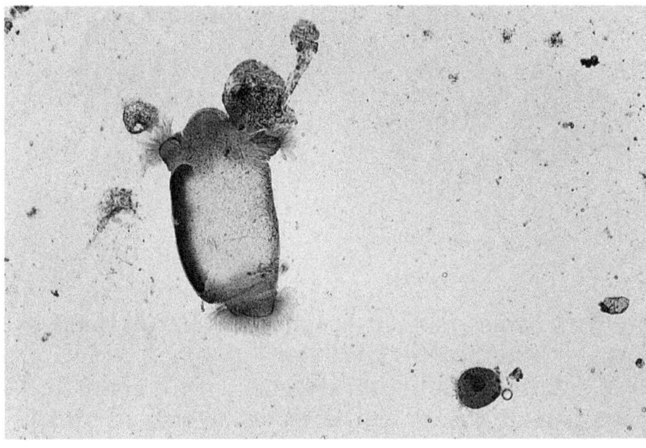

Fig. 6-11 Abdominal fluid from horse with chronic cecal impaction.
Two ciliated protozoa have marked difference in size. No evidence of intestinal rupture was found. (Wright-Giemsa stain)

lethargy, intermittent colic, intermittent fever, and variable fecal consistency. Clinical laboratory findings can include malabsorption (decreased glucose and d-xylose absorption), hypoalbuminemia, hypergammaglobulinemia, anemia (hemorrhage and chronic disease), and hypercalcemia (lymphoma and squamous-cell carcinoma). Peritoneal fluid frequently has an increased nucleated cell count (neutrophilic inflammation), increased protein, and, sometimes, exfoliated neoplastic cells. Microorganisms from the gut lumen may invade gastrointestinal neoplasms, resulting in abscessation and secondary septic peritonitis.

Lymphoma is the most common malignant neoplasm of the equine gastrointestinal tract.[8,13] It occurs most frequently in the small intestines and may be a primary alimentary lymphoma or a multicentric lymphoma that involves the intestines in addition to peripheral lymph

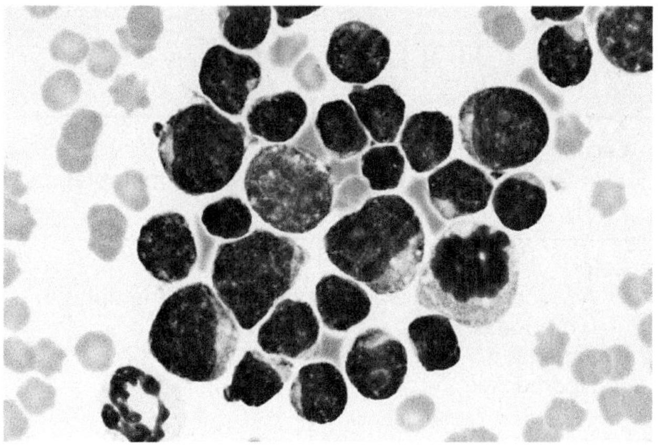

Fig. 6-12 Equine intestinal lymphoma.
Note mixed population of large, intermediate, and small lymphocytes with coarse chromatin pattern, indistinct nucleoli, and scant cytoplasm. (Wright-Giemsa stain)

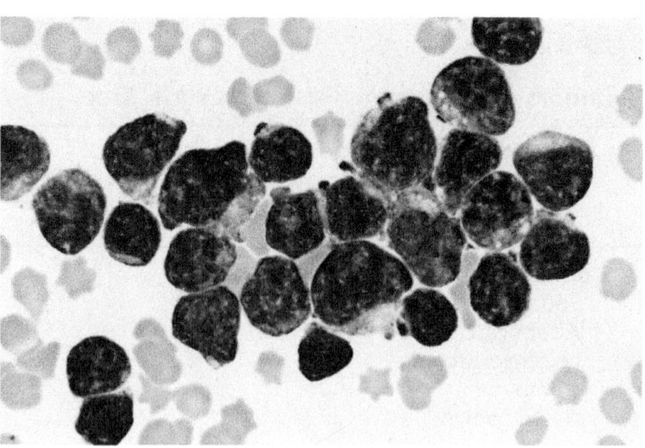

Fig. 6-13 Equine intestinal lymphoma.
Note pleomorphic population of large, immature lymphocytes with round to irregularly shaped nuclei, clumped chromatin pattern, one to four small nucleoli, and a scant to narrow rim of moderately basophilic, sometimes vacuolated cytoplasm. (Wright-Giemsa stain)

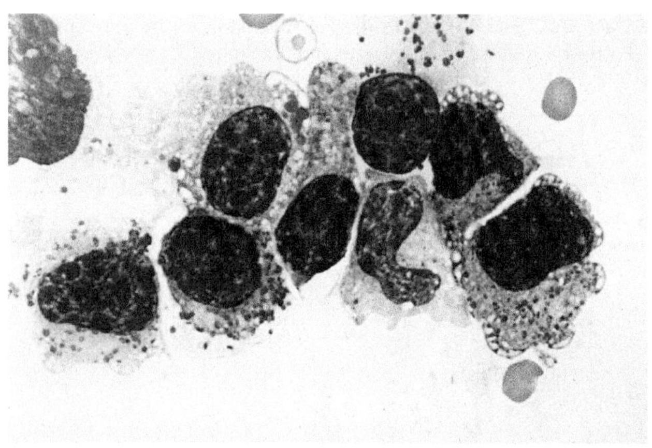

Fig. 6-14 Large granular lymphoma from intestine of horse with multicentric lymphoma.
Neoplastic cells are large cells with oval nuclei, clumped chromatin pattern, chromocenters, moderate amount of pale blue cytoplasm that contains cytoplasmic vacuoles, and numerous small to moderately large azurophilic granules. (Wright-Giemsa stain)

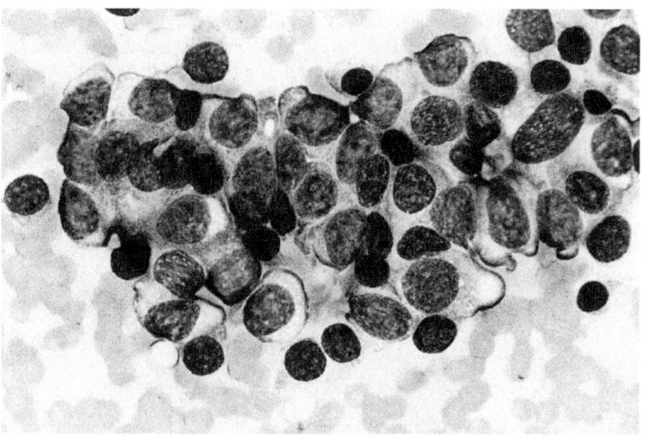

Fig. 6-15 Granular lymphoma.
Horse with granular lymphoma having lymphocytes with round to oval nuclei, coarsely stippled chromatin, and moderate amounts of pale blue cytoplasm that contains very small, eosinophilic cytoplasmic granules. Cytoplasmic granules were not obvious on histologic specimens. Small lymphocytes are interspersed among the granular lymphocytes. (Wright-Giemsa stain)

nodes and/or the thoracic cavity. Alimentary lymphoma is associated with local to diffuse thickening of the gut wall and marked enlargement of the mesenteric lymph nodes.[14] Neoplastic infiltrates can extend from the lamina propria and submucosa to the serosal surface. The lymphocyte population can vary from sheets of lymphoblasts or granular lymphocytes to a mixed population of large and small lymphocytes (Figs. 6-12 to 6-15).[14-18] Cytoplasmic granules in granular lymphoma cells are readily seen on cytology but may be poorly visible on histopathology.[15] Plasmacytoid cells and plasma cells can be abundant, and giant cells can occasionally be seen in the gut wall and lymph node of horses with lymphoma.[13,14]

A recent study of equine malignant lymphomas found that 77% (24/31) were high-grade tumors composed of large, atypical cells of B-cell origin.[16] The only intestinal lymphoma in this study was classified as a multicentric T-cell lymphoma, and all lymphomas with thymic masses were of T-cell origin. Forty-six percent (11/24) of the B-cell lymphomas were T-cell–rich,

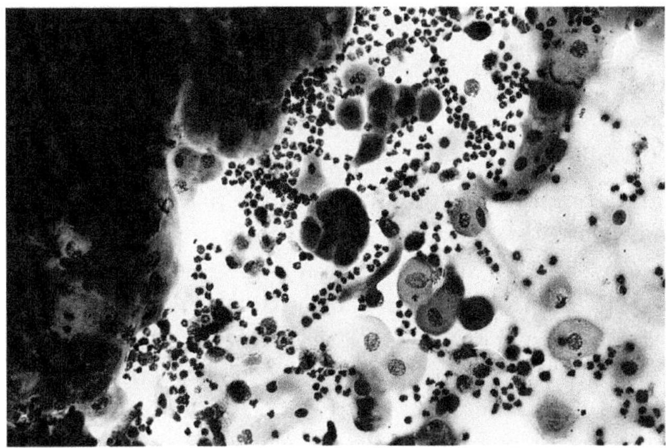

Fig. 6-16 Gastric squamous-cell carcinoma. Fine-needle aspiration biopsy from gastric squamous-cell carcinoma from horse. Cells exfoliating in large sheets tend to be more uniform than the cells that are in small clusters or individualized. Cells vary from round to spindloid with very basophilic to pale basophilic cytoplasm. Neutrophils are numerous. (Wright-Giemsa stain)

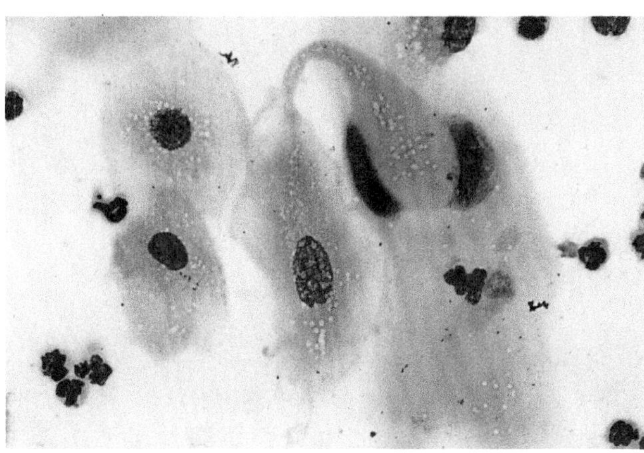

Fig. 6-17 Gastric squamous-cell carcinoma. Higher magnification of cells from an equine gastric squamous-cell carcinoma illustrates two cells with cytoplasmic tails. (Wright-Giemsa stain)

large B-cell lymphomas that contained a mixed lymphoid infiltrate of nonneoplastic, normal-appearing T-cells and large atypical B-cells with large, irregularly shaped nuclei, coarse chromatin, and atypical mitotic figures. Lymphocyte markers are necessary to differentiate mixed small- and large-cell lymphoma from T-cell–rich, large B-cell lymphoma. A mixed lymphoma composed of both small and large neoplastic B-cells has occurred in the stomach of a horse.[17] Additionally, a B-cell lymphoma was diagnosed in a horse with Sezary-like cells in the peripheral blood, cutaneous nodules, heart, abdominal cavity, and ventral colon.[18] Paraneoplastic hypereosinophilia, although uncommon, has been reported in a horse with intestinal lymphoma.[19]

Squamous-cell carcinoma, which is the second most common malignant neoplasm of horses, is the most common tumor of the equine esophagus and stomach.[13,20,21] Cytologically, squamous-cell carcinoma has been classified into three groups[20]:

1. Well-differentiated (>50% well-differentiated squamous cells called flakes and up to 30% round or oval squamous cells)
2. Moderately differentiated (>50% round or oval squamous cells and lesser numbers of flakes)
3. Poorly differentiated (round or oval pleomorphic cells with rare flakes)

Neoplastic cells frequently occur in thick cell clusters or sheets (Fig. 6-16). Thinner areas or individualized cells must be scrutinized to evaluate cellular details (Figs. 6-17 to 6-19). Marked variation in cell size, nuclear size, nucleolar size and shape, and number of perinuclear or large cytoplasmic vacuoles may be present. Cells from well-differentiated squamous-cell carcinoma are large polyhedral to spindle-shaped squamous cells with low nuclear to cytoplasmic ratios and abundant pale blue cytoplasm that forms angular borders. Cells may also appear dendritic, round, elongated, or caudate and have several colorless, refractile, or minute deep pink to purple cytoplasmic granules or a diffuse pink- to reddish-tinged cytoplasm. The nucleus is small, oval to round to irregular, with coarse chromatin. Irregularly shaped chromocenters and nucleoli, presence of cytoplasmic rings (dyskeratosis),

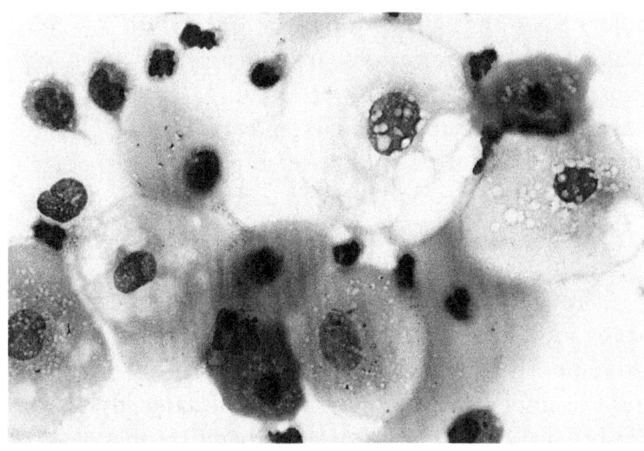

Fig. 6-18 Gastric squamous-cell carcinoma. Higher magnification of cells from an equine gastric squamous-cell carcinoma illustrating anisocytosis, anisokaryosis, and variability in cytoplasmic vacuolization and keratinization. (Wright-Giemsa stain)

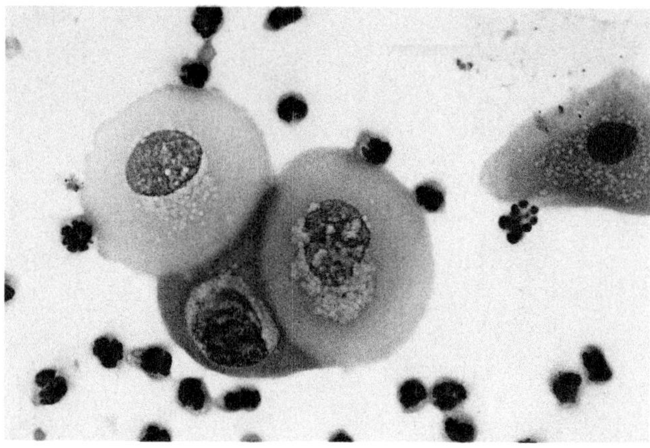

Fig. 6-19 Gastric squamous-cell carcinoma. Note cluster of three large immature squamous cells with oval nuclei, coarsely stippled chromatin, indistinct nucleoli, and fine perinuclear cytoplasmic vacuolization that is a dyskeratotic feature of squamous neoplasia. (Wright-Giemsa stain)

hyperchromasia, anisokaryosis, anisocytosis, caudate cells with extremely long cytoplasmic processes (tadpole cells), and intracytoplasmic migration of cells (emperipolesis) are features of dysplasia and neoplasia. Papanicolaou's stain is the best stain to evaluate keratinization, dyskeratotic changes, and cytologic features of thick cellular clusters. Cytoplasmic orangeophilia correlates to cellular keratinization. An extensive inflammatory reaction is frequently associated with squamous-cell carcinomas, especially with superficial ulceration.

Cells from well-differentiated squamous-cell carcinoma look like normal squamous epithelium, and cells from poorly differentiated squamous-cell carcinomas may be difficult to distinguish from reactive/dysplastic mesothelial cells or cells from poorly differentiated adenocarcinomas. Therefore, for the best cytologic interpretation, other causes for the presence of squamous cells in the sample must be ruled out. Two conditions that might be associated with squamous cells are ruptured gastric ulcers (possible dysplasia and neutrophilic inflammation) and inadvertent aspiration of amniotic fluid from a pregnant mare. Esophageal-gastric ulcers usually occur in foals or young horses whereas squamous-cell carcinomas usually occur in older horses (6 to 18 years of age).[21] Endoscopy and ultrasonography are helpful in confirming a cytologic opinion. Squamous-cell carcinomas have a propensity to seed organ surfaces and metastasize extensively throughout the pleural and peritoneal cavities, similar to mesothelioma, resulting in pleural and peritoneal fluids containing carcinoma cells. Most horses with gastric squamous-cell carcinoma have abundant peritoneal fluid that is characterized by a neutrophilic inflammation, hemosiderophages, and erythrophagia.[21] Sediment concentration and cytospin preparations increase the probability of finding squamous epithelium and evidence of neoplastic cytologic features in these samples.

Adenocarcinomas of the equine intestinal tract are rare.[13,22,23] Most frequently they are reported in the large intestine as solitary, nodular masses with low metastatic potential but a high tendency to undergo osseous metaplasia.[23] Tumor cells are round to columnar, with moderate to abundant amphophilic to basophilic cytoplasm and large nuclei with prominent nucleoli. Occasional signet ring cells, extracellular eosinophilic mucin, and rare acinar formation may be observed.[22] Histologically, these tumor cells vary from well-differentiated columnar cells forming glandular structures that contain goblet cells to anaplastic cells forming clusters or irregular glandular structures.[22,23]

Adenomatous polyposis was reported in a young, adult quarter horse gelding that presented with protein-losing enteropathy, extensive subcutaneous ventral edema, and severe hypoproteinemia.[24] Numerous polypoid, papillary, and glandular masses comprised of pseudostratified tall columnar cells with interspersed goblet cells were found in the small intestines.

Carcinoid tumors arising from the endocrine or paracrine cells in the mucosal lining of the stomach and intestine are rare in horses.[25] These endocrine cells are uniform, round to oval cells with oval, vesicular nuclei that lack prominent nucleoli but have abundant finely granular eosinophilic cytoplasm that is often stripped from the cell, leaving a pale eosinophilic background and naked nuclei. Special stains for argentaffin and argyrophilic properties or electron microscopy to identify secretory cytoplasmic granules are necessary to confirm the diagnosis.

Leiomyomas and *leiomyosarcomas* are smooth muscle tumors of the intestine in old horses. These tumors may occur in the small intestine, form encapsulated masses on the serosal surface, or cause pedunculated tumors protruding into the lumen of the rectum.[13] The cytologic appearance is similar to that of smooth muscle tumors in other sites. Cells are individualizing spindle-shaped cells with oval to elongated, cigar-shaped nuclei, lacy chromatin pattern, one or two indistinct nucleoli, and moderate amounts of pale blue cytoplasm. Cells become more pleomorphic and less spindle-shaped with malignant transformation. Cytologic differentials for well-differentiated mesenchymal cells from the gastrointestinal tract of horses include intestinal fibrosis, disseminated peritoneal leiomyomatosis, omental fibrosarcoma, and fibroplasia secondary to inflammation.[26,27] Intestinal fibrosis is characterized by diffuse thickening of the small intestine, arteriole sclerosis, capillary endothelial-cell hypertrophy, and hypertrophy and degeneration of smooth muscle nuclei. Disseminated peritoneal leiomyomatosis is a rare nonmalignant, multicentric proliferation of smooth muscle tissue that develops in the abdomen of females.[26,27]

Pedunculated lipomas associated with the intestinal mesenteric adipose tissue are well documented but infrequent causes of intestinal obstruction in aged horses.[28] Neither these tumors nor lipomatosis (uncommon benign infiltrative form of lipoma) can be definitively diagnosed by cytology.[8]

Inflammatory Lesions

Equine inflammatory gastrointestinal disorders are common.[13] Results of rectal biopsies in 105 horses revealed pathologic changes in 60 (57%).[11] Proctitis was the most frequent diagnosis and was classified as simple (neutrophilic inflammation), chronic (lymphocytes and plasma cells), or chronic suppurative (neutrophils, lymphocytes, and plasma cells). Proctitis in this study was often nonspecific and best reflected disease in the proximal gut rather than a morphologic entity.[11] However, even with their limitations, rectal biopsies and histopathology (and likely cytologic biopsies) are a useful adjunct for evaluating intestinal diseases in the horse. Neutrophilic inflammation and neutrophils on fecal smears have been observed with bacterial diseases such as salmonellosis.

Bacterial Enterocolitis: Bacterial gastrointestinal infections can be deadly, especially in the foal or the immunocompromised horse. Culture and sensitivity are always recommended to make a specific diagnosis and choose the best therapeutic approach. However, cytology can be helpful in quickly confirming a change in gastrointestinal flora and tentatively identifying the type of bacteria or the etiologic agent so that the appropriate therapy and diagnostics can be undertaken. Romanowsky stain is preferred over Gram's stain for the initial screening of fecal cytologic smears. With Romanowsky stains, bacteria (except negatively staining *Mycobacterium* spp.) appear dark blue, and morphologic differences such as rod or coccoid shape are readily distinguishable. Also, and very importantly, cellular morphology of inflammatory cells and epithelial cells is superior with Romanowsky stains.

The inflammatory reaction of bacterial infections not only varies with the specific bacterial agent but also with the duration of the bacterial infection. For example, *Rhodococcus (Corynebacterium) equi*, a gram-positive coccobacillus that causes enterocolitis in foals, initially causes a neutrophilic inflammation that progresses to a chronic inflammatory process with macrophages containing intracellular coccoid organisms and multinucleated giant cells infiltrating into the lamina propria. Equine salmonellosis can clinically manifest itself as a septicemic, acute, chronic, or asymptomatic carrier stage with differing cellular changes that may reflect the stage of the disease. *Clostridium* spp. are potential causes of diarrhea, especially in the foal. Although *Campylobacter jejuni* and enterotoxigenic *E. coli* have been isolated from foals with diarrhea, their significance is unclear.[13]

Equine monocytic ehrlichiosis *(E. risticii)* causes Potomac horse fever, a condition characterized by diarrhea, leukopenia, fever, and depression. Lesions in the intestines include hyperemia, congestion, hemorrhage, ulcers, and superficial necrosis. *Ehrlichia* spp. are obligate intracellular bacterial pathogens that replicate within the phagosomes of host cells. *E. risticii*, unlike *E. equi*, has not been identified on peripheral blood smears. The organisms are also not evident in hematoxylin and eosin–stained tissue but appear as small clusters of 10 to 15 fine brown dots (less than 1 μ in diameter) in epithelial cells and macrophages with modified Steiner silver stain.[13]

Proliferative enteritis characterized by small intestinal thickening, crypt epithelial-cell hyperplasia, curved intracellular bacteria, and severe enteritis has been described in several foals. *Lawsonia intracellularis* was identified as the etiologic agent.[29]

Chronic Inflammatory Bowel Disease: Chronic inflammatory bowel disease is characterized by focal or diffuse infiltration of leukocytes into the intestinal wall. Several equine diseases are in this group and include equine granulomatous gastroenteritis, eosinophilic gastroenteritis, intestinal tuberculosis, histoplasmosis, and lymphoproliferative disorders.[30-34] Cytologic features of granulomatous inflammation include macrophages, epithelioid cells, multinucleated giant cells, lymphocytes, and plasma cells. Specimens having granulomatous inflammatory cells should be scrutinized for fungal hyphae (Plates 5B and 5C), *Histoplasma* organisms (Plate 4C), *Mycobacterium* (Plates 4A and 4B), and parasitic larva.

Granulomatous gastroenteritis: Although granulomatous gastroenteritis and eosinophilic gastroenteritis are considered to be two distinct syndromes, there are some similarities, such as enteric as well as nonenteric granuloma formation.[32] Equine granulomatous enteritis is a focal to multisystemic granulomatous disease primarily affecting the small intestine.[35] Granulomas are composed of macrophages, lymphocytes, epithelioid cells and giant cells. Young horses appear to be at higher risk. Although the etiology of equine granulomatous gastroenteritis is unknown, an immunologic mechanism and an association with aluminum have been postulated.[31,35,36]

Eosinophilic gastroenteritis: Equine chronic eosinophilic gastroenteritis has been described as part of a distinct multisystemic epitheliotropic syndrome associated with eosinophilic dermatitis and eosinophilic granulomatous pancreatitis.[13,33,35] Diffuse or focal inflammatory infiltrates occur in the esophagus, stomach, small and large intestine, and mesenteric lymph nodes. The gut wall is infiltrated by eosinophils, mast cells, macrophages,

TABLE 6-2

Inflammatory Disorders of the Equine Gastrointestinal Tract

Infectious disorders

Parasites

Stomach *Gasterophilus* spp., *Habronema* spp., *Draschia megastoma, Trichostrongylus axei*

Small intestine *Strongyloides westeri, Parascaris equorum, Anoplocephala magna, Eimeria leuckarti, Cryptosporidia*

Large intestine larval Cyanthostomiasis (encysted small strongyle larvae), small strongyles (*Strongylus vulgaris, Strongylus edentatus, Strongylus equinus*), *Triodontophorus* spp., *Anoplocephala perfoliata, Oxyuris equi, Probstymayria vivipara, Tritrichomonas equi, Giardia, Cryptosporidia*

Bacteria (nongranulomatous)

Small intestine *Clostridium perfringens, Clostridium welchii, Lawsonia intracellularis*

Large intestine *Salmonella* spp., *Clostridium perfringens, Clostridium welchii, Ehrlichia risticii*

Bacteria (granulomatous)

Small intestine *Mycobacterium avium, Mycobacterium paratuberculosis, Rhodococcus equi*

Fungus/yeast

Candida, Histoplasma, Pythium, Aspergillus

Viruses

Small intestine rotavirus, coronavirus, adenovirus, equine herpesvirus-1 (adult horses)

Noninfectious disorders

Equine granulomatous enteritis
Equine eosinophilic gastroenteritis
Equine basophilic gastroenteritis
Lymphocytic/plasmacytic gastroenteritis
Chemical gastroenteritis blister beetle poisoning
Uremic gastritis
Amyloid

lymphocytes, and plasma cells. Peripheral eosinophilia is not observed, but diarrhea and hypoalbuminemia occur. The cause is unknown but immune-mediated etiology is likely.[13] Marked eosinophilic infiltration of the rectum may be of low diagnostic significance unless accompanied by pathologic lesions of equine eosinophilic gastroenteritis. Eosinophils were common finding in rectal biopsies from healthy horses.[11]

Basophilic enterocolitis: Basophilic enterocolitis, which may be a variant of eosinophilic gastroenteritis, has been described in a horse. Basophils were prominent in the inflammatory infiltrate of the ileum, cecum, and colon along with lymphocytes, plasma cells, macrophages, and eosinophils.[13,37]

Lymphocytic-plasmacytic enteritis: The etiopathogenesis of lymphocytic-plasmacytic enteritis is unknown, but it causes a protein-losing enteropathy and hypoalbuminemia.[13,33,34] Normal fecal consistency indicates that the protein-losing enteropathy primarily involves the small intestine and that the major portion of the large intestine is still functional. Therefore, small intestinal biopsies are more likely to be diagnostic than more readily obtainable rectal biopsies. Increased numbers of well-differentiated lymphocytes and plasma cells infiltrate the lamina propria. In the horse and dog, submucosal or transmural lymphocytic-plasmacytic infiltrates may signal a precursor to lymphoma.[13] Also, a differential for lymphocytic and eosinophilic infiltrates must include parasitic invasion.[13]

Viral Enteritis: Adenovirus, coronavirus, and rotavirus cause diarrhea in foals, and equine herpesvirus-1 can cause a necrotizing enterocolitis in the adult horse.[13] Unfortunately, cytology is not very helpful for diagnosing equine viral gastrointestinal diseases. Serology, molecular testing, viral cultures, and/or electron microscopy are necessary to document a viral etiology.

Fungus/Yeast: See granulomatous inflammation. Fungi and *Histoplasma* can cause gastroenteritis/enteritis in horses. *Candida* spp., budding yeast that are normal mucosal flora of the alimentary tract, can become opportunistic invaders with changes in the microenvironment. Branching, filamentous pseudohyphae and hyphae can replace the yeast forms. Gastroesophageal candidiasis occurs most frequently in foals and is associated with ulceration of the squamous epithelium.[13]

Parasitic Agents: Equine gastrointestinal parasites are listed in Table 6-2.[13,38] Encysted small *Strongylus* larvae (cyanthostomes) have become the principal parasitic pathogen of horses.[39,40] These encysted larvae, unlike small and large strongyles, are resistant to most modern anthelmintics. These small *Strongylus* larvae enter the large intestinal mucosa where they may arrest for years and accumulate to massive numbers. Clinical disease is associated with the simultaneous emergence of these encysted larvae. Risk factors for cyathostomosis are young horses, early spring, and recent anthelmintic treatment.[39] Acute-onset diarrhea and acute weight loss are the most common signs of this syndrome. Diagnosis is facilitated by finding excysted larvae on a rectal sleeve following rectal examination. Other laboratory findings may include peripheral neutrophilia and hypoalbuminemia.[39,40]

Equine cestodiasis (*Anoplocephala perfoliata* infections) also appear to be increasing.[39,41] Infections have been associated with colic, intestinal perforations, and intussusceptions at the ileocecocolic junction. Development of a serologic assay for *A. perfoliata* has enhanced diagnosis. Difficulties with fecal flotation relate to resistance of cestode eggs to float and passage of intact tapeworm segments without the release of eggs.[39]

Ciliated protozoa are abundant in the large intestine of the horse. Little is know about their function but many are bizarre nonpathogenic organisms (see Figs. 6-9 to 6-11). Chronic diarrhea has been associated with the presence of many fecal flagellates, especially *Tritrichomonas*; however, the pathogenicity is uncertain.[38]

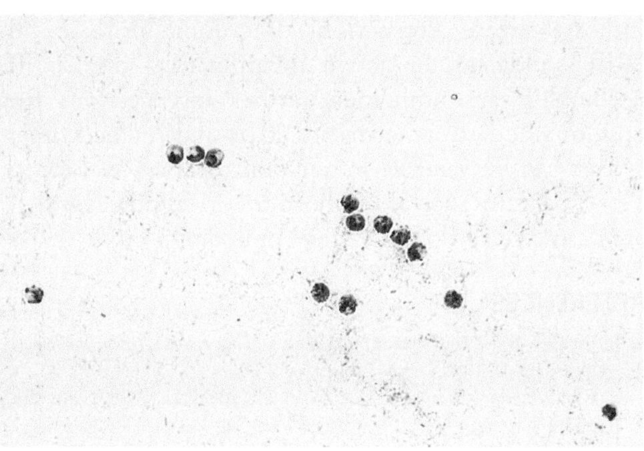

Fig. 6-20 Fecal smear with numerous small red staining *Cryptosporidia*.
Oocysts are slightly smaller than erythrocytes. (Acid-fast type stain)

Ciliated protozoa can invade the intestinal tract, but they can be postmortem invaders of colonic mucosa in enteric and nonenteric disorders.[13,42] Another protozoan, *Eimeria leuckarti*, may be frequently found in foal feces, but its pathogenicity is also questionable.[13,38]

The interpretation of infections with *Giardia* and *Cryptosporidia* are not straightforward, but newer more sensitive and specific tests such as immunofluorescent tests and fecal enzyme-linked immunosorbent assays are available to diagnose *Cryptosporidium* and *Giardia*.[43] In foals, infection rates with either *Cryptosporidium* or *Giardia* can be high (about 15% to 35%), even in foals without clinical signs (Fig. 6-20).[43]

Other Causes: Amyloid-associated gastroenteropathy is rare but when present is associated with malabsorption and enteric protein loss.[44] On cytologic preparations, amyloid appears as a homogenous pink extracellular staining matrix. Cytology is of limited help in diagnosing blister beetle poisoning or uremic gastritis/gastroenteritis, which are associated with nonspecific hemorrhagic lesions.[45]

Cytologic Features of Fecal Smears

Direct fecal smears can be valuable in horses with enteric disease. Normally, fecal smears contain large numbers of a mixed bacterial population, mucus, plant material, a few epithelial cells, and a lack of inflammatory cells. Feces in sick horses should be examined for occult blood, sand, clostridial organisms, *Salmonella* organisms, giardial cysts, cryptosporidial oocysts, ciliated protozoa, parasitic ova, parasitic larva, and WBCs. Ciliated protozoa should be present in normal fresh feces. Absence or massive numbers of ciliate protozoa indicate severe alternations of colonic flora. Fecal WBCs indicate an active inflammatory disease. If eosinophils are numerous, further investigations for eosinophilic gastroenteritis should be undertaken. Direct smears can be valuable in addition to flotation tests to detect parasites such as trophozoites or cestode eggs that are destroyed or do not levitate in flotation fluids.

REFERENCES

1. Pfeiffer and MacPherson: in White: *The Equine Acute Abdomen.* Philadelphia, 1990, Lea & Febiger, pp 2-24.
2. Reef: *Equine Diagnostic Ultrasound.* Philadelphia, 1998, Saunders, pp 321-346.
3. Byars and Bain: in Rantanen and McKinnon: *Equine Diagnostic Ultrasonography.* Baltimore, 1998, Williams & Wilkins, pp 595-602.
4. Tucker: in Rantanen and McKinnon: *Equine Diagnostic Ultrasonography.* Baltimore, 1998, Williams & Wilkins, pp 649-653.
5. Klohnen et al: Use of diagnostic ultrasonography in horses with signs of acute abdominal pain. *JAVMA* 209:1597-1601, 1996.
6. Traub-Dargatz and Brown: *Equine Endoscopy,* ed 2. St Louis, 1997, Mosby.
7. Pearson et al: in Cowell and Tyler: *Cytology and Hematology of the Horse.* Goleta, CA, 1992, American Veterinary Publications, pp 89-95.
8. East and Savage: Abdominal neoplasia (excluding urogenital tract). *Vet Clin North Am (Equine Pract)* 14:475-493, 1998.
9. Murray: Pathophysiology of peptic disorders in foals and horses: a review. *Equine Vet J Suppl* 29:14-18, 1999.
10. Ochoa et al: Hemosiderin deposits in the equine small intestine. *Vet Pathol* 20:641-643, 1983.
11. Lindberg et al: Rectal biopsy diagnosis in horses with clinical signs of intestinal disorders: a retrospective study of 116 cases. *Equine Vet J* 28:275-284, 1996.
12. Mackie and Wilkins: Enumeration of anaerobic bacterial microflora of the equine gastrointestinal tract. *Appl Environ Microbiol* 54:2155-2160, 1988.
13. Barker et al: in Jubb et al: *Pathology of Domestic Animals,* ed 4, Vol 2. San Diego, 1993, Academic Press, pp 33-317.
14. Platt: Alimentary lymphomas in the horse. *J Comp Pathol* 97:1-10, 1987.
15. Grindem et al: Large granular lymphocyte tumor in a horse. *Vet Pathol* 26:86-88, 1989.
16. Kelley and Mahaffey: Equine malignant lymphomas: morphologic and immunohistochemical classification. *Vet Pathol* 38:241-252, 1998.
17. Asahina et al: An immunohistochemical study of an equine B-cell lymphoma. *J Comp Pathol* 11:445-451, 1994.
18. Polkes: B-cell lymphoma in a horse with associated Sezary-like cells in the peripheral blood. *J Vet Intern Med* 13:620-624, 1999.
19. Duckett and Matthews: Hypereosinophilia in a horse with intestinal lymphosarcoma. *Can Vet J* 38:719-720, 1997.
20. Garma-Avina: The cytology of squamous cell carcinomas in domestic animals. *J Vet Diagn Invest* 6:238-246, 1994.
21. McKenzie: Gastric squamous cell carcinoma in three horses. *Aust Vet J* 75:480-483, 1997.
22. Fulton et al: Adenocarcinoma of intestinal origin in a horse: diagnosis by abdominocentesis and laparoscopy. *Equine Vet J* 22:447-448, 1990.
23. Kirchhof et al: Equine adenocarcinomas of the large intestine with osseous metaplasia. *J Comp Pathol* 114:451-456, 1996.
24. Patterson-Kane et al: Small intestinal adenomatous polyposis resulting in protein-losing enteropathy in a horse. *Vet Pathol* 37:82-85, 2000.
25. Orsini et al: Intestinal carcinoid in a mare: an etiologic consideration for chronic colic in horses. *JAVMA* 193:87-88, 1988.
26. Traub-Dargatz et al: Intestinal fibrosis with partial obstruction in five horses and two ponies. *JAVMA* 201:603-607, 1992.
27. Johnson et al: Disseminated peritoneal leiomyomatosis in a horse. *JAVMA* 205:725-728, 1994.
28. Blikslager et al: Pedunculated lipomas as a cause of intestinal obstruction in horses: 17 cases (1983-1990). *JAVMA* 201:1249-1252, 1992.
29. Smith: Identification of equine proliferative enteropathy. *Equine Vet J* 30:452-453, 1998.
30. Schumacher et al: Effects of intestinal resection on two juvenile horses with granulomatous enteritis. *J Vet Intern Med* 4:153-156, 1990.
31. Lindberg: Pathology of equine granulomatous enteritis. *J Comp Pathol* 94:233-247, 1984.
32. Sweeney et al: Chronic granulomatous bowel disease in three sibling horses. *JAVMA* 186:1192-1194, 1986.
33. Platt: Chronic inflammatory and lymphoproliferative lesions of the equine small intestine. *J Comp Pathol* 96:671-684, 1986.
34. MacAllister et al: Lymphocytic-plasmacytic enteritis in two horses. *JAVMA* 196:1995-1998, 1990.
35. Fogarty et al: A cluster of equine granulomatous enteritis cases: the link with aluminum. *Vet Hum Toxicol* 40:297-305, 1998.
36. Collery et al: Equine granulomatous enteritis linked with aluminum? Letter to the editor. *Vet Human Toxicol* 41:49-50, 1999.
37. Pass et al: Basophilic enterocolitis in a horse. *Vet Pathol* 21:362-364, 1984.
38. Bowman: *Georgi's Parasitology for Veterinarians,* ed 6. Philadelphia, 1995, Saunders.
39. Hutchens et al: Treatment and control of gastrointestinal parasites. *Vet Clin North Am (Equine Pract)* 15:561-573, 1999.
40. Love et al: Pathogenicity of cyathostome infection. *Vet Parasitol* 85:113-122, 1999.
41. Proudman et al: Tapeworm infection is a significant risk factor for spasmodic colic and ileal impaction colic in the horse. *Equine Vet J* 30:194-199, 1998.
42. Gregory et al: Tissue-invading ciliates associated with chronic colitis in a horse. *J Comp Pathol* 96:109-114, 1986.
43. Xiao and Herd: Epidemiology of equine *Cryptosporidium* and *Giardia* infections. *Equine Vet J* 26:14-17, 1994.
44. Hayden et al: AA: amyloid-associated gastroenteropathy in a horse. *J Comp Pathol* 98:195-204, 1988.
45. Helman and Edwards: Clinical features of blister beetle poisoning in equids: 70 cases (1983-1996). *JAVMA* 211:1018-1021, 1997.

CHAPTER 7

Lymph Nodes

Rick L. Cowell, Ronald D. Tyler, Karen E. Dorsey, and M.A. Guglick

Cytology is a useful tool for evaluating peripheral lymphadenopathy. Cytologic examination of lymph node aspirates provides a quick, easy, and inexpensive way to gain insight into the cause of the lymphadenopathy without significant risk to the patient. Lymph node cells exfoliate easily, resulting in highly cellular aspirates that allow for reliable cytologic interpretation. Cytology may yield a definitive diagnosis (eg, lymphosarcoma, some infectious lymphadenopathies) or may indicate the process causing lymphadenopathy (eg, immune stimulation, purulent inflammation).

Lymphadenopathy can be localized or generalized and primary or secondary in nature. Causes of lymphadenopathy include hyperplasia, lymphadenitis (neutrophilic, purulent, eosinophilic, granulomatous), immune stimulation, lymphosarcoma, and metastatic neoplasia. An algorithmic approach to lymph node aspirate evaluation and interpretation is presented in Fig. 7-1.

Sample Collection and Preparation

Aspiration Technique: When one is aspirating peripheral lymph nodes, the site of aspiration is prepared as for an injection. Suitable fine-needle aspirates can be collected using a 21- to 25-gauge needle attached to a 5-ml or larger syringe. Small (5-ml) syringes can be used when aspirating lymph nodes because lymph node cells exfoliate easier than those of many other body tissues. For collection, the lymph node is held stationary between the operator's thumb and forefinger. With syringe attached, the needle is inserted into the enlarged lymph node. The syringe plunger is rapidly withdrawn two thirds to three fourths of the barrel length to create sufficient negative pressure to aspirate lymphoid cells.

If the node is large enough to redirect the needle without fear of the needle's exiting the node, negative pressure is maintained while the needle is redirected. Otherwise, negative pressure should be released before the needle is redirected and then negative pressure reapplied. If the needle exits the node while negative pressure is being applied, artifacts (eg, aspiration of subcutaneous fat and/or various skin layers) may be seen on cytologic smears. Also, if only a small sample is collected, it may be aspirated into the syringe barrel and lost for cytologic evaluation.

When tissues are aspirated for cytologic evaluation, the tissue of least resistance is aspirated into the needle and/or syringe. If a vessel is ruptured and blood is aspirated, continued aspiration results in excessive blood contamination. This dilutes the sample and impairs cytologic evaluation. Therefore, once blood enters the syringe and/or needle, negative pressure should be released and the needle redirected, or the aspiration procedure should be repeated with a new syringe and needle, depending on the degree of blood contamination.[1]

When the sample appears in the hub of the needle or if the needle has been redirected three or four times but the sample is still not visible in the syringe or hub of the needle, negative pressure is released and the needle is withdrawn from the node. The needle is removed from the syringe and a few milliliters of air (2 to 4) is drawn into the syringe barrel. The needle is replaced on the

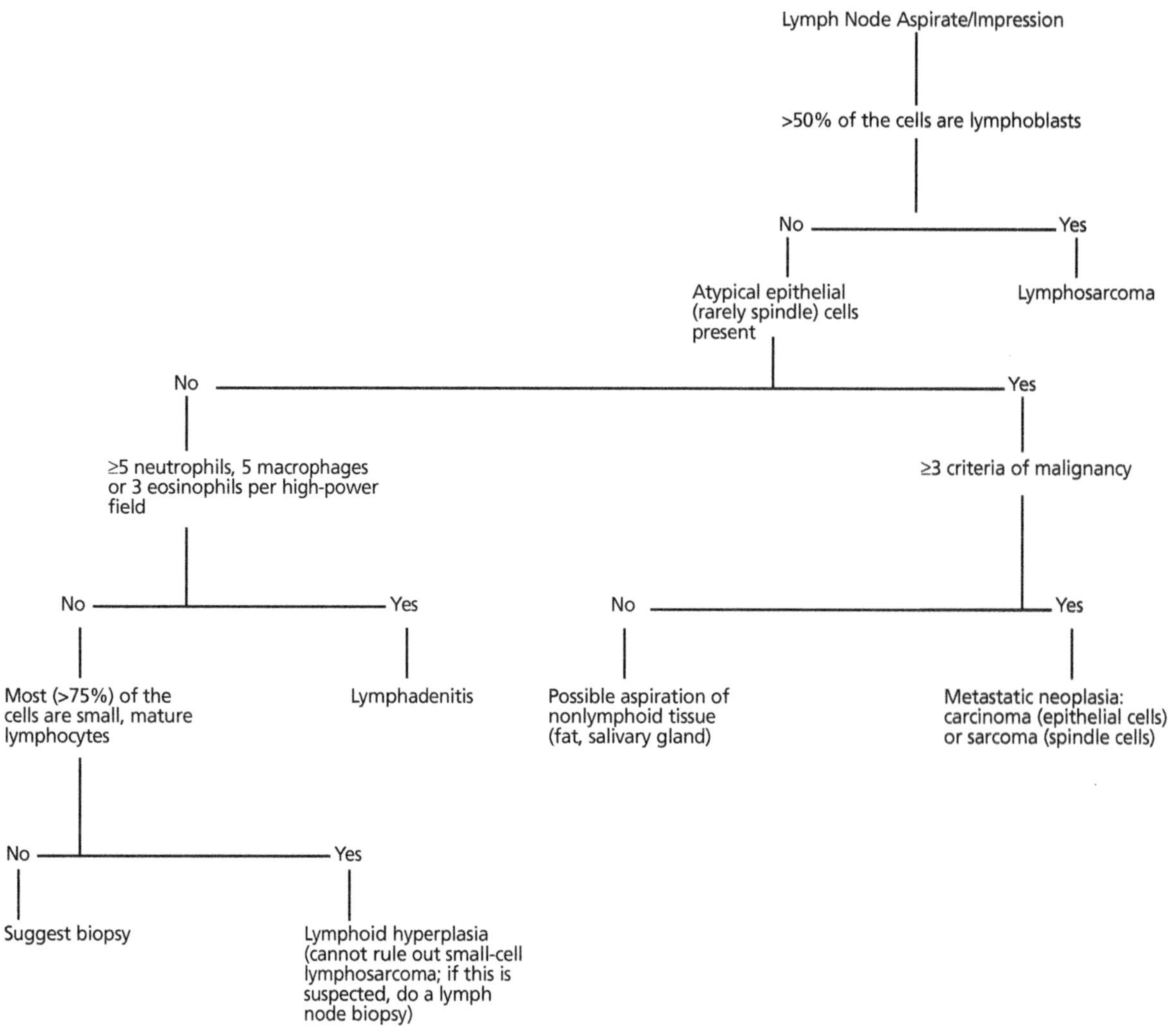

Fig. 7-1 Algorithmic approach to cytologic evaluation of lymph node aspirates. (Courtesy Oklahoma State University, Clinical Pathology teaching files.)

syringe and the plunger is rapidly depressed, forcing some of the aspirated contents onto a clean, dry glass slide. The sample must be smeared into a monolayer without causing excessive cell rupture (Fig. 7-2). Because lymphocytes, especially lymphoblasts, are fragile and rupture easily, special care must be taken. A combination smear procedure is depicted in Fig. 1-2. This requires some technical skill but can be mastered easily with minimal practice.

Nonaspiration Technique (Capillary Technique, Stab Technique): A 22-gauge needle is attached to a 3- to 10-ml syringe that has been prefilled with air. The node to be sampled is held firmly to aid penetration and to help direct the needle. The needle/syringe apparatus is grasped as if holding a throwing dart. The needle (attached to the syringe) is introduced into the mass. The needle is moved rapidly back and forth through the mass and along the same plane five to six times. There is no need to aspirate, since the cells are collected by shearing and capillary action. The needle is removed from the mass, and the material is expelled onto a clean glass microscope slide by rapidly depressing the plunger. Smears are made by one of the techniques described in Chapter 1.

Generally, one collects only enough material to make one smear. Therefore, the procedure should be repeated two or three times in different sites of the node or in

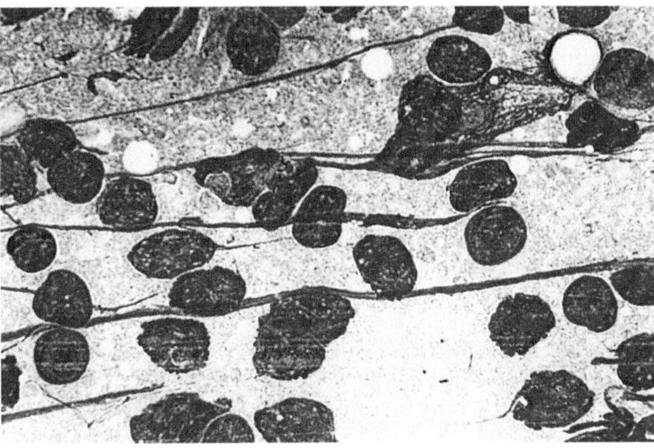

Fig. 7-2 Lymph node aspirate with all nucleated cells stripped of cytoplasm.
Nuclear chromatin of many cells forms strands across the slide. Smears with excessive cell rupturing cannot be evaluated cytologically. (Wright's stain; original magnification 250X)

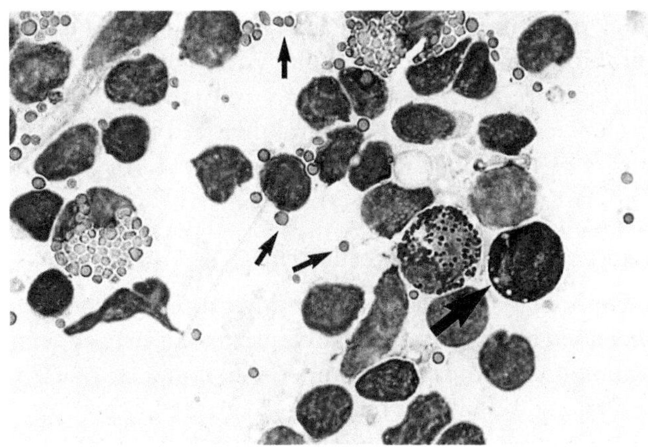

Fig. 7-3 Lymph node aspirate.
Note numerous small lymphocytes, a plasma cell (*broad arrow*), a basophil, and eosinophils. Free granules from ruptured eosinophils also are present (*narrow arrow*). (Wright's stain; original magnification 330X)

different nodes to have adequate slide numbers and areas to evaluate.

Staining

Several types of stains have been used for cytologic examination of lymph node aspirates. The most commonly used are the Romanowsky stains (Wright's, Giemsa, Diff-Quik). These stains are inexpensive, readily available to the practicing veterinarian, and easy to prepare, maintain, and use. They stain organisms and the cytoplasm of cells excellently. Nuclear and nucleolar detail usually is sufficient for differentiating neoplasia from inflammation and for evaluating neoplastic cells for cytologic evidence of malignancy.

Smears to be stained with Romanowsky stains should be air dried. Air drying partially preserves ("fixes") the cells and causes them to adhere to the slide so they do not fall off the slide during the staining procedure.

Commercially available Romanowsky stains include Diff-Quik, Dip-Stat, and various other "quick" Wright's stains. Most, if not all, Romanowsky stains are acceptable for staining lymph node preparations. The variations among the different Romanowsky stains should not cause a problem once the evaluator has become familiar with the stain used routinely.

The staining procedure recommended by the stain's manufacturer should be followed in general but adapted to the type and thickness of smear being stained and to the evaluator's preference. In general, the thinner the smear, the less immersion time needed in the stain. The thicker the smear, the more immersion time needed in the stain. For this reason, thick smears, such as smears of neoplastic lymph nodes, may require the recommended immersion time in stain be doubled or tripled. Each person tends to have different preferred staining characteristics. By trying variations in the recommended time intervals for the stains, the evaluator can establish immersion times to produce the preferred staining characteristics.[1]

Lymph Node Cell Types

A variety of cell types can be seen in lymph node aspirates. These include small lymphocytes, medium lymphocytes, large lymphocytes (lymphoblasts), plasma cells, macrophages, mast cells, neutrophils, eosinophils, inflammatory giant cells, and metastatic cancer cells. These cell types are identified by their morphologic characteristics.

Small Lymphocytes

Small lymphocytes are ≤9 μ in diameter (recognizably smaller than neutrophils) and have a scanty amount of clear to light blue cytoplasm that may contain a few azurophilic (red-purple) granules (Fig. 7-3). The nucleus is round to oval, usually indented, with dense clumps of nuclear chromatin in a coarse, smudged pattern. Nucleoli are not visible.

Medium Lymphocytes

Medium lymphocytes are 9 to 12 μ in diameter (about the same size as neutrophils), with a moderate amount of bluish cytoplasm that sometimes contains a few azurophilic granules. The nucleus is oval to irregularly shaped, with a stippled to granular chromatin pattern. Normal prolymphocytes may not have recognizable nucleoli or may have indistinct to prominent nucleoli. However, with prolymphocytic lymphosarcoma, nucleoli are usually single, large, and prominent. The presence of nucleoli in a nontraumatized lymphocyte indicates that it is either a prolymphocyte or a lymphoblast (large lymphocyte).

Large Lymphocytes (Lymphoblasts)

Lymphoblasts are larger than neutrophils, have an increased amount of bluish cytoplasm that may appear somewhat granular, and sometimes contains one to several azurophilic granules. A clear area in the cytoplasm representing the Golgi apparatus may be evident. The nucleus is oval, cleaved, notched, or irregular, with a finely stippled to granular chromatin pattern. Multiple small to large nucleoli are generally evident. While the cytoplasm is increased in volume, it typically is not recognizable all the way around the nucleus but tends to run confluent with the nucleus in one or more areas (see Figs. 7-9 and 7-10).

Plasma Cells

Plasma cells are oval, with an eccentric, round nucleus and coarse, cordlike nuclear chromatin (see Fig. 7-3). The cytoplasm stains deep blue, and a clear area representing the Golgi apparatus is recognizable between the nucleus and the greatest volume of cytoplasm. A plasma cell whose cytoplasm is filled with clear or pale-staining vacuoles (Russell bodies) is occasionally seen. These cells are sometimes referred to as *Mott cells*.

Macrophages

Macrophages tend to be larger than lymphoblasts and have a round, oval, or irregular nucleus with a loose or lacy chromatin pattern. The cytoplasm is blue-gray and frequently contains vacuoles and/or phagocytic debris.

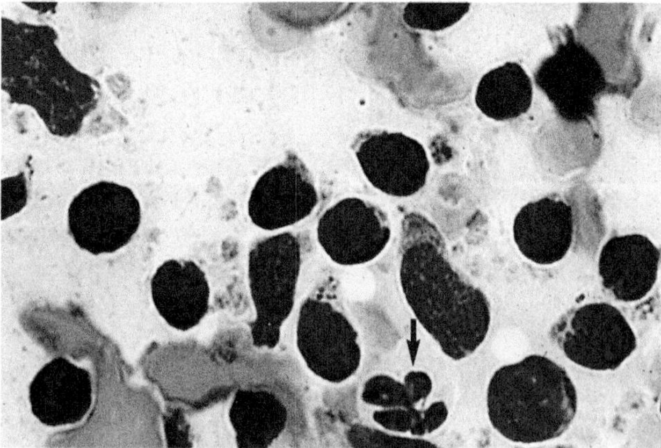

Fig. 7-4 Aspirate from hyperplastic lymph node. Small lymphocytes are the predominant cell type. The neutrophil (*arrow*) is larger than the small lymphocytes. (Wright's stain; original magnification 250X)

Mast Cells

Mast cells (Plate 7D) are readily recognized by their metachromatic (red-purple) intracytoplasmic granules. They are round cells with a round to oval nucleus and a moderate to abundant amount of cytoplasm.

Neutrophils

Neutrophils have clear cytoplasm and a segmented nucleus, with coarsely clumped nuclear chromatin (Fig. 7-4).

Eosinophils

Eosinophils are slightly larger than neutrophils and have a segmented nucleus with coarsely clumped nuclear chromatin (see Fig. 7-3). Large, round, eosinophilic intracytoplasmic granules are characteristic of eosinophils.

Inflammatory Giant Cells

Inflammatory giant cells are very large (several to many times the size of a neutrophil) and multinucleated, with a moderate amount of bluish cytoplasm. They may contain phagocytized organisms, cells, or debris.

Metastatic Cancer Cells

Tumor metastasis to lymph nodes is identified by recognizing cell types that are not normally present in lymph node aspirates or by recognizing a significant increase in numbers of a cell type that is normally present in only small numbers. Most metastatic cancer cells found in lymph node aspirates are carcinoma or adenocarcinoma (epithelial) cells. Metastatic tumor cells somewhat resemble the tumor of origin. In general, *metastatic carcinoma cells* are very large; tend to have a high nucleus to cytoplasm ratio, coarse nuclear chromatin, large angular nucleoli, and blue cytoplasm; and may contain cytoplasmic vacuoles (Plates 6A, 6C). *Metastatic sarcoma cells* generally are medium sized, with blue cytoplasm that tends to taper away from the nucleus in one or two directions, forming tails in some cells (see Table 1-3) (Plate 7C). They tend to have a high nucleus to cytoplasm ratio, fine to coarse nuclear chromatin patterns, and large (often angular) nucleoli and may contain cytoplasmic vacuoles.

The proportions and significance of the preceding cell types for various common conditions are discussed in the following material.

Cytologic Evaluation

Knowledge of normal cytologic characteristics of lymph node aspirates enables the evaluator to recognize abnormal findings. Some diagnoses that can be reliably made by cytologic examination of lymph node aspirates include the following.

Lymphosarcoma: >50% of the cells in the smear are lymphoblasts (large lymphocytes) and/or prolymphocytes.

Lymphadenitis: Though lymphadenitis may be present and sometimes can be recognized by experienced cytologists when smaller numbers of inflammatory cells are present than are listed below, the cell concentrations given are suggested for inexperienced cytologists in an effort to prevent "overdiagnosis."

Neutrophilic lymphadenitis: ≥5 neutrophils/100× objective (oil-immersion) field

Purulent lymphadenitis: ≥20 neutrophils/100× objective (oil-immersion) field

Eosinophilic lymphadenitis: ≥3 eosinophils/100× objective (oil-immersion) field

Chronic (macrophagic) lymphadenitis: ≥5 macrophages/100× objective (oil-immersion) field

Granulomatous lymphadenitis: Inflammatory giant cells present

Immune stimulation: ≥3 plasma cells/100× objective (oil-immersion) field

Metastatic neoplasia: Metastatic cancer cells are observed. These may be recognized as cell types not normally present in lymph node aspirates, with three or more criteria of malignancy, or as significantly increased numbers of a cell type that is normally present in lymph node aspirates in very small numbers.

Because cytology collects the sample from only a few, small, discrete foci of a lymph node, recognition of one or more of the above processes does not totally rule out the possibility of other processes occurring at an unsampled site.

However, lymphadenitis is nearly always diffuse throughout the node, and lymphosarcoma generally is sufficiently diffuse to be reliably identified when the affected lymph node is enlarged. On the other hand, metastatic tumor cells may be focal or diffuse.

Normal Lymph Nodes

The small lymphocyte is the predominant cell type (about 75% to 95% of cells present) in normal lymph nodes (Figs. 7-4 and 7-5).[2] The remaining cell types are an admixture, consisting primarily of medium-sized lymphocytes and lymphoblasts, with lesser numbers of macrophages, plasma cells, and neutrophils. Small, roundish, basophilic structures called *lymphoglandular bodies* (cytoplasmic fragments of lymphoid cells) are common findings in all lymph node aspirates (see Fig. 7-10). These lymphoglandular bodies must not be confused with an organism or parasite.

Lymphoid Hyperplasia

Hyperplastic lymph nodes consist primarily of small lymphocytes and generally appear cytologically very similar to normal lymph nodes (Figs. 7-4 and 7-5). Increased numbers of plasma cells, indicating immune stimulation, may be present. Even in the absence of increased numbers of plasma cells, the term *lymphoid hyperplasia* (as opposed to compatible with normal lymphoid tissue) is used if the lymph node is enlarged clinically. Lymphoid hyperplasia is usually caused by a localized reaction. However, lymphoid hyperplasia associated with generalized lymphadenopathy may occur. Hyperplasia occurs when antigens reach the lymph node and stimulate an immune response. If antigenemia is strong or if the lymph node itself is infected, neutrophilic, purulent, pyogranulomatous, or granulomatous lymphadenitis is the usual reaction.

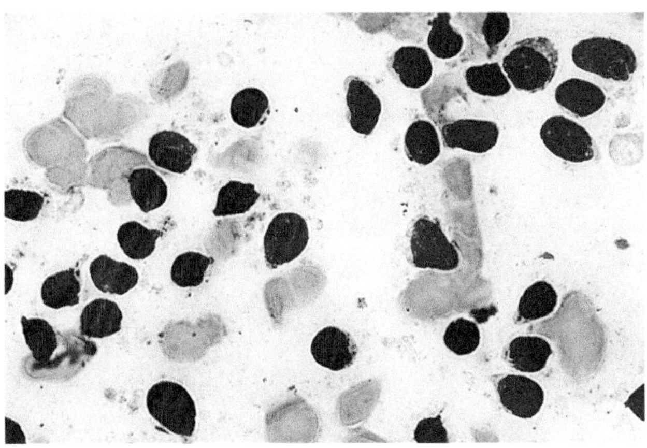

Fig. 7-5 Hyperplastic lymph node. Small lymphocytes predominate in this aspirate. (Wright's stain; original magnification 330X)

Lymphadenitis

Lymphadenitis may be neutrophilic (Fig. 7-6), purulent (Fig. 7-7), eosinophilic (Figs. 7-8 and 7-9), chronic (macrophages), granulomatous, or any combination of these reactions. Lymphadenitis may be primary or secondary. With *primary lymphadenitis*, the node itself is infected. A good example is strangles, caused by *Streptococcus equi*. Typically, in this disease, the mandibular, submaxillary, and retropharyngeal lymph nodes become heavily infiltrated with neutrophils (purulent lymphadenitis) with subsequent abscess formation.[3-5] In *secondary lymphadenitis*, the node itself is not infected but is draining a site(s) of inflammation (does not have to be an infection) distant from the node. Secondary lymphadenitis is usually neutrophilic and/or eosinophilic. Increased numbers of plasma cells, indicating immune stimulation, are often present with any cause of lymphadenitis. When evidence of purulent lymphadenitis, chronic lymphadenitis, granulomatous lymphadenitis, or pyogranulomatous lymphadenitis is present, a careful search for organisms and

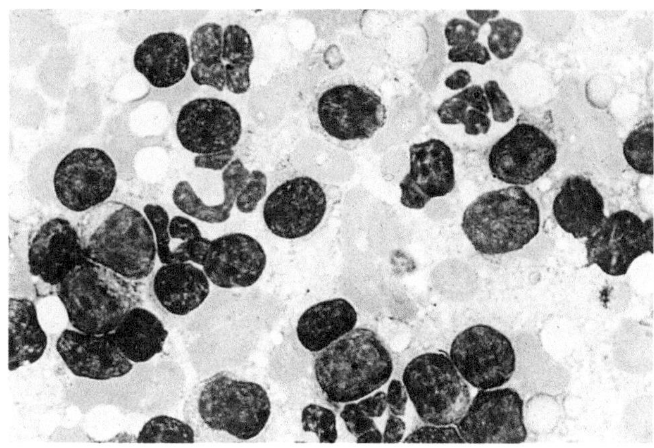

Fig. 7-6 Neutrophilic lymphadenitis.
Small lymphocytes and neutrophils predominate in this aspirate from a lymph node with neutrophilic lymphadenitis. Small lymphocytes are smaller than neutrophils and have a scanty amount of clear to slightly blue cytoplasm and a round to oval nucleus, with smudged nuclear chromatin. (Wright's stain; original magnification 250X)

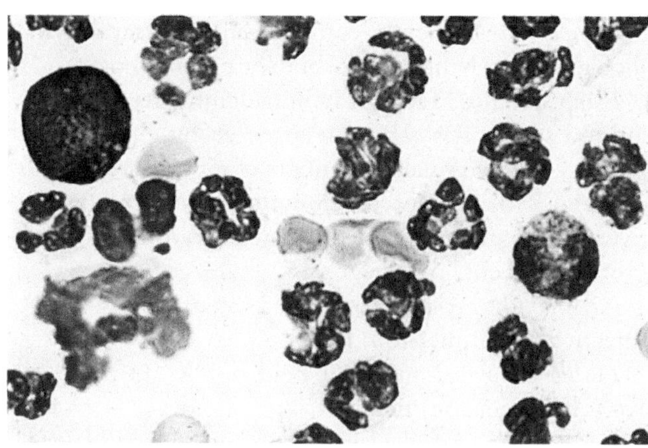

Fig. 7-7 Aspirate from infected lymph node.
Large numbers of neutrophils and intracellular bacterial rods characterize this as septic purulent lymphadenitis. (Wright's stain; original magnification 250X). (Courtesy Oklahoma State University, Stillwater.)

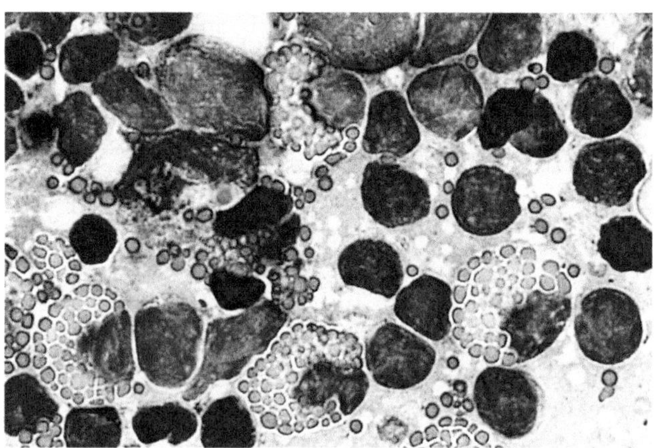

Fig. 7-8 Aspirate from lymph node of horse with eosinophilic lymphadenitis.
While small lymphocytes predominate, large numbers of eosinophils also are present. (Wright's stain; original magnification 330X)

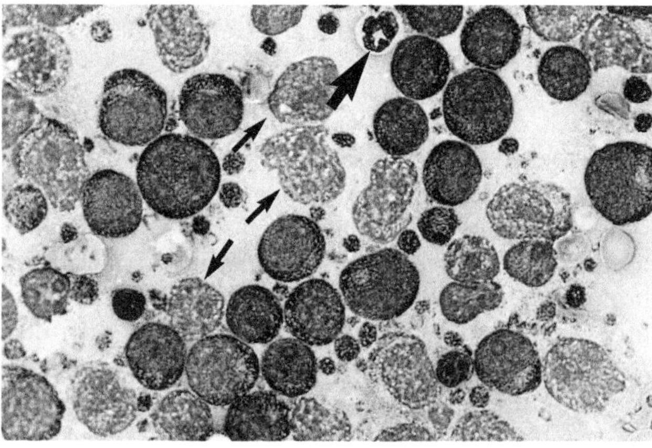

Fig. 7-9 Aspirate from lymph node of horse with lymphosarcoma.
Large lymphoblasts predominate. Lymphoblasts are larger than neutrophils (*broad arrow*) and must be differentiated from damaged cells (*narrow arrow*). (Wright's stain; original magnification 250X)

appropriate culture and sensitivity testing should be performed. Lymph nodes infected with bacteria manifest purulent lymphadenitis (Fig. 7-7), while nodes infected with systemic fungi, protozoa, or algae manifest granulomatous or pyogranulomatous lymphadenitis. However, some fungal infections, such as cutaneous phycomycosis (*Pythium, Basidiobolus haptosporus, Conidiobolus coronatus*), can cause marked eosinophilic infiltration of lymph nodes.[6] Eosinophilic lymphadenitis is common in lymph nodes draining the skin, respiratory tract, or digestive tract (Fig. 7-8). Any allergic inflammatory response can result in a secondary eosinophilic lymphadenitis.

Lymphosarcoma (Lymphoma)

Lymphosarcoma does not occur in horses as frequently as in other domestic animals.[7] However, in a survey of postmortem findings from 480 horses, lymphoma accounted

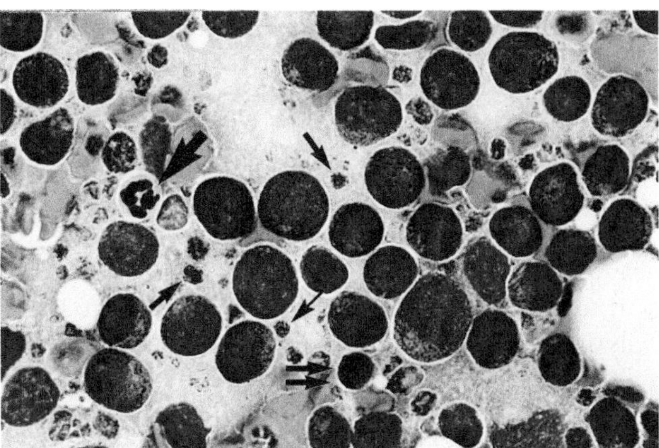

Fig. 7-10 Lymphosarcoma.
Lymphosarcoma is identified in this aspirate by the presence of large numbers of lymphoblasts. A neutrophil (*broad arrow*), small lymphocyte (*double arrow*), and numerous lymphoglandular bodies (*narrow arrow*) also are present. (Wright's stain; original magnification 330X)

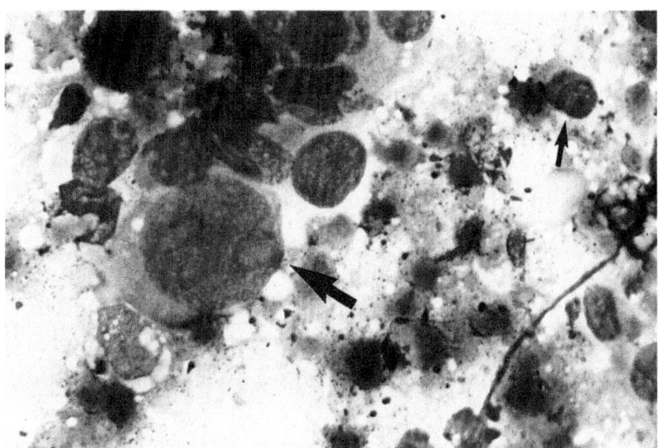

Fig. 7-11 Aspirate from lymph node containing metastatic carcinoma cells.
A single large carcinoma cell is present, with large angular nucleoli, coarse nuclear chromatin, and a high nucleus to cytoplasm ratio (*broad arrow*). A single intact small lymphocyte offers size comparison (*narrow arrow*). (Wright's stain; original magnification 100X) (Courtesy Oklahoma State University, Stillwater.)

for death in 2.5% of the cases.[8] Lymphosarcoma may be generalized or limited to one or two lymph nodes. Because lymph node architecture cannot be interpreted by cytology, lymphosarcoma is identified on cytologic smears by recognizing an abnormally increased proportion of lymphoblasts and/or prolymphocytes (large lymphocytes). Lymphosarcoma is characterized by lymphoblasts and/or prolymphocytes comprising >50% of the cell population (Figs. 7-9 and 7-10). When one is evaluating aspirates for lymphosarcoma, only intact lymphocytes should be examined. Lymphocytes ruptured during aspiration or slide preparation tend to spread out. Their nucleoli become visible, and these must not be mistaken for lymphoblasts. Usually these ruptured cells can be easily recognized by their loose nuclear chromatin, which stains much more eosinophilic than the nuclear chromatin of intact lymphocytes. Caution must be exercised when attempting to interpret smears in which a high percentage of the lymphocytes are ruptured. Lymphoblasts tend to be more fragile than small lymphocytes and rupture more easily. Therefore, lymphosarcoma may be masked because of a large number of ruptured cells in the smear.

Not all lymphosarcomas in horses are lymphoblastic. Lymphoplasmacytoid lymphosarcoma (plasmacytic lymphosarcoma) and lymphocytic (small lymphocyte) lymphosarcoma also occur in horses. Therefore, if lymphosarcoma is suspected clinically but cannot be recognized cytologically, excisional biopsy should be performed. The entire lymph node (incised at ¼-inch intervals) should be submitted in 10% buffered formalin for histopathologic evaluation. This allows the pathologist to evaluate the nodal architecture that is lost in cytologic smears.

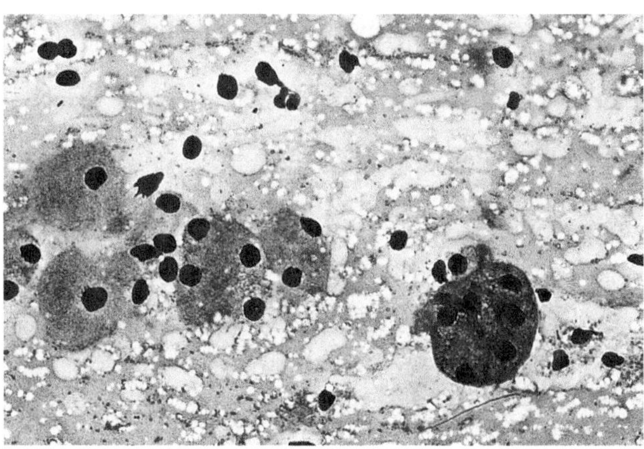

Fig. 7-12 Salivary epithelial cells in heavy eosinophilic background. (Wright's stain; original magnification 100X) (Courtesy Oklahoma State University, Stillwater.)

Nonlymphoid Neoplasia

Tumor metastasis to lymph nodes is characterized by moderate to large numbers of cells that either are not normally found in lymph nodes or are typically present only in very small numbers. Malignant epithelial-cell tumors (carcinomas, adenocarcinomas) are the most common type of nonlymphoid neoplasia seen in lymph node aspirates. They are recognized by the presence of large epithelial cells with coarse nuclear chromatin and large, prominent, frequently angular nucleoli. These cells may occur singly or in clusters and frequently show marked variation in cell and nuclear size (Fig. 7-11). Secretory products may be evident with adenocarcinomas.

Rarely, malignant spindle-cell tumors (sarcomas) may be identified in lymph node aspirates. Large numbers of cells exhibiting cytoplasm that trails away from the nucleus in one or two directions with nuclear criteria of malignancy indicate a malignant spindle-cell tumor (Plate 7C).

Mast-cell tumors rarely metastasize to the lymph nodes in horses. Only one case of metastatic mast-cell tumor has been reported in lymph nodes of the horse.[9] Metastatic mast-cell disease should be considered if a mast-cell tumor is present distal to the lymph node. Otherwise, when large numbers of mast cells are encountered in equine lymph node aspirates, conditions other than metastatic mast-cell neoplasia, such as phycomycotic lymphadenitis, parasitic lymphadenitis, and allergic lymphadenitis, are more likely.

Aspiration of Nonlymphoid Tissue

Subcutaneous fat is the most common nonlymphoid tissue accidentally aspirated when attempting to collect cytologic samples from lymph nodes. Fat is recognized grossly by its wet (oily) appearance on the slide and its failure to dry. Microscopically, intact fat cells are sometimes observed (Plate 6H). However, if only fat droplets (instead of intact fat cells) are aspirated, material may not be identified cytologically because most hematologic stains contain alcohol that dissolves fat droplets.

Also, salivary gland tissue may be accidentally aspirated when mandibular lymph node aspirations are attempted. Smears made from salivary gland aspirates usually consist of salivary cells in a background of heavy eosinophilic material (Fig. 7-12). Salivary gland cells are recognized as uniform, medium-sized to large cells that usually occur in clumps or clusters. They have abundant, slightly blue, foamy cytoplasm. Their nuclei are usually of uniform size and round, with dense chromatin. Care should be taken to not confuse these cells with neoplastic cells.

REFERENCES

1. Tyler et al: *Diagnostic Cytology of the Dog and Cat.* Goleta, CA, 1989, American Veterinary Publications, pp 1-19.
2. Perman et al: *Cytology of the Dog and Cat.* Denver, 1979, American Animal Hospital Association, pp 11-13.
3. Muhktar and Timoney: Chemotactic response of equine polymorphonuclear leucocytes to *Streptococcus equi. Res Vet Sci* 45:225-229, 1988.
4. Nara et al: Experimental *Streptococcus equi* infection in the horse: correlation with in vivo and in vitro immune responses. *Am J Vet Res* 44:529-534, 1983.
5. Yelle: Clinical aspects of *Streptococcus equi* infection. *Equine Vet J* 19:158-162, 1987.
6. Miller and Campbell: The comparative pathology of equine cutaneous phycomycosis. *Vet Pathol* 21:325-332, 1984.
7. Schalm: Lymphosarcoma in the horse. *Equine Pract* 13(2):23-27, 1981.
8. Baker and Ellis: A survey of post-mortem findings in 480 horses, 1958 to 1980. *Equine Vet J* 13:43-46, 1981.
9. Riley, Yovich, and McChowell: Malignant mast cell tumours in horses. *Aust Vet J* 68 (10): 346-347, 1991.

CHAPTER 8

Pleural Fluid

Heather L. DeHeer, Bruce W. Parry, and Carol B. Grindem

Thoracentesis is diagnostically indicated when there is physical, radiographic, or ultrasonographic evidence of pleural effusion or pleural neoplasia. Within the United States, pleuropneumonia is the most common cause of equine pleural effusion (termed *parapneumonic* effusions).[1,2] For this reason, thoracentesis may be a useful part of the clinical evaluation of horses with lower respiratory tract disease.[3,4] Occasionally, other underlying systemic disease results in development of pleural effusion; such effusions are termed *nonparapneumonic* effusions. Rarely, no underlying etiology is identified (called *idiopathic pleural* effusions). Both nonparapneumonic and idiopathic effusions are generally associated with a poorer prognosis.[1,5]

Clinical signs associated with pleural effusions vary, depending on the severity and duration, and may be fairly nonspecific. These include anorexia, depression, weight loss, exercise intolerance, pneumonia, dyspnea, dependent edema of the brisket and forelegs, and colic. Signs of colic may be attributable to actual concurrent gastrointestinal disorders or to severe *pleurodynia* (pleural pain) mimicking colic.[6] Pleurodynia signs may also mimic exertional rhabdomyolysis or laminitis. There may be a history of recent stress such as travel, training, or hospitalization. Thoracentesis may be a worthwhile procedure when findings from physical examination (including rectal palpation), hematologic examination, serum biochemistry assays, fecal examination, and abdominocentesis have not indicated a diagnosis.

The dynamics of pleural fluid production in horses are thought to be different from those in dogs, cats, and people.[7] In dogs and cats, the parietal pleura is supplied by systemic arteries, while the visceral pleura is supplied by pulmonary arteries, which are at a lower pressure. As a result, there is a net flow of pleural fluid from the parietal to visceral pleura. In horses, both pleurae are supplied by the systemic circulation. For the parietal surface this is mainly from intercostal arteries, while for the visceral surface, it is from bronchial, esophageal, and internal thoracic arteries.[7,8] Hence, there is no net flow of pleural fluid from one surface to the other in horses, and pleural fluid is removed by the numerous lymphatic vessels of the pleurae. Most of the parietal surface is drained through the sternal lymph nodes, while the mediastinal and diaphragmatic portions are drained through the mediastinal lymph nodes. The visceral pleura is drained through the tracheobronchial lymph nodes.[7,8]

As with peritoneal fluid, normal pleural fluid is essentially a dialysate of plasma, with low cellularity and total protein concentration. The amount of fluid in the thoracic cavity is just sufficient to ensure adequate lubrication of the parietal and visceral pleurae. Consequently, the volume, cellularity, and biochemical composition of the fluid often reflect the pathophysiologic status of the parietal and visceral pleural surfaces.

An increase in fluid volume results when the rate of fluid formation exceeds that of fluid removal. Pleural effusions have been reported in horses with a variety of conditions, including heart failure, chronic hepatic disease, hypoalbuminemia, diaphragmatic rupture, pleuritis, pneumonia, pulmonary abscesses, thoracic neoplasia, traumatic injury, parasitism, and hemothorax[3,8-11] (Table 8-1).

TABLE 8-1
Differential Diagnosis for Pleural Effusion in the Horse*

Bacterial pleuropneumonia
Neoplasia
Penetrating chest wound
Hemothorax
Esophageal perforation
Concurrent peritonitis
Diaphragmatic hernia
Pulmonary granuloma
Coccidioidomycosis
Cryptococcosis
Viral pneumonia
Fibrosing pneumonia
Hypoalbuminemia
Pericarditis
Excessive fluid therapy
Uroperitoneum
Septicemia
Equine infectious anemia
Aberrant metacestodes
Liver failure
Congestive heart failure
Mycoplasma felis
Chylothorax
Pulmonary embolism
Pulmonary hydatidosis
Idiopathic pleuritis

*From Chaffin: Thoracentesis and pleural drainage in horses. *Equine Vet Ed* 10(2):106-108, 1998.

Specimen Collection

Thoracentesis may be performed in the standing horse with minimal restraint. Specific collection techniques have been detailed elsewhere.[2,12,13] A bridle, halter, and stocks are usually adequate. If necessary, additional manual restraint and/or tranquilization may be used. Aseptic technique is employed. Most horses have a fenestrated mediastinum, and so fluid from either side is anticipated to be similar in the healthy horse. In disease conditions of the thorax, mediastinal fenestrations may become obstructed with fibrin; consequently, the two sides may not be affected to the same degree. It is therefore advisable to tap both sides, beginning with the more severely affected hemithorax. On the right side this is usually done at the sixth or seventh intercostal spaces, up to 10 cm dorsal to the level of the olecranon or the costochondral junction.[3,7,11,14] On the left side this is usually done at the sixth to ninth intercostal spaces, 4 to 6 cm dorsal to the level of the olecranon or just dorsal to the costochondral junction.[7,14] Entry just cranial to the rib margin prevents laceration of the intercostal vessels and nerves that course along the caudal aspect of the rib.[13] Care should be taken to avoid the lateral thoracic vein.[6,15] Thoracic auscultation, percussion, radiography, and/or ultrasonography may be useful to determine the location(s) of an effusion in many cases.[7,14,16,17] This may influence the site selected for thoracentesis.

Pleural fluid can usually be readily obtained on the first attempt when an effusion is present. However, if no fluid is collected, another site should be selected. If this is also unsuccessful, a 30-cm bitch catheter can be used.[11] Such difficulty in collecting a sample probably means the volume of fluid present is not increased. However, it could also mean that the effusion is loculated rather than diffuse. Radiography and (particularly) ultrasonography are useful ancillary techniques to visualize such loculation and to guide thoracentesis.[17]

Using standard techniques, 2 to 8 ml of pleural fluid can be obtained from most normal horses.[11] Only 1 or 2 ml of fluid is usually required for a total nucleated cell count, cytologic examination, total protein measurement, and bacteriologic testing (if necessary).

Complications of Thoracentesis

Complications of thoracentesis are considered uncommon,[14] and no undesirable sequelae were observed in one study of 18 clinically normal horses.[11] Improper technique may result in pneumothorax, lung laceration, hemothorax, cardiac arrhythmia, or puncture of bowel, liver, or heart.[6,13] Mild pneumothorax resulting from aspiration of air through the cannula is commonly asymptomatic, and any free air within the thoracic cavity is rapidly reabsorbed.[5] Occasionally, localized cellulitis surrounding the thoracentesis site requires symptomatic treatment.[15]

When draining a large volume of effusion, intravenous fluid support should be provided to prevent hemoconcentration. Unless severe respiratory distress warrants rapid drainage, fluid removal should be slow to prevent development of pulmonary edema.[5]

Specimen Handling Considerations

Pleural fluid from healthy horses contains a negligible quantity of fibrinogen and will not clot. However, mild blood contamination often occurs as the cannula is forced through intercostal muscles during thoracentesis. In addition, protein exudation is a common feature of inflammatory reactions, which are the most frequent cause of thoracic effusions. Both of these situations will increase fluid fibrinogen content, and as a result, the sample may clot.

Fluid should be collected into an EDTA tube for cell counts, cytologic examination, and (refractometric) total protein measurement. With small sample size (EDTA tubes less than one quarter filled), erroneous results for fluid protein levels and cell counts may be obtained (see section on biochemical examination).[18] Aside from protein analysis, other biochemistry tests are only occasionally performed on pleural fluid in select diagnostic situations.

When necessary, both aerobic and anaerobic microbiologic studies are performed on the centrifuged sediment collected in a sterile clot tube and on fluid collected into special transport tubes. The reference laboratory should be contacted for recommendations on handling and transportation of microbiologic specimens.

If a delay is anticipated between sample collection and processing in the laboratory, the specimen is best refrigerated in the interim. In this situation, direct smear preps of turbid fluid (high cellularity) or concentrated smears of clear fluid (low cellularity), made soon after sample collection, serve as a reference point for cell morphology. When a delay of several hours occurs before smears are prepared, macrophages in the pleural fluid may become vacuolated in vitro or exhibit erythrophagia, thus complicating the distinction between true hemorrhagic effusions and peripheral blood contaminated specimens. Nucleated cells may start to exhibit aging changes such as hypersegmentation and pyknosis, thereby resembling more chronic processes. Neutrophil nuclear hyposegmentation artifact may also be observed following delayed processing of EDTA-anticoagulated specimens. Also, bacterial overgrowth may occur, of either pathogenic or contaminant organisms, clouding interpretation.

When utilizing outside laboratories, it is best to determine, in advance of specimen collection, any special requirements for specimen storage, shipment, and submission favored by that particular laboratory for the analyses requested. In most instances, air-dried, direct or concentrated, line smears of fluid, together with EDTA and clot tube aliquots and culture transport media as indicated, are sufficient.

Gross Fluid Examination

Gross visual inspection of fluid consists of noting fluid volume, color, turbidity, odor, and clot formation. Normal, nonhemodiluted pleural fluid will not clot, is of small volume, and is clear to slightly hazy, pale straw yellow, and odorless.[11,13]

Subjective assessment of the color, turbidity, odor, and volume (as assessed by the ease or rate of collection) of pleural fluid in the thoracic cavity may often provide a provisional diagnosis and thus allow initiation of therapy before complete laboratory results are obtained. If the pleural fluid is grossly normal in appearance, it is probably normal, since most pleural effusions of the equine are exudative and will be visibly abnormal.[1] However, when samples are moderately contaminated by peripheral blood at collection, such diagnostic inferences are more difficult. Evaluating the gross appearance of pleural fluid should not be a substitute for total nucleated cell counts, cytologic examination, and total protein determination. However, in many cases, particularly those without significant hemorrhage, such assessments allow the fluid to be broadly categorized as originating from a transudative or exudative process.

Volume

It is usually possible to obtain a few milliliters of pleural fluid from a healthy horse, though this may not be possible at the first attempt. Some normal horses may have no retrievable fluid.[13] Of 18 clinically normal horses, 17 yielded 2 to 8 ml of pleural fluid on thoracentesis.[11]

Odor, Color, and Turbidity

Normal pleural fluid is odorless and sterile. A foul odor may accompany tissue necrosis or anaerobic bacterial infection.[13] However, absence of foul odor does not rule out either of these possibilities.

In disease, specimen color can vary from colorless to yellow, orange, red, brown, gray, or white. Effusion color varies with the numbers and relative proportions of RBCs and nucleated cells present and biochemical constituents such as hemoglobin, or lipid. Erythrocytes, which often cause reddish discoloration of specimens, are usually the result of contamination by hemorrhage from intercostal muscles during collection. If blood contamination is avoided, the gross appearance of normal pleural fluid is very similar to that of peritoneal fluid. A discolored supernatant usually reflects damage to erythrocytes and sometimes to leukocytes that has occurred prior to collection. Turbidity ranges from clear to opaque and is related to the cellular, protein, and/or lipid content of the fluid. Flocculent material visible within the specimen may contribute to increased turbidity and can be strands of fibrin or rarely ingesta/plant material from either accidental enterocentesis or gastrointestinal rupture. The latter may occur with selection of ventral thoracentesis sites, with caudal orientation of the cannula, or with diaphragmatic herniation of an intestinal segment.

Normal pleural fluid and transudative effusions are clear and colorless to pale yellow because of their low cellularity. Exudative effusions are more likely to be discolored and turbid, attributable to their increased cellularity and protein content. In these circumstances, it is diagnostically useful to grossly examine the sample's sediment and supernatant. In the field situation, this can be done by allowing the fluid to sediment by gravity. In the laboratory, a microhematocrit centrifuge or a regular centrifuge can be used. The *height* of the sediment in the tube is usually proportional to the cellularity of the fluid, while its color varies with the relative numbers of RBCs and nucleated cells present. It may be red when RBCs predominate or brown to gray to off-white when most cells are WBCs. Red (hemolytic), port wine, amber, red-brown, or brown discoloration of the supernatant usually reflects damage to RBCs and sometimes WBCs that occurred before collection.

Shades of pink to red discoloration will occur with the presence of red cells or free hemoglobin in the specimen. Changes in red discoloration during specimen collection can alert the veterinarian to possible peripheral blood contamination. Uniformly red discolored specimens generally represent true hemorrhagic effusions and may be associated with bleeding diatheses, major vessel laceration, tumor or abscess rupture, traumatic injury, pulmonary infarction, or lung lobe torsion.[13,19] Pneumothorax may accompany some causes of hemothorax. When the specimen grossly resembles whole blood, determination of packed cell volume (fluid and venous) and clotting times, as well as cytologic appearance, may be useful. Failure of the specimen to clot or presence of significant erythrophagia upon microscopic examination suggests true hemothorax. Contaminated specimens most often have a packed cell volume significantly less than that of peripheral blood, and platelet clumps may be visualized microscopically.

Reddish brown, port wine, or muddy effusions may be associated with ischemic tissue injury/necrosis or neoplasia.[13] Presence of degenerative leukocyte changes (loss of nuclear segmentation, indistinct nuclear margins) with concurrent presence of bacterial organisms is compatible with sepsis.

Milky, whitish, or opalescent discoloration may occur with increased leukocyte numbers or elevated lipid content (cholesterol and/or triglycerides). The terms *chylous* and *pseudochylous* are traditionally used to describe such fluid specimens. The turbidity and color change in chylous effusions are the result of increased fluid triglyceride content, with or without a concurrent increase in leukocytes. Pseudochylous effusions have a grossly similar appearance due to high cellularity and cholesterol content. Microscopic evaluation of chylous and pseudochylous effusions are discussed later.

Cytologic Examination

Subjective assessment of the color, turbidity, odor, and volume (as assessed by the ease or rate of collection) of pleural fluid in the thoracic cavity may often provide a provisional diagnosis and thus allow initiation of therapy before laboratory results are obtained. However, when samples are moderately contaminated by peripheral blood at collection, such diagnostic inferences are more difficult. Evaluating the gross appearance of pleural fluid should not be a substitute for cell counts and cytologic examination. However, in many cases, particularly those without significant hemorrhage, such assessments allow the fluid to be broadly categorized as originating from a transudative or exudative process.

A cell count, total protein determination, and cytologic evaluation can be performed in the laboratory. Such tests require little equipment and yield much useful information. The method by which smears are prepared in the laboratory for cytologic evaluation varies with the specimen's cellularity and the equipment available. Fluids with a total nucleated cell count less than 5000/μl are most readily examined if smears are made after cells are concentrated by some means. In diagnostic laboratories, special cytocentrifuges are often used for this purpose. A 100-μl aliquot yields ideal cell morphology for cytospin examination of most fluid specimens. (See Figs. 9-1 and 9-2.) Transudative, very-low-cellularity effusions may require up to 200 μl to improve cellularity for microscopic examination. Extremely high-cellularity, exudative effusions may require a reduced volume aliquot (25 to 50 μl) or specimen dilution to achieve cytospin preparations with ideal cell morphology and numbers.

In the practice laboratory without a cytocentrifuge, specimen concentration is achieved by centrifugation of up to 10 ml of pleural fluid in a tube for about 5 minutes at 1000 to 1500 rpm. The resultant supernatant is removed and saved for total protein measurement. The sedimented cells are then gently resuspended in about 0.25 to 0.5 μl of pleural fluid and smears prepared, often using a line smear technique to concentrate cells at the leading edge of the smear (see Chapter 1). Romanowsky-type stains are usually used, such as Wright's, May-Grünwald, Giemsa, or Diff-Quik. Fluids with a total nucleated cell count of 5000 to 10,000/μl may be prepared from centrifuged or uncentrifuged specimens, depending on the examiner's preference. (Cytospin preparations or line smears from centrifuged sediments yield more cellular and therefore more easily scanned smears in these situations.) When the total nucleated cell count is >10,000/μl and the fluid's turbidity is therefore greater than normal, direct smears of uncentrifuged specimens are usually satisfactory.

Cell Counts and Cytologic Examination

Total nucleated cell and erythrocyte counts of pleural fluid are performed as for a blood sample. Depending on laboratory resources, this can vary from manual dilution with microscopic enumeration to the use of automated cell counters. Reference values are detailed in Table 8-2. Small-volume specimens (EDTA tube less than one quarter filled) may be sufficiently diluted to mildly decrease cell counts.[18]

Though RBCs are present in pleural fluid collected from clinically normal horses, they are considered to be

TABLE 8-2
Reference Values for Equine Pleural Fluid*

Measurement	Observed range	Comments
RBC count	22,000–540,000/μl 22–540 x 10^9 L	≤ 370,000/μl (≤ 370 x 10^9 L) in 94% of horses
Total nucleated cell count	800–12,100/μl 0.8–12.1 x 10^9 L	≤ 8000/μl (≤ 8.0 x 10^9 L) in 94% of horses
Differential cell count		
Neutrophils	450–10,290/μl 0.5–10.3 x 10^9 L 32%–91%	450–7120/μl (≤ 0.5–7.1 x 10^9 L) in 94% of horses
Lymphocytes	0–680/μl 0–0.7 x 10^9 L 0%–22%	0%–10% in 94% of horses
Large mononuclear cells	50–2620/μl 0.1–2.6 x 10^9 L 5%–66%	
Eosinophils	0–170/μl 0–0.2 x 10^9 L 0%–9%	No eosinophils observed in 89% of horses; 0%–1% in 94% of horses
Specific gravity	1.008–1.031	
Total protein	0.2–4.7 g/dl 2–47 g/L	≤ 2.5 g/dl (25 g/L) in 83% of horses; ≤ 3.4 g/dl (≤ 34 g/L) in 94% of horses

*Values derived from 18 clinically normal horses. From Wagner and Bennett: Analysis of equine thoracic fluid. *Vet Clin Pathol* 11(1):13-17, 1982.

the result of contamination by minor hemorrhage from intercostal muscles. Accordingly, erythrophagocytosis is not a feature of normal pleural fluid.[11] The fluid supernatant is also clear and nonhemolyzed in normal specimens. Erythrocyte counts are not often performed on pleural fluid unless automated techniques are used that routinely include red cell number determination.

Nucleated cells are generally categorized as neutrophils, lymphocytes, large mononuclear cells (including monocytes, macrophages, and mesothelial cells), eosinophils, basophils, or mast cells. Differential counts are usually performed on 100 to 200 cells. Though the numbers of each cell type are usually expressed as a percentage value, these figures must be related to the total nucleated cell count,

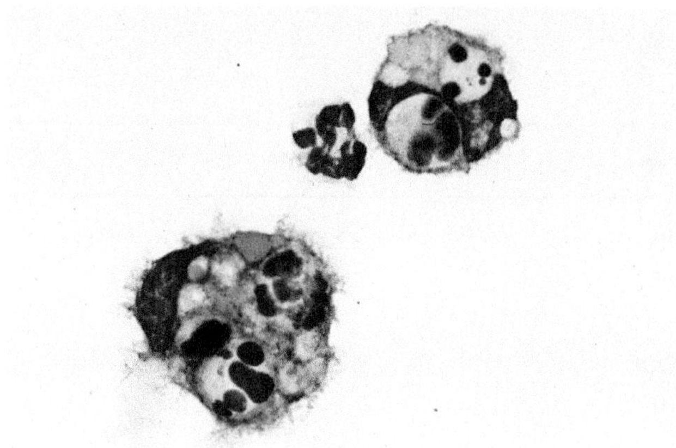

Fig. 8-1 Equine pleural fluid.
Cytophagic pleural macrophages may be infrequently observed in fluid collected from clinically normal horses but are a more common finding with mild inflammation. (Wright-Giemsa stain)

total protein concentration, and volume of fluid present for accurate interpretation. Assessment of cell morphology is a very important part of cytologic examination. General comments pertaining to peritoneal fluid leukocyte morphology are probably applicable to pleural fluid, though there is a paucity of such information readily available.

Neutrophils: Neutrophils that enter the thoracic cavity (as with neutrophils entering other body cavities or tissues) do not return to the bloodstream. Consequently, cell aging and death are normal events. Aged neutrophils are often moderately hypersegmented to pyknotic,[20-23] and leukophagocytosis of senescent neutrophils by macrophages may be infrequently observed (Fig. 8-1). This finding may be difficult to distinguish from occult or mild inflammation. Neutrophils in normal pleural fluid do not exhibit phagocytic activity per se.

The presence of band neutrophils or more immature granulocytic cells suggests acute inflammation and mobilization of the neutrophil storage and maturation pools. Presence of degenerative changes (such as cell swelling, loss of nuclear segmentation, and indistinct nuclear margins)[24] suggests a harsh pleural environment. This may occur secondary to the presence of bacterial cytotoxins within the thoracic cavity. Toxic changes (such as increased cytoplasmic basophilia, vacuolation, or Dohle bodies) may also be observed in septicemia or enterotoxemia. Such toxic change is considered to be "preexisting," occurring during myelopoiesis, rather than subsequent to migration into the pleural cavity. These changes, accompanied by visualization of phagocytized bacterial organisms (Figs. 8-2, 9-13, and 9-14) are compatible with septic pleuritis.

Large Mononuclear Cells: The category of large mononuclear cells incorporates nonreactive (tissue) macrophages of blood monocyte origin, reactive (tissue) macrophages, and mesothelial cells (see Figs. 9-2 and 9-4 to 9-6). As in peritoneal fluid, these cells are often difficult to distinguish morphologically.[11] They are conveniently grouped together and often referred to collectively as mononuclear phagocytes, since all have phagocytic potential (Figs. 8-1 and 8-3). All of these cells are large, usually with a moderate to high nuclear to cytoplasmic ratio, and abundant, somewhat basophilic cytoplasm (see Figs. 9-2 and 9-4). The nucleus is their most distinctive feature, but even that is not particularly characteristic, and subclassification of large mononuclear cells is quite subjective.

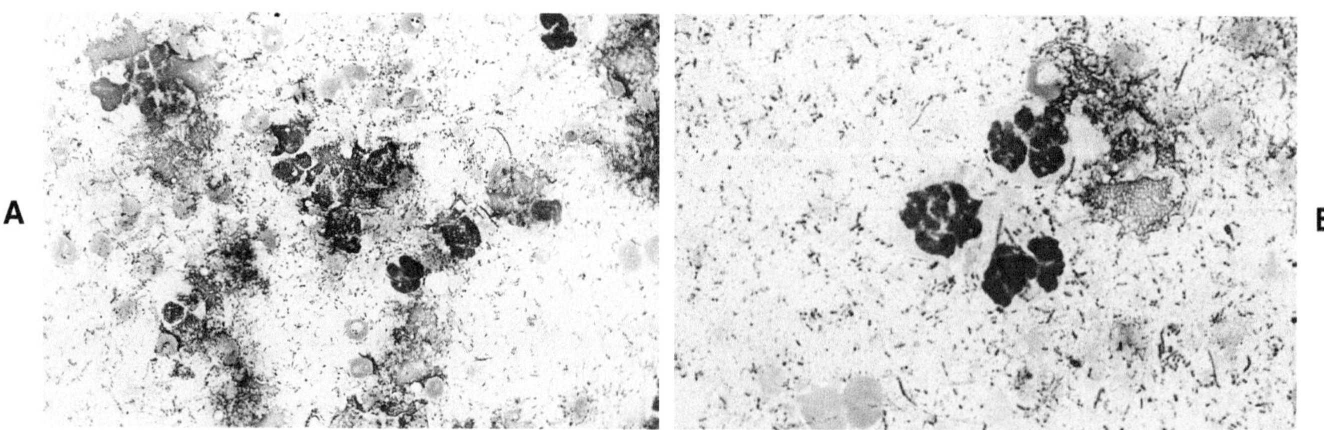

Fig. 8-2 Equine septic pleuritis.
A, Degenerate neutrophils, smudged cells, and low numbers of RBCs are present within a background of mixed bacterial organisms. **B,** Higher magnification view. (Wright-Giemsa stain)

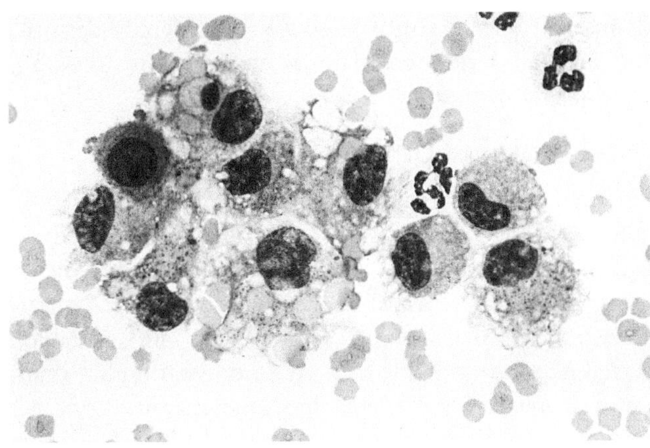

Fig. 8-3 Erythrophagocytic macrophages suggest previous or ongoing diapedesis or intrathoracic hemorrhage. (Wright-Giemsa stain)

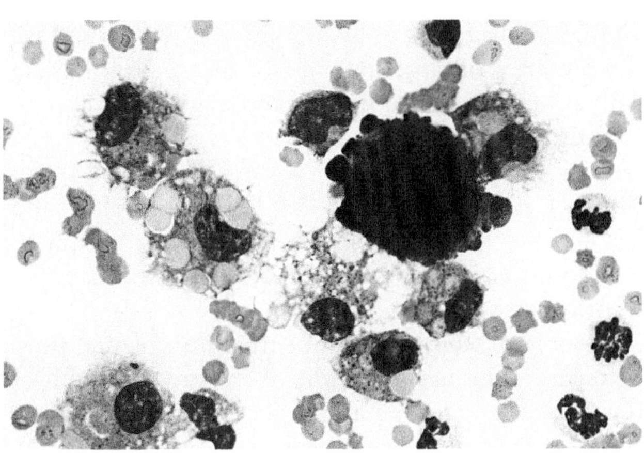

Fig. 8-4 Erythrophagocytic macrophages, nondegenerate neutrophils, and a single, deeply basophilic, reactive mesothelial cell are present. Reactive mesothelial changes may accompany inflammatory effusions and may begin to mimic neoplastic transformation. (Wright-Giemsa stain)

Mesothelial cells usually have an oval nucleus with a finely reticular chromatin pattern. When individualized, a fine eosinophilic "corona" or halo of glycocalyx may be evident along the cell margin (Fig. 8-5). In transudative effusions, they may occur in sheets or rafts, have a uniform appearance, and have a polygonal to rhomboid shape. In exudative effusions, mesothelial cells may become *reactive* or *transformed* and exhibit features suggesting increased proliferation, including increased cytoplasmic basophilia, multinucleation, prominent nucleoli, and mitotic activity (Figs. 8-4 and 8-5). Hyperplastic/dysplastic features can begin to mimic neoplasia in severe inflammatory conditions. Large numbers of mesothelial cells should raise suspicions of mesothelioma.[13]

Nonreactive macrophages (or monocytic cells) typically have an indented oval nucleus with a more homogeneous chromatin pattern. Its nucleus, however, can be quite pleomorphic, varying from elongated, round, convoluted, or lobulated.

Reactive cells tend to have more abundant, more basophilic cytoplasm. Reactive macrophages often have ruffled cytoplasmic margins, prominent cytoplasmic vacuoles, and/or inclusions (phagosomes). The latter may be unidentifiable debris or degenerating inflammatory cells or RBCs (see Figs. 8-1 and 8-3). Reactive large mononuclear cells were not observed in pleural fluid samples of 18 clinically normal horses.[11] In acute inflammatory effusions, the relative percentage of monocytes/macrophages decreases with increasing granulocytic cell numbers. In more chronic effusions, mononuclear/macrophages are typically present in increased percentages and may exhibit reactive changes.

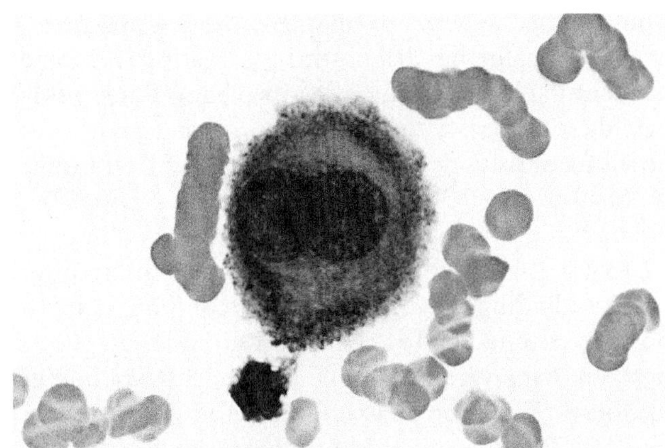

Fig. 8-5 Equine pleural fluid.
A single mesothelial cell is present. Note the increased cytoplasmic basophilia, binucleation, and ruffled cytoplasmic border, all of which support reactive transformation. (Wright-Giemsa stain)

Lymphocytes: Lymphocytes in normal pleural fluid are usually small to medium-sized cells, similar to lymphocytes in the peripheral blood. They recirculate into the bloodstream via the pleural lymphatics.

An increased lymphocyte percentage may occur in chronic inflammatory conditions, chylothorax (particularly acutely), or neoplasia. Lymphoblasts are not observed in normal pleural fluid. These cells have a densely staining, coarsely clumped chromatin pattern, possibly with obvious nucleoli, and intensely basophilic cytoplasm that may contain small to large vacuoles.

Cytologic diagnosis of lymphoma is usually based on the presence of large numbers of such cells.[13] Plasma cells are not a normal finding and may reflect chronic antigenic stimulation.

Other Cells: The morphology of eosinophils and basophils is the same in pleural fluid as in a peripheral blood smear, while that of mast cells is the same as in other tissues.

Neoplastic cells may be identified on pleural fluid cytology, although the relative diagnostic yield of this procedure for all tumor types may be low.[1,25] Neoplastic round cells (most commonly lymphoblasts), mesothelial cells (mesotheliomas), and epithelial cells (carcinomas and adenocarcinomas) are those most commonly encountered[25] (see Figs. 8-8 to 8-17). Criteria of malignancy include anisocytosis, anisokaryosis, variation in nucleus to cytoplasm ratio, increased cell size, nuclear gigantism, multinucleation, prominent/large/angular/multiple nucleoli, and increased/abnormal mitotic activity. Presence of concurrent inflammation may cloud distinction from reactive hyperplasia/dysplasia in some instances, necessitating further diagnostic investigation. Absence of identifiable neoplastic cells on pleural fluid cytology does not rule out neoplasia, since tumor cells do not consistently exfoliate into pleural effusions. In one study of 38 horses with thoracic neoplasia, pleural fluid cytologic diagnosis was achieved in only 12 (32%), 10 of which had lymphoma.[25] In another study evaluating only horses with lymphoma, 12 of 13 horses examined had pleural effusion, and fluid cytology was diagnostic in 10.[26] This suggests that a higher diagnostic yield for pleural fluid cytology is possible in cases of lymphoma than for other types of thoracic neoplasia. Given the fact that lymphoma accounts for over half of thoracic neoplasias in the equine[25,26] and that concurrent pleural effusion is common,[26,27] thoracentesis and pleural fluid cytology remain a valuable diagnostic tool.

Biochemical Examination

Biochemical analyses of pleural fluid routinely involve only determination of protein content and specific gravity. A variety of additional biochemical parameters may be measured in unique diagnostic circumstances or in research applications. Triglyceride and cholesterol concentrations are helpful in distinguishing chylous from pseudochylous effusions. Analysis of glucose, lactate, and fluid pH may aid in distinguishing *complicated* (septic) from *uncomplicated* parapneumonic effusions. Additionally, pleural fluid partial pressures of oxygen and carbon dioxide, as well as bicarbonate concentrations, have been infrequently compared with simultaneously collected venous and arterial blood gas data as a means of assessing pleural environment.[28]

Total Protein Content

For total protein measurements, pleural fluid is usually collected into an EDTA tube (as for cytologic examination). Concentrations are usually measured using a refractometer. Chemical methods, such as the biuret reaction (as for a blood sample), are also suitable. Reference values (Table 8-2) are somewhat higher than for peritoneal fluid. Nevertheless, as a generalization, the total protein concentration of normal pleural fluid is <2.5 g/dl, which is usually the lowest reading on the protein scale of most refractometers.

When sample volume is small (EDTA tube less than one quarter filled), fluid protein measurements, as determined by refractive index, may be artificially increased (solute effect of the EDTA), whereas biuret protein concentration results may be artificially decreased (dilutional effect).[18] Although, the artifactual effect is generally mild, it may reach diagnostic significance in distinguishing borderline modified transudates from either pure transudates or mild exudates.

Specific Gravity

Specific gravity is the density of a fluid as compared with distilled water, which has a value of 1.000. Periodic refractometer calibration using distilled water is recommended. Specific gravity is a reflection of the amount of dissolved solutes in the fluid, such as total protein, glucose, urea, bilirubin, and electrolytes. Reference values are given in Table 8-2. Total protein values are more commonly reported than specific gravity measurements.

Glucose and Lactate Concentrations

Water-soluble substances of low molecular weight, such as glucose and lactate, readily diffuse between the bloodstream and the thoracic cavity. Pleural fluid glucose concentrations in the healthy equine is reported to be similar to that of plasma.[29] Increased anaerobic glycolysis by metabolically active cells (leukocytes or neoplastic cells) or bacterial organisms may decrease fluid glucose concentrations. Decreased pleural fluid glucose concentrations (<40 mg/dl) are therefore useful in predicting sepsis, even in horses with negative pleural fluid cultures.[2,5,6] Pleural fluid glucose concentrations >60 mg/dl suggest an uncomplicated pleural effusion.[6]

Increased anaerobic glycolysis would be expected to increase fluid lactate concentrations. Detection of fluid lactate concentrations greater than a paired blood specimen (or fluid lactate dehydrogenase activity >1000 IU/L) lends further support to suspicion of sepsis.[28]

Unless specimens are processed immediately, tubes containing fluoride-oxalate are required for accurate

TABLE 8-3

Classification of Types of Thoracic Effusion

Effusion	Total Nucleated Cell Count	Total Protein Concentration*	Causes
Reference range (adult)	< 8000 cells/µl	< 2.5 g/dl	N/A
Transudate†	< 5,000 cells/µl (usually < 1500 cells/µl)	< 2.5 g/dl (usually <1.5 g/dl)‡	↓colloid osmotic pressure: Hypoalbuminemia ↑capillary hydrostatic pressure: Congestive heart failure; Lymphatic obstruction
Modified transudate	5000–15,000 cells/µl	2.0–5.0 g/dl	↑capillary hydrostatic pressure: Congestive heart failure; Lymphatic obstruction; Neoplasia; Lung lobe torsion; Acute esophageal perforation
Exudate	> 10,000–15,000 cells/µl	> 3.0–3.5 g/dl	↑capillary permeability: Inflammation/vasculitis; Ischemia/infarction/thromboembolism; Tissue necrosis; Lymphatic obstruction; Inflammation; Neoplasia; Acute to subacute esophageal perforation

*Determined by refractive index.
†Transudate may differ from normal thoracic fluid by increased volume alone.
‡Determined biochemically.

results. The fluoride arrests cell metabolism, thus preventing in vitro glucose depletion and lactate formation by cells and bacteria after collection.

Triglyceride and Cholesterol Concentrations

Fluid triglyceride and cholesterol concentrations are useful in distinguishing chylous from pseudochylous effusions. Chylous effusions are characterized by triglyceride concentrations greater than and cholesterol concentrations less than paired serum values.[30] Conversely, elevated fluid cholesterol and low triglyceride values are expected in pseudochylous effusions.

Pathologic Changes in Pleural Fluid

Classification of Pleural Fluid Findings

When the volume of fluid in the pleural space is increased, an effusion is present. An effusion develops when pleural fluid is produced at a faster rate than it is removed. This may be by increased transudation and/or exudation. The former produces an ascitic type of effusion, characterized by low (normal) cellularity and protein concentration. Common causes include increased capillary hydrostatic pressure, such as in congestive heart

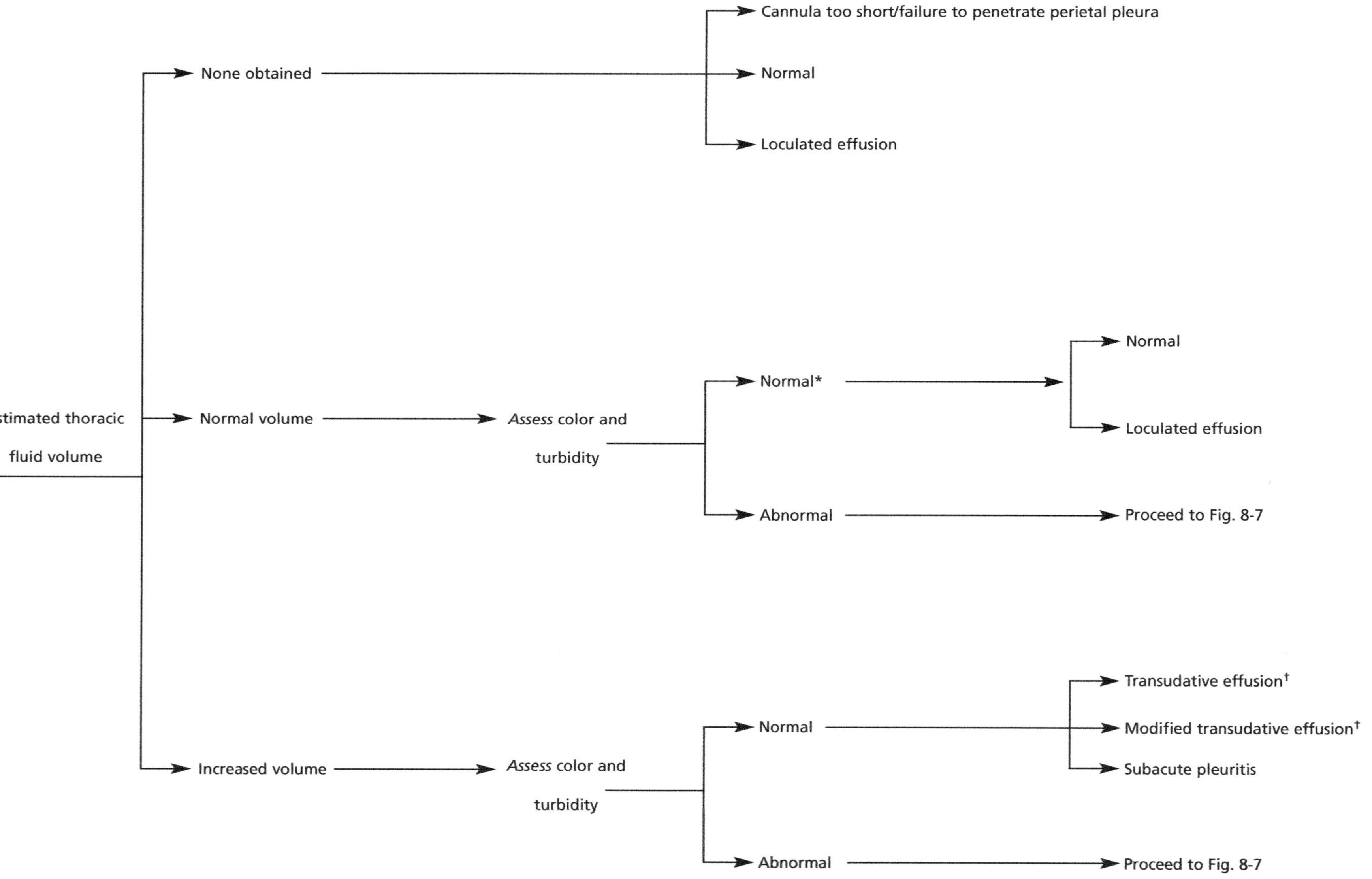

*Normal pleural fluid is light yellow to reddish yellow and clear to hazy.
†Cytologic examination is recommended, including total nucleated cell count and total protein measurement.

Fig. 8-6 Algorithm for initial approach to assessing pleural fluid specimens.

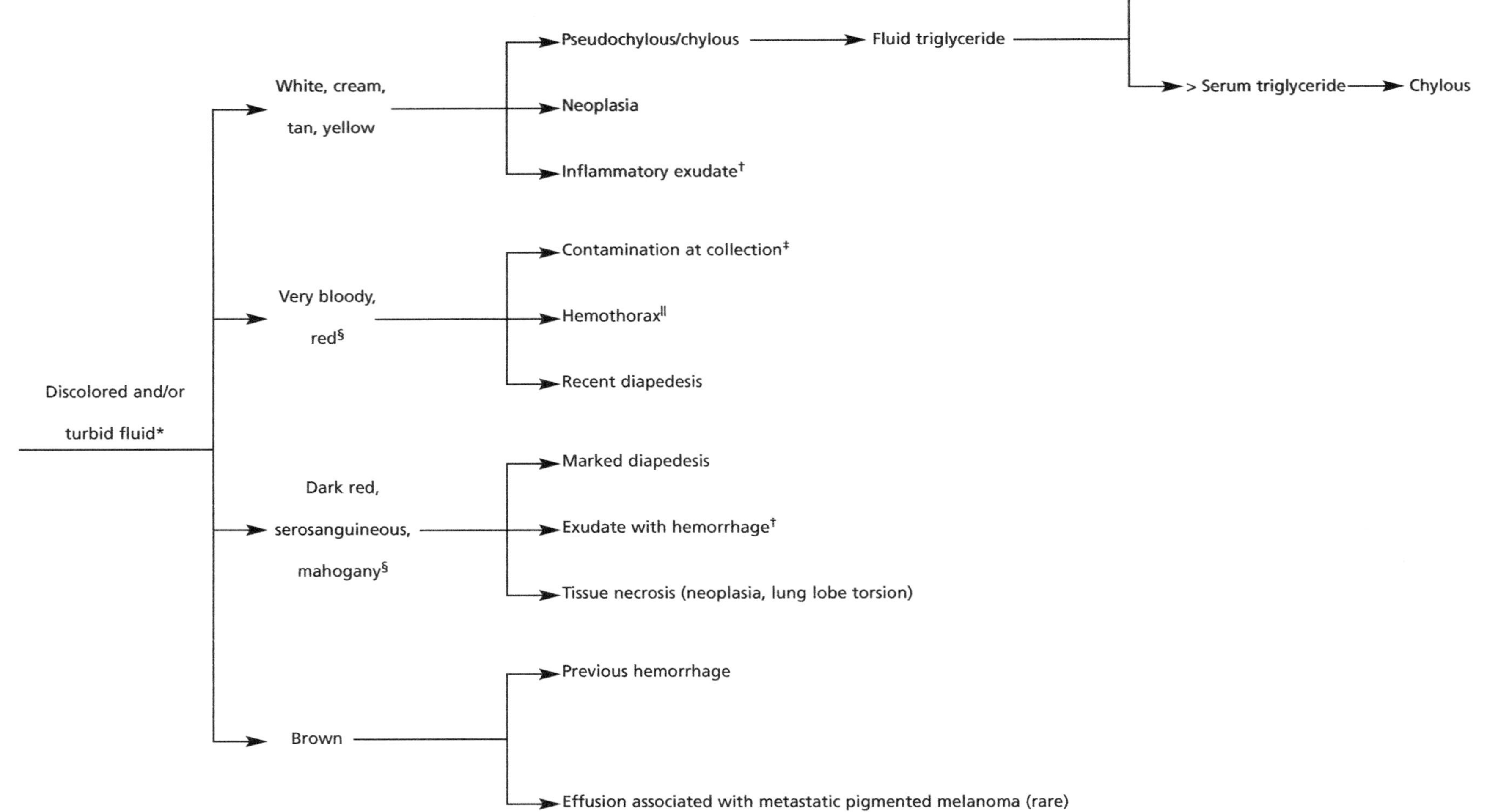

*Cytologic examination is recommended, including total nucleated cell count and total protein measurement. Neoplasia may be underlying cause of exudative or hemorrhagic effusion.

†Exudates have increased cellularity and total protein concentration. They may be subdivided into suppurative, chronic-suppurative, and chronic inflammatory reactions. Neutrophil morphology and phagocytic activity of macrophages should also be assessed (see text). Presence of bacteria denotes sepsis.

‡May be obvious during collection. May result in platelets on cytologic smears. Supernatant usually is not hemolyzed. No erythrophagocytosis.

§When pleural fluid has reddish discoloration, supernatant should be assessed for hemolysis. Hemolytic or port wine–colored supernatant suggests chronic hemorrhage or diapedesis. This may be associated with pulmonary parenchymal damage, including severe pleuritis.

||Specimen uniformly bloody throughout collection. Erythrophagocytosis may be apparent. Supernatant may be nonhemolyzed or hemolyzed. Total nucleated cell count is not greatly increased.

Fig. 8-7 Algorithmic approach to assessment of pleural fluid specimens with an abnormal gross appearance.

failure, and low plasma colloid osmotic pressure, as a result of hypoalbuminemia. In contrast, increased pleural capillary permeability and compromised lymphatic drainage, which occur in inflammation (pleuritis) and possibly in neoplasia involving the pleura, result in a fluid with increased nucleated cellularity and/or protein content.

Effusions have been classically grouped as transudates, modified transudates, exudates, or hemorrhagic effusions (Table 8-3). Though these are reasonably distinct groups, often with common pathophysiologic mechanisms linking various diseases within each category, this classification system has some limitations. For example, thoracic neoplasia and chylothorax produce effusions that do not fall neatly into any one of these categories. Furthermore, these conditions are important in their own right and do not really require classification in the above schema.

Another shortcoming of the classic classification system is that it suggests the separate categories are mutually exclusive. Such an assumption is incorrect. For example, the characteristics of transudates and modified transudates tend to merge, and these effusions often have common causes. Similarly, the distinction between some modified transudates and mild inflammatory exudates may also be quite subjective.

Finally, because pleural fluid reflects the status of the thoracic cavity and its viscera, it may change as the course of disease progresses. For example, a horse with acute pleuritis may have normal pleural fluid on thoracentesis, whereas horses with more long-standing disease usually have an obvious effusion that is exudative in character.[31,32] Despite these shortcomings, the four main categories are clinically relevant in most cases. Even if a sample does not fall neatly into a particular category, the result may still be diagnostically useful.

The following pages consider common alterations in volume, color, and turbidity of pleural fluid in various general disease processes and differentiation of pleural effusions. Figs 8-6 and 8-7 present an algorithmic approach to the interpretation of pleural fluid samples.

Transudates: Transudative (or ascitic) effusions have an increased volume with low cellularity and low total protein concentration. Because there is no lower limit to the cellularity and total protein content of normal pleural fluid, an estimate of the *volume* of fluid in the thoracic cavity is very important to classify a fluid as a transudative effusion (see Table 8-3).

Cytologic findings of transudative effusions are usually unremarkable, with neutrophils, lymphocytes, and large mononuclear cells often present in normal proportions. Cell morphology is also usually normal, except that reactive mesothelial cells may be noted (see Figs. 9-5, 9-6, 9-10, and 9-11). The latter cells may occur in any long-standing effusion and are therefore not pathognomonic for a transudative process. They are thought to result when the parietal and visceral mesothelial surfaces are separated by an excessive amount of fluid. These surfaces are usually closely apposed, resulting in contact inhibition of cellular proliferation.

Transudative effusions are uncommon in the thoracic cavity. They accounted for up to 7% of effusions in published surveys.[3,8,10,11] Causes included decreased plasma oncotic pressure secondary to hypoalbuminemia and increased venous or lymphatic pressure, such as in congestive heart failure and chronic liver disease. Other clinical and laboratory results must be considered to differentiate these causes.

Modified Transudates: Pleural fluid classified as a modified transudate has an increased volume, usually with a grossly normal appearance, a total nucleated cell count of 5000 to 15,000/µl (5.0 to 15.0 x 10^9/L), and a total protein concentration of 2.0 to 5.0 g/dl (20 to 50 g/L). Neutrophils, with normal morphology, tend to be the most numerous cells present. The exception to this generalization concerns chylous effusions, which may be opaque whitish pink, with a predominance of small lymphocytes.

Pleural effusions are seldom classified as modified transudates. They usually fall more neatly into the transudate or exudate categories. Modified transudates are most likely to result from increased venous or lymphatic pressure, as in congestive heart failure and chronic hepatic disease (see Table 8-3).

Exudates: Inflammatory exudates are the most frequent cause of pleural effusion in horses, accounting for 53% to 91% of abnormal pleural fluid specimens in published surveys.[1,3,8,10,11] Exudates have increased cellularity and total protein concentration, usually with a greatly increased volume. Their gross appearance varies with the number and relative proportions of RBCs and inflammatory cells present and can vary from reddish brown to gray or off-white in color.

The total nucleated cell count may be underestimated in some exudate fluid specimens because of cell clumping, associated with fibrin deposition, or because of marked karyolytic degeneration. These features are obvious when the smear is examined microscopically. The total nucleated cell count may also be influenced by the volume of fluid present in the thoracic cavity. For example, in resolving pleuritis, the volume of fluid in the thoracic cavity may decrease faster than the total nucleated cell count and total protein content. Consequently, though the rate of exudation may be slowing, the total nucleated cell count and protein concentration may actually increase transiently, even as the total number of cells in the pleural cavity is decreasing. It is therefore advisable to mentally adjust the total nucleated cell count and protein concentration of a specimen for the volume of fluid thought to be present in the cavity, particularly when performing serial thoracenteses to monitor the progress of disease or the response to treatment.

Exudates are classically subcategorized as either septic or nonseptic. In the horse, exudative thoracic effusions are usually the result of aerobic and/or anaerobic bacterial infection. The most common route of invasion is thought to be through the respiratory tract and lungs. Pneumonia and pulmonary abscessation are thus common concurrent findings and were noted in 39% to 77% of horses with pleuritis in four published surveys.[3,8,9,10] Predisposing factors include strenuous workouts/racing, recent respiratory viral disease, prolonged transportation with close confinement (particularly with other horses), and recent general anesthesia/surgery. The right apical lobe of the lung and right hemithorax are most frequently affected.[9,31,32] Inhaled or ingested foreign bodies and external thoracic trauma may also cause pleuropneumonia or pleuritis.[2,33-35] The former may perforate the respiratory tract or esophagus. Other infectious agents that may cause pleuritis include fungi (*Coccidioides* spp. and *Blastomyces dermatitidis*) and mycoplasmas.[3,23,36,37] Nonseptic exudates may be associated with neoplasia (see following).

Based on the proportion of neutrophils and large mononuclear cells, inflammatory reactions have been broadly grouped as follows.[38]

Suppurative (also called neutrophilic), when there are ≥70% neutrophils and ≤30% large mononuclear cells.

Chronic-suppurative (also called pyogranulomatous), when there are 50% to 70% neutrophils and 30% to 50% large mononuclear cells.

Chronic (also called granulomatous), when there are <50% neutrophils and >50% large mononuclear cells and lymphocytes.

These categories do not reflect the duration of the inflammatory process as much as the potential inciting cause. A suppurative inflammatory reaction may be very recent or may have existed for days to weeks. In contrast, chronic-suppurative and chronic inflammatory reactions tend to have been present for some period of time (days or more). Exudates of some duration often reveal increased phagocytic activity by macrophages, with ingested nucleated cells, RBCs, and unidentifiable debris. Cytoplasmic vacuolation is also relatively common in such situations. The numbers of lymphocytes may also increase in chronic inflammatory reactions and in the resolving stages of septic pleuritis. Most of these cells have a normal appearance (see Fig. 9-12), but occasionally large lymphoblastic-like cells may be observed.

Inflammatory exudation of proteins results in a high fibrinogen content in the pleural fluid, which may sometimes be observed on the cytologic smear. Nevertheless, the fluid may or may not clot when placed in a clot tube. Lack of coagulation suggests mechanical defibrinization or fibrinolysis by leukocytic or bacterial enzymes.

Assessing cell morphology is important when evaluating exudates. Bacterial cytotoxins may rapidly damage inflammatory cells in vivo, particularly neutrophils. Such sudden cell injury causes nuclear degeneration, noted as swollen, pale-staining nuclei (karyolysis) that may fragment (karyorrhexis). Karyolysis may be subjectively graded as mild (or slight), moderate, or marked (see Fig. 8-2). Whenever karyolysis is observed, the smear should be carefully examined for bacteria. The more marked the karyolysis, the greater the suspicion of sepsis. If bacteria are not found (or cultured) in such fluids, they are still the most likely cause of the exudative process but may be restricted to the pleura or to an abscess or loculated pocket elsewhere in the cavity.

Normal neutrophil morphology (possibly with evidence of some pyknotic degeneration) does not exclude a bacterial etiology. If the inciting microorganisms are walled off from the area of pleural cavity sampled, if they produce scant amounts of cytotoxins, or if antimicrobial therapy is initiated, cell morphology may remain normal despite a marked inflammatory response. Bacteria in a smear may be free and/or phagocytized. Mixed populations of organisms may be present. Both gram-positive and gram-negative microbes stain basophilically with Romanowsky stains.

Aerobic and anaerobic bacterial cultures are recommended for all pleural exudates, even if organisms are not observed microscopically. Anaerobic bacteria are common respiratory pathogens.[32,39] Their culture requires special transport media and careful handling. Because many are sensitive to cold, samples should not be refrigerated.

Commonly isolated aerobic organisms include *Escherichia coli*, *Rhodococcus* (*Corynebacterium*) *equi*, and species of *Pasteurella*, *Pseudomonas*, *Staphylococcus*, and *Streptococcus*.[3,9,32,39] Commonly isolated anaerobic species include *Bacteroides*, and *Clostridium*.[3,9,32,39] Mixed infections are common. Not all infected horses yield positive pleural fluid cultures, though bacteria are the most likely cause of the exudate. Of these horses with negative pleural fluid cultures, some may yield bacterial isolates from tracheobronchial aspirates.[9,32,39] It is therefore worthwhile to also culture tracheobronchial aspirates.

Findings Associated with Various Conditions

Pleuropneumonia

From a clinical perspective, four stages of pleuropneumonia have been suggested: subacute, acute, chronic, and end-stage.[31] These categories are not mutually exclusive and represent a continuum of the disease process. Though they do not have precise cytologic corollaries, analysis of pleural fluid helps to separate them.

Subacute pleuropneumonia describes the pathologic changes about 1 to 4 days after infection. Clinical signs are related to pneumonitis; with appropriate (symptomatic) therapy, the disease may be self-limiting, with minimal pleural involvement.[31,40]

Acute pleuropneumonia refers to the period about ½ to 2 weeks after infection, when the pneumonic condition has continued or worsened.[31,40] Though an exudative pleural effusion becomes apparent, bacteria may not have invaded the thoracic cavity per se.

Chronic pleuropneumonia refers to cases of 2 to 4 weeks' duration. By this time, a septic fibrinopurulent pleuritis has developed.[31,41]

End-stage pleuropneumonia refers to cases of a month or more in duration. By this time abscessation, loculation of fluid within the thoracic cavity, bronchopleural fistulas, and pleural scarring (fibrosis) have developed.[31,41] The prognosis for survival and return to work may be good to guarded in the subacute and acute stages but is poor to grave as the disease progresses.

Pleural fluid volume, total nucleated cell count, and total protein concentration are not good guides to prognosis.[9,13,42] Though small volumes of fluid suggest that an effusion is not present, limited quantities may also be related to obstruction of the cannula portals with either fibrin or lung tissue, incomplete insertion of the cannula through the parietal pleura, or centesis into an inappropriate location. Ultrasonography is useful to discern the reason for poor sample recovery and identify a suitable area for subsequent centesis attempts.[13,17] In contrast, large volumes of fluid are more easily interpreted and denote marked effusion. The total nucleated cell count, total protein content, and cellular composition of pleural fluid are useful to confirm pleuritis and (often) sepsis. There is, however, no relationship between total nucleated cell count or total protein concentration and survival.[9,13]

Whether a differing prognosis exists between horses with aerobic infections versus those with anaerobic infections is unclear. Some authors have found significantly greater survival rates for horses with aerobic infections over those with anaerobic infections,[32,39] while another detected no such difference.[41] Many horses with anaerobic infections (about 62%) have a putrid odor to their pleural fluid and/or breath (or tracheal wash).[32] Aerobes do not typically cause such a fetid smell. Hence, in the field situation, if the specimen has a putrefactive aroma, anaerobes are almost certainly involved. Note that lack of such an odor does not rule out anaerobic infection.

Neutrophils are the predominant leukocyte in most parapneumonic effusions; however, some effusions associated with anaerobic infections may contain numerous bacterial organisms and virtually no identifiable cells. In cellular effusions, neutrophil degenerative changes are common[1,13] (see Fig. 8-2). Large mononuclear cells may be plentiful and reactive. In effusions of longer duration, mesothelial cell hyperplasia and reactivity may mimic neoplastic change. There are usually few (if any) lymphocytes in an exudative effusion, and their morphology is generally normal. Large atypical lymphoblastic cells are sometimes present and may be confused with neoplastic lymphocytes. Cytologic diagnosis of lymphoma (see later) is usually based on the presence of large numbers of such cells. Plasma cells might also be expected to occur in pleural fluid in response to chronic antigenic stimulation. This has been described in peritoneal fluid.[43] Eosinophils are very uncommon in inflammatory pleural effusions but have been reported.[11]

Hemorrhagic Effusions

Hemorrhagic effusions have a uniformly bloody appearance during collection. A specimen that is initially nonhemorrhagic but becomes discolored with RBCs likely contains iatrogenic contamination from intercostal blood vessels. If the fluid is uniformly bloody throughout collection, iatrogenic contamination may have occurred, but previous hemorrhage into the thoracic cavity should also be considered.

Hemorrhage (RBCs) in a pleural fluid sample may be the result of iatrogenic contamination at collection, hemorrhagic diapedesis, or intrathoracic hemorrhage.

Iatrogenic Contamination: A small amount of hemorrhage from intercostal blood vessels is common in pleural fluid samples. If the specimen becomes less bloody or actually clears of blood during collection, contamination at collection is obvious. Iatrogenic hemorrhage should also be considered in specimens that are uniformly bloody throughout the collection process. Recent hemorrhage (during or a few hours before collection) usually produces a clear to plasma-like supernatant upon centrifugation, rather than one that is hemolyzed. Microscopy may reveal platelets, often pale staining and clumped, with negligible erythrophagocytosis.

Hemorrhagic Diapedesis: Hemorrhagic diapedesis may be associated with pleuritis or neoplasia. The gross appearance of the fluid varies, depending on the relative amounts of RBCs and inflammatory cells. The supernatant may appear hemolyzed. Actual RBC counts seldom exceed 750,000/µl (750 × 10^9/L).[11] Erythrophagocytosis may be observed (see Figs. 8-3 and 8-4). Other cytologic findings depend on the underlying cause.

Intrathoracic Hemorrhage: Few cases of hemothorax are described in the literature.[8,11,19] Hemothorax may occur with trauma, bleeding diatheses, major vessel laceration, tumor or abscess rupture, pulmonary infarction, or lung lobe torsion.[13,19] The pleural fluid PCV and total protein concentration is generally less than that of peripheral blood but might be comparable in cases of severe hemorrhage. As in cases of hemoperitoneum, cytologic examination would probably reveal leukocytes in proportions similar to those in peripheral blood and few (if any) platelets. The fluid may not clot because of rapid defibrination in the pleural cavity. Hence, lack of coagulation after collection in a clot tube would not necessarily indicate coagulopathy. If the fluid has a clear, plasma-like supernatant and there is no cytologic evidence of erythrophagocytosis, the hemorrhage probably occurred recently. A hemolyzed supernatant and/or erythrophagocytosis suggests a more long-standing disorder (see Figs. 8-3 and 8-4).

Chylothorax

Chylothorax is very rare in horses. Such effusions have been described in foals to be associated with congenital diaphragmatic hernia, meconium impaction, and idiopathic causes.[44-46] No reports of chylothorax in adult horses exist in the literature.

Grossly, the fluid of chylothorax is whitish pink and milky opaque. Pseudochylous effusions of severe chronic inflammation may be grossly similar in appearance. Upon standing or with centrifugation, the numerous leukocytes of pseudochylous effusions tend to form sediment topped by clear supernatant. In contrast, true chylous effusions fail to clear with centrifugation. With standing or refrigeration, the lipids of chylous effusions tend to form a cream layer on the surface of the specimen. Alkalization and the addition of ether cause dissolution of chylomicrons and clearing of chylous specimens.

Fluid triglyceride and cholesterol concentrations are the most reliable tests in distinguishing chylous from pseudochylous effusions. Chylous effusions are characterized by triglyceride concentrations greater than and cholesterol concentrations less than paired serum values. Conversely, elevated fluid cholesterol and low triglyceride values are expected in pseudochylous effusions.

Microscopically, chylous effusions may be observed to contain a high percentage of small lymphocytes in the acute stages, and a circulating lymphopenia may be present. In longer standing effusions, however, mixed inflammatory reactions can occur. Sudan III, Sudan IV, or Oil Red O stain for lipid can be used on air-dried fluid smears to assess the presence of chylomicrons, characteristic of chylous effusion.[38] In our experience, residual stain and stain precipitant may be difficult to discern from chylomicrons, and tiny refractive bodies representing chylomicrons may more readily be visualized on unstained wet mounts (lowered condenser, reduced light).

Neoplasia

Neoplasia involving the chest cavity may produce an effusion. Thoracic neoplasia accounted for 5% to 38% of pleural effusions in four published reviews.[3,8,10,11] Lymphoma was the most frequent cause, accounting for 33% to 100% of these tumors. Pleural fluid cytology can be useful in establishing the diagnosis of intrathoracic neoplasia, but the diagnostic yield of this procedure is variable.[1,25,26,47] Successful cytologic diagnosis appears to be more frequent for lymphoma than for other types of neoplasia.[26,47] This may be related to more frequent incidence, greater likelihood of pleural involvement, higher degree of neoplastic cell exfoliation, and lesser extent of concurrent inflammation diluting the neoplastic cell population. Mesotheliomas, carcinomas, and adenocarcinomas may also be encountered.[25]

The following points should be kept in mind when evaluating pleural effusions from horses with suspected intrathoracic neoplasia:

1. *Intrathoracic tumors* may not exfoliate cells into the pleural fluid. This would preclude diagnosis by thoracentesis. Pleuroscopy may be useful to visualize intrathoracic masses and pleural metastases.[48]
2. *Tumors that obstruct lymph flow* from the pleural cavity may produce a voluminous effusion, characteristic of a modified transudate.
3. *Tumors involving serosal surfaces*, especially those that erode serosal blood vessels, may cause hemorrhagic diapedesis or hemothorax.
4. *Necrosis or infection of a tumor* may result in pleuritis. Such an inflammatory exudate may overshadow the presence of tumor cells.
5. *Reactive mesothelial cells* may be mistaken for neoplastic cells, especially by the novice cytologist. Such cells may arise in any effusion.

Examination of multiple fluid aliquots is suggested to enhance the likelihood of a cytologic diagnosis of neoplasia in suspect cases.[5] Concentration of fluid for cytologic examination by some means (either cytocentrifugation or sediment smears) may facilitate identification of neoplastic cells when they constitute only a small percentage of total nucleated cells.

Lymphoma: Lymphoma has been categorized into four main forms: alimentary, cutaneous, mediastinal (thymic), and multicentric.[27,49,50] A thoracic effusion may occur in the alimentary and multicentric forms of the disease. It may have characteristics of a modified transudate or a hemorrhagic effusion. Though neoplastic cells are not always observed in such fluids, when present they may allow diagnosis.[3,47,51,52] Neoplastic lymphocytes are frequently lymphoblasts. They are usually large cells, with a high nuclear to cytoplasmic ratio, and basophilic cytoplasm (Figs. 8-8 to 8-13). They exhibit variable, often

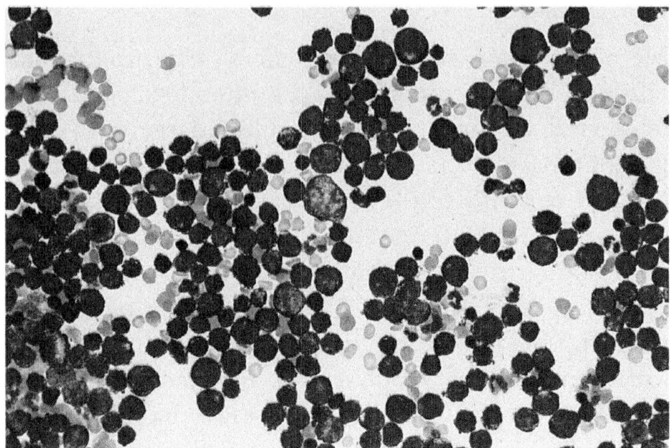

Fig. 8-8 Pleural effusion from equine lymphoma.
Note the heterogeneous population of lymphocytic cells. The diagnosis of lymphoma in the horse may be complicated by the presence of both mature lymphocytes and neoplastic lymphoblasts. (Wright-Giemsa stain)

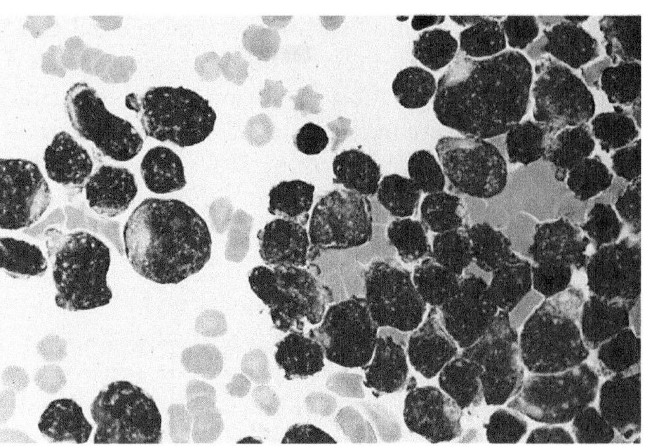

Fig. 8-9 Equine lymphoma.
Higher magnification view of a neoplastic effusion similar to the one in Fig. 8-8 from another horse with thoracic lymphoma. Lymphoid cells vary from blastic to mature in morphology. (Wright-Giemsa stain)

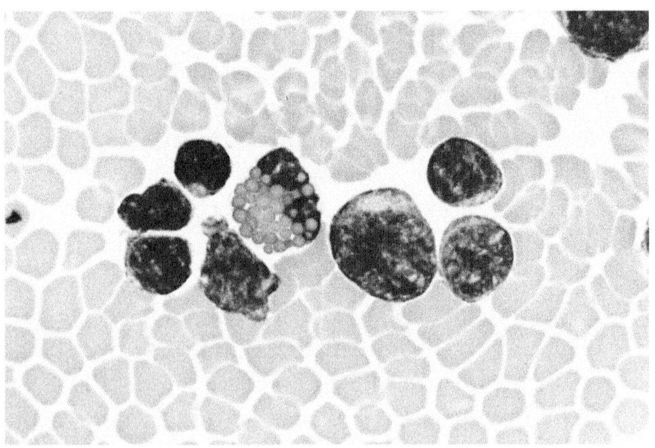

Fig. 8-10 Mixed-cell lymphoma.
A single eosinophil is seen at the center of the field. Eosinophils may be increased in lymphoma as part of a paraneoplastic reaction. (Wright-Giemsa stain)

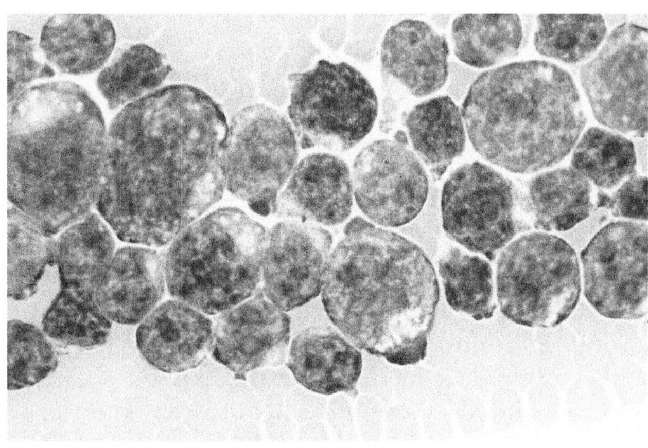

Fig. 8-11 Equine lymphoma.
Note the different morphologic appearance. Characteristic features include paler staining nuclear chromatin and more prominent nucleoli. Again a mixed-size lymphoid-cell population is observed. (Wright-Giemsa stain)

marked anisokaryosis and anisocytosis. Their nucleus is usually round to oval but may be indented or cleaved. The chromatin pattern is generally fairly uniform and delicate. Nucleoli are often prominent and may vary in number, size, and shape within and between cells. A few mitotic figures may be seen, some with abnormal spindle formation. Mitotic activity is not diagnostic of lymphoma and may occur in other tumors and in some nonneoplastic disorders.

Other forms of lymphoma involving pleural fluid, such as the histiocytic and lymphocytic types, have not been described in the literature. Based on findings in other specimens, histiocytic lymphoma is characterized by large cells, with considerable anisokaryosis, anisocytosis, and variable nuclear to cytoplasmic ratio. These cells frequently have abundant, slightly to moderately basophilic cytoplasm (see Fig. 9-26). In lymphocytic (small-cell) lymphoma, lymphocytes are well differentiated and therefore have normal morphology. Differential diagnoses for effusions with an increased percentage of small lymphocytes include chylothorax and lymphocytic inflammation associated with antigenic

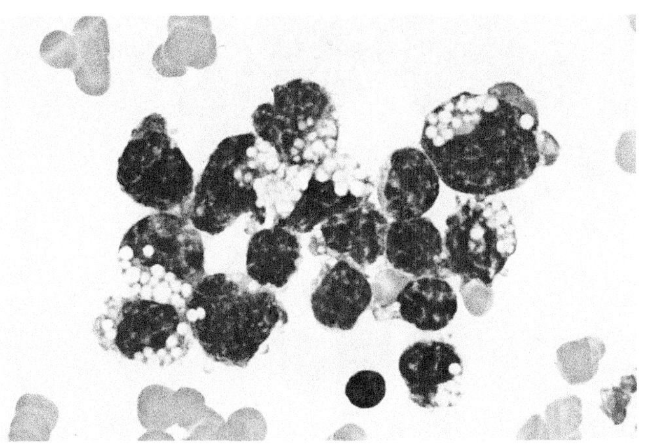

Fig. 8-12 Equine lymphoma.
Yet another morphologic appearance of equine lymphoma. These neoplastic lymphoblasts exhibit cytoplasmic vacuolation, giving them a vaguely histiocytic appearance. (Wright-Giemsa stain)

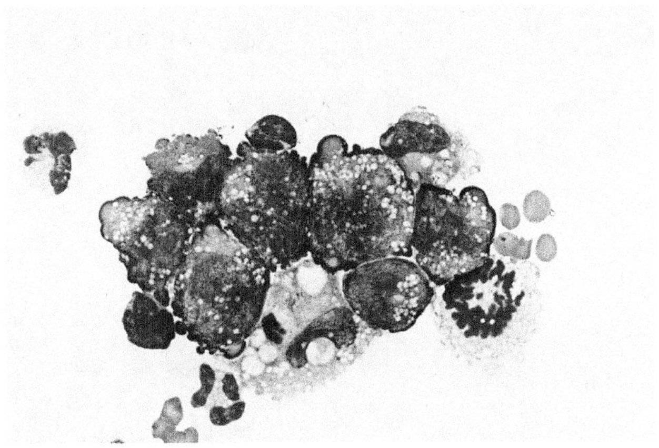

Fig. 8-13 Equine lymphoma.
Note vacuolated morphologic appearance of lymphoma from another horse. These cells feature round to indented, eccentric nuclei having irregularly clumped chromatin and one or more indistinct nucleoli. Cytoplasm is moderately basophilic, mildly increased in volume, with ruffled margins and frequent cytoplasmic vacuolation. Special stains and immunophenotyping were necessary to distinguish lymphoid from histiocytic or other tissue origin. A mitotic cell, mildly degenerate neutrophils, and a cytophagic macrophage are also present. (Wright-Giemsa stain) (Courtesy Dr. Christine A. Stanton, North Carolina State University, Raleigh.)

stimulation (see Fig. 9-12). Eosinophils have been reported to accompany lymphoma in the horse as part of a paraneoplastic process[53] (Fig. 8-10).

Immunophenotyping of equine lymphoma into B-cell, T-cell, or nonimmunoreactive categories is possible using antibodies to cell surface antigens. In one study of 31 cases of equine lymphoma, 24 (77%) were found to be of B-cell origin. Many of these tumors (11/24, 46%), however, contained a heterogeneous mixture of both B- and T-lymphocytes, with nonneoplastic T-cells constituting 40% to 80% of nucleated cells.[54]

Squamous-Cell Carcinoma: Squamous-cell carcinomas occasionally metastasize to the pleural cavity.[55-57] Most frequently, these metastases originate from primary gastric squamous-cell carcinoma, arising less often from other sites including prepuce, vulva, penis, oral cavity, or eye.[47] In metastatic gastric squamous-cell carcinoma, clinical signs of thoracic involvement are uncommon but may include tachycardia, dyspnea, ventral thoracic edema, and diminished ventral lung sounds. Radiographic evidence of pleural effusion is common, and fluid cytology is most often consistent with a suppurative exudate.[47]

Neoplastic cells may exfoliate into the pleural fluid as clusters or as individual cells, with quite variable morphology (see Figs. 9-30 and 9-31). Well-differentiated tumors have large squamous-type cells with a medium-sized to large nucleus, a reticular to coarsely clumped chromatin pattern, indistinct nucleoli, and a moderate to low nuclear to cytoplasmic ratio. Cytoplasm is abundant and pale blue when Romanowsky stains are used, may be slightly vacuolated (particularly perinuclearly), and may possibly be partly cornified. The last imparts a smooth, glassy, homogeneous appearance to the cytoplasm. Less-well-differentiated tumors may exhibit greater anisokaryosis and anisocytosis with variable (often high) nuclear to cytoplasmic ratios. Nuclei are irregularly round and nucleoli may be prominent and variable in size, shape, and number within and between cells.

Adenocarcinoma: Metastatic adenocarcinomas are reported to constitute 43% of metastatic thoracic neoplasia.[47] Primary sites include kidney, ovary, uterus, mammary gland, pancreas, thyroid gland, and undetermined.[47,58] Effusions resulting from metastatic involvement can vary in classification from transudates to exudates. Only infrequently do such effusions contain identifiable neoplastic cells. Cytologic features supporting a diagnosis of adenocarcinoma would include the presence of neoplastic epithelial cell clusters, with cells organized into ducts, tubules, or acinar structures (Figs. 8-14 and 8-15). Additionally, the cytoplasm may contain clear vacuoles or vacuoles containing secretory product. Special stains may enhance the cytologic diagnosis of adenocarcinoma when frequent cytoplasmic vacuolation is present. PAS stain will aid in distinguishing glycoprotein secretory material, particularly when coupled with diastase to rule out cytoplasmic glycogen.[13]

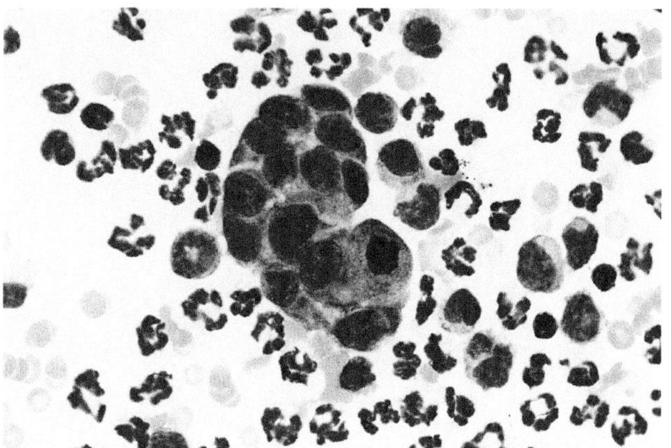

Fig. 8-14 Adenocarcinoma.
A single cluster of uniform epithelial cells are present within a background of chronic suppurative inflammation in equine pleural fluid. Only mild variation in cell size and nuclear size are evident to support a diagnosis of neoplasia. These neoplastic cells would be difficult to distinguish cytologically from reactive mesothelial cells; however, the subtle acinar formation supports a diagnosis of adenocarcinoma. (Wright-Giemsa stain)

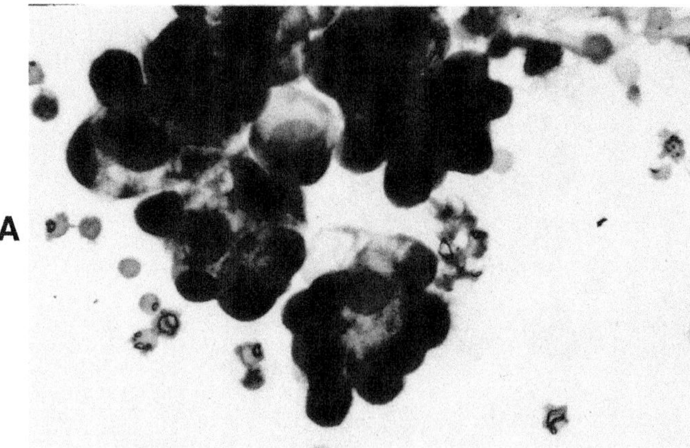

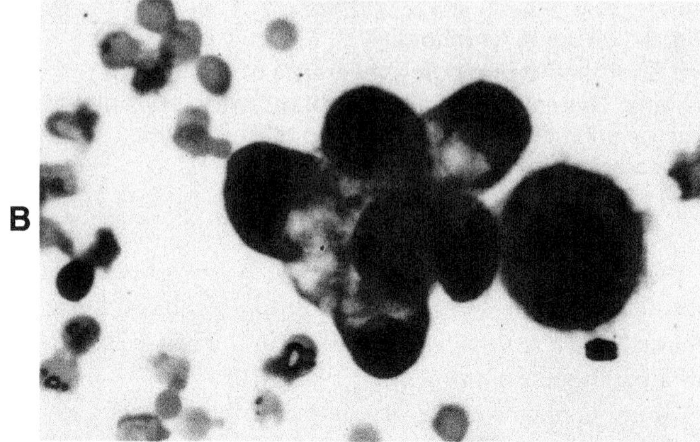

Fig. 8-15 Metastatic mammary adenocarcinoma.
A, Note acinar clusters of cells with moderate anisokaryosis. **B,** Note marked anisokaryosis and anisocytosis and varied nucleus to cytoplasm ratio. (Wright's stain; original magnification 400X)

Mesothelioma: Pleural mesothelioma may occur as a primary tumor, when arising from the visceral or parietal pleura, or less frequently as a metastatic tumor arising from the mesothelium of the pericardial or peritoneal cavities.[47] Pleural effusion is commonly observed, and cytologic examination frequently reveals numerous individual and clustered, pleomorphic mesothelial cells.[47] The distinction between reactive and neoplastic mesothelial cells may not be easy, particularly in the presence of concurrent inflammation. Neoplastic mesothelial cells are characterized by a pleomorphic appearance, with mild to marked anisokaryosis and anisocytosis. The nuclear to cytoplasmic ratio is likewise variable. Cells may be arranged in small aggregates of a few cells to large clusters of more than 50. Larger aggregates resemble polyps, pseudomembranes, solid spheres, or chains of cells. Cell borders are distinct. Nuclei are round to oval, and multinucleation is common (3-4 nuclei/cell) (Fig. 8-16). Mitoses may be readily observed. Cytoplasmic volume may vary widely between cells and may contain clear vacuoles. Vacuoles vary from multiple small to medium-sized vacuoles to single very large vacuoles that displace the nucleus marginally and greatly distended the cell (signet ring formation). Such vacuolation may also be seen with adenocarcinomas, but acinar arrangements of cells favor a diagnosis of adenocarcinoma.

Electron microscopy and/or immunohistochemistry may be necessary to confirm mesothelial cell lineage.[58]

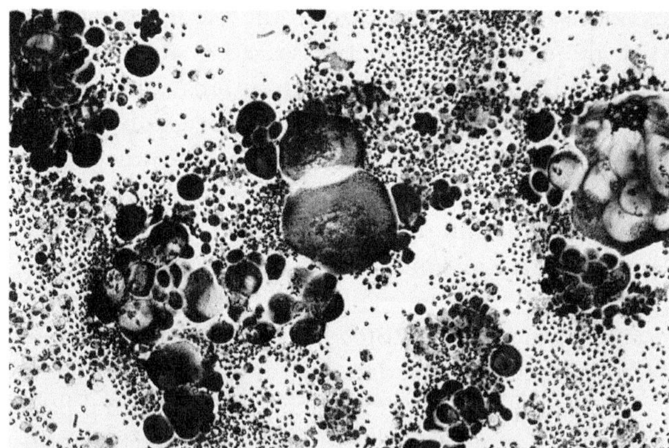

Fig. 8-16 Equine pleural malignant mesothelioma.
Numerous clusters of neoplastic mesothelial cells are present within a background of chronic suppurative inflammation. Criteria of malignancy include giant cell size, marked anisocytosis and anisokaryosis, marked variation in N:C ratio, and multiple/prominent/angular nucleoli. Signet ring forms, cytoplasmic vacuolation, and emperipolesis are also observed. (Wright-Giemsa stain)

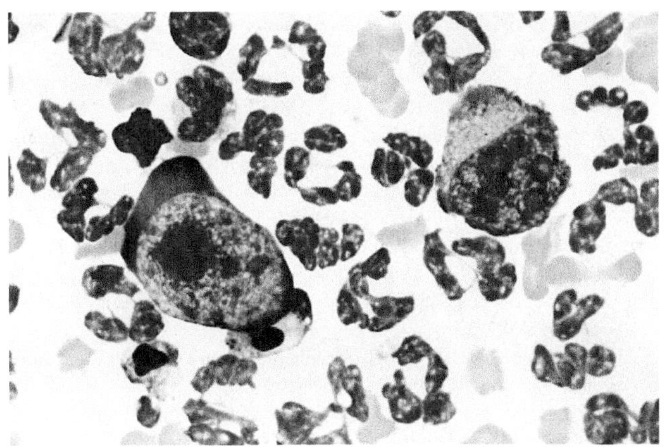

Fig. 8-17 Undifferentiated round-cell neoplasia from thoracic cavity of horse.
Neoplastic discrete cells are present within a background of suppurative inflammation. These cells are large, with irregularly round, eccentric nuclei, having clumped chromatin, and several, variably sized, sometimes large nucleoli. Cytoplasm is scanty and varies from moderately to deeply basophilic staining. Differential diagnoses would include lymphoma, other round-cell neoplasia, mesothelioma, or undifferentiated carcinoma. (Wright-Giemsa stain)

Other Tumors: Hemangiosarcoma, either arising within or metastasizing to the thoracic cavity, is an uncommon cause of thoracic effusion in the equine.[47] Hemothorax may be associated with presence of thoracic hemangiosarcoma (see Fig. 9-32). Neoplastic cells were not noted in fluid specimens from previously reported cases but would be anticipated to resemble neoplastic endothelial cells in other tissues.

A variety of carcinomas have been reported to occur rarely within the thoracic cavity of the equine and result in formation of an effusion. These include primary lung carcinomas and metastatic renal carcinoma, melanoma,[25] and pancreatic adenocarcinoma.[58] Neoplastic cells may or may not be identified on fluid cytology (Fig. 8-17).

Metastatic fibrosarcoma of the thorax has been reported to produce a voluminous pleural effusion containing numerous to no neoplastic cells.[47,59] Omental fibrosarcoma has been reported in a horse with both thoracic and abdominal exudative effusions; however, neoplastic cells were not identified.[58] A single case report of gastric leiomyosarcoma documented concurrent exudative thoracic and abdominal effusions.[58] Similarly, metastatic rhabdomyosarcoma of the thorax was reported to result in thoracic effusion in one of two cases.[47] Fluid was blood tinged but contained a normal nucleated cell distribution and protein content.

Hepatoblastoma with pleural metastasis was reported to cause a hemorrhagic type of effusion.[60] Neoplastic cells were not observed in the fluid, however.

Incidental Findings

Glove powder (corn starch) may occasionally contaminate pleural fluid specimens. Microscopically it appears as variably sized, round to hexagonal particles with a central fissure or cross (see Fig. 9-37). They are usually clear (nonstaining) with Romanowsky stains but may have a bluish hue. A central fissure or cross is prominent when examined under polarized light (see Fig. 9-38).

Cornified squamous epithelial cells, presumably from superficial skin contamination, are occasionally observed.[42] Rarely, adherent bacterial cocci are associated with their surface.

REFERENCES

1. Schott and Mansmann: Management of pleural effusion in the horse. *Proc Am Assoc Equine Pract* 35:439-449, 1990.
2. Byars and Becht: Pleuropneumonia. *Vet Clin North Am (Equine Pract)* 7(1):63-78, 1991.
3. Smith: Pleuritis and pleural effusion in the horse: a study of 37 cases. *JAVMA* 170:208-211, 1977.
4. Raphel and Beech: Pleuritis secondary to pneumonia or lung abscessation in 90 horses. *JAVMA* 181:808-810, 1982.
5. Schott and Mansmann: Thoracic drainage in horses. *Compend Contin Ed Pract Vet* 12(2):251-261, 1990.
6. Chaffin et al: Equine bacterial pleuropneumonia. Part II. Clinical signs and diagnostic evaluation. *Compend Contin Ed Pract Vet* 16(3):362-378, 1994.
7. Smith: Diseases of the pleura. *Vet Clin North Am (Equine Pract)* 1:197-204, 1979.
8. Mair: Pleural effusions in the horse. *Vet Annual* 27:139-146, 1987.
9. Raphel and Beech: Pleuritis secondary to pneumonia or lung abscessation in 90 horses. *JAVMA* 181:808-810, 1982.
10. Raphel and Beech: Pleuritis and pleural effusion in the horse. *Proceedings of the 27th Annual Convention AAEP*, 1981, pp 17-25.
11. Wagner and Bennett: Analysis of equine thoracic fluid. *Vet Clin Pathol* 11(1):13-17, 1982.
12. Parry: in Cowell and Tyler: *Cytology and Hematology of the Horse*. Goleta, CA, 1992, American Veterinary Publishers, pp 107-120.
13. Beech: in Beech: *Equine Respiratory Disorders*. Philadelphia, 1991, Lea & Febiger, pp 27-40, 63-68, 215-222.
14. Derksen: in Robinson: *Current Therapy in Equine Medicine*. Philadelphia, 1987, Saunders, pp 579-581.
15. Chaffin: Thoracentesis and pleural drainage in horses. *Equine Vet Ed* 10(2):106-108, 1998.
16. Roudebush and Sweeney: Thoracic percussion. *JAVMA* 197:714-718, 1990.
17. Reimer: Diagnostic ultrasonography of the equine thorax. *Comp Cont Ed Pract Vet* 12:1321-1327, 1990.
18. Knoll and MacWilliams: EDTA-induced artifact in abdominal fluid analysis associated with insufficient sample volume. *Proceedings of the 24th Annual Meeting, American Society of Veterinary Clinical Pathology*, p 13, 1989.
19. Perkins et al: Hemothorax in 2 horses. *J Vet Intern Med* 13:375-378, 1999.
20. Bach: Exfoliative cytology of peritoneal fluid in the horse. *Vet Annual* 13:102-109, 1973.
21. Bach and Ricketts: Paracentesis as an aid to the diagnosis of abdominal disease in the horse. *Equine Vet J* 6:116-121, 1974.
22. Brownlow et al: Reference values for equine peritoneal fluid. *Equine Vet J* 13:127-130, 1981.

23. Toribio et al: Thoracic and abdominal blastomycosis in the horse. *JAVMA* 214(9):1357-1360, 1999.
24. Barrelet: Peritoneal fluid: part 2—cytologic exam. *Equine Vet Ed* 5(3):126-128, 1993.
25. Mair and Brown: Clinical and pathological features of thoracic neoplasia in the horse. *Equine Vet J* 25(3):220-223, 1993.
26. Garber et al: Sonographic findings in horses with mediastinal lymphosarcoma—13 cases (1985-1992). *JAVMA* 205(10):1432-1436, 1994.
27. Mair et al: Clinicopathological features of lymphosarcoma involving the thoracic cavity in the horse. *Equine Vet J* 17(6):428-433, 1985.
28. Brumbaugh and Benson: Partial pressures of oxygen and carbon dioxide, pH, and concentrations of bicarbonate, lactate, and glucose in pleural fluid from horses. *Am J Vet Res* 51(7):1032-1037, 1990.
29. Schott and Mansmann: Glucose concentration in equine pleural effusion. *Proceedings of the 7th Veterinary Respiratory Symposium, Comp Respiratory Society*, p 32, 1988.
30. Meadows and MacWilliams: Chylous effusions revisited. *Vet Clin Pathol* 23(2):54-62, 1994.
31. Mansmann: The stages of equine pleuropneumonia. *Proceedings of the 29th Annual Convention AAEP*, 1983, pp 61-63.
32. Sweeney et al: Diseases of the lung: diagnostic approach and management of horses with anaerobic pleuropneumonia. *Proceedings of the 30th Annual Convention AAEP*, 1984, pp 263-273.
33. Collins et al: Pleural effusion associated with acute and chronic pleuropneumonia and pleuritis secondary to thoracic wounds in horses: 43 cases (1982-1992). *JAVMA* 205(12):1753-1758, 1994.
34. Hultgren et al: Pleuritis and pneumonia attributed to a conifer twig in a bronchus of a horse. *JAVMA* 189:797-798, 1986.
35. O'Brien: Septic pleuritis associated with an inhaled foreign body in a pony. *Vet Record* 119:274-275, 1986.
36. Hoffman et al: Mycoplasma felis pleuritis in two show-jumper horses. *Cornell Vet* 82(2):155-162, 1992.
37. Rosendal et al: Detection of antibodies to *Mycoplasma felis* in horses. *JAVMA* 188:292-294, 1986.
38. Rebar: *Handbook of Veterinary Cytology*. St Louis, 1980, Ralston Purina, pp 29-36.
39. Sweeney et al: Aerobic and anaerobic bacterial isolates from horses with pneumonia or pleuropneumonia and antimicrobial susceptibility patterns of the aerobes. *JAVMA* 198(5): 839-842, 1991.
40. Arthur: Subacute and acute pleuritis. *Proceedings of the 29th Annual Convention AAEP*, 1983, pp 65-69.
41. Mansmann: Chronic pleuropneumonia. *Proceedings of the 29th Annual Convention AAEP*, 1983, pp 71-73.
42. Bennett: Evaluation of pleural fluid in the diagnosis of thoracic disease in the horse. *JAVMA* 188:814-815, 1986.
43. Brownlow: Abdominal paracentesis in the horse. A clinical evaluation. MVSc thesis. Sydney, 1979, University of Sydney.
44. Mair et al: Chylothorax associated with a congenital diaphragmatic defect in a foal. *Equine Vet J* 20:304-306, 1988.
45. Scarratt et al: Chylothorax and meconium impaction in a neonatal colt. *Equine Vet J* 29:77-79, 1997.
46. Schumacher et al: Chylothorax in an Arabian filly. *Equine Vet J* 21(2): 132-134, 1989.
47. Scarratt and Crisman: Neoplasia of the respiratory tract. *Vet Clin North Am (Equine Pract)* 14(3):451-471, 1998.
48. Mackey and Wheat: Endoscopic examination of the equine thorax. *Equine Vet J* 17:140-142, 1985.
49. van den Hoven and Franken: Clinical aspects of lymphosarcoma in the horse: a clinical report of 16 cases. *Equine Vet J* 15:49-53, 1983.
50. Theilen and Madewell: *Veterinary Cancer Medicine*. 2nd ed. Philadelphia, 1987, Lea & Febiger, pp 431-437.
51. Schalm: Lymphosarcoma in the horse. *Equine Pract* 3(2):23-27, 1981.
52. Mair et al: Clinicopathological features of lymphosarcoma involving the thoracic cavity in the horse. *Equine Vet J* 17:428-433, 1985.
53. Duckett and Matthews: Hypereosinophilia in a horse with intestinal lymphosarcoma. *Can Vet J* 38:719-720, 1997.
54. Kelley and Mahaffey: Equine malignant lymphomas: morphologic and immunohistochemical classification. *Vet Pathol* 35(4):241-252, 1998.
55. Meuten et al: Gastric carcinoma with pseudohyperparathyroidism in a horse. *Cornell Vet* 68:179-195, 1978.
56. Wrigley et al: Pleural effusion associated with squamous cell carcinoma of the stomach of a horse. *Equine Vet J* 13:99-102, 1981.
57. Vaala: Pleuritis and pleural effusion in a mare secondary to disseminated squamous cell carcinoma. *Comp Cont Ed Pract Vet* 9:674-677, 1987.
58. East and Savage: Abdominal neoplasia (excluding urogenital tract). *Vet Clin North Am* (*Equine Pract*) 14(3): 475-492, 1998.
59. Jorgensen et al: Lameness and pleural effusion associated with an aggressive fibrosarcoma in a horse. *JAVMA* 210(9):1328-1331, 1997.
60. Prater et al: Pleural effusion resulting from malignant hepatoblastoma in a horse. *JAVMA* 194:383-385, 1989.

CHAPTER 9

Peritoneal Fluid

Heather L. DeHeer, Bruce W. Parry, and Carol B. Grindem

Peritoneal fluid evaluation is a diagnostically useful adjunct to history, physical examination, and routine CBC and biochemical evaluation of abdominal disease in both the horse and the foal. Abnormalities in peritoneal fluid may be associated with a variety of disorders affecting the equine, including colic, peritonitis, traumatic injury, and neoplasia. Serial evaluation of peritoneal fluid is useful in discerning the need for surgical intervention, monitoring progression of disease and response to therapy, and determination of prognosis.

Normal peritoneal fluid represents an ultrafiltrate of plasma and has a low volume, low cellularity, and low total protein concentration. Its function is to lubricate the organ surfaces and reduce friction. The volume, cellularity, and biochemical composition of peritoneal fluid is a reflection of (1) the pathophysiologic status of the parietal and visceral mesothelial surfaces, (2) capillary hydrostatic pressure, (3) plasma colloidal oncotic pressure, and (4) conditions affecting vascular permeability and lymphatic flow. An increase in fluid volume results when the rate of fluid formation exceeds that of fluid removal. Rupture of a hollow viscus or vessel may also contribute exogenously to increased peritoneal fluid volume. Under normal circumstances, peritoneal fluid is drained from the abdominal cavity by specialized lymphatic lacunae in the diaphragm, which connect with the right lymphatic duct. Such drainage is critical for recirculation of protein entering the peritoneal cavity.

Peritoneal fluid can be readily collected via abdominocentesis in the minimally restrained, standing horse by the veterinarian in the field. Abdominocentesis may also be performed in laterally recumbent horses. This technique is most commonly employed in fluid collection from foals. Various collection techniques have been thoroughly detailed elsewhere.[1-3] Equipment requirements are minimal and include clippers, surgical scrub, local anesthetic agent, sterile gloves, scalpel, teat cannula, gauze sponges, and collection tubes. Use of aseptic technique is essential. Tranquilizers may be required if the horse is intractable. Analgesics may be required if colic causes severe abdominal pain, so the operator can safely attempt fluid collection. Unless drainage of large volumes of abdominal effusion is medically indicated, a specimen of 3 to 5 ml is generally adequate for complete fluid analysis. The specimen may be divided among collection tubes containing transport media suitable for microbiologic culture, sterile clot tubes or heparin-containing anticoagulant tubes suitable for biochemical analysis, and EDTA anticoagulant tubes for cell counts, preservation of cell morphology, and cytologic examination.

Potential Complications of Abdominocentesis

Blood Contamination

Blood in the abdominocentesis specimen may be the result of peripheral blood contamination such as occurs with superficial hemorrhage from skin incision, perforation of abdominal muscles when the cannula or needle strays from the midline, perforation of a blood vessel on the serosal surface, or perforation of an abdominal organ (especially the spleen). Conversely, hemorrhagic diapedesis from a lesion in the peritoneal cavity or hemoperitoneum represent causes of true hemorrhagic effusions. Discerning contamination from true hemorrhage is important for accurate interpretation of fluid analysis results. A variety of gross and microscopic findings may aid in distinction of these processes. During specimen collection, if the peritoneal fluid flowing from the cannula or needle is initially free of hemorrhage and then becomes bloody, contamination at collection is obvious. Similarly, if the peritoneal fluid is initially bloody and then *clears* of hemorrhage as it is collected, contamination is likely. Such observations should be noted on the animal's case record and/or on the clinical pathology request form, as appropriate. When the specimen is uniformly bloody or discolored throughout collection, and at different sites, hemorrhagic diapedesis or hemoperitoneum is likely. Estimation of peritoneal fluid quantity and comparison of fluid and whole blood packed cell volume (PCV) may assist in differentiating hemorrhage from contamination. Large volumes of grossly bloody peritoneal fluid are more compatible with true intraperitoneal hemorrhage; a high PCV is useful to confirm this suspicion. Further microscopic differentiation of these possibilities are discussed later (see section on hemorrhagic effusions).

Peripheral blood contamination can be minimized by using several precautions during specimen collection. When one is selecting an abdominocentesis site, obvious superficial veins must be avoided. Nevertheless, cutaneous incision frequently causes minor hemorrhage. Consequently, the stab wound should be *blotted* with a sterile gauze sponge immediately before the cannula or needle is inserted through the abdominal wall. Whenever possible, a sterile, blunt-tipped teat cannula is preferred over needles for specimen collection, because it minimizes the risk of vessel or organ laceration. Walking or rocking the animal to try to increase the amount of peritoneal fluid in the ventral abdominal cavity during abdominocentesis is not recommended, especially when a needle is used for sample collection, because of the increased risk of intestinal laceration.[4]

Enterocentesis

Occasionally during abdominocentesis, the cannula or needle accidentally perforates the intestine. Contamination of peritoneal fluid with intestinal contents is frequently evident grossly. A green to brown fluid color, fermentative odor, and flocculent appearance suggest penetration of the gastrointestinal tract, particularly in a horse not exhibiting clinical signs consistent with rupture. Enterocentesis fluid may be grossly normal in appearance, so microscopic examination is essential to rule out of this potential complication.[5]

The reported frequency of accidental enterocentesis has varied from 2% to 5%, without any significant clinical sequelae. Another author attributed severe complications to accidental enterocentesis in three animals (0.4% of abdominocenteses over a 2-year period).[4] Complications most frequently occurred in horses with preexisting gastrointestinal compromise secondary to a distended viscus.

Despite the infrequency of serious clinical complications following enterocentesis, one study demonstrated (by serial abdominocenteses) that peritonitis was evident within 4 hours.[5] Total nucleated cell counts within the peritoneal fluid peaked 2 days after enterocentesis, with a mean nucleated cell count of 113,333/μl and maximum observed count of 540,000/μl. Neutrophils comprised the overwhelming majority of these cells and commonly showed *toxic change*; however, bacteria were not observed. The total nucleated cell count had decreased considerably by day 4 (when the study ended), with a mean nucleated cell count of 8650/μl and a maximum observed count of 25,400/μl. Nevertheless, all nine horses were clinically normal throughout the study, with the exception of one animal that was febrile on day 1. Peripheral blood total and differential leukocyte counts did not alter significantly at any stage.

Effects of Repeat Abdominocentesis or Laparotomy

In some cases, abdominocentesis may need to be repeated on several occasions to monitor changes in peritoneal fluid, and the changes observed may be critical in determining the need for surgical intervention. Serial, uncomplicated abdominocenteses in normal horses cause little change in peritoneal fluid composition.[8,9] The total nucleated cell count and total protein concentration may increase slightly but do not typically exceed reference values.[5] Differential cell counts also remain unchanged. Cell morphology remains normal, possibly with some hypersegmentation of neutrophils and some leukophagocytosis. With mild blood contamination, a small increase in red blood cell (RBC) numbers may be noted, with evidence of erythrophagocytosis.

Peritoneal fluid analysis may be useful in the postceliotomy patient for early detection of complications such as hemorrhage or sepsis and to monitor for resolution of underlying disease. Postoperative changes in peritoneal fluid values have been well documented[10-12] and may be difficult to discern from pathologic alterations when conventional reference ranges are used. In such circumstances, use of specialized reference ranges[10,11] is necessary for meaningful interpretation of fluid analysis results.

Specimen-Handling Considerations

Fluid should be collected into an EDTA tube for cell counts, cytologic examination, and (refractive index) total protein measurement. With small sample size (EDTA tubes less than one-quarter filled), erroneous results for fluid protein levels and cell counts may be obtained (see section on biochemical examination later in this chapter).[13]

If a delay is anticipated between sample collection and processing in the laboratory, the specimen is best refrigerated in the interim. In this situation, direct smear preparations of turbid fluid (high cellularity) or concentrated smears of clear fluid (low cellularity), made soon after sample collection, serve as a reference point for cell morphology. When delay of several hours occurs before smears are prepared, macrophages in the peritoneal fluid may become vacuolated in vitro or exhibit erythrophagia, thus complicating the distinction between true hemorrhagic effusions and peripheral blood–contaminated specimens. Nucleated cells may start to exhibit aging changes such as hypersegmentation and pyknosis, thereby resembling more chronic processes. Also, bacterial overgrowth may occur, of either pathogenic or contaminant organisms, clouding interpretation.

When one is using outside laboratories, it is best to determine, in advance of specimen collection, any special requirements for specimen storage, shipment, and submission favored by that particular laboratory for the analyses requested. In most instances, air-dried, direct or concentrated, line smears of fluid, together with EDTA and clot tube aliquots and culture transport media as indicated, are sufficient.

Gross Fluid Examination

Gross visual inspection of fluid consists of noting fluid volume, color, turbidity, and odor. Normal peritoneal fluid is of small volume, clear to slightly turbid or opalescent, pale yellow to straw colored (depending on diet),[14] and odorless. Much useful information may be gained by assessing the ease with which the fluid is obtained and by visually appraising the turbidity and color of the sample. A total nucleated cell count, cytologic examination, and total protein measurement should be performed on all specimens. Caution must be exercised to resist the temptation to limit fluid analysis simply to gross visualization, since grossly "normal-appearing" peritoneal fluid is sometimes observed with accidental enterocentesis,[5] as well as with disease conditions such as ruptured bladder.[15]

Volume

There is little free peritoneal fluid in the abdominal cavity of a healthy horse, the quantity being only sufficient to ensure lubrication of the parietal and serosal mesothelial surfaces.[16,17] Nevertheless, in 20 clinically normal horses examined at necropsy, about 100 to 300 ml of free peritoneal fluid was found.[18] These estimates are probably below the actual amount of fluid bathing the mesothelium of the abdominal cavity, but they reflect the approximate quantity of fluid potentially available for sampling by abdominocentesis. In an unpublished study of six clinically normal horses with peritoneal fluid cell counts, cytologic findings, and total protein concentration within published reference values, 580 to 2050 ml of fluid was estimated to be present based on a dye dilution technique.[19]

It is important for the veterinarian to adopt a standard technique for abdominocentesis, since this permits subjective estimation of the volume of fluid within the abdominal cavity, based on the ease of collection and rate of flow. Over a 5- to 10-minute interval, 10 to 100 ml of peritoneal fluid may be collected from most normal horses, with 50 to 60 ml commonly collected in 10 minutes.[6,14] However, collection of such large volumes is not necessary for routine analysis of peritoneal fluid. Usually 3 to 5 ml can be easily collected from most animals and is adequate for laboratory purposes.[7] If abdominocentesis is nonproductive or if samples are bloody, additional attempts can be made in alternate locations remote from the initial abdominocentesis site. Several such attempts should be made before the abdominocentesis is considered to be a *dry tap* (no fluid collected despite several attempts at different locations). This may occur when:

The needle or catheter fails to enter the peritoneal cavity. This is mainly a problem in fat ponies when a 5-cm needle is used. Penetration of the falciform ligament impedes the flow of fluid.[20]

The volume of peritoneal fluid is not increased. Such a finding does not exclude the possibility of a pathologic process involving the abdominal viscera. Early in the course of intestinal obstructions, dislocations, or incarcerations, there may be minimal changes in peritoneal fluid. Consequently, it can be very useful to perform repeated abdominocenteses to detect changes. Retroperitoneal lesions do not necessarily cause a peritoneal effusion. Further, intestinal intussusceptions or extraabdominal incarcerations, such as diaphragmatic and inguinal hernias, do not necessarily cause a peritoneal effusion.

The ventral colon is distended and thus excludes peritoneal fluid from the ventral abdominal area. In a similar fashion, compartmentalization of fluid by the omentum or disrupted fluid flow secondary to formation of adhesions can impede movement of fluid to the ventral midline.[20]

The horse is dehydrated, as from grass sickness.[14] Even when the volume of peritoneal fluid collected does not appear to be excessive, it is still important to observe the specimen's color, turbidity, and odor.

Occasionally no peritoneal fluid can be collected from a normal horse, despite several attempts.[7,14,18]

When the volume of peritoneal fluid collected is subjectively increased, an effusion is most probably present and/or the peritoneal fluid is under increased pressure from distended loops of bowel. A peritoneal effusion develops when the rate of peritoneal fluid production exceeds the rate of fluid removal. Increased peritoneal fluid quantity may be produced by both transudation and/or exudation. Transudation results in an ascitic (low-cellularity, low-protein-content) effusion, while exudation results in a fluid of high cellularity and high protein concentration.

Color and Clarity

Visual appraisal of peritoneal fluid, together with assessment of the volume (as above), can often provide a provisional diagnosis. This may be used to guide initial therapy until laboratory results are available. Specimen color can vary from colorless to yellow, orange, red, brown, green, gray, or white. Effusion color varies with the numbers and relative proportions of RBCs and nucleated cells present and biochemical constituents such as hemoglobin, bilirubin, or lipid. A discolored supernatant usually reflects damage to erythrocytes and sometimes to leukocytes that occurred prior to collection. Turbidity ranges from clear to opaque and is related to the cellular, protein, and/or lipid content of the fluid. Flocculent material visible within the specimen contributes to increased turbidity and can represent fibrin clots associated with inflammation, hemorrhage, or ingesta/plant material from either accidental enterocentesis or gastrointestinal rupture.

Normal peritoneal fluid and ascitic effusions have a clear, colorless to pale yellow-orange appearance because of their low cellularity. Exudative effusions are more likely to be discolored and turbid because of their increased cellularity and protein content. In these circumstances, it is diagnostically useful to grossly examine the sample's sediment and supernatant. In the field situation, this can be done by allowing the fluid to sediment by gravity. In the laboratory, a microhematocrit centrifuge or a regular centrifuge can be used. The *height* of the sediment in the tube is usually proportional to the cellularity of the fluid, while its color varies with the relative numbers of RBCs and nucleated cells present.

Shades of pink to red discoloration will occur with the presence of red cells or free hemoglobin in the specimen. Changes in red discoloration during specimen collection can alert the veterinarian to possible peripheral blood contamination. Uniformly red discolored specimens generally represent true hemorrhagic effusions and may be associated with bleeding diatheses, tumor rupture, traumatic injury, or devitalized bowel.

When the specimen grossly resembles whole blood, estimation of specimen quantity, determination of fluid PCV, clotting times, and cytologic appearance may be useful in distinguishing contamination or splenic tap from hemoperitoneum. A small-volume specimen having a PCV similar to or greater than peripheral blood, without cytologic evidence of erythrophagia, is characteristic of a splenic tap.[1,2] Contaminated specimens most often have a PCV significantly less than that of peripheral blood, and platelet clumps may be visualized microscopically. Increased fluid volume, failure of the specimen to clot, or presence of significant erythrophagia upon microscopic examination suggests true hemoperitoneum. Specimen color may aid in differentiating previous from recent/ongoing hemorrhage: a bright red color suggests recent or ongoing hemorrhage, while a reddish brown to brown color may be compatible with previous hemorrhage.

Reddish brown, port wine, or muddy effusions are also frequently associated with ischemic tissue injury/necrosis and suggest a poor prognosis.[1,2] Presence of degenerative leukocyte changes (loss of nuclear segmentation, indistinct nuclear margins) with concurrent presence of bacterial organisms is compatible with devitalized bowel. Additionally, a brown or golden brown peritoneal fluid may rarely occur in peritoneal effusions associated with metastatic pigmented melanoma.

Dark green fluid color is compatible with the presence of free bile as a result of damage to the bile duct or rupture of the duodenum.[1] Additionally, observation of bright orange bilirubin crystals or a positive Ictotest on the fluid specimen would support bile peritonitis. A bright green fluid color is more compatible with enterocentesis of the large colon or cecum. Mixed bacterial organisms and/or plant material would aid in the distinction of enterocentesis from bile peritonitis.

Milky, whitish discoloration may occur with increased leukocyte content or elevated lipid content (cholesterol and/or triglycerides). The terms *chylous* and *pseudochylous* are traditionally used to describe such fluid specimens. The turbidity and color change in chylous effusions are the result of increased fluid triglyceride content, with or without a concurrent increase in leukocytes. Pseudochylous effusions have a grossly similar appearance due to high cellularity and cholesterol content. Microscopic evaluation of both chylous and pseudochylous effusions is discussed later.

Cytologic Examination

A cell count, total protein determination, and cytologic evaluation can be performed in the laboratory. Such tests require little equipment and yield much useful information. The method by which smears are prepared in the laboratory for cytologic evaluation varies with the specimen's cellularity and the equipment available. Fluids with a total nucleated cell count <5000/μl are

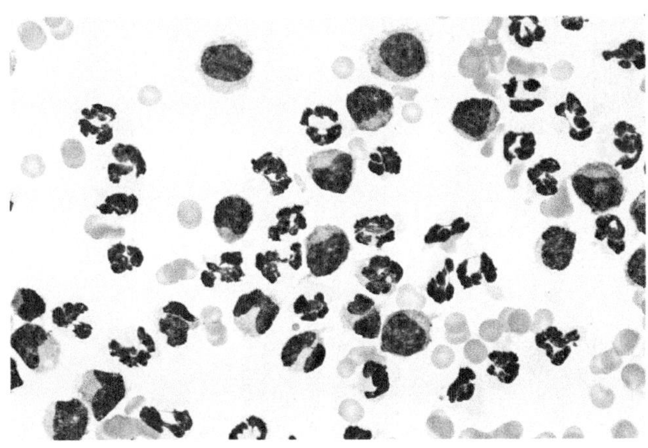

Fig. 9-1 Cytocentrifugation of normal equine abdominal fluid for cytologic examination.
Concentration of cellularity in this fashion yields the ideal cell density and morphology for microscopic examination of most fluid specimens. A 100-μl aliquot is sufficient for most samples. In this fluid, nondegenerate neutrophils are the predominant cell type. (Wright-Giemsa)

most readily examined if smears are made after cells are concentrated by some means. In diagnostic laboratories, special cytocentrifuges are often used for this purpose. A 100-μl aliquot yields ideal cell morphology for cytospin examination of most fluid specimens (Figs. 9-1 and 9-2). Transudative, very-low-cellularity effusions may require up to 200 μl to improve cellularity for microscopic examination. Extremely high-cellularity, exudative effusions may require a reduced volume aliquot (25 to 50 μl) or specimen dilution to achieve cytospin preparations with ideal cell morphology and numbers.

In laboratories lacking a cytocentrifuge, specimens may be concentrated for cytologic examination with centrifugation of up to 10 ml of peritoneal fluid in a tube for about 5 minutes at 1000 to 1500 rpm. The resultant supernatant is removed and saved for total protein measurement. The sedimented cells are then gently resuspended in about 0.25 to 0.5 ml of peritoneal fluid and smears prepared, often using a line smear technique to concentrate cells at the leading edge of the smear (see Chapter 1). Romanowsky-type stains are usually used, such as Wright's, May-Grünwald, Giemsa, or Diff-Quik. Fluids with a total nucleated cell count of 5000 to 10,000/μl may be prepared from centrifuged or uncentrifuged specimens, depending on the operator's preference. (Line smears from centrifuged sediments yield more cellular and therefore more easily scanned smears in these situations.) When the total nucleated cell count is >10,000/μl and the fluid's turbidity is therefore greater than normal, direct smears of uncentrifuged specimens are usually satisfactory.

Cell Counts

Total nucleated cell counts of peritoneal fluid are performed as for a blood sample. This can vary from manual dilution with microscopic enumeration to the use of automated cell counters. Reference values for peritoneal fluid of mature aged horses and of foals are summarized in Table 9-1. Small volume specimens (EDTA tube less than one-quarter filled) may be sufficiently diluted to mildly decrease cell counts.[13]

As a generalization, the total nucleated cell count is typically less than 10,000/μl (10.0×10^9/L) and often below 5000/μl (5.0×10^9/L) in mature or aged horses.[9,21,22] Foals appear to have appreciably lower values.[20,23] When a microhematocrit centrifuge is used to sediment cells from peritoneal fluid so that total protein content can be measured on the supernatant, the packed nucleated cell volume is less than 1%.[6]

Similarly, there is a negligible packed RBC volume. Normal peritoneal fluid contains very few RBCs (see Table 9-1) and negligible erythrophagocytosis. Erythrocyte counts are not often performed on peritoneal fluid unless automated techniques are employed that routinely include red cell number determination.

Nucleated cells are generally categorized as neutrophils, lymphocytes, large mononuclear cells (including monocytes, macrophages, and mesothelial cells), eosinophils, basophils, or mast cells. Differential cell counts are usually performed on 100 to 200 cells and are expressed as percentage values. Peritoneal fluid differential cell count results must not be interpreted alone. For accurate assessment, these percentages must be related to the total nucleated cell count, total protein concentration, and volume of fluid present.

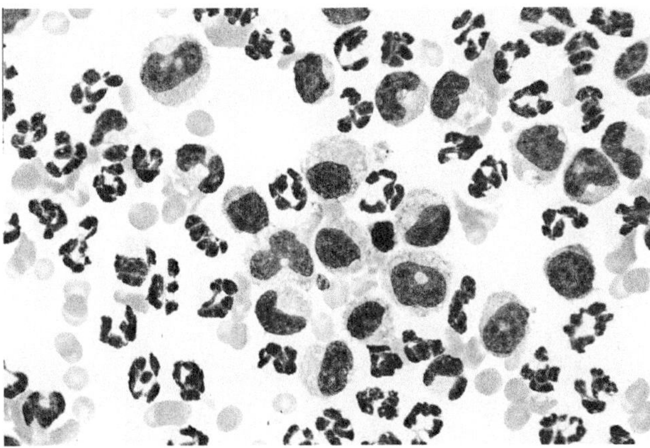

Fig. 9-2 Cytocentrifugation of normal equine abdominal fluid showing a greater percentage of large mononuclear cells than in Fig. 9-1.
A range of nuclear morphology is characteristic of this cell type. Nuclei may vary from round to oval to bean-shaped to lobulated. (100-μl aliquot, Wright-Giemsa)

TABLE 9-1

Reference Values for Cell Counts and Refractometer Total Protein and Specific Gravity in Equine Peritoneal Fluid

Number of animals	25 Horses[5,a]	20 Horses[30]	20 Horses[6]	20 Horses and Ponies[15]	13 Horses[1]	17 Foals[22]	32 Foals[19h]	15 Horses[20h]	10 Horses[8h]	8 Horses[21h]
Clinical findings	Normal	Normal	Normal	Normal	Normal	Normal	Normal	Normal	Normal	Normal
Necropsy of peritoneal cavity	Normal	—	—	Normal	—	—	—	Normal	—	—
Total erythrocyte count (/µL)	—	200-5400	—	—	—	—	0-42,500	—	—	0-43,200
Total nucleated cell count (/µL)	200-9000	50-4600	1900-4700	500-10,100[d]	1890-4610	60-1420	0-3572	1400-3000	1100-2560	486-2114
Differential cell count										
Neutrophils (%)	36-78	80-98	48-80	22-82	24-62	2-94	0-56	14-100[i]	58.4-72.8	—
Lymphocytes (%)	0-29	1-11	9-34	1-19	5-36	0-7	0-71.3	b	2.0-6.0	—
Large mononuclear cells (%)	3-50	1-17	0-4	19-68	17-50	5-98	0-92	0-86	22.8-36.0	—
Mesothelial cells (%)	b	Occasional	5-22	b	b	b	b	b	b	—
Eosinophils (%)	0-3	0-7	0	0-5[d]	1-6	0-4[f]	—	—	.1-.9	—
Other cells (%)	—	Occasional mast cell	0	Rare basophils[e]	—	g	—	—	—	—
Refractometer										
Total protein (g/dl)	0.1-3.4	0.1-2.5	—	0.2-1.5	0.7-1.1	1.4-1.9	0.4-3.2	3.8-13.8	—	<2.5
Specific gravity	1.000-1.093	1.006-1.030	—	1.008-1.012	1.000-1.015	1.012-1.015	—	1.006-1.104	1.010-1.014	—

Data from Bach and Ricketts: Paracentesis as an aid to the diagnosis of abdominal disease in the horse. *Equine Vet J* 6:116-121, 1974; Behrens et al: Reference values of peritoneal fluid from healthy foals. *J Equine Vet Sci* 10(5):348-352, 1990; Malark et al: Effect of blood contamination on equine peritoneal fluid analysis. *J Am Vet Med Assoc* 201(10):1545-1548, 1992; Milne et al: Analysis of peritoneal fluid as a diagnostic aid in grass sickness (equine dysautonomia). *Vet Record* 127:162-165, 1990; Morley and Desnoyers: Diagnosis of ruptured urinary bladder in a foal by identification of calcium carbonate crystals in the peritoneal fluid. *J Am Vet Med Assoc* 200(8):1515-1517, 1992; Nelson: Analysis of equine peritoneal fluid. *Vet Clin North Am* (*Large Anim Pract*) 1:267-274, 1979; Olson: Squamous cell carcinoma of the equine stomach: a report of five cases. *Vet Record* 131(8):170-173, 1992; Parry et al: Unpublished data, 1985; Schneider et al: Response of pony peritoneum to four peritoneal lavage solutions. *Am J Vet Res* 49:889-894, 1988; Schumacher et al: Effects of enterocentesis on peritoneal fluid constituents in the horse. *J Am Vet Med Assoc* 186:1301-1303, 1985.

[a] Bach reported virtually identical results in 1973, with the exception that the total nucleated cell count was 200 to 11,000/µL and neutrophils were 36% to 91%.
[b] Included in large mononuclear cell group.
[c] Assumed to be a refractometer method.
[d] 19 horses (95%) had total nucleated cell count of 1500 to 7600/µL and eosinophils 0% to 3%.
[e] Basophils (1%) were observed in only one horse (5%).
[f] 16 foals (94%) had 0% eosinophils.
[g] No degenerative cellular changes were noted. Rare cytophagia observed.
[h] Values are for mean ± 2SD.
[i] Total granulocytes (including neutrophils and eosinophils).

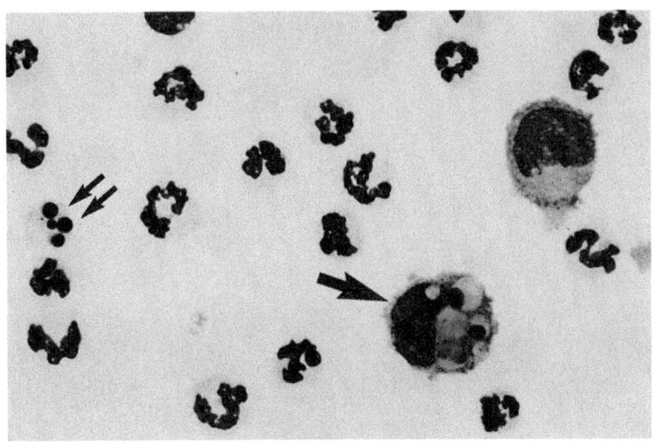

Fig. 9-3 Neutrophil morphology.
Neutrophils entering the peritoneal cavity do not return to the systemic circulation but age and die in the peritoneal fluid. Under normal circumstances, aging is noted as hypersegmentation of the nucleus and then pyknosis (the nucleus condenses and fragments) *(double arrow)*. Such cells are removed (phagocytosed and digested) by macrophages *(arrow)*. (Original magnification X950; May-Grunwald-Giemsa)

Reference values for peritoneal fluid cytologic composition are listed in Table 9-1. The predominant cells usually are neutrophils, followed by large mononuclear cells and then lymphocytes. Eosinophils are uncommon. Basophils and mast cells are rarely observed.

Cell Morphology

Assessment of cell morphology is a very important part of the cytologic examination of peritoneal fluid. In addition to total cell numbers and differential counts, morphologic features suggesting cell age, activity, and peritoneal cavity environmental conditions can aid in prioritizing differential diagnosis, assessing response to treatment, and determining prognosis.

Neutrophils: Neutrophils entering the peritoneal cavity (like neutrophils entering other body cavities or tissues) do not return to the bloodstream. Consequently, neutrophil aging and death are normal events. Aged neutrophils are often moderately hypersegmented to pyknotic cells[14,16,18] (Fig. 9-3). Leukophagocytosis of senescent neutrophils by macrophages (Fig. 9-3) may be observed in peritoneal fluid collected from clinically healthy animals.[6,14,16,18] Neutrophils in normal peritoneal fluid do not exhibit phagocytic activity per se.[6,14,16,18]

The presence of band neutrophils or more immature granulocytic cells suggests acute inflammation and mobilization of the neutrophil storage and maturation pools. Frequently, observation of immature granulocytic cells is associated with poor prognosis.[24]

The presence of degenerative changes (such as cell swelling, loss of nuclear segmentation, and indistinct nuclear margins)[25] suggests a harsh peritoneal environment. This may occur secondary to the presence of bacterial cytotoxins or chemical irritants (bile or urine) within the abdominal cavity. Toxic changes (such as increased cytoplasmic basophilia, vacuolation, or Dohle bodies) may also be observed in septicemia or enterotoxemia. Such toxic change is considered to be "preexisting," occurring during myelopoiesis, rather than subsequent to migration into the peritoneal cavity. These changes, accompanied by visualization of phagocytized bacterial organisms (see Figs. 9-13 to 9-15) are compatible with septic peritonitis.

Relatively hyposegmented neutrophils in a bloody peritoneal fluid specimen may support peripheral blood contamination, since circulating neutrophils are expected to be less aged than tissue neutrophils. Neutrophil nuclear hyposegmentation artifact may also be observed following delayed processing of EDTA anticoagulated specimens.

Large Mononuclear Cells: The category of large mononuclear cells encompasses nonreactive (tissue) macrophages of blood monocyte origin, reactive (tissue) macrophages, and mesothelial cells. Because these cells are often difficult to distinguish morphologically, they are commonly grouped together.[7,16,18,26] They are also often referred to collectively as mononuclear phagocytes, since all are potentially phagocytic. All of these cells are large, usually with a moderate to high nucleus to cytoplasmic ratio and abundant, somewhat basophilic cytoplasm (Fig. 9-4). The nucleus is their

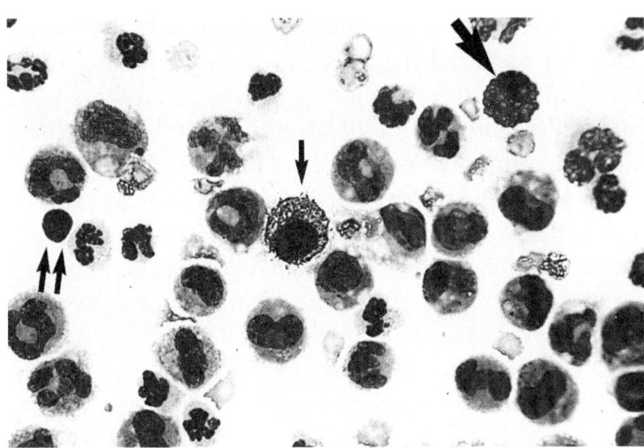

Fig. 9-4 Numerous large mononuclear cells (probably macrophages), several neutrophils, a small mature lymphocyte *(double arrows)*, an eosinophil *(large arrow)*, and a mast cell *(small arrow)* in peritoneal fluid. Note that several macrophages appear to be reactive, with somewhat vacuolated basophilic cytoplasm. (Original magnification X950; May-Grunwald-Giemsa)

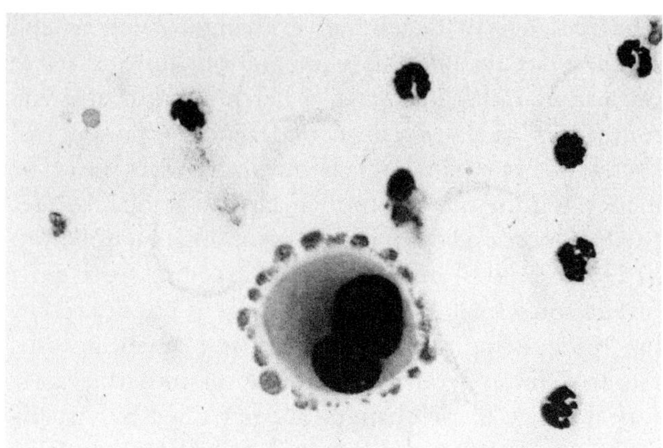

Fig. 9-5 Large reactive binucleate mesothelial cell in peritoneal fluid.
Note the apparent pseudopodia, which are an artifact of drying. (Original magnification X950; May-Grunwald-Giemsa)

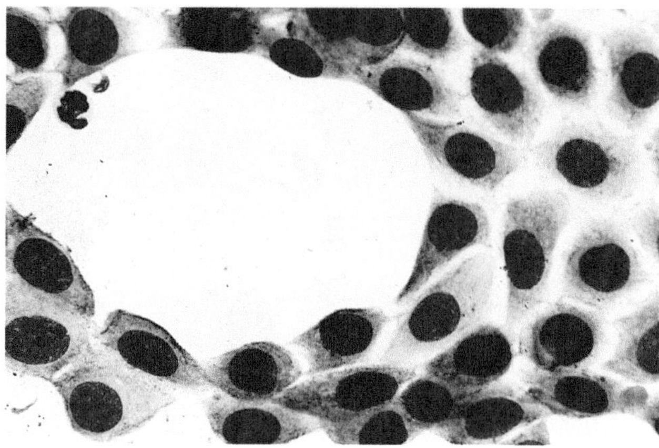

Fig. 9-6 Sheet of mesothelial cells in peritoneal fluid of horse with transudative effusion.
Sheets of cells may also be seen as a postmortem artifact in fluid collected several hours after death. (Original magnification X950; May-Grunwald-Giemsa)

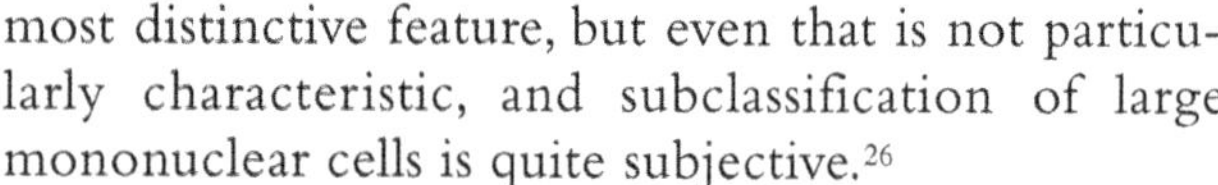

most distinctive feature, but even that is not particularly characteristic, and subclassification of large mononuclear cells is quite subjective.[26]

Mesothelial cells usually have an oval nucleus with a finely reticular chromatin pattern. They occur in the highest proportions in low-cellularity, high-volume effusions (transudates). When individualized, a fine eosinophilic "corona" of glycocalyx may be evident along the cell margin. In normal peritoneal fluid, they frequently occur in sheets or rafts, are uniform in appearance, and polygonal to rhomboid in shape. Transudative effusions may be associated with mesothelial proliferation resulting from loss of contact inhibition subsequent to fluid separation of mesothelial surfaces, and tufts or balls of mesothelial cells may be observed. In exudative effusions, mesothelial cells become *reactive* or *transformed* and exhibit features suggesting increased proliferation, including increased cytoplasmic basophilia, multinucleation, prominent nucleoli, and mitotic activity[25] (Fig. 9-5). Hyperplastic/dysplastic features can begin to mimic neoplasia in severe inflammatory conditions,[1] and in rare instances, fine azurophilic cytoplasmic granulation has been reported.[24] Such cells are seen in very small numbers in normal peritoneal fluid.[6,14,16,18] Peritoneal fluid collected several hours after death often contains numerous sheets of exfoliated mesothelial cells, similar to those seen in some effusions (Fig. 9-6). Such a finding may thus be a postmortem artifact.

The nonreactive macrophage (or monocytic cell) typically has an indented oval nucleus with a more homogeneous chromatin pattern. However, the nucleus of the latter cell can be quite pleomorphic, varying in shape from elongated, to round, to convoluted or lobulated. These cells are reported to constitute anywhere from approximately 5% to 80% of normal peritoneal nucleated cell differential counts.[1] In acute inflammatory effusions, the relative percentage of monocytes/macrophages decreases with increasing neutrophil numbers. In more chronic effusions, mononuclear/macrophages are typically present in increased percentages and frequently exhibit reactive changes.[25] Reactive cells tend to have more abundant, more basophilic cytoplasm. Reactive macrophages often have ruffled cytoplasmic margins, prominent cytoplasmic vacuoles, and/or inclusions (phagosomes). The latter may be unidentifiable debris or degenerating inflammatory cells or RBCs (see Figs. 9-3 and 9-4). Such cells, though readily apparent in normal peritoneal fluid, are present in small numbers.[6,16,18] Cytophagia is rare in peritoneal fluid from foals.[23]

Lymphocytes: Lymphocytes in normal peritoneal fluid are usually small to medium-sized cells (see Fig. 9-4), similar to peripheral blood lymphocytes.[14,16,18] These cells constitute only a small percentage of normal peritoneal fluid nucleated cells and recirculate into the bloodstream via the diaphragmatic lymphatic lacunae. An increased lymphocyte percentage may occur in chronic inflammatory conditions, parasitism, chyloperitoneum (particularly acutely), or neoplasia.

Lymphoblasts are not observed in normal peritoneal fluid. These cells have a densely staining delicate chromatin pattern, often with obvious nucleoli and intensely basophilic cytoplasm that may contain small to large vacuoles. Cytologic diagnosis of lymphoma is usually based on the presence of large numbers of such cells. Other considerations include marked inflammation[24] or accidental aspiration of lymphoid tissue. Large granular lymphocytes have been observed in

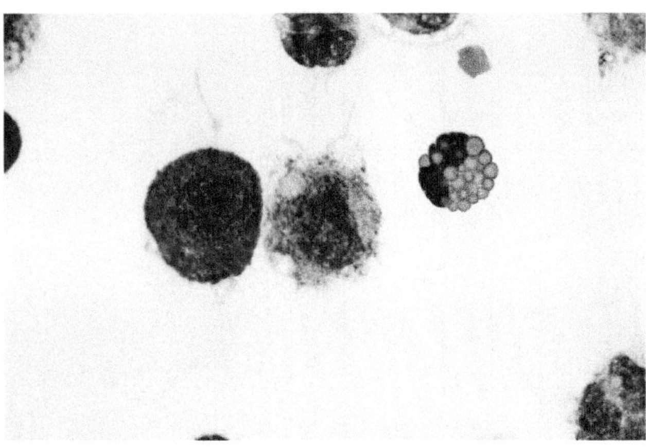

Fig. 9-7 Higher magnification of eosinophil *(left)*, large mononuclear cell *(center)*, and mast cell *(right)* in equine peritoneal fluid. Note that the large mononuclear cell has phagocytized an erythrocyte. (Wright-Giemsa)

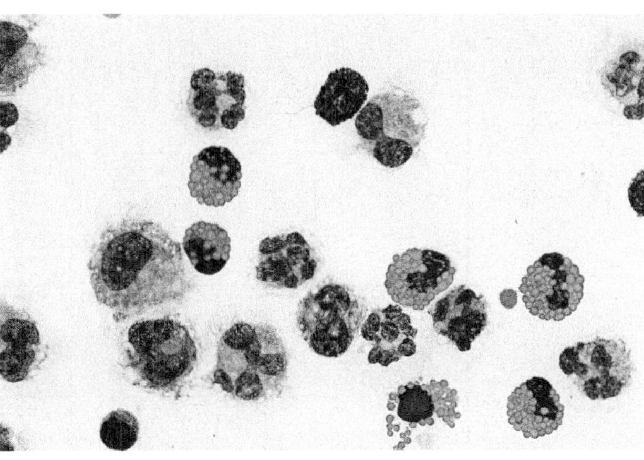

Fig. 9-8 Eosinophilia in abdominal fluid
Eosinophilia may be accompanied by the presence of basophils *(center bottom)*. (Wright-Giemsa)

peritoneal fluid with both inflammatory disease[24] and large granular lymphoma.[27] Plasma cells may also be observed in low numbers in inflammatory fluid specimens and reflect chronic antigenic stimulation.[16] Occasionally these cells may contain cytoplasmic vacuoles distended with immunoglobulin (Russell bodies).[24]

Other Cells: Eosinophils (Figs. 9-4, 9-7, and 9-8) and basophils have the same morphology as in a peripheral blood smear. Mast cells (Figs. 9-4 and 9-7) have the same morphology as in other tissue specimens and are an infrequent finding, even in inflammatory conditions. Increased eosinophil percentage (Figs. 9-8 and 9-9), possibly associated with a concurrent increase in basophils and mast cells, is inconsistently associated with intestinal parasitism or parasitic larval migration[6, 16, 24, 25] and may also accompany other septic or nonseptic causes of inflammation as well as neoplasia.[25,28] There is often an accompanying neutrophilic exudate.

Neoplastic cells are occasionally identified in peritoneal fluid cytology. Neoplastic round cells (most commonly lymphoblasts) and epithelial cells (mesotheliomas and carcinomas) are those most commonly encountered.[25] Criteria of malignancy include anisocytosis, anisokaryosis, variation in nucleus to cytoplasm ratio, increased cell size, nuclear gigantism, multinucleation, prominent/large/angular/multiple nucleoli, and increased/abnormal mitotic activity. Presence of concurrent inflammation may cloud distinction from reactive hyperplasia/dysplasia in some instances,[25] necessitating further diagnostic investigation. Absence of identifiable neoplastic cells on peritoneal fluid cytology does not rule out neoplasia, since tumor cells do not consistently exfoliate into peritoneal fluid, even in disseminated disease.[29,30]

Biochemical Examination

Biochemical analysis of peritoneal fluid routinely involves determination of protein content, specific gravity, and fibrinogen concentration. A variety of additional biochemical parameters may be measured in unique diagnostic circumstances or in research applications. For total protein, specific gravity, and fibrinogen measurements, peritoneal fluid is usually collected in an EDTA tube (as for cytologic examination). When sample volume is small (EDTA tube less than one-quarter filled), fluid protein measurements, as determined by refractive index, may be artificially increased (solute effect of sodium or potassium EDTA), whereas biuret

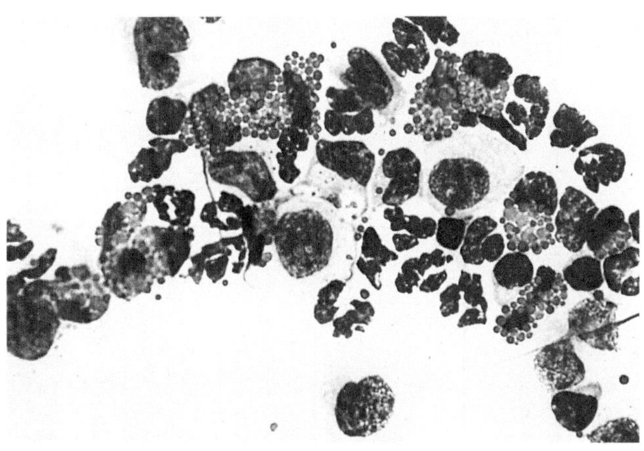

Fig. 9-9 Numerous eosinophils in peritoneal fluid of horse with parasitic hepatitis.
(Original magnification X950; May-Grunwald-Giemsa)

TABLE 9-2

Biochemistry Reference Values for Equine Blood and Peritoneal Fluid

	13 Horses[1,a]		20 Horses[17,b]		17 Horses[33,c]		32 Foals[19,b,h]		9 Horses[39,b]		15 Horses[20,b]	
	Blood	PF	Blood	PF	Blood	PF	Blood	PF	Blood	PF	Blood	PF
Albumin (g/dl)			1.7-3.9	0.3-1.0								
Globulin (g/dl)	3.9-4.6	0.7-1.4										
Total protein (g/dl)[d]	6.0-7.2	1.0-2.4	4.7-8.9	0.1-2.8								
Amylase (U/L) (37C)					14-35	0-14						
ALP (U/L)[e]	28-137	4-27	59-543	0-161			13.3-73.9	130.7-538.7			—	0-126.3
AST (U/L)[e]	133-225	4-27	59-543	0-161			12.2-87.8	94.2-277.4				
Total bilirubin (mg/dl)	0.8-1.5	0.3-0.8	0-5.3	0-1.2								
Creatinine (mg/dl)	1.5-1.8	0.3-0.8					.95-1.83	.91-1.87				
GGT (U/L) (37C)					9-29	0-6						
Glucose (mg/dl)	92-103	91-106	45-167	74-203	72-101	88-115	94.9-178.9	53.8-125				
Inorganic phosphorus (mg/dl)[f]	4.2-5.2	4.2-5.1	0.6-6.8	1.2-7.4					2.3-3.2	2.4-3.2		
Lactate (mg/dl)					6.3-15.3	3.6-10.8						
LDH (U/L)[e]	151-214	62-108	182-590	0-355			2.5-90.5	174.9-478.1				
Lipase (U/L) (37C)					23-87	0-36						
Urea (BUN) (mg/dl)[g]	11.0-15.5	12.7-21.8	8.1-24.9	10.9-23.2								
Fibrinogen (mg/dl)							<200-400	200-800				

Data from Behrens et al: Reference values of peritoneal fluid from healthy foals. *J Equine Vet Sci* 10(5):348-352, 1990; Broome et al: Evaluation of peritoneal fluid and serum creatine kinase isoenzyme concentrations as indicators of small intestinal surgical disease in horses (abstract). *Vet Surg* 23(5):397, 1994; Brownlow et al: Abdominal paracentesis in the horse—basic concepts. *Aust Vet Pract* 11:60-68, 1981; May et al: Chyloperitoneum and abdominal adhesions in a miniature horse. *J Am Vet Med Assoc* 215(5):676-678, 1999; Nelson: Analysis of equine peritoneal fluid. *Vet Clin North Am (Large Anim Pract)* 1:267-274, 1979; Parry et al: Unpublished data, 1985.

ALP, alkaline phosphatase; AST, aspartate aminotransferase (also called glutamate oxaloacetate transaminase, GOT); GGT, gamma glutamyltransferase; LDH, lactate dehydrogenase.

[a]Figures are ranges.
[b]Figures are mean ± 2 SD.
[c]Figures are ranges.
[d]See also Table 9-1.
[e]Temperature not stated.
[f]Reference values (ranges) for 9 horses:[39] Blood- 1.8-3.7 mg/dl (0.58-1.19mmol/L); PF- 1.6-3.7 mg/dl (0.52-1.19mmol/L)
[g]Reference values (ranges) for 10 foals:[22] Blood- 2.3-7.0 mg/dl (0.8-2.5mmol/L); PF- 2.3-7.8 mg/dl (0.8-2.8mmol/L)
[h]Peritoneal fluid Na, K, and Cl values determined to be similar to concurrent serum values.

protein concentration results may be artificially decreased (dilutional effect).[13] Although the artifactual effect is generally mild, it may reach diagnostic significance in distinguishing early, low-volume exudates from normal or borderline modified transudates from either pure transudates or mild exudates.

For most other biochemical tests, specimens may be collected in heparin or clot tubes. The exceptions are glucose measurement (when there will be a delay between collection and processing) and lactate measurements. Tubes containing fluoride-oxalate are required for the latter tests. The fluoride arrests cell metabolism, thus preventing in vitro glucose depletion and lactate production by cells and bacteria after collection. All biochemistry tests are usually performed on the peritoneal fluid supernatant after centrifugation. Possible exceptions are glucose and lactate measurements, which can also be done on uncentrifuged (whole) peritoneal fluid.

Total Protein Content

Total protein concentration is measured using a refractometer or by a biochemical method such as the biuret reaction (as for a blood sample). Refractive index is rapid, easy, and inexpensive; however, it is less accurate at low protein concentrations than biochemical methods. Reference values are given in Tables 9-1 and 9-2. As a generalization, the total protein concentration of normal peritoneal fluid is <2.5 g/dl (25 g/L), which is usually the lowest reading on the protein scale of most refractometers. Some authors report that any value >1.5 g/dl, as measured by the biuret reaction, indicates pathologic change.[24]

Specific Gravity

Because of the low total protein content of peritoneal fluid, specific gravity is commonly measured. Specific gravity is the density of a fluid as compared with distilled water (which has a value of 1.000). It is a reflection of the amount of dissolved solutes in the fluid, such as total protein, glucose, urea, and bilirubin. Reference values are given in Table 9-1. Total protein values are more commonly reported than specific gravity measurements.

Fibrinogen Content

Normal peritoneal fluid contains a negligible amount of fibrinogen and therefore does not clot. Using a heat precipitation method, fibrinogen concentrations <50 mg/dl (0.5 g/L) and <100 mg/dl (1 g/L) have been reported.[18,31] These figures are probably overestimated because the heat precipitation method is not very sensitive to low fibrinogen concentrations.

Increased fluid fibrinogen concentration may occur iatrogenically with blood contamination during specimen collection or pathologically with exudation. Causes of hemoabdomen may also transiently elevate fluid fibrinogen; however, it is quickly consumed by defibrinization within the peritoneal cavity, so such specimens often fail to clot.

Other Biochemical Tests

Reference values for paired blood and peritoneal fluid concentrations of the following analytes are presented in Table 9-2. Reference values for other biochemical tests have been published, including calcium, alanine aminotransferase (ALT), α-2-antiplasmin, antithrombin III (ATIII), creatine phosphokinase (CPK), chloride, fibrin(ogen) degradation products (FDP), pH, plasminogen, protein C, potassium, and sodium.[1,18,20,32,33] The diagnostic merit of these assays has not been confirmed.

- Albumin
- Alkaline phosphatase (ALP)
- Amylase
- Aspartate aminotransferase (AST, SGOT)
- Bilirubin
- Creatinine
- Fibrinogen
- Gamma glutamyltransferase (GGT)
- Globulins
- Glucose
- Inorganic phosphorus
- Lactate
- Lactate dehydrogenase (LDH)
- Lipase
- Urea

Water-soluble substances of low molecular weight, such as electrolytes (Na, K, Cl), glucose, phosphate, and urea, readily diffuse between the bloodstream and the peritoneal cavity. Consequently their concentrations in blood and peritoneal fluid are quite similar and well correlated.[16,18] In contrast, substances of high molecular weight, such as enzymes, most proteins, and substances that are partly or primarily attached to carrier proteins, such as calcium and unconjugated bilirubin, are usually found in lower concentration in peritoneal fluid than in blood and take longer to equilibrate when there is an abrupt change in their concentration in either blood or peritoneal fluid. Consequently, serum and peritoneal fluid values of these substances are often poorly correlated.

Creatinine and Urea: Comparison of creatinine and urea concentration in the peritoneal fluid with that of serum values aids in the diagnosis of uroperitoneum. In health, peritoneal fluid values approximate serum values for both analytes. With acute uroperitoneum, concentrations of urea and creatinine in the peritoneal fluid will exceed those of serum, usually by a ratio of greater than 2:1.[1,2,15,20,23] With time, equilibration of fluid and serum concentrations can occur, with diffusion of analytes from the fluid to the vascular space as well as with development of effusion secondary to chemical peritonitis. The former effect affects fluid urea concentrations more rapidly than creatinine concentrations because urea's smaller molecular weight facilitates diffusion.

Glucose, Lactate, LDH, and pH: Water-soluble substances of low molecular weight, such as glucose and lactate, readily diffuse between the bloodstream and the peritoneal cavity. Peritoneal fluid glucose concentration in the healthy equine is reported to be similar to or slightly greater than that of serum.[1,34,35] Increased anaerobic glycolysis by metabolically active cells (leukocytes or neoplastic cells) or bacterial organisms may decrease fluid glucose concentrations. Peritoneal fluid glucose concentrations <40 mg/dl or serum-to-fluid glucose differences of >50 mg/dl may be useful in predicting sepsis, particularly in horses with negative or pending fluid bacterial cultures.[35]

Additionally, increased anaerobic glycolysis would be expected to increase fluid lactate concentrations, thus lowering fluid pH. Detection of fluid lactate concentrations greater than those of paired blood specimens or fluid pH <7.3 lends further support to suspicion of sepsis.[1,35]

Unless specimens are processed immediately, tubes containing fluoride-oxalate are required for accurate results. The fluoride arrests cell metabolism, thus preventing in vitro glucose depletion and lactate formation by cells and bacteria after collection.

LDH catalyzes the oxidation of pyruvate to lactate during anaerobic glycolysis, and peritoneal fluid LDH activity would be anticipated to increase in parallel with decreasing fluid glucose concentration, increasing fluid lactate levels, and decreasing pH. In one study comparing peritoneal fluid LDH activities in horses with nonseptic and septic peritonitis, however, a significant difference was *not* detected between the groups.[35] The authors hypothesized that tissue injury associated with celiotomy in the nonseptic peritonitis group may have contributed to elevated peritoneal fluid LDH activity. LDH activity may be of diagnostic utility in assessing likelihood of sepsis in the presurgical patient, however.

Cholesterol and Triglycerides: Chylous and pseudochylous effusions are grossly similar in appearance, and biochemical testing is frequently useful in distinguishing these fluids.[36-39] Chylous effusions are characterized by a high triglyceride content, and fluid values will greatly exceed serum values. Conversely, fluid cholesterol levels remain low, less than paired serum values. In contrast, pseudochylous effusions typically have cholesterol concentrations greater than and triglyceride concentrations less than serum values.

Amylase and Lipase: Peritoneal fluid amylase and lipase activity are less than paired serum values in the healthy horse.[34] Inversion of this relationship may occur with pancreatitis, cholelithiasis, small intestinal mucosal injury, or rupture of the small intestine.[34]

Phosphate: Peritoneal fluid phosphate concentrations have been suggested to be useful in detection of major intestinal injury.[40,41] Horses requiring surgical resection of necrotic bowel associated with severe colic had significantly greater peritoneal fluid phosphate concentrations than either normal horses or horses with medical causes of colic.[40] Peritoneal fluid phosphate levels >3.6 mg/dl predicted the need for surgical intervention with a sensitivity of 77% and a specificity of 76%.[40] This same report suggested that serum phosphate levels alone may be of value when peritoneal fluid specimens are unavailable. It is critical to use age-appropriate reference ranges, since foals may have greater serum and peritoneal fluid phosphate values, attributable to increased osseous metabolism.

ALP and AST: Activities of ALP and AST in equine peritoneal fluid are significantly less than that of serum activities in health. Because of the high tissue activity of these enzymes in liver and intestinal mucosa, elevated peritoneal fluid values have been suggested to potentially reflect damage to these organs. Lack of tissue specificity limits diagnostic reliability, however, and studies have shown that much of the ALP activity in adult equine peritoneal fluid is granulocytic in origin.[20]

Another potential application of fluid ALP activity is in the diagnosis of equine dysautonomia (grass sickness).[2,21] This condition may mimic surgical causes of colic both in clinical signs and in peritoneal fluid abnormalities. In a study comparing fluid ALP activities in normal horses with those from horses with grass sickness and either medical or surgical causes of colic, significantly greater ALP activity was detected in peritoneal fluid from surgical cases of colic.[21] Peritoneal fluid ALP activity from grass sickness cases was greater than that of normal horses but much less than that of surgical colic cases, aiding in differentiating these disorders. Peritoneal fluid values for ALP and AST in clinically normal foals and adult horses are reported in Table 9-2.

Pathologic Changes in Peritoneal Fluid

The constituents of peritoneal fluid reflect the pathophysiologic state of the intraabdominal mesothelium and viscera. This state may change during the period of observation of an animal, so repeated abdominocentesis may yield greater insight in to the progression of disease or response to therapy than an isolated fluid specimen.

TABLE 9-3

Classification of Peritoneal Effusion

Effusion	Total Nucleated Cell Count	Total Protein Concentration[c]	Causes
Reference range (adult)	< 10,000/μl	< 2.5 g/dl	N/A
Transudate[a]	< 5,000/μl (often < 1500/μl)	< 2.5 g/dl (often <1.5 g/dl)[b]	↓colloid osmotic pressure: hypoalbuminemia ↑capillary hydrostatic pressure: congestive heart failure portal hypertension Lymphatic obstruction
Modified transudate	1,500–10,000/μl	2.5–3.5 g/dl	↑capillary hydrostatic pressure: congestive heart failure portal hypertension Lymphatic obstruction Neoplasia Uroperitoneum Chyloperitoneum Peracute rupture of viscus
Exudate	> 10,000/μl (may have clumped cells)	> 3.0–3.5 g/dl	↑capillary permeability: inflammation/vasculitis ischemia/infarction/ thromboembolism tissue necrosis Lymphatic obstruction: inflammation neoplasia Subacute rupture of viscus

[a]Transudate may differ from normal peritoneal fluid by increased fluid volume alone.
[b]If determined biochemically
[c]Determined by refractive index

For example, early in the course of intussusception or strangulation-obstruction, peritoneal fluid values may be within reference limits or indicative of a transudative effusion. These values would be similar to those in the peritoneal fluid from a horse with an enteric foreign body. However, as the affected gut becomes more compromised by poor vascular perfusion and poor venous return, the peritoneal fluid would become more abnormal, with increasing hemorrhagic diapedesis of RBC and development of neutrophilic peritonitis. The latter would become progressively more severe as the mucosal barrier to enteric macromolecules and microorganisms deteriorated. Eventually, septic peritonitis would develop and the horse would go into endotoxemic shock. In contrast, peritoneal fluid from a horse with an enteric foreign body would tend to remain unchanged.

Successful medical therapy of primary peritonitis may be reflected by a decreasing inflammatory reaction before clinical improvement is noted. Serial abdominocenteses may thus be useful to document a lack of change, a deterioration, or an improvement in peritoneal disorders. The following pages consider common alterations in volume, color, and turbidity of

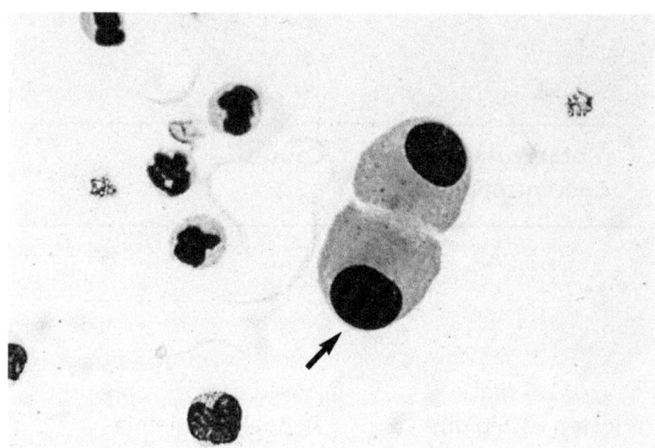

Fig. 9-10 Dividing mesothelial cells *(arrow)* in long-standing effusion.
Horse had resolving peritonitis. An effusion had been present for about a week. (Original magnification X950; May-Grunwald-Giemsa)

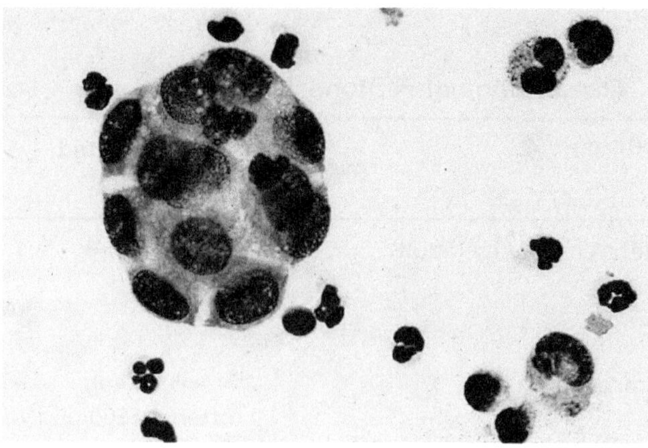

Fig. 9-11 Raft of mesothelial cells in peritoneal fluid.
Same horse as in Fig. 9-10. (Original magnification X950; May-Grunwald-Giemsa)

peritoneal fluid in various general disease processes and differentiation of peritoneal effusions.

Interpreting Peritoneal Fluid Findings

Effusions have been classically grouped as transudates, modified transudates, exudates, or hemorrhagic effusions (Table 9-3). Though these are reasonably distinct groups, often with common pathophysiologic mechanisms linking various diseases within each category, this classification system has some limitations. For example, abdominal neoplasia, chyloperitoneum, and uroperitoneum produce effusions that do not fall neatly into any one of these categories. Furthermore, these conditions are important in their own right and do not really require classification in the above schema.

Another shortcoming of this classification system is that it suggests that the separate categories are mutually exclusive. Such an assumption is incorrect. For example, the characteristics of transudates and modified transudates tend to merge, and these effusions often have common causes. Similarly, the distinction between some modified transudates and mild inflammatory exudates may also be quite subjective. Finally, because peritoneal fluid is a dynamic medium and reflects the status of the abdominal cavity and its contents, it may change as the course of disease progresses. For example, early in the course of an intestinal strangulation/obstruction, peritoneal fluid may be a modified transudate (or even a transudate in the very early stages of the dislocation). As the degree of intestinal ischemia worsens, the peritoneal fluid becomes an exudative and hemorrhagic effusion.

Despite these limitations, the four main categories are clinically relevant in most cases. Clinicians are, however, reminded that if a fluid does not neatly fall into a particular classification, the result may still be diagnostically useful. Finally, as emphasized previously, because peritoneal fluid constituents may change in the period of a few hours, serial abdominocenteses may be diagnostically useful in some cases.

Transudates

Ascitic or transudative effusions have an increased volume with a pale to colorless appearance because of their low cellularity and low total protein concentration. Therefore, since there is no lower limit to the cellularity and total protein content of normal peritoneal fluid, estimation of increased fluid volume in the peritoneal cavity is very important to classify a fluid as a pathologic transudative effusion.

Cytologic findings of these effusions are usually unremarkable, with neutrophils, lymphocytes, and large mononuclear cells present in normal proportions. Cell morphology is also usually normal, but increased numbers of reactive mesothelial cells may be noted (Figs. 9-5, 9-6, 9-10, and 9-11). These mesothelial cells are not pathognomonic for transudative effusions. They may occur in any long-standing effusion and are thought to arise from decreased contact inhibition as a result of separation of the parietal and visceral mesothelia by the excessive amount of fluid bathing these surfaces.

Transudative effusions have been commonly associated with chronic diarrhea, protein-losing gastroenteropathy, and weight loss or failure to gain weight.[42] Such ascitic effusions may also be seen in other conditions associated with marked hypoalbuminemia (and thus decreased plasma oncotic pressure) and/or intestinal vascular or lymphatic stasis/obstruction. Possible causes include protein-losing glomerulopathy, chronic hepatopathy, and early intestinal obstruction, especially from an intraluminal foreign body, impaction, or intussusception. Obviously other clinical and laboratory findings must be incorporated into the case database to differentiate which of these causes is most likely.

Modified Transudates

"Modified transudates" tends to be an awkward category of effusions with respect to the clinicopathologic characterization and clinical interpretation, and for this reason, its elimination as an effusion type has been proposed.[24]

A key feature of modified transudates is their *increased volume* within the peritoneal cavity, since their cell counts and protein concentrations greatly overlap equine normal reference ranges. Occasionally, however, the total protein concentration may be somewhat increased. Modified transudates are thus distinguished from pure transudates because they are more cellular and have a higher protein concentration. Though their total nucleated cell counts and protein values may be above reference limits, they are not as increased as exudates.

Modified transudates usually have a grossly normal appearance. At most they have mildly increased turbidity with minimal discoloration, the exception being chylous effusions, which may be opaque whitish pink. Neutrophils with normal morphology tend to be the prominent cells in modified transudates.[42]

Modified transudates have a wide variety of causes.[42] They usually result from increased hydrostatic pressure within the intestinal venous or lymphatic systems. They have been reported in horses with congestive heart failure, neoplasia, diarrhea, and chronic weight loss. Other causes for development of modified transudative effusions include peracute/acute rupture of a hollow viscus, early chemical peritonitis (uroabdomen, pancreatitis), or chyloperitoneum.

Modified transudates are often detected in horses with colic. In such cases they indicate that any intestinal lesion present has not likely resulted in severe intestinal ischemia, infarction, or necrosis.[42] Such an observation is commonly made in cases involving the large bowel.[43,44] However, in severe, peracute inflammatory conditions such as necrotizing enterocolitis, peritoneal fluid values may remain within normal limits even immediately prior to death in up to 50% of cases.[45] As the degree of intestinal ischemia increases in severity, hemorrhagic diapedesis occurs and the peritoneal fluid becomes progressively more sanguineous, provided the affected segment of bowel is within the peritoneal cavity.[44]

Modified transudates occasionally have a moderately to markedly increased total protein concentration, with low to normal total nucleated cell count. Conditions in which this has been seen include proximal enteritis, weight loss, endocarditis (without congestive heart failure), splenomegaly, and chronic hepatic fibrosis.[31,42,46] In the last, the peritoneal fluid bilirubin concentration was also markedly increased.

Exudates

Exudates have an increased volume, cellularity, and total protein concentration. Therefore, they have an abnormal gross appearance that, as described earlier, varies with the number and relative proportions of RBC and inflammatory cells present.

Total nucleated cell count of exudates may be underestimated in specimens because of cell clumping associated with fibrin deposition or because of marked karyolytic degeneration. For this reason, automated methods of cell enumeration may be highly inaccurate. This is obvious when the smear is examined microscopically. Total nucleated cell count may also be influenced by volume of fluid present in the peritoneal cavity. For example, in a horse with resolving peritonitis, the volume of peritoneal fluid within the abdominal cavity may decrease faster than the total nucleated cell count and total protein content. Consequently, though the rate of exudation may be decreasing, initially the total nucleated cell count and total protein concentration may actually increase, even though the total numbers of cells in the peritoneal cavity are also declining. Thus, particularly when one is performing repetitive abdominocenteses to monitor a horse's progress, it is advisable to mentally adjust the total nucleated cell count and total protein concentration for the volume of fluid thought to be present in the cavity. Additionally, improvement in neutrophil morphology may aid in substantiating resolution of peritoneal disease in such situations.

Exudates are classically subcategorized as nonseptic and septic. This distinction is easy to make when bacteria are observed. However, the absence of bacteria on a smear and the inability to culture organisms from peritoneal fluid do not necessarily imply a nonseptic cause.[47] Assessing neutrophil morphology is very important in evaluating exudates.[31,42,48,49] Bacterial cytotoxins may rapidly damage inflammatory cells in vivo, especially neutrophils. Such acute cell injury causes cellular disruption and nuclear degeneration. *Karyolysis* (swollen, palely stained nuclei) suggests sepsis and the smear should be carefully scrutinized. The more marked the karyolysis, the greater the suspicion of sepsis. Even if bacteria are not found (or cultured) in such fluids, they are still the most likely cause of the exudative process.

Normal neutrophil morphology (possibly with evidence of some pyknotic degeneration) does not exclude a bacterial etiology. If the inciting microorganisms produce scant amounts of cytotoxins, the inflammatory response may be marked while cell morphology remains normal. A striking example is the peritonitis produced by *Actinobacillus equuli*.[16,50,51] The total nucleated cell count in these cases may be extremely high (possibly >150,000/µl; 150 × 10^9/L), comprising 70% to 90% neutrophils with good morphology and 10% to 30% large mononuclear cells with some leukophagocytosis. Organisms are infrequently observed on these smears, but positive cultures are virtually always obtained.

Based on the proportion of neutrophils and large mononuclear cells, inflammatory reactions have been broadly grouped as follows.[52]

Suppurative (also called neutrophilic), when there are ≥70% neutrophils and ≤30% large mononuclear cells

Chronic-suppurative (also called pyogranulomatous), when there are 50% to 70% neutrophils and 30% to 50% large mononuclear cells

Chronic (also called granulomatous), when there are <50% neutrophils and >50% mononuclear cells (including both large and small mononuclear cells)

These categories do not reflect the duration of the inflammatory process as much as the potential inciting cause. A suppurative inflammatory reaction may be very recent or may have existed for days to weeks. In contrast, chronic-suppurative and chronic inflammatory reactions tend to have been present for some period of time (days or more). Exudates of some duration often reveal increased phagocytic activity by macrophages, with ingested nucleated cells, RBCs, and unidentifiable debris.[26] Cytoplasmic vacuolation is also relatively common in such situations. The numbers of lymphocytes may also increase in chronic inflammatory reactions and in the resolving stages of septic peritonitis.[16] Most of these cells have a normal appearance (Fig. 9-12), but occasionally large lymphoblastic-like cells may be observed.

Inflammatory exudation of proteins results in a high fibrinogen content in the peritoneal fluid, which may sometimes be observed on the cytologic smear. Nevertheless, the fluid often does not clot when placed in a clot tube.[42,49] Lack of coagulation suggests mechanical defibrinization or fibrinolysis by leukocytic or bacterial enzymes.

Classification of a fluid as an exudate documents peritonitis. The next diagnostic challenge is to determine the cause of peritonitis and to then proceed with the appropriate therapy. Broadly speaking, peritonitis may be considered in nonseptic and septic categories.

Nonseptic Peritonitis: Spontaneous causes of nonseptic peritonitis include peritoneal neoplasia (particularly if the tumor has ischemic or necrotic foci), bile peritonitis, chyloabdomen (particularly long-standing cases),[36,37] seminoperitoneum, and uroperitoneum. Laparoscopy, accidental enterocentesis, uncomplicated abdominal surgery, and routine open castration can lead to nonseptic postoperative peritonitis within 24 hours.* The magnitude of the response tends to be directly related to the invasiveness and duration of the procedure. Neutrophilic leukocytosis and hyperfibrinogenemia may also occur within the first few days after surgery, but the peritonitis is usually subclinical. Cell morphology is generally normal, though occasionally some degeneration may be noted. Bacteria are absent. The total nucleated cell count usually returns to reference limits in about 1 week but may still be increased 14 days postoperatively. Postoperative reference ranges for peritoneal fluid parameters have been established and are reported in Table 9-4.

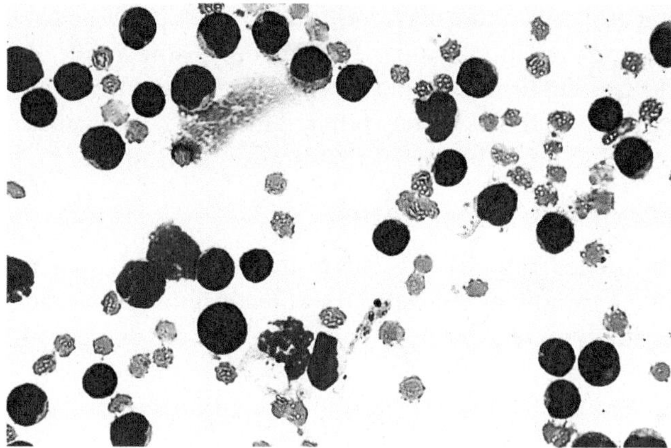

Fig. 9-12 Numerous small to medium-sized lymphocytes in peritoneal fluid sample.
These cells were often reactive (basophilic cytoplasm). Severe bot infestation and cholangitis were found on necropsy. (Original magnification X950; May-Grunwald-Giemsa)

Septic Peritonitis: Causes of septic peritonitis includes peritonitis per se (spontaneous peritonitis for which no underlying cause is identified), encapsulated and ruptured abdominal abscesses, accidental enterocentesis, complicated abdominal surgery, and gastrointestinal or genitourinary tract rupture following trauma or necrosis.[16,47,50,55-63] Peritoneal fluid alterations are commonly accompanied by a circulating neutrophilic leukocytosis, inflammatory hyperglobulinemia, and hyperfibrinogenemia. Encapsulated abscesses, as expected, often produce only mild peritonitis, whereas ruptured abscesses may cause a marked inflammatory exudate. Bacteria may be observed in peritoneal fluid in both situations.

When present in peritoneal fluid specimens, bacteria may vary in numbers, types, and location. In general, the prognosis is better when these organisms are few and phagocytosed by neutrophils or, less commonly, macrophages.[42,48,49] When organisms are numerous and many are free (nonphagocytosed), the prognosis is more

*See references 5, 10-12, 21, 33, 53, and 54.

TABLE 9-4
Reference Values for Peritoneal Fluid Cell Counts and Protein Concentrations in Horses Following Abdominal Surgery

Number of Horses	10 Ponies[11a]	10 Horses[10a]	5 Horses[10a]
Procedure	Exploratory celiotomy	Small colon resection & anastomosis with drain placement	Exploratory celiotomy & drain placement
WBC # (10^3/μl)			
Days post op - 1	110-165	84-177	98-235
3	35-330	43-86	21-83
5	62-101	37-58	28-60
7	—	28-63	28-59
%Neutrophils			
Days post op - 1	79-100	69-86	86-92
3	80-96	82-92	78-88
5	64-100	73-88	72-86
7	—	75-85	60-88
%Monocytes			
Days post op - 1		15-32	6-13
3	NA	7-16	6-16
5		11-25	12-22
7		13-22	10-34
%Lymphocytes			
Days post op - 1		0-1	1-3
3	NA	0-2	2-7
5		0-4	0-5
7		1-4	1-7
RBC # (x10^3/μl			
Days post op - 1		0-19,900	122-467
3	NA	125-298	0-90
5		38-117	0-25
7		0-202	0-36
TP (g/dl)			
Days post op - 1	2.7-6.7	3.3-4.0	3.3-5.5
3	3.6-6.2	4.0-4.5	3.7-4.4
5	3.8-4.8	4.0-5.0	3.6-4.4
7	—	3.9-4.9	0-8.3
SG			
Days post op - 1	1.021-1.037		
3	1.025-1.037	NA	NA
5	1.020-1.036		
7	—		
Fibrinogen[b] (mg/dl)			
Days post op - 1	<100-570	140-250	110-250
3	<100-280	210-320	100-250
5	120-280	170-260	140-260
7	—	<100-240	<100-170

Data from Hanson et al: Evaluation of peritoneal fluid following intestinal resection and anastomosis in horses. *Am J Vet Res* 53(2):216-221, 1992; Malark et al: Equine peritoneal fluid analysis in special situations (abstract). *Proceedings of the 36th Annual Convention of the AAEP*, 1990, p 645.

[a] Values are mean ± 2 standard deviations.

[b] 100 mg/dl lower limit of detection.

NA - Not analyzed

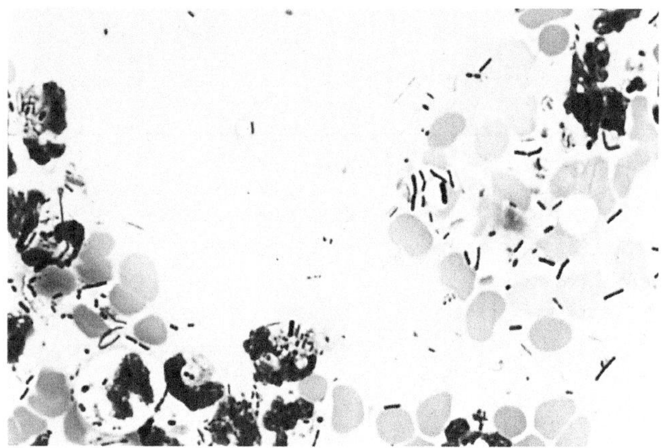

Fig. 9-13 This peritoneal fluid sample from a horse with septic peritonitis shows mild to moderate karyolytic degeneration of neutrophils and large numbers of bacteria. The population of organisms is mixed, with some free and some phagocytosed. (Original magnification X950; May-Grunwald-Giemsa)

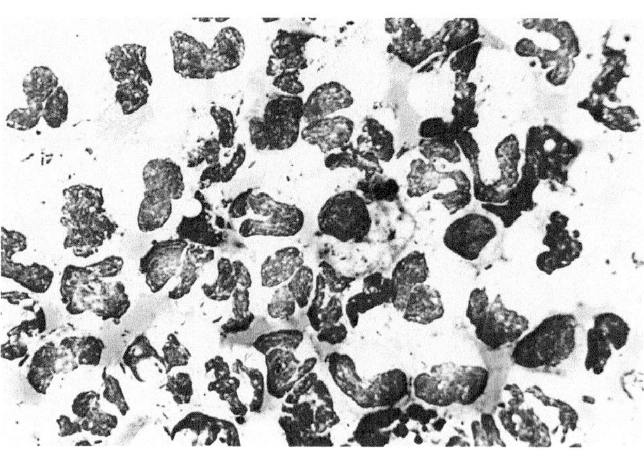

Fig. 9-14 This peritoneal fluid sample from a horse with septic peritonitis shows marked karyolytic degeneration of neutrophils and bacteria. (Original magnification X950; May-Grunwald-Giemsa)

Fig. 9-15 This peritoneal fluid sample from a horse with septic peritonitis has a mixed population of bacteria and markedly degenerate cells (cell ghosts). The horse had a ruptured stomach. (Original magnification X950; May-Grunwald-Giemsa)

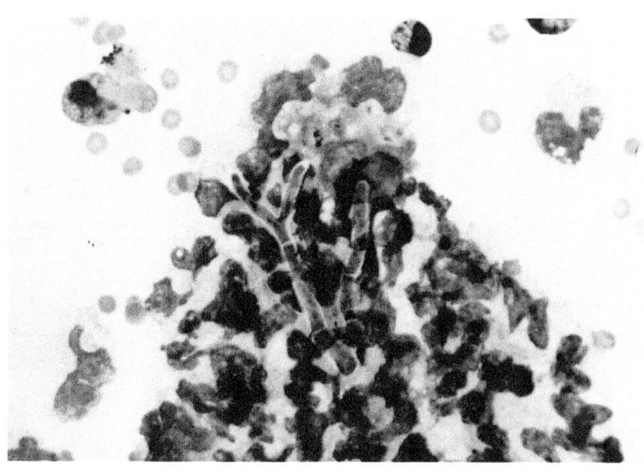

Fig. 9-16 Equine abdominal fluid.
A basophilic staining, septate, fungal hyphae exhibiting dichotomous branching is present within a background of chronic suppurative inflammation. (Wright-Giemsa) (Courtesy Dr. Mary Jo Burkhard, North Carolina State University, Raleigh.)

guarded. An extreme example of this is the septic peritonitis associated with gastrointestinal or abscess rupture. In such cases there may be very few (if any) intact inflammatory cells and marked karyolytic degeneration evidenced by very pale-staining *smudged* nuclei (Figs. 9-13 to 9-15). Cell counts may be erroneously elevated in fluid specimens from rupture cases if determined by automated means because of inclusion of plant debris and bacterial clumps in the cell count. Results should be verified by microscopic examination. Bacteria may be present in large numbers, represented by a mixed population of organisms. It should be noted that all gram-positive and gram-negative microbes stain basophilic with Romanowsky stains.

The site of the rupture in the gastrointestinal tract often influences the type of fluid obtained by abdominocentesis.[16,42] Gastric and cecal (large intestinal) ruptures generally result in widespread contamination of the peritoneal cavity and marked cellular disruption. In some cases, especially with gastric rupture, smears are almost acellular (see Fig. 9-15). These fluids often have a turbid brown granular appearance, with a brownish

TABLE 9-5

Typical Equine Peritoneal Fluid Analysis Results for Various Conditions

Condition	Color/ Turbidity	Total Nucleated Cell Count	Differential Cell Count	Protein[a]
Healthy Impaction Diarrhea Peracute volvulus	Pale yellow / clear	<10,000/μl[b]	~50:50 ratio of mononuclear cells and neutrophils	<2.5 gm/dl
Lymphoma	Yellow-white / cloudy	Elevated	Lymphoblasts	Elevated
Chylous / pseudochylous	White - pink / coudy	Normal to elevated	Small lymphocytes	
Excess EDTA	Pale yellow / clear	Low - normal	Normal	Elevated
Acute volvulus	Yellow-red / clear	Normal - elevated	Normal - ↑ neutrophils	
Subacute volvulus	Yellow-red /cloudy	Elevated	↑ Neutrophils	
Postenterocentesis	Yellow / cloudy	Elevated	↑ Neutrophils	
Peritonitis Postsurgery	Yellow-white to Reddish-brown / cloudy	Marked elevation	↑ Neutrophils	Elevated
Strangulated volvulus[c]	Wine colored / cloudy	Elevated	↑ Neutrophils RBC's, macrophages	Elevated
Enterocentesis	Brown-green / cloudy	Low to normal	↑ Neutrophils, extracellular bacteria, plant debris, protozoa	Low - normal
Rectal Tear[d]		Elevated	↑ Neutrophils - degenerative, intra and extracellular bacteria	Elevated
Blood contamination	Red / cloudy	Normal	↑ Neutrophils, lymphocytes platelets, RBCs	Elevated
Hemoperitoneum			↑ Neutrophils, RBCs, macrophages containing pigment, erythrophagia	

[a]Refractive index.
[b]Foals < 1,500 – 3,600/μl.
[c]With tissue necrosis.
[d]Peracutely, peritoneal fluid may be normal to hemorrhagic, progressing to inflammatory.

supernatant. However, in one retrospective study of 50 cases of gastric rupture, 6 of 33 horses from which peritoneal fluid was obtained for analysis had no plant material or bacterial organisms identified on cytologic examination.[64] Of these, only one had an elevated cell count. Distinguishing such gastrointestinal ruptures from an accidental enterocentesis is discussed later (see section on accidental enterocentesis).

In contrast, small intestinal and rectal ruptures usually result in less peritoneal contamination by gut contents because the omentum can more effectively isolate the affected bowel from the rest of the peritoneal cavity. Nevertheless, septic peritonitis with a marked neutrophilic exudate still occurs.

Rectal palpation, percutaneous and transrectal ultrasonography, and exploratory laparotomy may aid diagnosis of intraabdominal abscesses.[16,55-61] Aerobic and anaerobic microbial cultures are recommended. To improve the chances of a positive culture, various transport media and systems are available. The clinician should ascertain which methods are preferred by the referral laboratory. Commonly isolated organisms include *Corynebacterium pseudotuberculosis, Rhodococcus equi, Streptococcus zooepidemicus,* and *Streptococcus equi.*[56,57] *Actinobacillus equuli, Escherichia coli, Corynebacterium pyogenes, Bacteroides* sp., and other *Streptococcus* species have also been reported to cause peritonitis.[16,47,50,55,65] Microbial culture is variably successful in cases of abdominal abscessation.[55,56,66] Therefore, a negative culture does not exclude sepsis as a cause of peritonitis, especially if karyolytic degeneration of cells is noted on a smear.[16,47] Rarely, septic peritonitis is associated with disseminated fungal infections (Fig. 9-16).

Findings Associated with Various Conditions

Table 9-5 summarizes anticipated peritoneal fluid analysis results for a variety of conditions affecting the horse. These conditions are discussed at greater length in the following pages.

Accidental Enterocentesis

As noted earlier, occasionally the intestine is accidentally punctured during abdominocentesis. This provokes an inflammatory reaction in the peritoneal cavity but is usually without obvious clinical signs or sequelae. In such situations the specimen contains gut contents. It generally has a greenish brown turbid and granular appearance, with a characteristic somewhat fermentative odor. Analysis often reveals a low protein concentration, low specific gravity, and low cell count. Microscopically there are very few (if any) identifiable cells and a mixed population of bacteria (Figs. 9-17 and 9-18). Ciliated protozoa and plant fibers may also be obvious (Fig. 9-19).

During specimen collection, the veterinarian may feel the needle or cannula *pop* into the viscus. If this sensation has not been appreciated during collection, the specimen must be distinguished from gastrointestinal rupture. If the horse's cardiovascular status is good to fairly good, a ruptured gut is most unlikely. Horses with gastrointestinal ruptures quickly develop cardiovascular collapse.

Hemorrhagic Effusions

Hemorrhage (RBCs) into a peritoneal fluid sample may be the result of iatrogenic contamination at collection, hemorrhagic diapedesis (usually from a compromised segment of the gastrointestinal tract), intraabdominal hemorrhage, or splenic paracentesis (Fig. 9-20).

Iatrogenic Contamination: When bleeding is observed from superficial blood vessels or when the peritoneal fluid is initially nonbloody but becomes hemorrhagic (or vice versa) during collection, iatrogenic contamination is likely. Microscopic examination of such fluid may reveal platelets, often pale staining and clumped together. Unless a delay occurs between sample collection and processing, no significant amount of erythrophagocytosis would be anticipated. Contamination should also be considered in specimens that are uniformly bloody throughout collection. Centrifugation should reveal a clear, plasma-like supernatant and sedimented red cells rather than a uniformly hemolyzed appearance.

Effects of peripheral blood contamination on peritoneal fluid RBC counts, WBC counts, and total protein were examined in peritoneal fluid specimens from eight clinically healthy horses.[22] Although RBC counts increased significantly with increasing blood contamination, no significant change was observed in WBC, WBC differential, or total protein values.

Hemorrhagic Diapedesis: Hemorrhagic diapedesis frequently occurs in sections of intestine with compromised vascular supply and venous return. It results in peritoneal fluid that appears blood-tinged, (sero)sanguineous, turbid amber, cloudy reddish brown, muddy brick red to turbid brown, or various other hues of red or brown.[7,42,46,67] Often the supernatant of these fluids is also abnormal and may be described as hemolyzed or red to port wine in color. Such findings are common in horses with severe intestinal ischemia or infarction, and they generally indicate the need for surgical intervention if the horse is to have a chance of survival.[7,67] Hemorrhagic diapedesis may also occur with some neoplasms and in some cases of primary peritonitis.

Erythrophagocytosis is often seen in horses with hemorrhagic diapedesis (see Fig. 9-20). Other cytologic findings vary with the underlying cause.

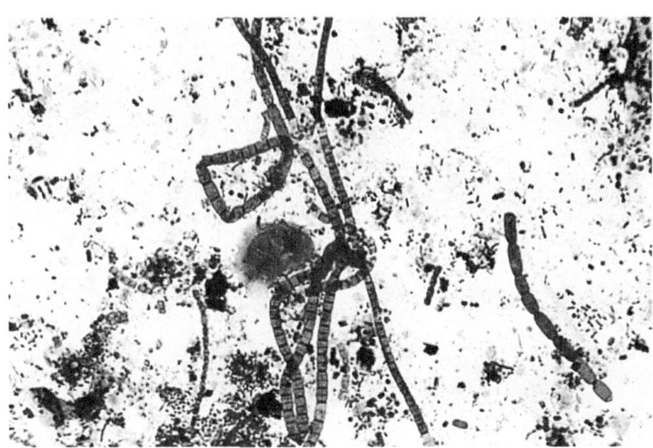

Fig. 9-17 Accidental enterocentesis produced fluid with a mixed population of bacteria and no identifiable cells. (Original magnification X950; May-Grunwald-Giemsa)

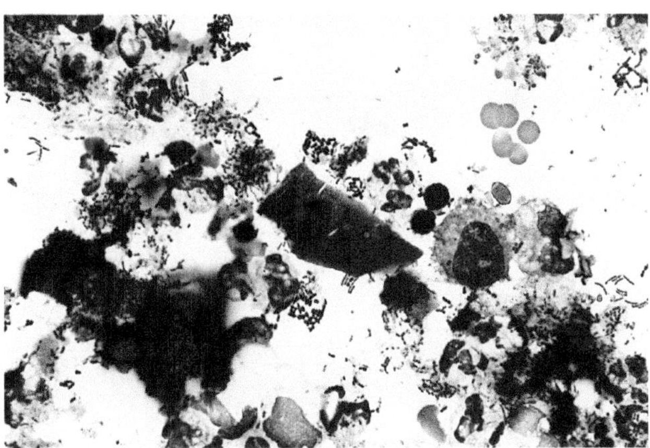

Fig. 9-18 Intestinal rupture produced fluid with mixed organisms, plant debris, few erythrocytes, and degenerative leukocytes sometimes containing phagocytized bacterial organisms. (Wright-Giemsa)

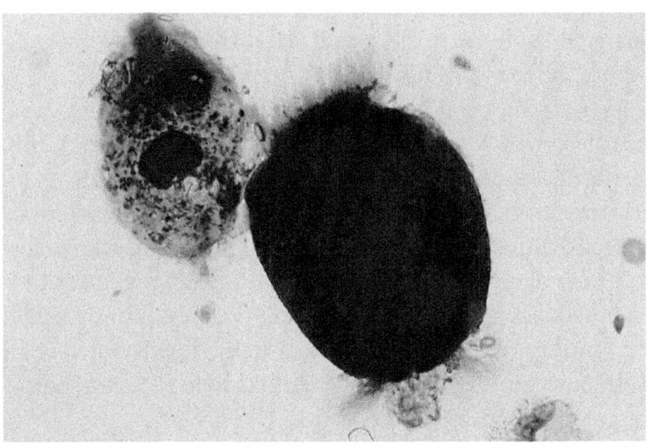

Fig. 9-19 Ciliated protozoa may be seen in either accidental enterocentesis or gastrointestinal rupture. (Wright-Giemsa)

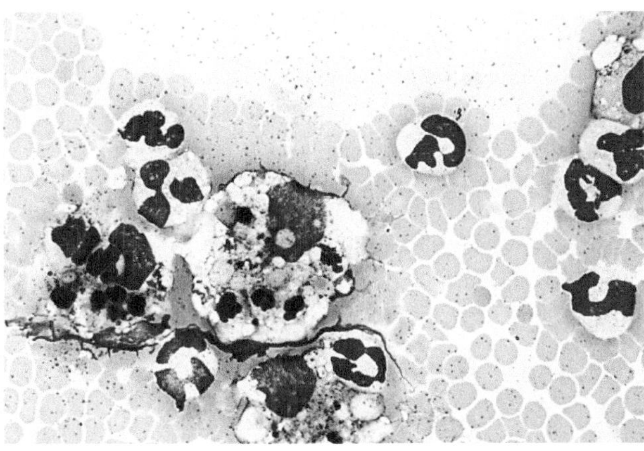

Fig. 9-20 Phagocytic macrophages are evident in this sample from a horse with hemorrhagic diapedesis associated with congestive heart failure. Note the erythrophagocytosis and leukophagocytosis. The former indicates that at least some of the hemorrhage preceded abdominocentesis. (Original magnification X950; May-Grunwald-Giemsa)

Intraabdominal Hemorrhage: In contrast to hemorrhagic diapedesis, actual hemorrhage into the peritoneal cavity is uncommon.[42] It may occur following severe blunt external trauma, penetrating wounds, rupture of the uterine artery or uterine body at foaling, or erosion of blood vessels by a neoplasm or as the result of a coagulation defect. In such cases, the peritoneal fluid PCV and total protein concentration is typically less than but approaching those of peripheral blood. Cytologic examination often reveals leukocytes in proportions similar to those in peripheral blood. Platelets are usually absent, and the fluid may have a low fibrinogen concentration due to rapid defibrinization in the peritoneal cavity. Therefore, this fluid often does not clot. Absence of clot formation in vitro does not necessarily indicate coagulopathy as the cause of hemoperitoneum. If the peritoneal fluid has a clear, plasma-like supernatant and there is no cytologic evidence of erythrophagocytosis, the hemorrhage probably occurred very recently. A hemolyzed supernatant and/or erythrophagocytosis suggests a more long-standing disorder. Mahogany to brown supernatants may be associated with extensive devitalized bowel and carry a poor prognosis.

Splenic Paracentesis: Inadvertent puncture of the spleen may occur during abdominocentesis, especially in horses

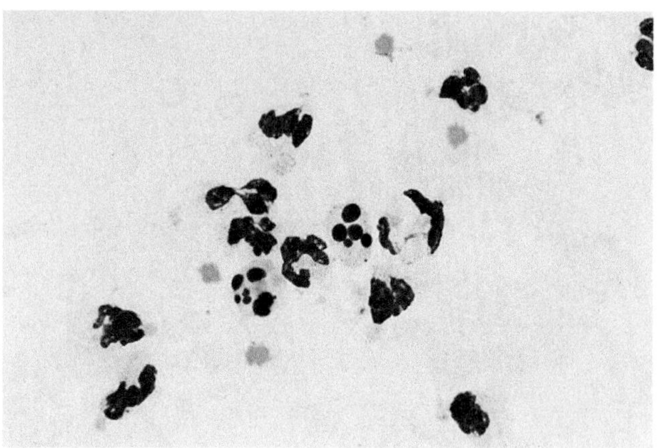

Fig. 9-21 Low magnification of seminoperitoneum. Pale basophilic sperm heads can be seen phagocytized within neutrophils. (Courtesy Dr. Peter S. MacWilliams, University of Wisconsin.)

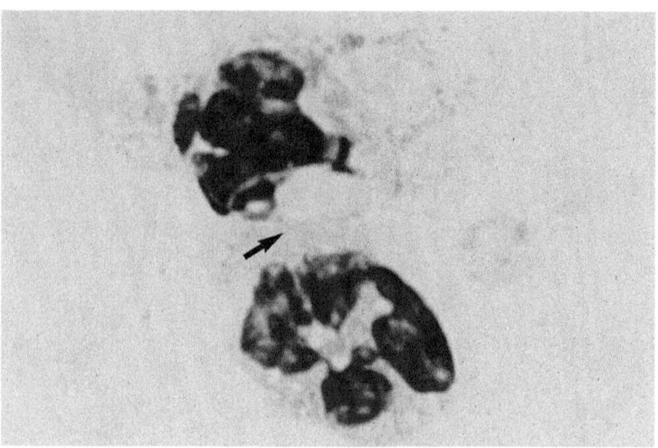

Fig. 9-22 In this peritoneal fluid sample from a mare with seminoperitoneum, a neutrophil contains phagocytosed sperm heads *(arrow)*. (Wright's-Giemsa, X1500) (Courtesy Dr. Peter S. MacWilliams, University of Wisconsin.)

with splenomegaly. No untoward sequelae have been reported.[6] The needle or cannula is often felt to penetrate the organ. The fluid subsequently obtained usually has a thick, very dark red appearance.[6,42] It may have a PCV greater than that of peripheral blood, if not diluted with peritoneal fluid, and contain numerous small mature lymphocytes and platelets. Nonreactive monocytic macrophages and neutrophils are also present. The fluid readily clots.

Seminoperitoneum

Perforation of the vagina during coitus or artificial insemination is uncommon in mares. It may result in septic and nonseptic peritonitis or seminoperitoneum.[16,67,68] With seminoperitoneum, neutrophils and macrophages contain phagocytosed sperm heads (Figs. 9-21 and 9-22). It is postulated that the associated mild neutrophilic exudate probably results from exposure of the peritoneum to seminal fluid.

Uroperitoneum

Rupture of the urinary bladder is seen most frequently in neonatal foals and is usually thought to be the result of parturient trauma.[15,69] Male foals are more commonly affected than females. Cystorrhexis may also occur in adult males, usually secondary to urolithiasis, and in adult females, usually associated with trauma at parturition.

Uroperitoneum in foals is often associated with neutrophilic leukocytosis in the peripheral blood and with marked hyponatremia, hypochloremia, and hyperkalemia.[15,69,70] However, these electrolyte abnormalities occurred in only about 40% of affected foals in another survey and should not be considered essential for diagnosis of uroperitoneum.[71]

Analysis of peritoneal fluid in these animals reveals an increased volume of clear, pale yellow fluid with a low cell count and low specific gravity.[15,69] A mild neutrophilic exudate may be observed, especially with concurrent gastrointestinal tract disease.[71] In normal foals and adults, the peritoneal fluid urea and creatine concentrations are similar to but usually slightly lower than corresponding blood values. Ratios >1:1 are strongly suggestive of, and ratios >2:1 are diagnostic for, uroperitoneum, provided the fluid sampled was not from accidental cystocentesis of distended bladder. Azotemia, particularly in the foal, is not as reliable an indicator of uroperitoneum as fluid to serum ratios of creatinine and urea.

Creatinine ratios are more reliably increased in bladder rupture than urea nitrogen ratios. Urea is a much smaller and therefore more readily diffusible molecule than creatinine. Consequently, it has been shown that in cattle with uroperitoneum, immediately after the bladder ruptures the peritoneal fluid urea and creatinine concentrations are much higher than corresponding blood values.[72] However, urea more rapidly equilibrates across the peritoneum, so the difference between blood and peritoneal fluid values decreases faster for urea than for creatinine. Eventually, concentrations of both substances in blood and peritoneal fluid are comparable but increased. In horses with chronic renal failure, fluid to serum ratios of creatinine and urea will also approach 1:1; however, fluid values will usually remain less than that of serum.

Calcium carbonate crystals have been identified on peritoneal fluid cytology on rare instances[15] and are considered diagnostic of ruptured bladder (Fig. 9-23).

Chyloabdomen

Chylous abdominal effusions are very rare in horses. In foals, such effusions have been reported to be associated with intraabdominal abscessation[61] and congenital

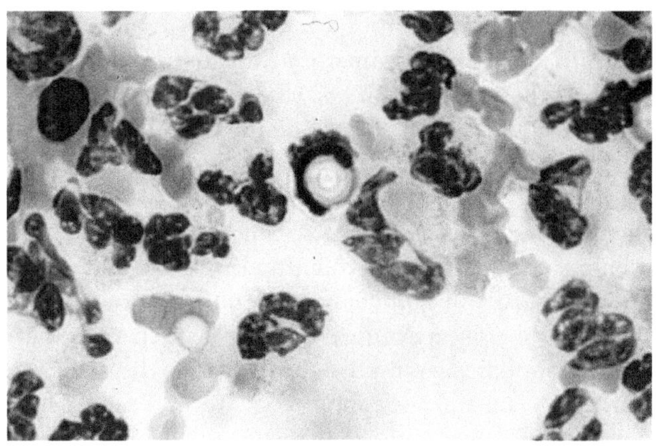

Fig. 9-23 Calcium carbonate crystal (intracytoplasmic) from abdominal fluid of foal with uroperitoneum.
A single refractile crystal can be identified within a mildly degenerative neutrophil. Mild suppurative inflammation with toxic change may accompany chemical (urine) peritonitis. (Wright-Giemsa) (Courtesy Dr. Mary Jo Burkhard, North Carolina State University, Raleigh.)

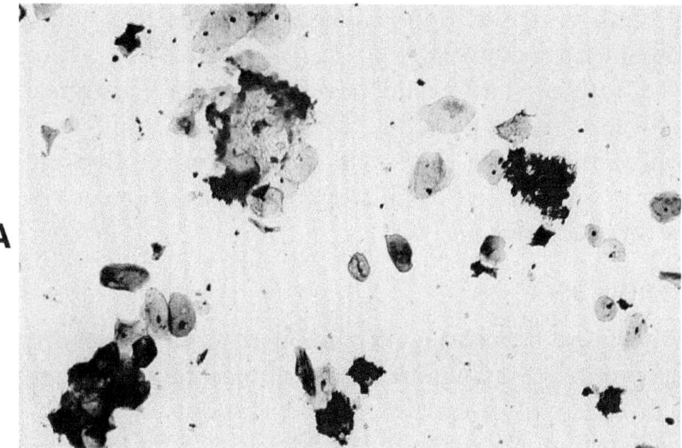

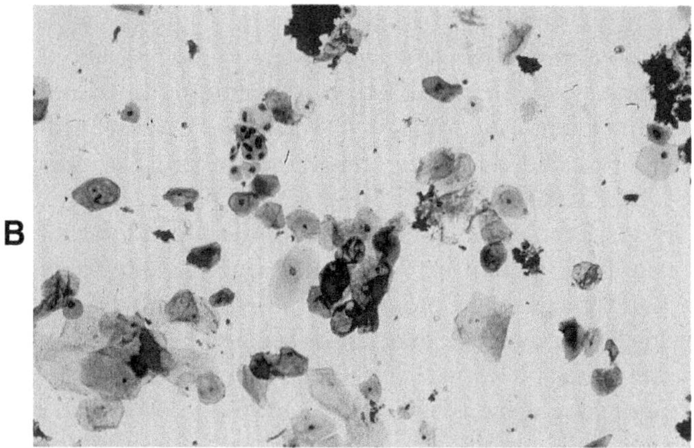

Fig. 9-24 Amniocentesis fluid from bovine.
Equine amniocentesis fluid is of similar cytologic appearance. (Wright-Giemsa) **A,** Well-differentiated squamous epithelial cells are seen intermingled with golden green aggregates of meconium. **B,** More numerous squamous epithelial cells.

malformation of the mesenteric lymphatics.[37] In mature horses, chylous effusions have been reported to occur secondary to severe cestode infection of the ileum and chronic peritonitis,[36] large colon torsion,[38] and abdominal adhesions.[39]

Grossly, the fluid of chyloabdomen is whitish pink and milky opaque. Pseudochylous effusions of severe chronic inflammation may be grossly similar in appearance. Upon standing or with centrifugation, the numerous leukocytes of pseudochylous effusions tend to form sediment topped by clear supernatant. In contrast, true chylous effusions fail to clear with centrifugation. With standing or refrigeration, the lipids of chylous effusions tend to form a cream layer on the surface of the specimen. Alkalization and the addition of ether cause dissolution of chylomicrons and clearing of chylous specimens.

Fluid triglyceride and cholesterol concentrations are useful in distinguishing chylous from pseudochylous effusions. Chylous effusions are characterized by triglyceride concentrations greater than, and cholesterol concentrations less than, paired serum values. Conversely, elevated fluid cholesterol and low triglyceride values are expected in pseudochylous effusions.

Microscopically, chylous effusions may be observed to contain a high percentage of small lymphocytes in the acute stages, and a circulating lymphopenia may be present. In longer standing effusions, however, a mixed inflammatory reactions can occur. Sudan III, Sudan IV, or Oil Red O stain for lipid can be used on air-dried fluid smears to assess the presence of chylomicrons, characteristic of chylous effusion.[73]

Pregnancy and Postpartum

Results of fluid analysis performed on abdominal fluid collected from 15 healthy mares in late gestation (10 days prior to foaling) were within reference ranges for adult horses.[74] Abdominocentesis should be performed in a cranial location during advanced pregnancy to avoid accidental amniocentesis. Fluid obtained is seen to contain low numbers of individualized, mature squamous epithelial cells and a variable quantity of golden/green/brown meconium debris microscopically (Fig. 9-24).

Following routine foaling, peritoneal fluid nucleated cell counts and protein concentrations may increase slightly but remain within reference ranges for adult horses.[41,74] Increased neutrophil percentage has been noted following routine foaling and following uncomplicated and complicated dystocias. An elevated fluid protein concentration has been observed following complicated dystocias.[41]

Uterine rupture and development of peritoneal effusion were reported to occur as postpartum complications in two mares.[75] Effusions from both were septic suppurative exudates; one had evidence of recent hemorrhage.

Neoplasia

Abdominal neoplasia is uncommon in horses, and reports of cytologic findings are few. Peritoneal fluid cytology can be useful in establishing the diagnosis of intraabdominal neoplasia, but the diagnostic yield of this procedure is variable.[76] In one report of 25 horses with intraabdominal neoplasia, lymphoma was diagnosed in 12 horses, gastric squamous-cell carcinoma in 9, and various adenocarcinomas in 4.[55] Cytology of peritoneal fluid revealed neoplastic cells in approximately half of the lymphoma and squamous-cell carcinoma groups. Even when a specific diagnosis beyond that of "neoplasia" cannot be determined cytologically, valuable diagnostic and prognostic information is gained with the knowledge that tumor seeding has occurred within the abdominal cavity. Such information carries a poor prognosis.

The following points should be kept in mind when evaluating peritoneal effusions from horses with suspected intraabdominal neoplasia.

- Intraabdominal tumors may not exfoliate cells into the peritoneal fluid. This would preclude their diagnosis by abdominocentesis.
- Tumors involving serosal surfaces, especially those that erode serosal blood vessels, may cause hemorrhagic diapedesis or hemoperitoneum.
- Necrosis or infection of a tumor may result in peritonitis. Such an inflammatory exudate may overshadow the presence of tumor cells.
- *Reactive mesothelial cells* may be mistaken for neoplastic cells, especially by the novice cytologist.

Lymphoma: Lymphoma has been classified into alimentary, mediastinal (thymic), multicentric, and cutaneous forms.[22] In alimentary and multicentric forms, there may be an abdominal effusion, which may vary from a modified transudate to a hemorrhagic effusion.[42,77] Neoplastic lymphoid cells are not always evident in peritoneal fluid specimens[77-80]; however, when present they suggest the diagnosis.

Neoplastic lymphocytes are frequently lymphoblasts. These are large cells, usually with a high nucleus to cytoplasm ratio and basophilic cytoplasm (Figs. 9-25 to 9-29). They exhibit variable, often marked anisokaryosis and anisocytosis. They usually have an irregularly round nucleus with a fairly uniform, delicate chromatin pattern and prominent nucleoli. The nucleoli may vary in number, size, and shape within and between cells. Hence, one to five small to large, round, oval, or angular nucleoli may be seen in each nucleus.

Mitotic figures, sometimes revealing abnormal spindle formation, may be visible in some cases of lymphoma. Mitotic activity may also be noted with other tumors, as well as in nonneoplastic conditions (such as mesothelial hyperplasia), and is therefore not diagnostic of lymphoma. Histiocytic lymphocytes may be the main cell type in some cases (see Figs. 9-26 and 9-28). As their name implies, morphology of these cells resembles abnormal mononuclear phagocytes. Features include large cell size but with greater variation in nuclear morphology and

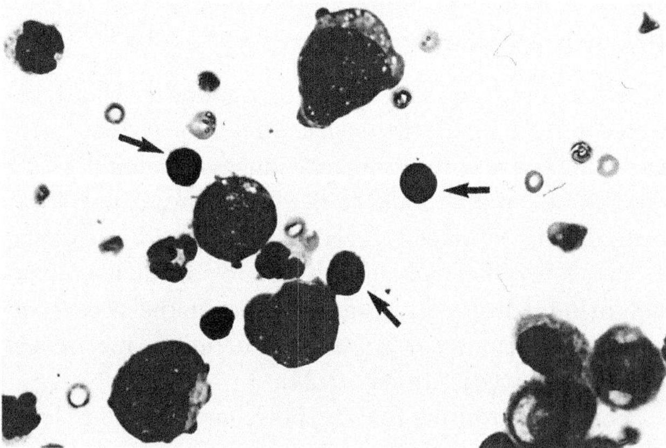

Fig. 9-25 This peritoneal fluid sample from a horse with lymphoblastic lymphosarcoma contains large lymphoblasts and small mature lymphocytes (*arrows*). (Original magnification X950; May-Grunwald-Giemsa)

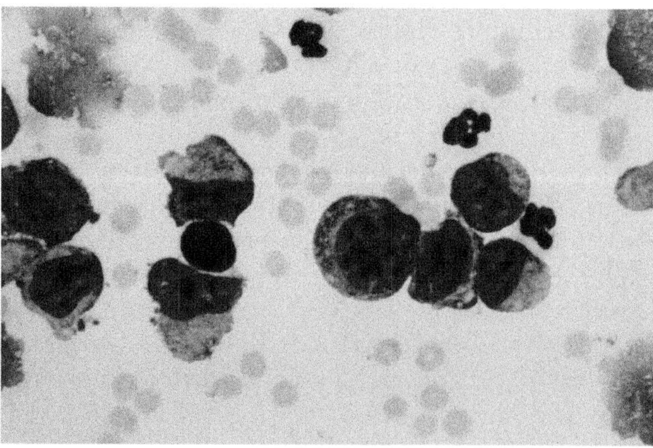

Fig. 9-26 Peritoneal fluid sample from horse with histiocytic lymphosarcoma.
Note the large neoplastic lymphocytes. (Original magnification X950; Wright's-Giemsa)

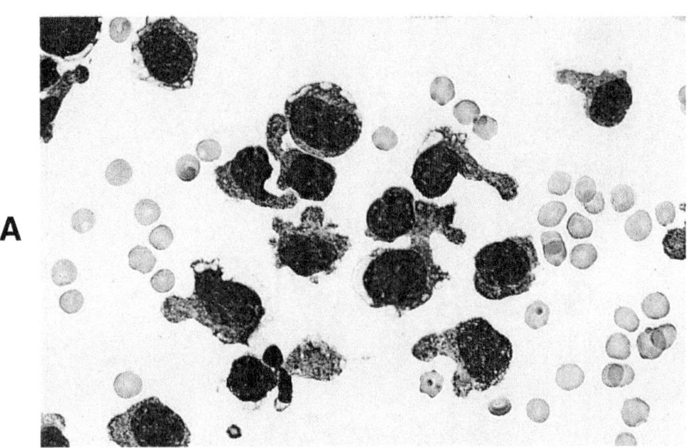

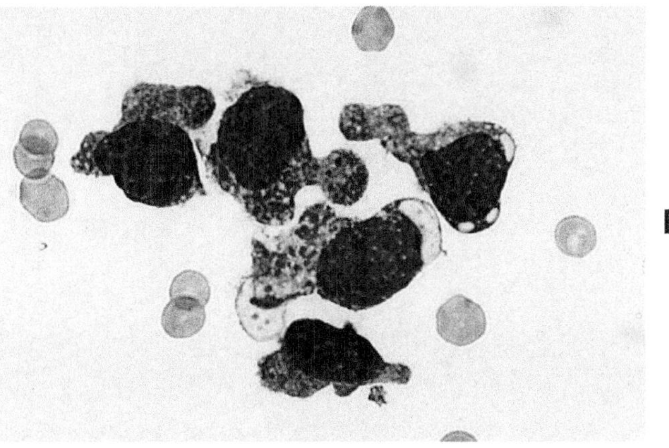

Fig. 9-27 Equine large granular lymphoma.
A, Lower magnification of pleomorphic neoplastic discrete cells. Characteristic features include round eccentric nuclei with irregularly clumped chromatin. Cytoplasm is grainy in texture and contains numerous dispersed magenta-staining granules. Pseudopodia are prominent. **B,** Higher magnification view. (Wright-Giemsa)

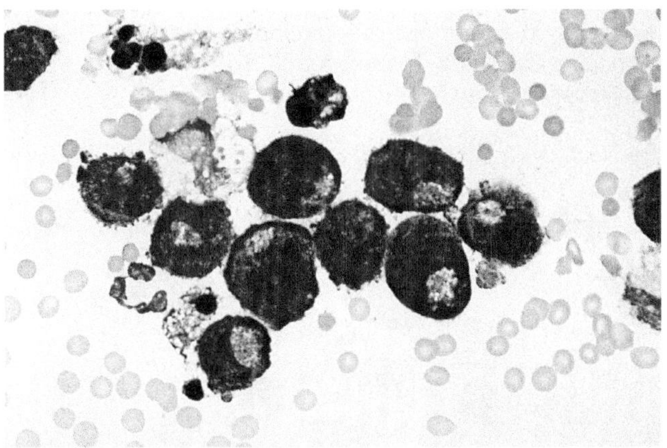

Fig. 9-28 Equine lymphoma.
Another morphologic appearance of lymphoma. These cells are darkly staining and feature eccentric bean-shaped nuclei with coarsely clumped chromatin. Cytoplasm is more abundant and has a prominent perinuclear Golgi and ruffled borders. A single large mononuclear cell and neutrophil are also present. (Wright-Giemsa)

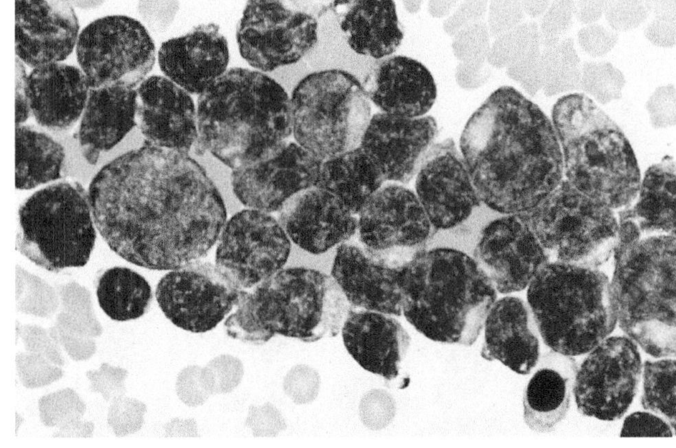

Fig. 9-29 Equine lymphoma.
Yet another morphologic appearance of lymphoma. These cells are paler staining and feature round to slightly indented nuclei with delicate chromatin and multiple prominent nucleoli. Cytoplasm is scantly and lightly basophilic. (Wright-Giemsa)

nucleus to cytoplasmic ratio. Their cytoplasm tends to be more abundant and less basophilic than that of normal lymphocytes. The neoplastic lymphocytes of large granular lymphoma (LGL) may be similar in morphology, with the exception that few to numerous, fine to coarse, magenta-staining granules are dispersed or clustered within their cytoplasm[27] (see Fig. 9-27).

Well-differentiated (small-cell) lymphoma is more difficult to diagnose by cytologic examination, since these cells have normal morphology. Differential diagnoses in such cases include chyloabdomen and lymphocytic inflammation associated with antigenic stimulation (see Fig. 9-12). Flow cytometric analysis for identification of cell surface markers may aid in confirmation of a clonal lymphocyte population in well-differentiated lymphoma.[81,82] Meaningful results are most often obtained when peritoneal fluid cell counts are high and neoplastic cells constitute a substantial proportion of the nucleated cell population.

Gastric Squamous-Cell Carcinoma: Gastric squamous-cell carcinoma is the most common neoplasm of the equine stomach, arising from the esophageal region.[29,30] Gastric squamous-cell carcinomas have

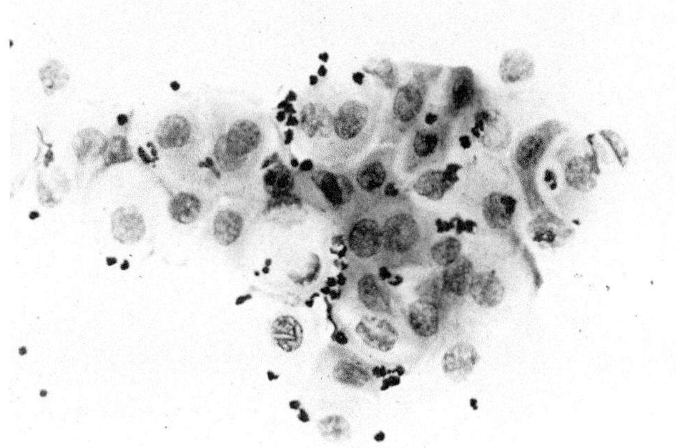

Fig. 9-30 Equine squamous-cell carcinoma, well-differentiated morphology.
Cluster of relatively uniform, large nonkeratinized squamous epithelial cells with abundant pale blue cytoplasm, oval nuclei with indistinct nucleoli. Smaller more basophilic cells have more criteria of malignancy. Neutrophils are infiltrating into the cell cluster. (Wright-Giemsa) (Courtesy Dr. Mary Jo Burkhard, North Carolina State University, Raleigh.)

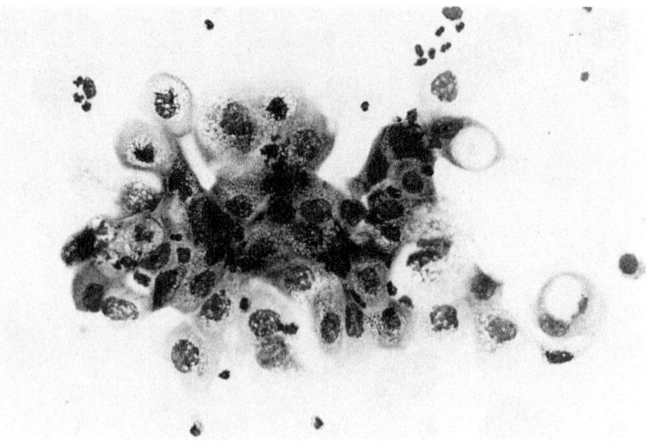

Fig. 9-31 Equine squamous-cell carcinoma, less well-differentiated morphology.
Neoplastic cells are differing in size, nucleus to cytoplasmic ratio, stain quality, and cytoplasmic vacuolization. Perinuclear vacuolization is a characteristic feature of squamous-cell malignancy. Vacuoles coalescing to form a clear ring around the nucleus, "tadpole-cell" formation, and emperipolesis are cytologic features supporting a diagnosis of squamous-cell carcinoma. (Wright-Giemsa) (Courtesy Dr. Mary Jo Burkhard, North Carolina State University, Raleigh.)

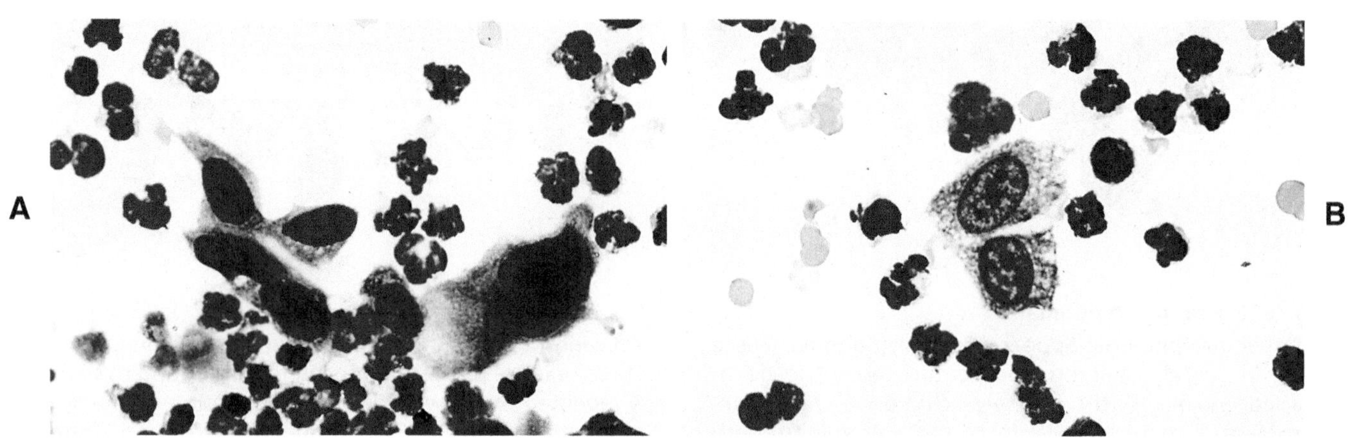

Fig. 9-32 Peritoneal fluid from horse with hemangiosarcoma.
A, Note the large spindloid cells, singly and in a cluster. **B,** Note the large oval nuclei and the prominent nucleoli of variable size and shape in the two central spindloid cells. (Original magnification X950; May-Grunwald-Giemsa)

been previously reported to metastasize more readily to the pleural cavity than to the peritoneal cavity.[83] In more recent reports, thoracic metastases were detected on postmortem examination in three of eight horses, whereas extensive abdominal metastasis was observed in all eight.[29,30]

In any event, gastric squamous-cell carcinomas may erode and perforate the stomach wall and implant on the peritoneum. Effusions from horses with gastric squamous-cell carcinoma are typically exudative and may or may not contain exfoliated neoplastic cells.[76] These cells may be present as clusters or as individual cells. Their morphology can be quite variable (Figs. 9-30 and 9-31). Well-differentiated tumors have large squamous-type cells, having a medium-sized to large nucleus, and abundant cytoplasm. Consequently, the nuclear to cytoplasmic ratio is moderate to low. Cytoplasm is pale blue with Romanowsky stains and may be slightly vacuolated (particularly perinuclearly) and possibly partly cornified. The latter imparts a

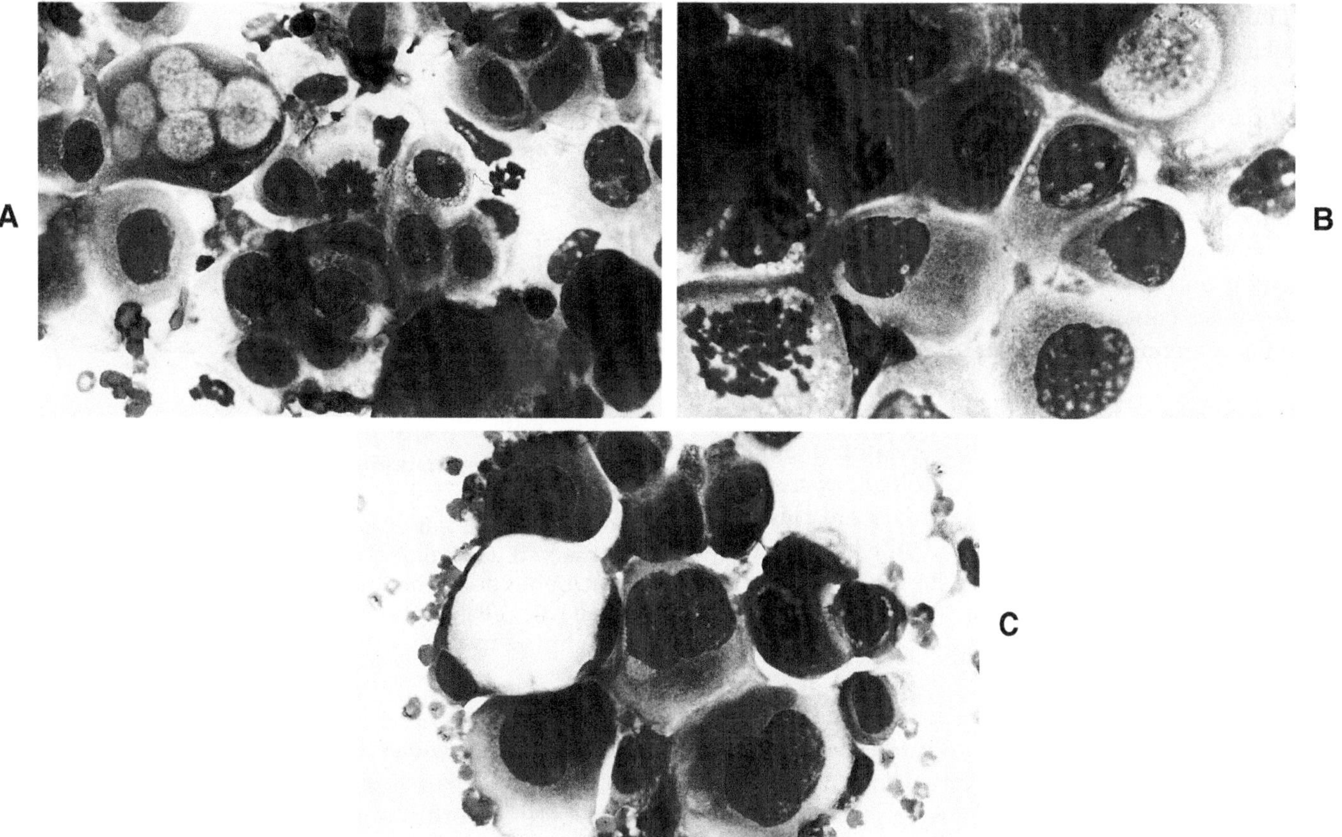

Fig. 9-33 Equine metastatic ovarian cystadenocarcinoma.
A, Numerous clusters of neoplastic epithelial cells are present and exhibit several criteria of malignancy, including marked variation in cell size, nuclear size, and nucleus to cytoplasmic ratio. A mitotic figure is present at the center of the field, and several cells contain one or more cytoplasmic vacuoles containing lightly stippled eosinophilic material. **B,** Higher magnification. Note the prominent cell junctions characteristic of epithelial neoplasms. An abnormal mitotic figure is located in the lower left field. A single large cytoplasmic vacuole containing eosinophilic material is seen in the upper right cell. **C,** Note the marked variation in cell and nuclear size. Numerous binucleated cells are seen. Perinuclear vacuolization is present in some cells. Signet ring formation is evident at the center left aspect of the cell cluster. (Abdominal fluid concentrated smear; Wright-Giemsa) (Courtesy Dr. Anne M. Barger, North Carolina State University, Raleigh.)

smooth, glassy, homogenous appearance to the cytoplasm. Less-well-differentiated tumors may exhibit greater anisokaryosis and anisocytosis with variable (often high) nuclear to cytoplasmic ratios. Nuclei are irregularly round and nucleoli may be prominent and variable in size, shape, and number within and between cells. The chromatin pattern may be reticular to coarsely clumped; nucleoli are not readily visible.

Other considerations for the presence of squamous cells on fluid cytologic examination include surface/cutaneous contamination, either from the horse or from the person handling the specimen. In advanced pregnancy, inadvertent amniocentesis may yield squamous cells on fluid cytology. Squamous cells in these instances would be mature and well-differentiated.

Hemangiosarcoma: Hemangiosarcoma is rare in horses[16,84] and may result in hemoperitoneum.[76] Neoplastic cells may rarely be present, in low numbers, in the peritoneal fluid (Fig. 9-32). These are large fusiform cells found individually or in clusters, having a large oval nucleus, often with a reticular to coarsely clumped chromatin pattern. Nucleoli are prominent, often multiple, and may vary in size and shape within and between cells. Criteria of malignancy include slight to marked anisokaryosis and anisocytosis. Neoplastic cells may have a moderate to high nuclear to cytoplasmic ratio and basophilic, somewhat vacuolated cytoplasm.

Adenocarcinoma: Adenocarcinomas arising from the gastrointestinal tract, mammary gland, pancreas, genitourinary tract, or unknown locations have been associated with abnormal peritoneal and sometimes pleural fluid effusions.[55,76,85] Effusions can vary in classification from transudates to exudates. Only infrequently do such effusions contain identifiable neoplastic cells. Cytologic features supporting a diagnosis of adenocarcinoma would include the presence of neoplastic epithelial cell clusters, with cells organized into ducts, tubules, or acinar structures. Additionally, the cytoplasm may contain clear vacuoles or vacuoles containing secretory product (Fig. 9-33).

Mesothelioma: Mesothelioma is rare in horses.[76,86] It usually produces a large volume of peritoneal fluid; up to 30 liters has been reported.[76] Cytologic examination frequently reveals numerous individual and clustered, pleomorphic mesothelial cells and an elevated leukocyte count (Figs. 9-34 and 9-35). The distinction between reactive and neoplastic mesothelial cells may not be easy, particularly in the presence of concurrent inflammation.

Neoplastic mesothelial cells are characterized by a pleomorphic appearance, with mild to marked anisokaryosis and anisocytosis. The nuclear to cytoplasmic ratio is likewise variable. Cells may be arranged in small aggregates of a few cells to large clusters of more than 50. Larger aggregates resemble polyps, pseudomembranes, solid spheres, or chains of cells. Cell borders are distinct. Nuclei are round to oval, and multinucleation is common (3 to 4 nuclei/cell). Mitoses may be readily observed. Cytoplasmic volume may vary widely between cells and may contain clear vacuoles. Vacuoles vary from multiple small to medium-sized vacuoles to single, very large vacuoles that displace the nucleus marginally and greatly distended the cell (*signet ring* formation). Such vacuolation may also be seen with adenocarcinomas, but acinar arrangement of cells favors a diagnosis of adenocarcinomas.

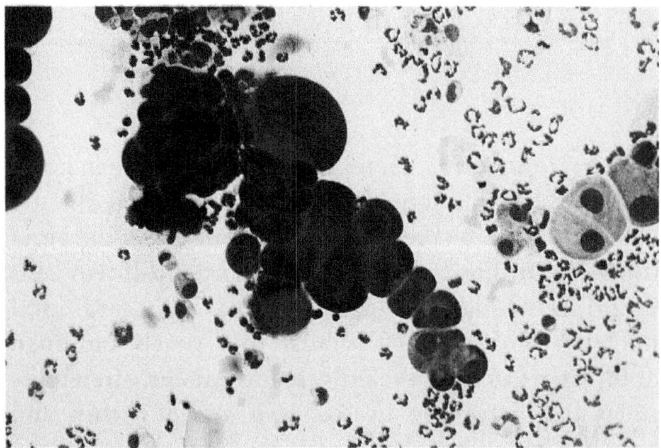

Fig. 9-34 Malignant mesothelioma from abdominal cavity of horse.
Peritoneal fluid. Note the clustering of variably sized but very large cells, within a background of inflammation. Intracellular bridging and infrequent magenta-staining, intercellular matrix are visible. (Wright-Giemsa)

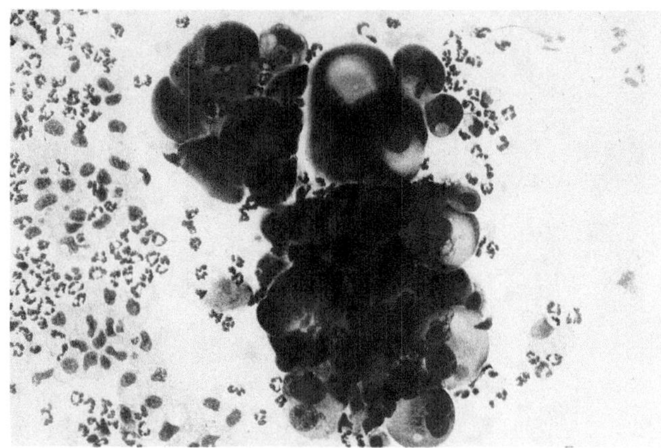

Fig. 9-35 Higher magnification of equine malignant mesothelioma.
Occasional vacuolation of neoplastic cell cytoplasm is observed, sometimes forming signet rings. Neutrophils are sometimes seen migrating within neoplastic cell cytoplasm; this is termed *emperipolesis*. (Wright-Giemsa)

Electron microscopy and/or immunohistochemistry may be necessary to confirm mesothelial-cell lineage.[76]

Malignant Melanoma: Melanophages were documented in the peritoneal fluid of two cases of malignant melanoma.[6,16] Malignant melanocytes may also be observed in varying numbers on peritoneal fluid cytology from horses with metastatic melanoma (our personal observation) (Fig. 9-36).

Other Neoplasia: Disseminated leiomyomatosis is a rare, benign, multicentric proliferation of smooth muscle tissue.[76,87] An underlying hormonal mechanism is postulated. A single case report exists in the equine, and peritoneal fluid collected from this horse was unremarkable with the exception of an elevated protein concentration.[87]

A single case report of gastric leiomyosarcoma documented concurrent exudative thoracic and abdominal effusions.[76] Omental fibrosarcoma has been reported in a horse with both thoracic and abdominal exudative effusion; however, neoplastic cells were not identified on cytologic examination.[76]

Hepatic neoplasms do not commonly metastasize to the peritoneal cavity but may be associated with nonseptic peritoneal exudate.[76] Pheochromocytoma has been reported in association with hemoperitoneum.[76]

Strangulating pedunculated lipomas are frequently associated with abnormal peritoneal fluid analysis results,

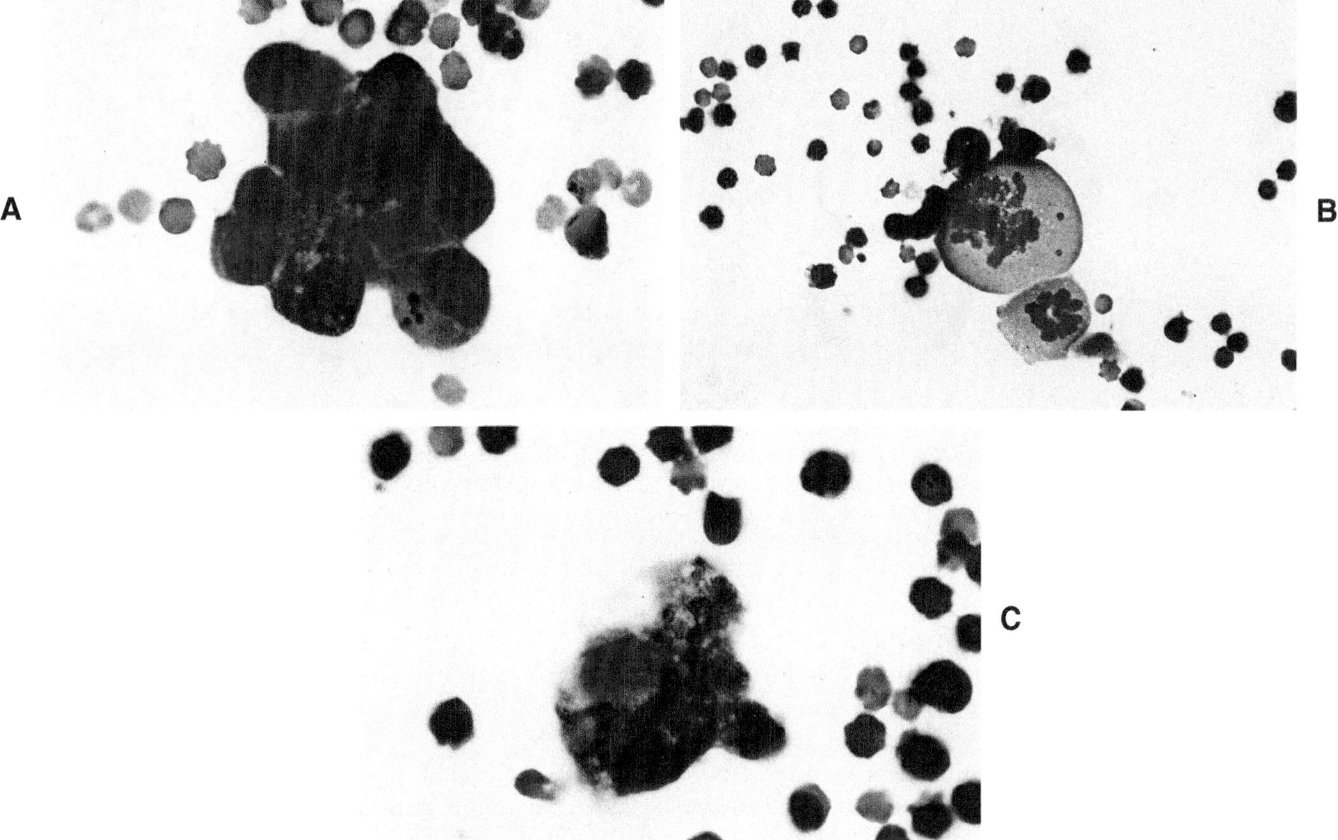

Fig. 9-36 Equine metastatic melanoma.
A, A single darkly staining cluster of neoplastic melanocytes is present and exhibits three-fold anisocytosis, two-fold anisokaryosis, and a variable nucleus to cytoplasmic ratio. Occasional cells contain scattered, coarse, golden brown cytoplasmic pigment granules consistent with melanin. **B,** Lower magnification of two giant cells in mitoses. **C,** A smaller cluster of neoplastic cells containing more abundant melanin pigment. (Abdominal fluid direct smear; Wright-Giemsa) (Courtesy Dr. Anne M. Barger, North Carolina State University, Raleigh.)

the degree of alteration depending on the duration and extent of bowel ischemia.[88]

Incidental Findings

Glove powder (corn starch) may occasionally contaminate peritoneal fluid specimens. Microscopically it appears as variably sized, round to hexagonal particles with a central fissure or cross (Fig. 9-37), which is prominent when examined under polarized light (Fig. 9-38). They are usually clear (nonstaining) with Romanowsky stains but may have a bluish hue.

Microfilariae (*Setaria* sp.) are occasionally observed in peritoneal fluid samples (Fig. 9-37). They are not considered diagnostically important.[89] Ciliated protozoa may be observed with accidental enterocentesis or with gastrointestinal rupture (see Fig. 9-19).

Cornified squamous epithelial cells, presumably from superficial skin contamination, are occasionally observed.[14] Rarely, adherent bacterial cocci are associated with their surface.

Carboxymethylcellulose, a high-molecular-weight polysaccharide administered intraperitoneally to decrease incidence of postoperative adhesions, has been shown to produce a granular, magenta precipitant on peripheral blood smears in a dose-dependent fashion. A similar precipitant was also observed in peritoneal fluid.[90]

Colic

Use of various clinical pathology tests, including peritoneal fluid analysis, for diagnosis, for determining the need for surgical intervention, and for assessing prognosis in colic cases (including septic and nonseptic peritonitis, gastroenteritis, diarrhea, bowel impactions, and strangulating and nonstrangulating organ displacements) has been reviewed.[55,67,91-95] Various mathematical models have been developed to attempt to objectively predict the

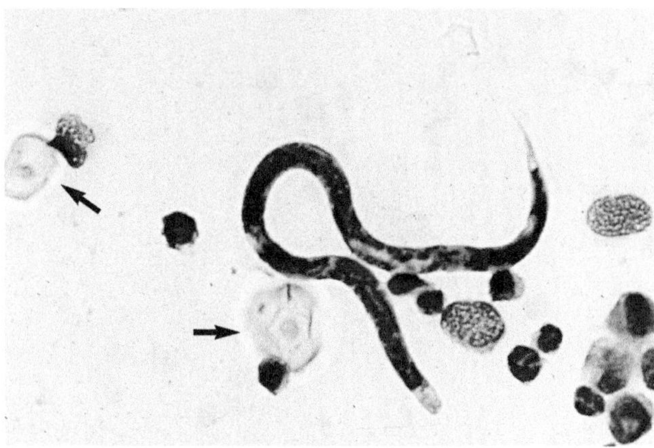

Fig. 9-37 Glove powder granules *(arrows)* and a microfilaria may be incidental findings in peritoneal fluid smears. (Original magnification X500; Wright's) (Courtesy Dr. Rick L. Cowell, Oklahoma State University, Stillwater.)

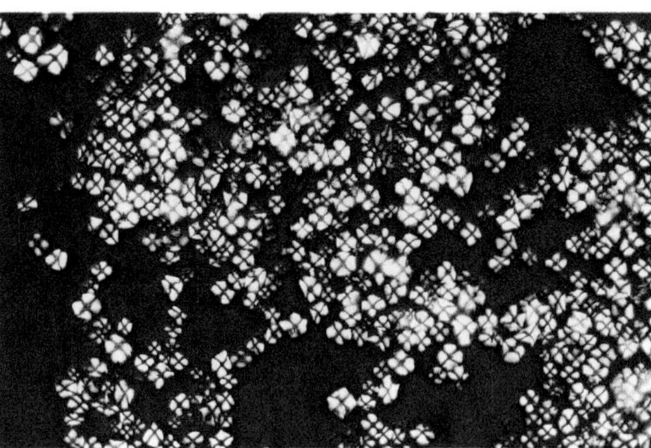

Fig. 9-38 Glove powder (corn starch) has a prominent central fissure or cross when viewed with polarized light.

short-term prognosis and the need for surgery in such cases.[96-101] Though it is apparent from these studies that such decisions do not require a definitive diagnosis of the cause of colic before treatment commences, the more data clinicians can gather about a case, the better informed they and their clients will be about such matters as long-term prognosis, type of lesion likely to be encountered in the abdomen in surgical cases, and type of intraoperative and postoperative care that may be required for a successful outcome. Consequently, a full clinical examination, including abdominocentesis, provides a good database for complete assessment of horses with colic.

Volume, Color, and Turbidity: Evaluation of the volume, turbidity, and color of peritoneal fluid, as discussed earlier, may facilitate decisions about initial treatment of a horse with colic before laboratory results are known (Figs. 9-39 and 9-40). When serosanguineous fluid is obtained, surgical intervention is supported.[7,42,67,101] This is particularly appropriate when such peritoneal fluid is associated with gross abdominal distention or rectal palpation of distended bowel.[101]

Erythrocyte Counts: Enumeration of erythrocytes is of dubious value in evaluating the peritoneal fluid of horses with colic. Studies recording peritoneal fluid erythrocyte counts in horses with colic report conflicting findings.[93,94,102,103] High peritoneal fluid erythrocyte counts may suggest the need for surgical intervention or convey a poor prognosis.

Nucleated Cell Counts: Peritoneal fluid findings show considerable overlap in quite diverse clinical conditions. While these findings may be very useful in diagnosing peritonitis, sepsis, and neoplasia as outlined earlier, cytologic variables alone have not consistently been valuable in predicting prognosis or the need for surgery.[91-94,96,100-105] In several retrospective studies, significantly elevated peritoneal fluid nucleated cell counts were more commonly associated with sepsis or failure to survive.[35,106]

Total Protein Concentration: Changes in peritoneal fluid total protein concentration tend to reflect the changes in the total nucleated cell count. Reports investigating the utility of peritoneal fluid protein concentrations for predicting the cause of colic, need for surgical intervention, likelihood of sepsis, or prognosis are conflicting. In one study of 36 horses having either septic or nonseptic peritonitis, significantly higher fluid protein concentrations were detected among horses with sepsis.[35] Another study evaluating 75 horses with duodenitis-proximal jejunitis, horses having peritoneal fluid protein concentrations >3.5 mg/dl were four times more likely not to survive.[94] And in a retrospective study of 147 cases of large colon impaction, nonsurvivors had significantly higher peritoneal fluid protein concentrations than survivors.[107] However, in another study of 122 horses with acute diarrhea, no significant difference in fluid protein concentrations were found between survivors and nonsurvivors.[92] And in a retrospective review of 218 colic cases, fluid protein concentration was not significantly associated with predicting cause of colic, need for surgery, or outcome of disease.[93]

Other Biochemical Measurements: Several biochemical tests have been considered as part of the assessment of peritoneal fluid in colic cases. In general, they have not been objectively compared with each other

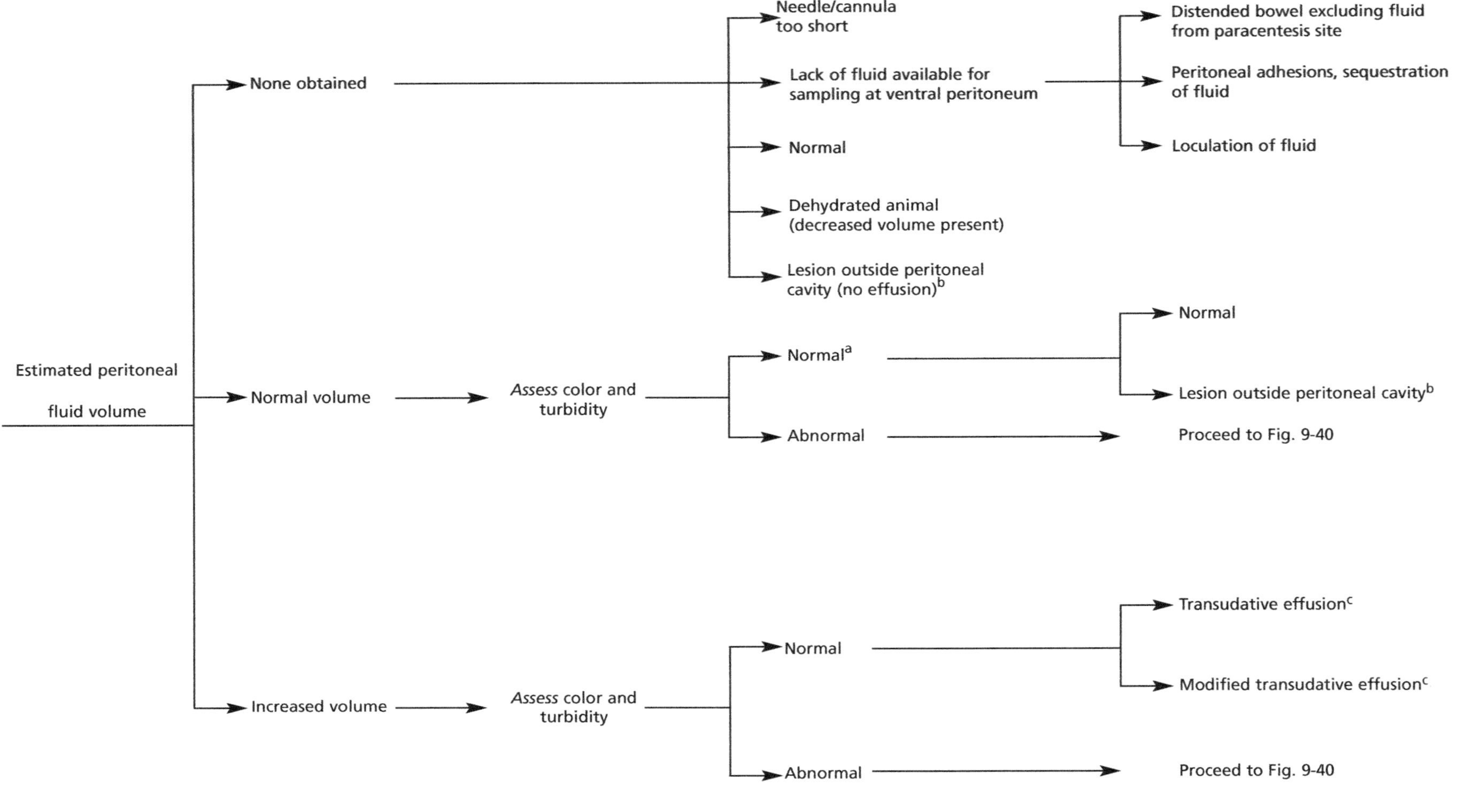

[a] Normal peritoneal fluid is clear to slightly turbid and colorless to pale yellow.

[b] For example, diaphragmatic hernia, scrotal hernia, enteric salmonellosis, and lesions involving kidney, bladder, uterus, etc. Several of these problems might actually produce increased amounts of peritoneal fluid in the transudate/modified transudate category.

[c] Cytologic examination is recommended, including total nucleated cell count and total protein measurement.

Fig. 9-39 Algorithm for initial approach to assessing peritoneal fluid specimens.

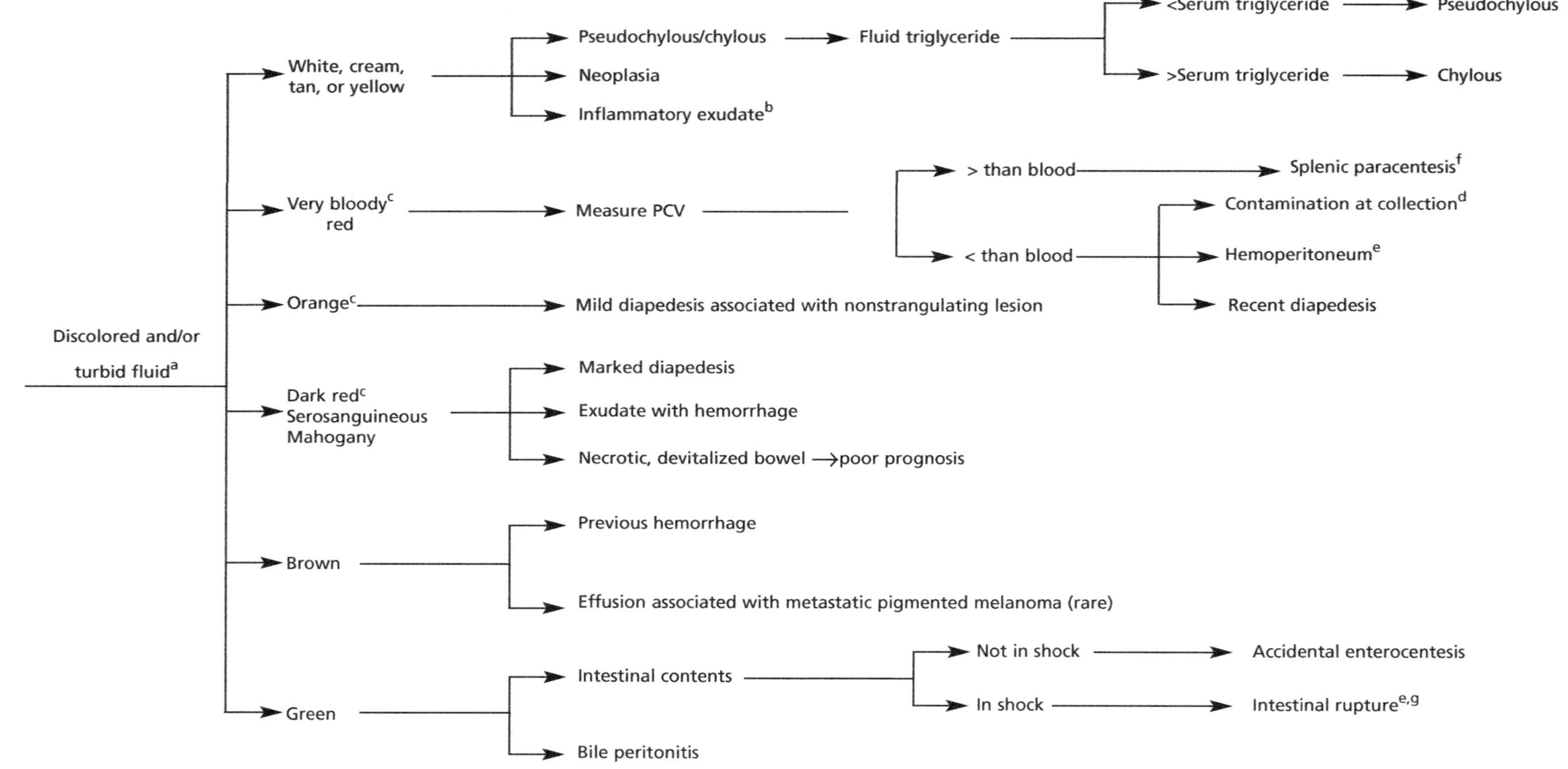

[a] Cytologic examination is recommended, including total nucleated cell count and total protein measurement.

[b] Exudates have increased cellularity and total protein concentration. They may be subdivided into suppurative, chronic-suppurative, and chronic inflammatory reactions. Neutrophil morphology and phagocytic activity of macrophages should also be assessed (see text). Presence of bacteria denotes sepsis.

[c] When peritoneal fluid has a reddish discoloration, the supernatant should be assessed for hemolysis. Hemolytic or port-wine-colored supernatant suggests intestinal infarction (but may be seen in some cases with severe peritonitis). Possibly also see erythrophagocytosis on cytologic smear.

[d] May be obvious during collection. May result in platelets on cytologic smears. The supernatant usually is not hemolysed. No erythrophagocytosis.

[e] Specimen uniformly bloody throughout collection. Erythrophagocytosis may be apparent. Supernatant may be nonhemolyzed or hemolyzed. The total nucleated cell count is not greatly increased.

[f] Numerous platelets and lymphocytes present. Clots readily.

[g] Could also be accidental enterocentesis in a horse with an infarcted bowel.

Fig. 9-40 Algorithmic approach to assessment of peritoneal fluid specimens with abnormal gross appearance.

as means of formulating a prognosis or determining the need for surgical intervention. With the exception of total protein measurement, the following tests are not widely used.

Enzyme Determinations: The activities of alkaline phosphatase, aspartate aminotransferase, and lactate dehydrogenase increased in the peritoneal fluid of horses with experimental colonic infarction.[108] However, the clinical usefulness of these changes to detect early intestinal ischemia was considered to be limited. In a later study comparing peritoneal fluid analysis results among normal horses, horses with medical causes of colic, surgical causes of colic, acute grass sickness, and subacute grass sickness, total and intestinal isoenzyme alkaline phosphatase levels were significantly higher in the surgical colic cases than in the other groups. A less substantial, but significant, increase from normal was observed among the horses affected with grass sickness.[21] Peritoneal fluid values among horses with medical causes of colic did not differ from normal. The degree of enzyme elevation appears well correlated with the extent of ischemic necrosis characteristic of these disorders. Caution should be exercised in interpretation of elevated fluid alkaline phosphatase activity in specimens with high nucleated cell counts and significant neutrophil degeneration, since a disruption of granulocytes may also elevate fluid alkaline phosphatase activity.

Another study reported fluid lactate dehydrogenase activity was not useful in distinguishing septic from nonseptic peritonitis.[35]

A significant increase in serum and peritoneal fluid creatine kinase isoenzyme levels was observed in horses with surgical small intestinal disorders compared to those with nonsurgical disorders or normal horses.[33]

Fibronectin Content: The fibronectin concentration of peritoneal fluid may be useful in indicating mesenteric thrombosis. Mean ± SD fibronectin values were significantly higher in 57 horses with exudative effusions not associated with mesenteric thrombosis (321 ± 82 μg/ml) than in 16 horses with exudative effusions and thrombosis (138 ± 57 μg/ml).[109] The total nucleated cell count, total protein concentration, and fibrinogen concentration of peritoneal fluid were similar in both groups.

Lactate and Glucose Content: Paired blood and peritoneal fluid lactate (lactic acid) and glucose concentrations are seldom determined in colic cases. Nevertheless, their assessment, combined with peritoneal fluid total nucleated cell count and total protein measurement, might provide valuable information regarding the degree of intestinal ischemia, cardiovascular status, and likelihood of sepsis (Fig. 9-41).[1,35,91] Increased anaerobic glycolysis of ischemic bowel with venous stasis results in increased lactate diffusing into the peritoneal fluid, increasing lactate concentration.

Lactate is removed from the bloodstream by the liver. Provided hepatic perfusion is adequate, blood lactate concentration does not increase. However, if acute circulatory failure (shock) develops because of dehydration, hypovolemia, and/or endotoxemia, blood lactate concentration also increases. This increase is exacerbated by peripheral tissue hypoxia particularly involving skeletal muscle.

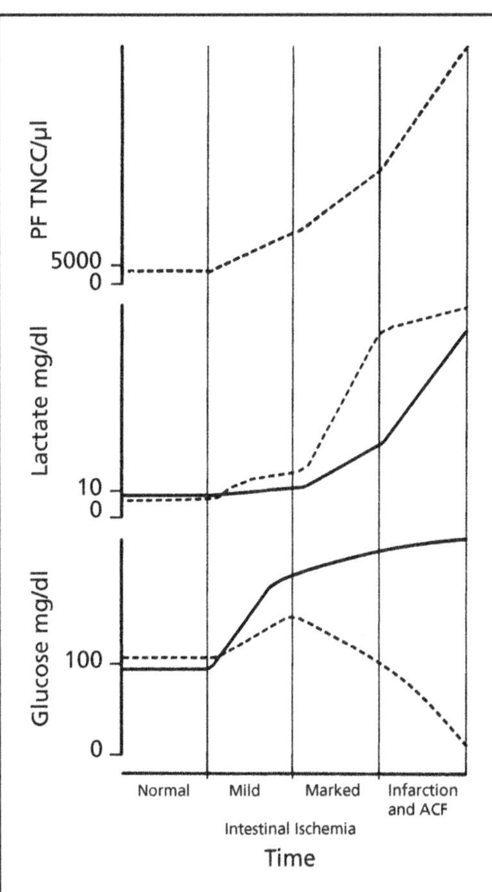

Fig. 9-41 Postulated relationship between peritoneal fluid total nucleated cell count (PF TNCC) and the concentrations of lactate and glucose in blood *(solid line)* and peritoneal fluid *(dashed line)* in horses with intestinal ischemia. Bacterial invasion across the bowel into the peritoneal cavity occurs during the infarction stage and exacerbates the inflammatory response and glucose depletion. Acute circulatory failure (ACF, shock) may be caused by hypovolemia, dehydration, or endotoxemia. Prognosis decreases with progressively increasing blood lactate and glucose concentrations.

Unfortunately, the situation in clinical cases is not always as uncomplicated as that outlined above. Lactate levels may be similarly elevated in both surgical and nonsurgical colic cases. Despite this limitation, in horses with elevated lactate levels destined for surgery, the veterinarian would be forewarned of the probable severity of intestinal ischemia and the likely need for resection.

The result of increased glycolysis due to peritoneal fluid leukocytosis or sepsis would be an anticipated decrease in the peritoneal fluid glucose concentrations. Concurrent with the above changes in blood and peritoneal fluid lactate concentrations, blood glucose values initially increase in response to adrenaline release associated at first with abdominal pain and later with cardiovascular compromise. Discrepancy between serum and fluid glucose levels may result from insufficient time for equilibration between blood and peritoneal fluid (if the hyperglycemia occurs rapidly) and/or from utilization of fluid glucose by inflammatory cells. As the intestine becomes more severely compromised, bacterial toxins and organisms enter the peritoneal cavity, causing more severe peritonitis and further decreasing the peritoneal fluid glucose concentration. Therefore increasing blood glucose and lactate concentrations are usually associated with more guarded prognoses.

Phosphate Determination: Measurement of blood and peritoneal fluid (inorganic) phosphate concentrations have been recommended as guides to the severity of intestinal ischemia.[40,41] In one study, peritoneal fluid phosphate levels >3.6 mg/dl predicted intestinal lesions requiring surgical intervention or euthanasia with a sensitivity of 77% and a specificity of 76%.[40] This same report suggested that serum phosphate levels alone may be of value when peritoneal fluid specimens are unavailable. It is critical to use age-appropriate reference ranges, since foals may have greater serum and peritoneal fluid phosphate values attributable to increased osseous metabolism.[40] Peritoneal fluid phosphate concentrations measured in six foals (aged 2 to 11 months) with signs of abdominal pain exceeded critical values for adult horses (range 3.9 to 7.2 mg/dl) in all cases, including two without intestinal lesions.[40]

REFERENCES

1. Nelson: Analysis of equine peritoneal fluid. *Vet Clin North Am (Large Anim Pract)* 1:267-274, 1979.
2. Barrelet: Peritoneal fluid: part 1—lab analyses. *Equine Vet Educ* 5(2):81-83, 1993.
3. Parry and Brownlow: In Cowell and Tyler: *Cytology and Hematology of the Horse*. Goleta, 1992, American Veterinary Publishers, pp 121-151.
4. Tulleners: Complications of abdominocentesis in the horse. *JAVMA* 182:232-234, 1983.
5. Schumacher et al: Effects of enterocentesis on peritoneal fluid constituents in the horse. *J Am Vet Med Assoc* 186:1301-1303, 1985.
6. Bach and Ricketts: Paracentesis as an aid to the diagnosis of abdominal disease in the horse. *Equine Vet J* 6:116-121, 1974.
7. Swanwick and Wilkinson: A clinical evaluation of abdominal paracentesis in the horse. *Aust Vet J* 52:109-117, 1976.
8. Schneider et al: Response of pony peritoneum to four peritoneal lavage solutions. *Am J Vet Res* 49:889-894, 1988.
9. Juzwiak et al: Effect of repeated abdominocentesis on peritoneal fluid constituents in the horse. *Vet Res Commun* 15(3):177-180, 1991.
10. Malark et al: Equine peritoneal fluid analysis in special situations (abstract). *Proceedings of the 36th Annual Convention of the AAEP*, 1990, p 645.
11. Hanson et al: Evaluation of peritoneal fluid following intestinal resection and anastomosis in horses. *Am J Vet Res* 53(2):216-221, 1992.
12. Santschi et al: Peritoneal fluid analysis in ponies after abdominal surgery. *Vet Surg* 17(1):6-9, 1988.
13. Knoll and MacWilliams: EDTA-induced artifact in abdominal fluid analysis associated with insufficient sample volume. *Proc 24th Ann Mtg Am Soc Vet Clin Pathol*, p 13, 1989.
14. Bach: Exfoliative cytology of peritoneal fluid in the horse. *Vet Annual* 13:102-109, 1973.
15. Morley and Desnoyers: Diagnosis of ruptured urinary bladder in a foal by identification of calcium carbonate crystals in the peritoneal fluid. *J Am Vet Med Assoc* 200(8):1515-1517, 1992.
16. Brownlow: Abdominal paracentesis in the horse. A clinical evaluation. MVSc thesis. University of Sydney, 1979.
17. Brownlow et al: Abdominal paracentesis in the horse—basic concepts. *Aust Vet Pract* 11:60-68, 1981.
18. Brownlow et al: Reference values for equine peritoneal fluid. *Equine Vet J* 13:127-130, 1981.
19. Parry et al: Unpublished data, 1985.
20. Behrens et al: Reference values of peritoneal fluid from healthy foals. *J Equine Vet Sci* 10(5):348-352, 1990.
21. Milne et al: Analysis of peritoneal fluid as a diagnostic aid in grass sickness (equine dysautonomia). *Vet Record* 127:162-165, 1990.
22. Malark et al: Effect of blood contamination on equine peritoneal fluid analysis. *J Am Vet Med Assoc* 201(10):1545-1548, 1992.
23. Grindem et al: Peritoneal fluid values from healthy foals. *Equine Vet J* 22(5):359-361, 1990.
24. Garma-Avina: Cytology of 100 samples of abdominal fluid from 100 horses with abdominal disease. *Equine Vet J* 30(5):435-444, 1998.
25. Barrelet: Peritoneal fluid: part 2—cytologic exam. *Equine Vet Educ* 5(3):126-128, 1993.
26. Brownlow: Mononuclear phagocytes of peritoneal fluid. *Equine Vet J* 14:325-328, 1982.
27. Grindem et al: Large granular lymphoma tumor in a horse. *Vet Pathol* 26:86-88, 1989.
28. Duckett and Matthews: Hypereosinophilia in a horse with intestinal lymphosarcoma. *Can Vet J* 38:719-720, 1997.
29. McKenzie et al: Gastric squamous cell carcinoma in 3 horses. *Aust Vet J* 75(7):480-483, 1997.
30. Olson: Squamous cell carcinoma of the equine stomach: a report of five cases. *Vet Record* 131(8):170-173, 1992.
31. McGrath: Exfoliative cytology of equine peritoneal fluid-an adjunct to hematologic examination. *Proc 1st Intl Symp Equine Hematol*, 1975, pp 408-416.
32. Baxter et al: Effects of exploratory laparotomy on plasma and peritoneal fluid coagulation/fibrinolysis in horses. *Am J Vet Res* 52 (7):1121-1127, 1991.
33. Broome et al: Evaluation of peritoneal fluid and serum Creatine Kinase isoenzyme concentrations as indicators of small intestinal surgical disease in horses (abstract). *Vet Surg* 23(5):397, 1994.
34. Parry and Crisman: Serum and peritoneal fluid amylase and lipase reference values in the horse. *Equine Vet J* 23(5):390-391, 1991.
35. Van Hoogmoed et al: Evaluation of peritoneal fluid pH, glucose concentration, and lactate dehydrogenase activity for detection of septic peritonitis in horses. *J Am Vet Med Assoc* 214(7):1032-1036, 1999.
36. Traub-Dargatz et al: Challenging cases in internal medicine: What's your diagnosis? (chylous abdomen). *Vet Med* 89(2):100-104, 1994.
37. Campbell-Beggs et al: Chyloabdomen in a neonatal foal. *Vet Record* 137:96-98, 1995.

38. Mair and Lucke: Chyloperitoneum associated with torsion of the large colon in a horse. *Vet Record* 131:421, 1992.
39. May et al: Chyloperitoneum and abdominal adhesions in a miniature horse. *J Am Vet Med Assoc* 215(5):676-678, 1999.
40. Arden and Stick: Serum and peritoneal fluid phosphate concentrations as predictors of major intestinal injury associated with equine colic. *J Am Vet Med Assoc* 193:927-931, 1988.
41. Fischer: Advances in diagnostic techniques for horses with colic. *Vet Clin North Am (Equine Pract)* 13(2):203-219, 1997.
42. Brownlow: Abdominal paracentesis as an aid in the diagnosis of abdominal disorders in the horse. *Proc 74 Equine Gastroenterol*, Postgrad Comm in Vet Sci, University of Sydney, 1985, pp 21-44.
43. Hackett: Nonstrangulated colonic displacement in horses. *JAVMA* 182:235-240, 1983.
44. Fischer and Meagher: Strangulating torsions of the equine large colon. *Comp Cont Ed Pract Vet* 8:S25-S30, 1986.
45. Saville WJ et al: Necrotizing enterocolitis in horses: a retrospective study. *J Vet Intern Med* 10(4):265-270, 1996.
46. Adams and Sojka: In Colahan et al: *Equine Medicine and Surgery*, ed. 5. St Louis, 1999, Mosby, pp 580-590.
47. Dyson: Review of 30 cases of peritonitis in the horse. *Equine Vet J* 15:25-30, 1983.
48. Adams et al: Cytologic interpretation of peritoneal fluid in the evaluation of equine abdominal crises. *Cornell Vet* 70:232-246, 1980.
49. Brownlow: Polymorphonuclear neutrophil leucocytes of peritoneal fluid. *Equine Vet J* 15:22-24, 1983.
50. Gay and Lording: Peritonitis in horses associated with *Actinobacillus equuli*. *Aust Vet J* 56:296-300, 1980.
51. Golland et al: Peritonitis associated with Actinobacillus equuli in horses: 15 cases (1982-1992). *J Am Vet Med Assoc* 205(2):340-343, 1994.
52. Rebar: *Handbook of Veterinary Cytology*. St Louis, 1980, Ralston Purina, pp 29-36.
53. Fisher et al: Diagnostic laparoscopy in the horse. *JAVMA* 189:289-292, 1986.
54. Blackford et al: Equine peritoneal fluid analysis following celiotomy. *Proc 2nd Equine Colic Res Symp*, 1985, pp 130-133.
55. Zicker et al: Differentiation between intra-abdominal neoplasms and abscesses in horses, using clinical and laboratory data: 40 cases (1973-1988). *J Am Vet Med Assoc* 196(7):1130-1134, 1990.
56. Rumbaugh et al: Internal abdominal abscesses in the horse: a study of 25 cases. *JAVMA* 172:304-309, 1978.
57. Hutchins et al: Intraabdominal abscessation in the horse. *Proc 74 Equine Gastroenterol*, Postgrad Comm in Vet Sci, University of Sydney, 1985, pp 97-102.
58. Clabough and Scrutchfield: Ruptured abdominal abscess in the horse. *Southwest Vet* 37:145-148, 1986.
59. Sanders-Shamis: Perirectal abscesses in six horses. *JAVMA* 187:499-500, 1985.
60. Prades et al: Surgical treatment of an abdominal abscess by marsupialisation in the horse: a report of two cases. *Equine Vet J* 21:459-461, 1989.
61. Hanselaer and Nyland: Chyloabdomen and ultrasonographic detection of an intra-abdominal abscess in a foal. *JAVMA* 183:1465-1467, 1983.
62. Hawkins et al: Peritonitis in horses: 67 cases (1985-1990). *J Am Vet Med Assoc* 203:284-288, 1993.
63. Clabough and Duckett: Septic cholangitis and peritonitis in a gelding. *J Am Vet Med Assoc* 200(10):1521-1524, 1992.
64. Kiper et al: Gastric rupture in horses: 50 cases (1979-1987). *J Am Vet Med Assoc* 196(2):333-336, 1990.
65. Lavoie et al: Aerobic bacterial isolates in horses in a university hospital. *Can Vet J* 32(5):292-294, 1991.
66. Schumacher et al: Effects of castration on peritoneal fluid in the horse. *J Vet Intern Med* 2:22-25, 1988.
67. Parry: Prognosis and the necessity for surgery in equine colic. *Vet Bulletin* 52:249-260, 1982.
68. Blue: Genital injuries from mating in the mare. *Equine Vet J* 17:297-299, 1985.
69. Richardson and Kohn: Uroperitoneum in the foal. *JAVMA* 182:267-271, 1983.
70. Behr et al: Metabolic abnormalities associated with rupture of the urinary bladder in neonatal foals. *JAVMA* 178:263-266, 1981.
71. Adams and Koterba: Exploratory celiotomy for suspected urinary tract disruption in neonatal foals: a review of 18 cases. *Equine Vet J* 20:13-17, 1988.
72. Sockett et al: Metabolic changes due to experimentally induced rupture of the bovine urinary bladder. *Cornell Vet* 76:198-212, 1986.
73. Meadows and MacWilliams: Chylous effusions revisited. *Vet Clin Pathol* 23(2):54-62, 1994.
74. Van Hoogmoed et al: Peritoneal fluid analysis in peripartum mares. *J Am Vet Med Assoc* 209(7):1280-1282, 1996.
75. Brooks et al: Uterine rupture as a postpartum complication in two mares. *J Am Vet Med Assoc* 187(12):1377-1379, 1985.
76. East and Savage: Abdominal neoplasia (excluding urogenital tract). *Vet Clin North Am (Equine Pract)* 14(3):475-492, 1998.
77. Mackey and Wheat: Reflections on the diagnostic approach to multicentric lymphosarcoma in an aged Arabian mare. *Equine Vet J* 17:467-469, 1985.
78. van den Hoven and Franken: Clinical aspects of lymphosarcoma in the horse. *Equine Vet J* 15:49-53, 1983.
79. Rebhun and Bertone: Lymphosarcoma in the horse. *JAVMA* 184:720-721, 1984.
80. Mair and Hillyer: Chronic colic in the mature horse: a retrospective review of 106 cases. *Equine Vet J* 29(6):415-420, 1997.
81. Kelley and Mahaffey: Equine malignant lymphomas: morphologic and immunohistochemical classification. *Vet Pathol* 35:241-252, 1998.
82. Savage: Lymphoproliferative and myeloproliferative disorders. *Vet Clin North Am (Equine Pract)* 16(3):563-579, 1998.
83. Wrigley et al: Pleural effusion associated with squamous cell carcinoma of the stomach of the horse. *Equine Vet J* 13:99-102, 1981.
84. Frye et al: Hemangiosarcoma in a horse. *JAVMA* 182:287-289, 1983.
85. Foreman et al: Pleural effusion secondary to thoracic metastatic mammary adenocarcinoma in a mare. *JAVMA* 197:1193-1195, 1990.
86. Ricketts and Peace: A case of peritoneal mesothelioma in a Thoroughbred mare. *Equine Vet J* 8:78-80, 1976.
87. Johnson et al: Disseminated peritoneal leiomyomatosis in a horse. *J Am Vet Med Assoc* 205(5):725-728, 1994.
88. Bilkslager et al: Pediculated lipomas as a cause of intestinal obstruction in horses: 17 cases (1983-1990). *J Am Vet Med Assoc* 201(8):1249-1252, 1992.
89. Cowell et al: Collection and evaluation of peritoneal and pleural effusions. *Vet Clin North Am (Equine Pract)* 3:543-561, 1987.
90. Burkhard et al: Blood precipitate associated with intra-abdominal carboxymethylcellular administration. *Vet Clin Pathol* 25(4):114-117, 1996.
91. Parry: Use of clinical pathology in evaluation of horses with colic. *Vet Clin North Am (Equine Pract)* 3:529-542, 1987.
92. Cohen and Woods: Characteristics and risk factors for failure of horses with acute diarrhea to survive: 122 cases (1990-1996). *J Am Vet Med Assoc* 214(3):382-390, 1999.
93. Freden et al: Reliability of using results of abdominal fluid analysis to determine treatment and predict lesion type and outcome for horses with colic: 218 cases (1991-1994). *J Am Vet Med Assoc* 213(7):1012-1015, 1998.
94. Seahorn et al: Prognostic indicators for horses with duodenitis-proximal jejunitis. 75 horses (1985-1989). *J Vet Intern Med* 6(6):307-311, 1992.
95. Cohen and Divers: Acute colitis in horses. Part 1. Assessment. *Compend Contin Educ Pract Vet* 20:92-98, 1998.
96. Parry et al: Prognosis in equine colic: a comparative study of variables used to access individual cases. *Equine Vet J* 15:211-215, 1983.
97. Puotenen-Reinhart: Study of variables commonly used in examination of equine colic cases to assess prognostic value. *Equine Vet J* 18:275-277, 1986.
98. Orsini et al: Prognostic index for acute abdominal crisis (colic) in horses. *Am J Vet Res* 49:1969-1971, 1988.
99. Reeves et al: Prognosis in equine colic patients using multivariable analysis. *Can J Vet Res* 53:87-94, 1989.
100. Reeves et al: A multivariable prognostic model for equine colic patients. *Prev Vet Med* 9:241-257, 1990.
101. Ducharme et al: A computer-derived protocol to aid in selecting medical versus surgical treatment of horses with abdominal pain. *Equine Vet J* 21:447-450, 1989.

102. Hunt et al: Interpretation of peritoneal fluid erythrocyte counts in horses with abdominal disease. *Proc 2nd Equine Colic Res Symp*, 1986, pp 168-174.
103. Parry et al: Assessment of the necessity for surgical intervention in cases of equine colic: a retrospective survey. *Equine Vet J* 15:216-221, 1983.
104. Mair et al: Peritonitis in adult horses: a review of 21 cases. *Vet Record* 126:567-570, 1990.
105. Morris and Johnston: Peritoneal fluid constituents in horses with colic due to small intestinal disease. *Proc 2nd Equine Colic Res Symp*, 1986, pp 134-142.
106. Cable et al: Abdominal surgery in foals: a review of 119 cases (1977-1994). *Equine Vet J* 29(4):257-261, 1997.
107. Dabareiner and White: Large colon impaction in horses: 147 cases (1985-1991). *J Am Vet Med Assoc* 206(5):679-685, 1995.
108. Turner et al: Biochemical analysis of serum and peritoneal fluid in experimental colonic infarction in horses. *Proc 1st Equine Colic Res Symp*, 1982, pp 79-87.
109. Feldman et al: Effusion fibronectin concentrations detect presence of mesenteric thrombosis: a preliminary prospective report. *Proc 2nd Equine Colic Res Symp*, 1986, pp 57-59.

CHAPTER 10

Synovial Fluid

Edward A. Mahaffey

Diseases of the legs and feet comprise a major segment of equine practice. Many diseases causing lameness involve joints, and synovial fluid analysis is often an important part of the diagnostic process in such cases.

Synovial fluid from a normal joint is a dialysate of plasma that is modified by secretion of hyaluronic acid, glycoproteins, and other macromolecules. Though smaller molecules found in plasma, such as glucose and electrolytes, also occur in synovial fluid in concentrations similar to those in plasma, proteins from plasma normally cross the "blood-synovial barrier" to a limited extent.

Synovial fluid has two functions. Articular cartilage receives its nutrition from synovial fluid. Synovial fluid also lubricates joint surfaces, limiting friction and wear between opposing articular cartilage surfaces. This lubrication has been attributed to glycoproteins in the fluid. Though hyaluronate has some lubricating properties, it is probably less important than glycoproteins in reducing friction between articular cartilage surfaces.

Normal synovial lining consists of fibrous and adipose connective tissues covered incompletely by a lining of intimal cells. Within the connective tissue is a highly vascular network of fenestrated capillaries. The lining cells are not true cells residing on a basement membrane. Instead, they rest directly on the fibrillar network of the underlying connective tissue. Two types of cells have been identified in synovial lining; these have been designated as type-A and type-B lining cells. Type-A cells are phagocytic and more numerous. Type-B cells are thought to secrete hyaluronic acid.[1]

Characteristics of Normal Synovial Fluid

Physical Characteristics

Normal equine synovial fluid is light yellow and clear, with no suspended particulate material. The volume of fluid that can be collected depends on the joint being sampled and the health of the joint. In general, the ability to collect synovial fluid samples of adequate volume for testing does not pose the problem in horses that it does in dogs and cats. At least 1 ml of fluid usually can be collected from the major limb joints of healthy horses.

Viscosity: Though techniques for quantifying viscosity have been described, viscosity can be quickly estimated by placing a drop between the thumb and forefinger, slowly pulling the fingers apart, and observing the strand of synovial fluid that forms between the fingers. Synovial fluid of normal viscosity forms a strand at least 2.5 cm long before it breaks. Another simple technique is to observe the length of the strand of synovial fluid that forms on the end of a needle before it drips from the needle. Again, normal synovial fluid forms a strand at least 2.5 cm long.

Thixotropism: Normal synovial fluid does not clot upon standing but often becomes gelatinous. This phenomenon is called thixotropism; the specimen can be returned to its fluid state by agitation.

Cellular Composition

Nucleated Cell Count: Total nucleated cell counts of normal equine synovial fluid have been reported to vary widely from one joint to another. Though counts over 2,000 cells/μl have been reported for fluid from the temporomandibular joints of clinically normal animals, fluid from the more commonly sampled limb joints of healthy horses usually contains less than 500 nucleated cells/μl.[2,3]

Erythrocytes: Normal synovial fluid is almost completely free of erythrocytes, and erythrocyte counts are seldom performed on synovial fluid specimens. Nevertheless, almost all specimens contain some erythrocytes due to contamination with blood during sample collection. Erythrocytes may also enter synovial fluid in a variety of diseases involving the joint. Physical and cytologic characteristics of synovial fluid help differentiate erythrocytes associated with sample contamination during collection from erythrocytes associated with joint disease. These characteristics are discussed later in this chapter.

Differential Cell Count: Published values regarding the relative proportions of the various cell types that occur in normal synovial fluid vary widely. One useful general guideline is that *the proportion of neutrophils in normal synovial fluid should not exceed 10%*, with the possible exceptions of some samples with very low total cell counts and samples with marked blood contamination.

The most obvious differences in reported values are in the proportions of mononuclear cells. Most mononuclear cells in normal synovial fluid are lymphocytes and large mononuclear cells. The latter include monocytes/macrophages and, probably, some synovial lining cells. It may be possible to distinguish synovial lining cells from macrophages in cytologic preparations. Some cells that have been classified as "clasmatocytes" are probably synovial lining cells. Intact clumps of synovial lining cells are occasionally aspirated (Fig. 10-1). In our laboratory, mononuclear cells in synovial fluid are routinely classified as lymphocytes or macrophages. Macrophages usually predominate, though the proportions of macrophages and lymphocytes vary from one joint to another.[4] The relative proportions of lymphocytes and macrophages seldom provide useful diagnostic information. Some laboratories routinely report all lymphocytes, macrophages, and synovial lining cells under the heading of "mononuclear cells." Eosinophils occur infrequently (<1% of total cells) in normal equine synovial fluid.

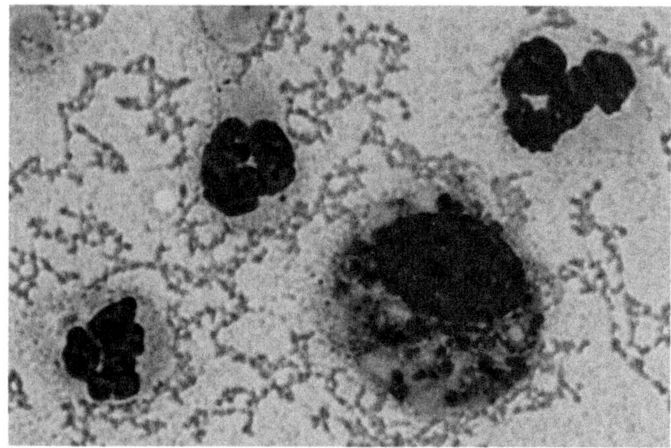

Fig. 10-2 Three neutrophils and a macrophage-containing metachromatic cytoplasmic granule in synovial fluid from a horse with degenerative joint disease.

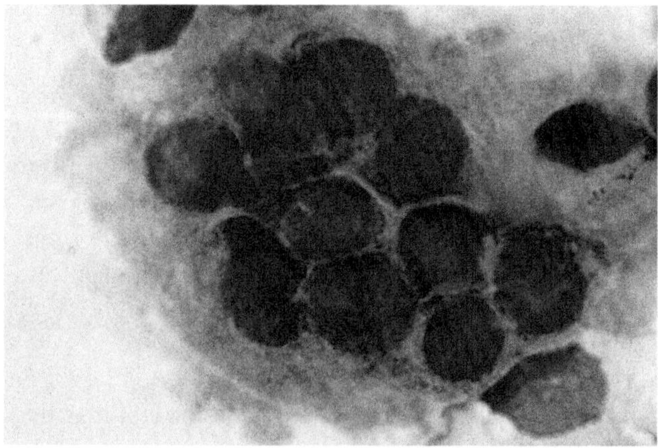

Fig. 10-1 Synovial lining fragment in synovial fluid from a horse. (Wright's stain)

The size of macrophages and degree of cytoplasmic vacuolation in synovial fluid vary widely. Some macrophages have relatively dark blue cytoplasm with few or no vacuoles. Other macrophages, often the larger ones, have numerous clear cytoplasmic vacuoles. Some of this vacuolation is an artifact caused by delayed processing of the fluid after collection. Another morphologic feature of some synovial fluid macrophages is the presence of few to many metachromatic cytoplasmic granules (Fig. 10-2).

Throughout the background of most synovial fluid smears is mucin, which appears as finely granular pink material. This mucin should not be confused with bacteria, which stain dark blue with Wright's stain.

Techniques for Examination of Synovial Fluid

Synovial Fluid Collection

Synovial fluid can be aspirated from most joints with a 1-inch, 18- to 20-gauge needle. The skin should be prepared by clipping the hair and performing a surgical scrub to avoid introducing bacteria into the joint. Ethyl chloride spray may be used, if needed, on the overlying skin to lessen the sensation of the needle penetration. Fluid for cytologic evaluation should be placed in an EDTA tube. Note, however, that EDTA interferes with the mucin clot test. If a mucin clot test is to be run, another aliquot of synovial fluid should be placed in a tube with no anticoagulant (*eg*, red-top tube) or one containing heparin.

Mucin Clot Test

The mucin clot test provides a semiquantitative index of the degree of polymerization of hyaluronic acid in synovial fluid. It should not be performed on samples collected in EDTA; samples collected in heparin or with no anticoagulant should be used. The test is performed by mixing about 1 part of the supernatant from centrifuged synovial fluid with 4 parts of 2.5% glacial acetic acid. The acid causes precipitation or clumping of synovial fluid mucin. After gently mixing, the clumped mucin is observed.

A four-level subjective grading scheme is used for recording results of mucin clot tests. The clot is classified as *good* if a single, compact clot forms in an otherwise clear solution. It is classified as *fair* if a single, soft clot forms in a slightly turbid solution. A *poor* clot is friable and may break apart if the tube is gently agitated. The surrounding fluid in such specimens is cloudy. A *very poor* clot should be recorded if the tube contains only flecks of precipitated mucin in an otherwise cloudy solution.

Hyaluronic acid content has been measured directly in synovial fluid, but this test is not performed in most clinical laboratories.[5]

Total Protein Concentration

Most plasma proteins, especially those with higher molecular weight, are excluded from synovial fluid by the dialyzing properties of the synovial membrane and hyaluronic acid in the perisynovial connective tissue. Some glycoprotein is synthesized by the synovial lining cells and secreted into the fluid. Values reported in the veterinary literature for the protein concentration of normal equine synovial fluid vary widely. One author, using the biuret technique, reported a reference range of 0.92 to 3.11 g/dl.[6] Another investigator reported a reference range of 0.5 to 1.0 g/dl using the Coomassie blue method. This latter author attributed the different results to methodologic differences.[7] In limited comparisons, we have found that the biuret and Coomassie blue methods yield very similar values and that these values are in the range reported above for the biuret method.

Refractometric measurements have also been used to qualify protein in equine synovial fluid.[8] While refractometry has been suggested by some to provide at least an index of synovial fluid protein concentration, others have criticized its use.[3,9]

Other Tests

In addition to direct measurement of hyaluronic acid content, other chemical tests that have been performed on equine synovial fluid include measurement of creatine kinase and lactate dehydrogenase total activity and isoenzyme activity, alkaline phosphatase activity, and glucose content.[6,10] None of these has been used widely in diagnosis of joint disease in animals.

Nucleated Cell Counts

Nucleated cell counts of synovial fluid can be determined manually with a hemacytometer or automatically with an electronic cell counter. The techniques give similar results with canine synovial fluid.[11] Because normal equine synovial fluid often has a much lower nucleated cell count than feline or canine synovial fluid, the validity of electronically determined counts on some equine specimens is open to question. Cell counts of synovial fluid from normal equine joints may be so low that they are below the background threshold level of electronic cell counters. Manual electronic counters can provide accurate counts on specimens with at least 500 cells/µl. If the electronically determined count is near the threshold level of the instrument, a manual count should be performed.

Manual cell counts should be performed by loading the hemacytometer chamber with undiluted synovial fluid if the total cell count is low. The number of nucleated cells in the four corner primary squares should be counted; the total number of cells in the four corners is multiplied by 2.5 to obtain the number of cells per microliter. Specimens with high cell counts must first be diluted with a white blood cell pipette in the same fashion as when performing manual white blood cell counts on blood. Saline should be used as the diluent for synovial fluid rather than the dilute acetic acid that is sometimes used as a diluent for blood. Acetic acid causes precipitation of the mucin in synovial fluid. A standard white blood cell pipette may be filled to the 0.5 mark with synovial fluid and then filled to the 11 mark with saline. After the diluted synovial fluid is mixed and the first few drops discarded, a hemacytometer chamber should be charged with fluid. Nucleated cells in the four corner squares should be counted as above. The total is then multiplied by 50 to obtain the number of cells per microliter of undiluted synovial fluid.

It may be difficult to obtain counts on markedly exudative specimens because of the presence of cell clumps, fibrin, and necrotic debris. Another potential technical difficulty is that cell counts of routinely diluted synovial fluid may be falsely low because the viscous synovial fluid does not mix evenly with the diluent in the pipette. Pretreatment of such synovial fluid with hyaluronidase reportedly causes an apparent increase in the cell count of more than twofold.[12] This technique is not routinely used in most clinical laboratories.

Cytologic Examination

Cytologic examination of synovial fluid is best accomplished on smears made from sediment of centrifuged specimens. Centrifugation at 500 to 1500 G for 5 to 10 minutes is adequate; most centrifuges used to separate plasma from blood cells can be used to concentrate synovial fluid cells. If the cell count is dramatically increased (>20,000/µl), direct smears may be preferable.

Wedge or coverslip smears may be prepared from synovial fluid sediment (see Chapter 1). It is very important that smears be as thin as possible. Because of the viscosity of synovial fluid, cells have a tendency not to flatten well on slides. When this happens, it can be difficult to identify individual nucleated cells. Even the normally simple task of distinguishing neutrophils from mononuclear cells can be almost impossible.

Synovial fluid is routinely stained with Romanowsky stains, such as Wright's. New methylene blue applied to air-dried smears has also been recommended.[13] Gram's stain can be useful for detecting gram-positive bacteria.

Another technique that has been advocated for cytologic evaluation of synovial fluid involves density gradient centrifugation followed by staining to demonstrate cartilage fragments in the fluid.[14] The number and morphology of the fragments are then evaluated microscopically.

Cytologic Classification of Joint Disease

The ways in which synovium responds to injury are limited and are reflected in a limited number of patterns of abnormal synovial fluid cytology. Though several attempts to classify joint disease in some detail solely on the basis of abnormalities in synovial fluid have been made, it is doubtful that such detailed classification is justified. Synovial fluid results must be interpreted in conjunction with all other available information. Historical information, physical examination findings, and radiographs are central to diagnosis of joint disease. Arthroscopy, culture, and synovial membrane biopsy can provide additional information in selected cases.

Most abnormal equine synovial fluids can be classified into one of two categories: those with normal to moderately increased cell counts (typically <5000/µl) and a predominance of mononuclear cells or those with markedly increased cell counts (typically >5000/µl) and a predominance of neutrophils. The first pattern occurs with degenerative and traumatic joint diseases, and the second pattern is usually associated with septic arthritis. Exceptions and less common patterns are discussed under miscellaneous conditions.

Degenerative and Traumatic Joint Disease

Horses may be affected by a variety of degenerative and traumatic joint diseases, and the characteristics of synovial fluid in those diseases are relatively consistent. Some authors have characterized these diseases as "nonpurulent inflammatory."[10] The severity of inflammation in these diseases varies widely and is often minimal. One limitation of synovial fluid analysis is that the fluid from some horses with degenerative or traumatic joint disease is indistinguishable from normal synovial fluid.

Physical and Chemical Characteristics: The volume of synovial fluid may be decreased, though it is more often normal in degenerative and chronic traumatic joint diseases. Volume may also be increased in such conditions as hydrarthrosis of the tarsus and stifle.[7] The color is normal (light yellow) or it may be blood tinged if joint disease is accompanied by significant hemorrhage. Distinguishing acute joint hemorrhage from contamination with blood during sample collection can be difficult and is often best accomplished by careful observation during aspiration of the fluid. In acute hemarthrosis, the red color is uniform throughout the specimen. If the fluid is streaked with blood as it is being collected, one can assume that contamination has occurred. Dark yellow (xanthochromic) synovial fluid may indicate previous hemorrhage into the synovium or joint cavity.

Fluid viscosity in these diseases varies from normal to decreased, with an inverse relationship between the volume of joint effusion and viscosity. Results of a mucin clot test may be graded as good to poor. When the synovial fluid is diluted by serous effusion (hydrarthrosis), as occurs in some degenerative joint diseases, poor mucin clots have been attributed to dilution of the synovial fluid macromolecular components.[10]

Protein concentration of synovial fluid in most degenerative and traumatic joint disease is unchanged to slightly increased.

Cellular Characteristics: The total nucleated cell count of synovial fluid from horses with degenerative and traumatic joint diseases varies from normal to moderately increased. In most cases, there are <5000 cells/µl.[10] Counts in the range of 1000 to 3000 cells/µl are typical.

Cytologic examination reveals a predominance of mononuclear cells, usually macrophages. Though some authors have stressed the need to distinguish between vacuolated, actively phagocytic macrophages and less

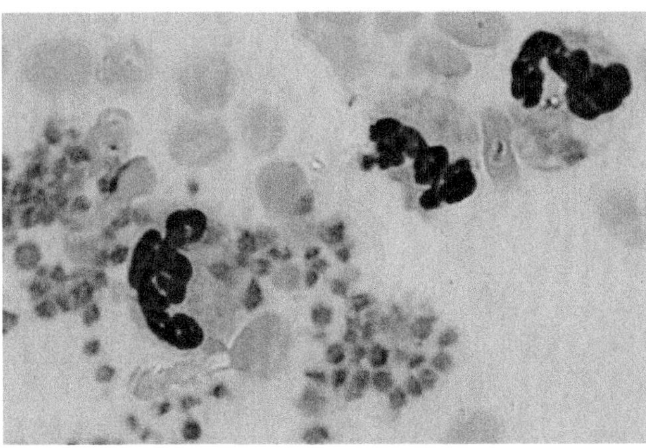

Fig. 10-3 Neutrophils, erythrocytes, and clumped platelets in equine synovial fluid. The presence of platelet clumps suggests that hemorrhage occurred during sample collection.

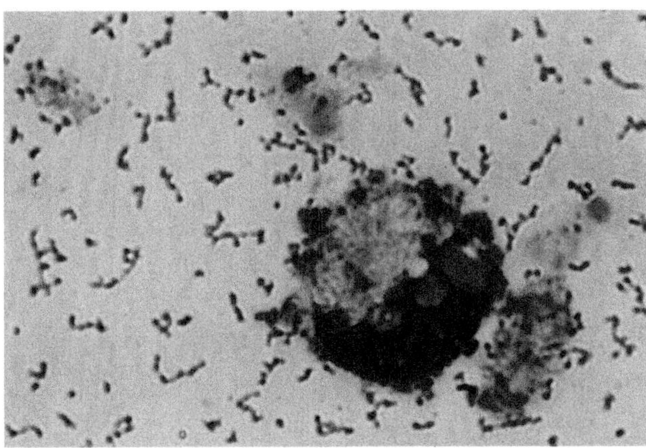

Fig. 10-4 Macrophage containing a phagocytosed erythrocyte in synovial fluid from a horse with acute traumatic joint disease.

active monocytes with few or no cytoplasmic vacuoles, there is actually a continuum of cells with differing degrees of cytoplasmic vacuolation. The extent of vacuolation is of little diagnostic significance. Some of the smaller cells with few vacuoles may be synovial lining cells. Occasional large mononuclear cells in synovial fluid contain pink cytoplasmic granules.

Neutrophils usually comprise <10% of the total cells in synovial fluid from horses with traumatic and degenerative joint diseases, as they do in fluid from normal joints. Possible exceptions include samples with very low total cell counts and samples from joints in which hemorrhage has occurred.

Cytologic diagnosis of acute traumatic joint disease with hemorrhage is complicated by the frequency with which blood is introduced into the synovial fluid specimens during sample collection. Though erythrocytes theoretically are not found in normal synovial fluid, the collection process almost inevitably introduces at least a few erythrocytes into the fluid. One indication of sample contamination is finding platelets or, more often, platelet clumps in the fluid (Fig. 10-3). Phagocytosis of erythrocytes by macrophages (erythrophagia) in a freshly collected and processed specimen suggests that erythrocytes were already in the fluid at the time it was collected (Fig. 10-4). One caveat is that erythrophagia can occur in vitro during sample transport. Hematoidin crystals and hemosiderin-laden macrophages in any synovial fluid sample indicate older hemorrhage (Fig. 10-5).

Cartilage fragments are more likely found in concentrated cytologic preparations from horses with degenerative or traumatic joint diseases than in similar preparations from healthy horses. Attempts have been made to relate the severity of joint disease to number and types of cartilage fragments found.[14] That technique, however, has not gained wide acceptance among clinical pathologists.

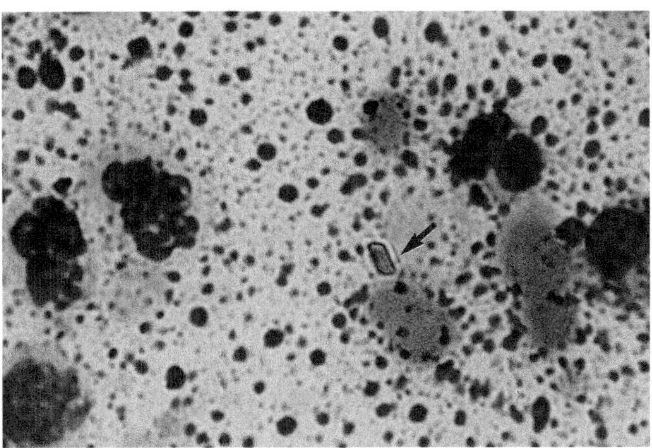

Fig. 10-5 Neutrophils and a hematoidin crystal *(arrow)* in synovial fluid from a horse with septic arthritis and joint hemorrhage. Hematoidin is a breakdown product of hemoglobin.

Inflammatory Joint Diseases

For the purposes of this discussion, inflammatory joint diseases are defined as those with markedly increased numbers of neutrophils in synovial fluid. The two major groups of diseases that classically are considered under this heading are septic arthritis and such immune-mediated joint diseases as rheumatoid arthritis and systemic lupus erythematosus. Differentiating the two groups is a common diagnostic problem in dogs. Though isolated case reports describe horses

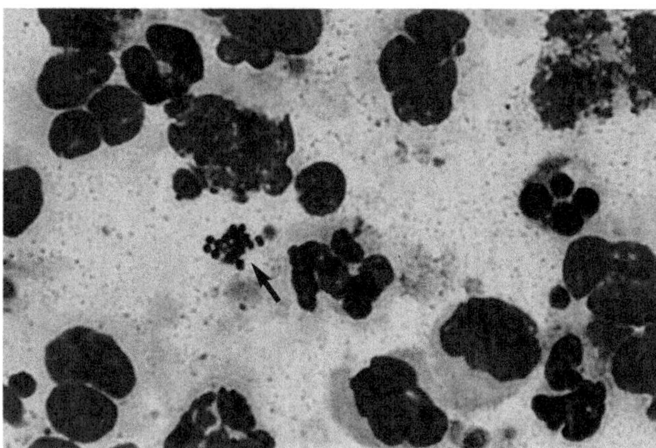

Fig. 10-6 Numerous neutrophils in synovial fluid from a horse with septic arthritis. Karyorrhexis affects one cell, and several others are karyolytic. Also present is a free cluster of cocci (*arrow*).

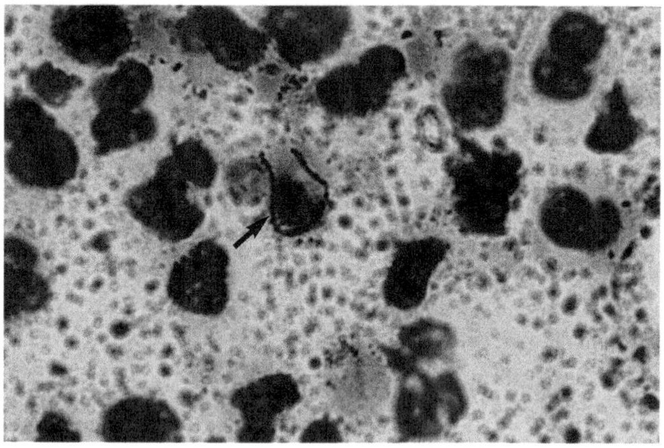

Fig. 10-7 Numerous karyolytic neutrophils and one chain of cocci (*arrow*) in synovial fluid from a horse with septic arthritis. Most of the pink granular material in the background is nucleic acid from necrotic exudative cells.

with clinical and laboratory features suggestive of systemic lupus erythematosus, the existence of immune-mediated arthritis is not well documented in horses.[15,16] Even if one accepts the existence of immune-mediated joint disease in horses, it must be rare. For that reason, septic arthritis should be the top differential diagnosis when purulent synovial fluid is encountered. Among the few noninfectious causes of neutrophilic exudation into synovial fluid of horses are acute traumatic joint disease and chronic hemarthrosis.

Physical and Chemical Characteristics: The volume of fluid may be normal to markedly increased. The fluid may vary from yellow to cream colored and may be cloudy to opaque. If blood is mixed with the fluid, it will be brown. Flocculent material is often suspended in the fluid.

The viscosity of purulent synovial fluid typically is decreased, often markedly so. The mucin clot is usually graded as poor or very poor. The poor mucin clot in septic arthritis is attributed to the action of bacterial hyaluronidase. Nonseptic neutrophilic synovial fluids also may have poor mucin clots for reasons that are incompletely understood.

The protein content of synovial fluid from horses with inflammatory joint disease is consistently increased. This is attributable to increased synovial vascular permeability as well as breakdown of cellular elements within the exudate.

Simultaneous measurement of plasma or serum glucose levels and synovial glucose content has been advocated for diagnosis of septic arthritis.[7] Synovial fluid glucose content that is markedly lower than the serum glucose level supposedly indicates septic arthritis. Because of the ability of neutrophils to consume glucose, any synovial fluid specimen containing numerous neutrophils is likely to have a low synovial fluid glucose content. Also, the glucose content of such specimens decreases rapidly after collection. Glucose measurements on synovial fluid are not performed routinely in most laboratories.

Cytologic Characteristics: The nucleated cell count in inflammatory joint disease usually is markedly increased (almost always >5000/μl) and may exceed 100,000/μl. Some specimens may contain so many cell clumps and so much cellular debris and fibrin as to make an accurate count impossible. The cell count can increase very rapidly in septic arthritis. In one experimental model in horses, the mean nucleated cell count increased to about 40,000 cells/μl within the first 24 hours of infection.[9]

Neutrophils are usually the predominant cells in synovial fluid from horses with inflammatory joint disease. Nuclear degeneration (karyolysis) may be evident in fluid from horses with septic arthritis but can be more difficult to assess in synovial fluid than in peritoneal and pleural fluids (Fig. 10-6). When synovial fluid mucin prevents neutrophils from flattening on a slide, the degree of nuclear degeneration may be underestimated.

Many different bacteria may cause septic arthritis in horses. Among the more common causes in young animals are *Actinobacillus equuli, Streptococcus* spp., and *Escherichia coli*. Detecting bacteria in synovial fluid from animals with septic arthritis is often difficult. There are often few bacteria in the fluid; they may be found within neutrophils or free in the synovial fluid (Fig. 10-7). Organisms are often more numerous in the synovial lining than in the synovial fluid. Gram's stain can be used to advantage in detecting gram-positive

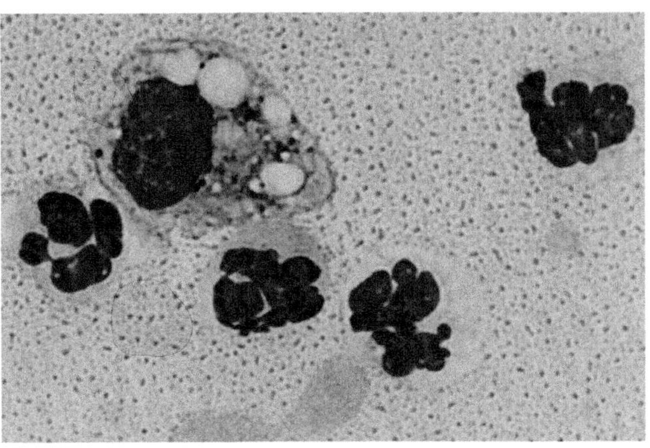

Fig. 10-8 Neutrophils and a macrophage in synovial fluid from a horse with acute traumatic joint disease.

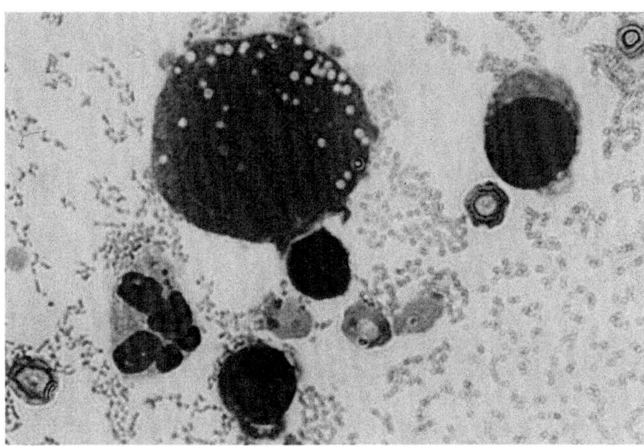

Fig. 10-9 Three lymphocytes, a macrophage, and a neutrophil in synovial fluid from a horse with lymphocytic synovitis.

bacteria in synovial fluid, but it is inferior to Wright's stain for detecting gram-negative bacteria.

Miscellaneous Conditions

Acute Traumatic Joint Disease: Though traumatic joint disease usually is associated with nucleated cell counts of <5000/µl and a predominance of mononuclear cells, acute trauma is mentioned occasionally as a cause of slightly increased synovial fluid neutrophil numbers.[17] Acute traumatic injury in horses infrequently is accompanied by marked neutrophilic exudation into the synovial fluid, with total cell counts >10,000/µl and >75% neutrophils (Fig. 10-8). Such cases present a diagnostic dilemma because the cytologic features may be difficult to distinguish from those of septic arthritis. An extremely high count (>40,000/µl) is unlikely to be caused by acute traumatic injury. Also, high cell counts attributable to trauma typically decrease within a few days to <5000 cells/µl.

Chronic Hemarthrosis: Chronic hemorrhage into joints can in itself incite inflammation. In hemophilia of people and dogs, such inflammation can be severe and destructive. The cellular reaction may vary widely, though it is often predominantly neutrophilic. Chronic hemarthrosis resulting from trauma has been described in a horse.[18] The synovial fluid characteristics were not described in detail, though hemosiderin-laden macrophages were found in synovial fluid. Other cytologic indicators of intraarticular hemorrhage include erythrophagia, which is associated with recent hemorrhage and hematoidin crystals. The latter may be found either free or within leukocytes.

Lymphocytic Synovitis: Rarely, equine synovial fluid specimens have cell counts >5000 cells/µl and a marked predominance of lymphocytes (Fig. 10-9). Rare plasma cells may also be found in such specimens (Fig. 10-10). A synovial biopsy from one affected horse revealed proliferative synovitis, with marked infiltration of the synovium by lymphocytes, resembling rheumatoid arthritis or chronic *Mycoplasma* arthritis in other species. A similar reaction was described in the synovium of a pony infected with *Borrelia burgdorferi*, though the synovial fluid characteristics in that pony were not described.[19] Lymphocytic synovitis should be viewed as one of the patterns of inflammatory response of the synovium rather than as an entity.

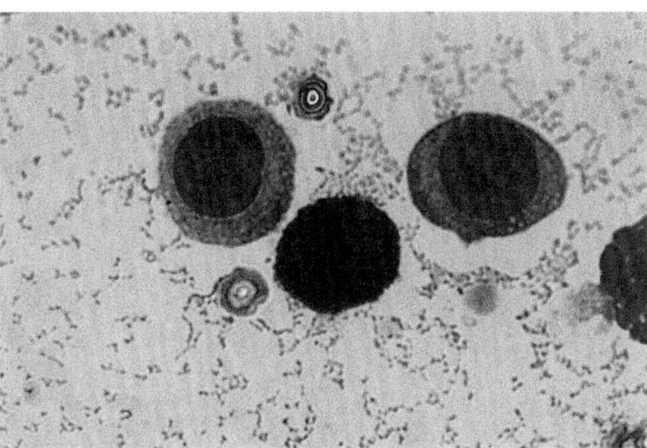

Fig. 10-10 Two lymphocytes and a plasma cell in synovial fluid from a horse with lymphocytic synovitis.

Eosinophilic Synovitis: A single equine case of eosinophilic synovitis, characterized by marked synovial hyperplasia with infiltration of the synovium by eosinophils, has been reported.[20] The total nucleated cell counts in affected joints were 8300/µl and 9200/µl, with 20% and 11% eosinophils, respectively. The cause of the synovitis was undetermined.

REFERENCES

1. Jubb et al: *Pathology of Domestic Animals*, 4th ed. New York, 1993, Academic Press, pp. 139-141.
2. Duncan et al: *Veterinary Laboratory Medicine*. 3rd ed. Ames, 1994, Iowa State University Press, pp. 214-216.
3. Davies: The cell content of synovial fluid. *J Anat* 79:66-73, 1945.
4. Van Pelt: Properties of equine synovial fluid. *JAVMA* 141:1051-1061, 1962.
5. Hilbert et al: Hyaluronic acid concentration in synovial fluid from normal and arthritic joints of horses. *Aust Vet J* 61:22-24, 1984.
6. Van Pelt: Interpretation of synovial fluid findings in the horse. *JAVMA* 165:91-95, 1974.
7. Tew: Synovial fluid analysis: applications in equine joint injury and disease. *Proc Ann Mtg AAEP*, 1983. pp. 121-127.
8. Bartone: Comparison of various treatments for experimentally induced equine infectious arthritis. *Am J Vet Res* 48:519-529, 1987.
9. Tew: Discussion on synovial fluid analysis. *Proc Ann Mtg AAEP*, 1983, pp. 141-144.
10. Yancik: Evaluation of creatine kinase and lactate dehydrogenase activities in clinically normal and abnormal equine joints. *Am Vet J Res* 48:463-466, 1987.
11. Atiola: A comparison of manual and electronic counting for total nucleated cell counts on synovial fluid from canine stifle joints. *Can J Vet Res* 50:282-284, 1986.
12. Palmer: Total leukocyte enumeration in pathologic synovial fluid. *Am J Clin Path* 49:812-814, 1968.
13. Perman: in Kaneko: *Clinical Biochemistry of Domestic Animals*. 3rd ed. New York, 1980, Academic Press, pp. 749-783.
14. Tew and Hackett: Identification of cartilage wear fragments in synovial fluid from equine joints. *Arthritis Rheum* 24:1419-1424, 1981.
15. Vrins and Feldman: Lupus erythematosus-like syndrome in a horse. *Equine Pract* 5(6):18-25, 1983.
16. Byars et al: Non-erosive polysynovitis in a horse. *Equine Vet J* 16:141-143, 1984.
17. Dyson: Synovial fluid and equine joint disease. *Equine Vet J* 16:79-80, 1984.
18. Dyson: Lameness associated with recurrent hemarthrosis in a horse. *Equine Vet J* 18:224-226, 1986.
19. Burgess: Arthritis and panuveitis as manifestations of *Borrelia burgdorferi* infection in a Wisconsin pony. *JAVMA* 189:1340-1344, 1986.
20. Turner et al: Acute eosinophilic synovitis in a horse. *Equine Vet J* 22:215-217, 1990.

CHAPTER 11

Cerebrospinal Fluid

Peter S. MacWilliams

Diagnosis and clinical management of nervous system disease involve a careful assessment of the history and environment, a complete physical examination, and a neurologic examination. Ancillary diagnostic procedures may include hematologic measurements, serum chemistry assays, serologic tests, toxicologic assays, radiographic procedures, and cerebrospinal fluid (CSF) analysis. These test results, in combination with the clinical findings, are used to formulate a differential diagnosis, make a definitive diagnosis, decide treatment, and determine a prognosis.

CSF is produced by ultrafiltration and active transport in the choroid plexus of the brain. The fluid circulates in the subarachnoid space and is absorbed by arachnoid villi associated with venous sinuses in the central nervous system (CNS).[1,2] CSF is in direct contact with the brain and spinal cord and functions to cushion, protect, and nourish these delicate tissues.

Collection of CSF is indicated when lesions in the brain or spinal cord are suspected. The procedure for CSF collection is relatively safe, with some prior experience, and requires minimal equipment. Collection of CSF from the atlanto-occipital space may be contraindicated in horses with acute cranial trauma. Relative risk should be carefully considered for horses that require sedation or anesthesia. Removal of CSF from horses with increased intracranial pressure is usually contraindicated because the cerebrum and cerebellum may herniate rapidly around bony prominences in the calvaria.

The usual laboratory analysis of CSF consists of gross inspection, cell counts, measurement of protein content, and cytologic examination. On the basis of these preliminary results and the differential diagnosis, additional tests may be indicated, such as cultures for bacteria and fungi. Other measurements include enzyme activities, electrolyte concentrations, glucose content, antibody titers, and polymerase chain reactions for detection of specific antigens.[3] The clinician can use alterations detected in the CSF to make a definitive diagnosis. CSF with abundant neutrophils, increased protein content, and numerous bacteria confirms a diagnosis of septic meningoencephalitis. In other cases, CSF results may be less conclusive but can help categorize the disease as infectious, inflammatory, metabolic, toxic, traumatic, degenerative, or neoplastic.

Sample Collection

CSF can be collected from either the atlanto-occipital or the lumbosacral region of the spine.[1,4] The neurologic examination and clinical condition of the horse determine the collection site.[5] Lesions localized to the brain and cervical spine are most likely to produce abnormalities in CSF collected from the atlanto-occipital site. Lumbosacral collection is most appropriate for lesions in the caudal segments of the spinal cord. For some horses, comparison of the results for CSF collected from both sites can be helpful in lesion localization. Collection of CSF from either site requires correct positioning, adequate restraint, appropriate needles, surgical preparation of the skin, and availability of specimen tubes. Atlanto-occipital collection is limited to comatose horses or those under general anesthesia because immobilization and lateral recumbency are necessary for collection. Collection of CSF from the lumbosacral site can be achieved in the standing adult horse. In foals, CSF can be collected from either site with the animal in lateral recumbency.[6] People involved in the collection and laboratory analysis should exercise extreme caution if rabies is being considered in the differential diagnosis.

CSF should be collected into sterile, clear-glass or plastic-capped vials. An aliquot can be removed aseptically from the tube and used for cell counts, total protein concentration, and cell identification. The remainder of the specimen can be used for microbial culture or chemistry assays if indicated. Although most CSF specimens do not clot, a tube containing EDTA should be readily available in case the fluid is bloody or purulent. If the fluid is bloody on initial penetration, several tubes should be available so that multiple aliquots can be collected to see if the fluid clears. A recent study in horses revealed that blood contamination diminished significantly as three or four 2-ml aliquots of CSF were removed sequentially from the lumbosacral site.[7]

Atlanto-Occipital Technique

For atlanto-occipital collection the horse is placed in lateral recumbency with the neck flexed such that the longitudinal axis of the head and cervical spine are at a right angle.[4,8] The nose is elevated to a horizontal plane. The subarachnoid space is located at a depth of 5 to 8 cm in adults and 2 to 4 cm in foals. A 9-cm, 18- to 20-gauge styletted spinal needle is used for adult horses. A 4-cm, 20-gauge disposable needle is appropriate for foals. The needle is inserted through the skin at the intersection of a line drawn between the cranial border of the wings of the atlas and the dorsal midline, which is identified by palpating the external occipital protuberance (Fig. 11-1). The needle is directed perpendicular to the cervical spine toward the rostral end of the mandible. Some resistance is encountered as the needle passes through the funicular part of the ligamentum nuchae. The needle is advanced until the atlanto-occipital membrane and dura mater are penetrated, which is perceived as a "popping" sensation or as a sudden absence of resistance. When either sensation is detected, the stylet is removed to allow CSF to flow. Position of the needle should not be adjusted without the stylet in place. The neck or head should not be moved while the needle is close to the subarachnoid space.

Lumbosacral Technique

The lumbosacral site can be accessed in most standing adult horses with a 15- to 20-cm, 18-gauge styletted spinal needle after infiltration of the skin and subcutis with local anesthetic. For large horses (12 to 17 hands tall) a 20-cm styletted spinal needle is suggested. A 20- to 23-cm needle may be required for draft horses over 17 hands tall.[4,8] Anatomic landmarks are the tuber sacrale of the ilium and the dorsal midline. The needle is inserted through a stab wound located at the intersection of a line drawn between the cranial edges of each tuber sacrale and the midline, which is localized by palpating the spinous processes of the sixth lumbar vertebra and the second sacral vertebra (Fig. 11-2). A depression in the skin is often located in this area. The needle is directed perpendicular to the long axis of the vertebral column and advanced with stylet in place until the interarcuate

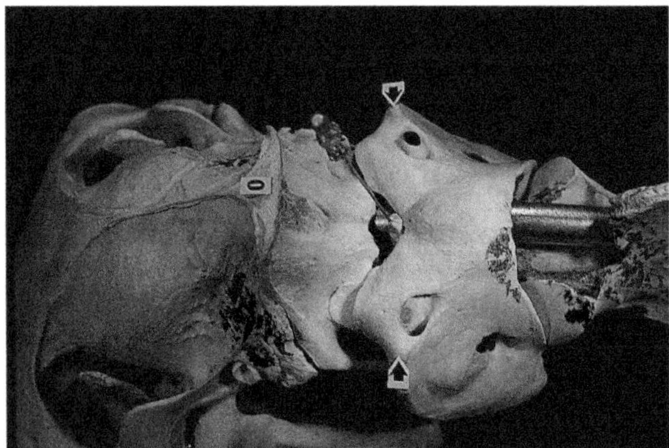

Fig. 11-1 Anatomic landmarks for collection of CSF from atlanto-occipital site. Needle is placed at the intersection of an imaginary line between the cranial border of the wings of the atlas *(arrows)* and the midline, which is designated by the external occipital protuberance *(O)*.

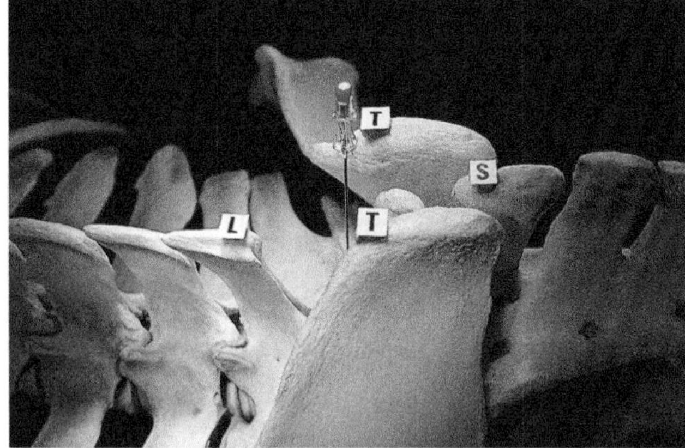

Fig. 11-2 Anatomic landmarks for collection of CSF from lumbosacral site. Needle is inserted perpendicular to the long axis of the spine, at the intersection of the midline and the cranial edges of the tuber sacrale *(T)* of each ilium. The midline is identified by the spinous processes of the sixth lumbar *(L)* and second sacral *(S)* vertebrae.

ligament, dura mater, and arachnoid membrane are penetrated, as identified by a popping sensation or decreased resistance. Average depth of the subarachnoid space is 13 cm in adults. Entry of the needle into the subarachnoid space may be accompanied by excitement, tail movement, flexion of the pelvic limbs, or contraction of the axial muscles.[1]

Laboratory Assessment

As with other body fluids, the laboratory analysis of CSF consists of inspection of gross appearance, cell counts, measurement of protein content, cell identification, and special chemistry assays.[9] Cells, especially neutrophils, degenerate and lyse rapidly in CSF because of its low protein content and its electrolyte concentrations, which are different from corresponding plasma values. Therefore, procedures for cell counts and preparation of smears on glass slides for cell identification should be done within 30 minutes of collection. Cells can be preserved for preparation of glass slides by mixing 8 to 10 drops (0.25 ml) of fresh CSF with 1 ml of 40% ethanol or by adding autologous serum to the sample. The addition of 1 drop of autologous serum to 0.25 ml of CSF will preserve cell morphology and differential counts for 48 hours when stored at 4° C.[10] Measurement of protein content and special assays can be done on CSF that is refrigerated or frozen without additives.

Macroscopic appearance

Visual inspection of the color and turbidity of CSF is best done by viewing the specimen through natural sunlight or against a white background.[8] A white index card with lines provides a background for accurate color assessment and fine lines to detect turbidity.

Normal CSF is clear, colorless, and watery and does not form a clot.[3,8] Any deviation in color or turbidity is considered abnormal, and the cause should be determined. Causes of CSF turbidity include elevated cell count, presence of microorganisms, or a marked increase in protein content.[1,8] Cell counts greater than 400 to 500 μl are necessary before CSF becomes turbid. The presence of myelographic contrast media or fat aspirated during collection may cause turbidity.[5] Abnormal colors encountered in the macroscopic assessment of CSF are red tinged, bright red, xanthochromic, and opaque white (Fig. 11-3). Cloudy CSF with a white tinge indicates a marked increase in nucleated cells. Red-tinged or bright-red fluid indicates pathologic or iatrogenic hemorrhage.[1,4,8]

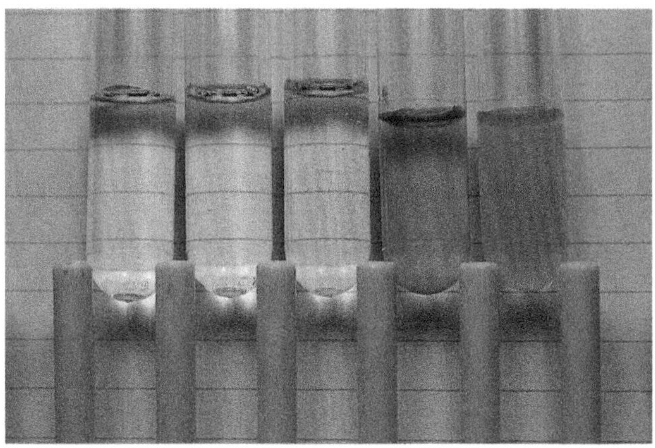

Fig. 11-3 Macroscopic examination of CSF. Tubes are viewed against a lined white index card to assess color and turbidity. *Left to right,* Normal CSF, mildly xanthochromic CSF, moderately xanthochromic CSF, red-tinged turbid CSF caused by hemorrhage, and cloudy red-tinged fluid from a horse with bacterial meningitis.

It is important to differentiate between hemorrhage caused during the collection procedure and that resulting from trauma or disease. *Iatrogenic hemorrhage* occurs when the spinal needle penetrates vessels in the meninges or surrounding tissue. This can be recognized by careful observation of the fluid as it drips from the needle and by gross and microscopic inspection of the specimen. CSF that is red tinged or bloody during initial collection, then clears as additional CSF is collected, indicates iatrogenic hemorrhage. In addition, red-tinged or bloody fluid that has a clear supernatant after centrifugation indicates iatrogenic hemorrhage. Microscopic assessment of stained films reveals platelets and noncrenated erythrocytes.

Subarachnoid hemorrhage resulting from disease is recognized by a red-tinged or bloody CSF that has a xanthochromic supernatant. *Xanthochromia* is a yellow-orange coloration of the CSF caused by erythrocyte breakdown products, oxyhemoglobin, and bilirubin.[8] Other causes include a marked increase in CSF protein (>400 mg/dl) and severe icterus, which allows plasma bilirubin to cross the blood-CSF barrier. Subarachnoid hemorrhage may cause release of oxyhemoglobin from lysed erythrocytes. Xanthochromia forms in 2 to 4 hours, peaks at 24 to 36 hours, and may persist for 4 to 8 days.

Bilirubin appears in CSF 48 hours after subarachnoid hemorrhage and may persist for 3 or 4 weeks. Microscopic features of pathologic hemorrhage include the presence of hemosiderin, hematoidin, and phagocytosed erythrocytes within macrophages. Xanthochromia in the CSF of a horse without a history of jaundice indicates prior hemorrhage, likely associated with trauma, neoplasia, vascular disorders, or infectious disease.

Protein concentration and refractive index

Normal equine CSF has a very low protein content compared with other body fluids (Table 11-1). Most of the protein in normal CSF is albumin. The usual

TABLE 11-1

Reference Values for CSF in Adult Horses[1,4]

Test	Reference
Appearance	Clear, colorless
WBC count	0–8 cells/μl
Protein	20–80 mg/dl
Refractive index	1.3347–1.3350
Differential count	Small lymphocytes ~ 70%
	Monocytes, macrophages ~ 30%

methods for measurement of serum proteins, such as biuret reagent or protein refractometer, are insensitive. Quantitative and qualitative methods are available for CSF protein analysis.

In the supernatant from a centrifuged sample, *refractive index* of CSF reflects protein content and the concentration of other solutes, such as electrolytes or glucose. Suspended particulates (*eg*, cells, bacteria) will increase refractive index.[3] Hemoglobin discoloration of the supernatant from lysed erythrocytes or the presence of radiographic contrast media may falsely increase the refractive index. For CSF that is clear and colorless, an increase in CSF refractive index is usually indicative of an elevated protein concentration.

Quantitative measurement of CSF protein is usually done by turbidimetric method using trichloroacetic acid or dye-binding methods using Coomassie brilliant blue or Ponceau S.[8] These methods require a spectrophotometer and measure both albumin and globulin in CSF. Some Coomassie blue methods underestimate globulin concentrations. Reference ranges for equine CSF protein are much higher than those reported for other animals (see Table 11-1). Values above this range must be interpreted in conjunction with the clinical signs, neurologic examination, and other laboratory results, since normal horses with CSF protein values in the range of 100 to 120 mg/dl have been identified.[3] Foals less than 1 week old have CSF protein values in the range of 90 to 180 mg/dl, which gradually decrease to adult levels within 2 weeks after birth.[6,11] Comparison of protein values between samples collected from the atlanto-occipital and lumbosacral sites can help localize lesions. When this difference in protein concentration is greater than 25 mg/dl, the lesion is closer to the site with the higher value.[12]

The Pandy and Nonne-Apelt tests can be used to detect increases in globulin levels in CSF.[1,8] Reagents for both methods cause precipitation of globulins that is visible grossly. Reagent for the *Pandy test* consists of 10 mg of carbolic acid crystals dissolved in 100 ml of distilled water. A few drops of CSF are added to 1 ml of reagent, and the solution is observed for turbidity. Reagent for the *Nonne-Apelt test* is a saturated solution of ammonium sulfate. Several drops of CSF are layered on the surface of 1 ml of reagent and observed for precipitation at the interface. For both tests the amount of precipitation is graded subjectively from zero to 3+. Normal CSF does not produce a visible precipitate in either test because albumin, the primary protein in normal CSF, does not react. The Pandy and Nonne-Apelt tests have been replaced by quantitative methods that measure globulins, specific immunoglobulins (IgG, IgM, IgA), and antibody titers for herpesvirus and protozoal myelitis.[3]

General causes of elevated CSF protein include increased permeability of the blood-CSF barrier, increased synthesis of immunoglobulins in the CNS, degeneration or necrosis of neural tissue, and obstruction of CSF circulation.[2,8,13] Protein values must be interpreted in conjunction with the total and differential cell counts. The highest protein values are observed in horses with a suppurative meningitis or encephalitis.[13] CSF from these horses has a marked increase in nucleated cell count, with a predominance of neutrophils and variable numbers of bacteria. Protein concentrations are increased frequently in horses with CNS neoplasia, but cell counts are usually normal or slightly increased, with a predominance of mononuclear cells.

Nonsuppurative inflammatory diseases are characterized by a marked increase in CSF protein but a normal cell count. Local production of immunoglobulins and vasculitis are probable mechanisms for the lack of correlation between the protein concentration and cell count. When the total protein content is elevated, quantitation of the albumin and globulin fractions by electrophoresis or measurement of immunoglobulin levels may be necessary to differentiate the causes, including intrathecal hemorrhage from necrosis or inflammation and iatrogenic hemorrhage during collection, as well as the causes previously cited.[14,15] Hemorrhage within the subarachnoid space contributes minimally to the total protein concentration but can influence immunoglobulin levels.

Cell Counts

Cell counts should be done within 30 minutes because nucleated cells in CSF deteriorate rapidly after collection. For most CSF specimens, red blood cell (RBC, erythrocyte) and white blood cell (WBC, leukocyte) counts can be obtained by adding undiluted CSF directly to a hemacytometer.[8] The counting chamber is allowed to stand for 5 minutes to permit cells to settle on the grid. RBCs and WBCs are counted in all nine squares. The total number of each cell type in all nine squares is multiplied by 1.1 to obtain numbers of RBCs and WBCs per microliter. In the hemacytometer chamber, erythrocytes can be recognized as small, refractile, and light tan, with a round, discoid, or crenated shape (Fig. 11-4). Leukocytes are larger than erythrocytes and have an irregular cell margin, granular cytoplasm, and a barely visible nucleus. Normal ranges for cell counts are listed in Table 11-1. If cell counts are high or identification of WBCs and RBCs is difficult, samples are diluted with a WBC pipette in 10% glacial acetic acid containing 0.2 g of crystal violet per deciliter.[3] This fluid stains WBC nuclei and lyses RBCs. Diluting fluid is drawn up to the 1 mark in the pipette, and the CSF is drawn up to the 11 mark. The pipette is agitated, the first few drops are discarded, and the chamber is filled. Cells in all nine large squares are enumerated, and the total is multiplied by 1.2 to obtain WBCs per microliter.

Formulas and factors have been used to correct the CSF WBC count and total protein value for contamination by peripheral blood during collection. The standard formula uses the RBC count in blood and CSF along with the WBC count in blood to correct the measured WBC count in CSF, as follows[2]:

Corrected WBC CSF = Measured WBC CSF – (WBC blood × RBC CSF/RBC blood)

Total protein values can be substituted for corresponding WBC values to calculate a corrected CSF total protein. A factor that has been applied frequently is that CSF protein content increases 1 mg/dl for every 1000 RBCs/µl in CSF and that CSF WBC count increases by 1 cell/µl for every 500 RBCs/µl of CSF. Studies with equine CSF indicate that these calculations or factors do not generate accurate results.[7]

Differential Cell Counts and Cell Identification

Normal CSF contains very few nucleated cells. Samples from horses with inflammatory disease rarely have WBC counts in excess of 1000 to 2000 cells/µl. Therefore, cells must be concentrated before microscopic examination. Cellular components in CSF can be concentrated by sedimentation, membrane filtration, or centrifugation in a standard laboratory centrifuge or a cytocentrifuge.[8,16] Whichever method is preferred, slides should be prepared within 30 minutes of collection unless the cells have been preserved by adding autologous serum or ethanol to fresh CSF, as previously described. Without some form of preservation, about one third of the cells disintegrate within 24 hours, and a preferential reduction appears to occur in neutrophils in animals with suppurative meningitis.[10] This indicates that the differential count may be skewed in samples that are not handled properly.

Concentrating cells by centrifugation or sedimentation are methods that use readily available equipment. Cells can be concentrated by spinning CSF in a centrifuge for 5 minutes at 200 x g (1000 rpm for most bench-top models). The supernatant is removed and saved for protein determination or other tests. After adding a few drops of serum or 7% bovine albumin solution, the sediment is resuspended, and smears are made

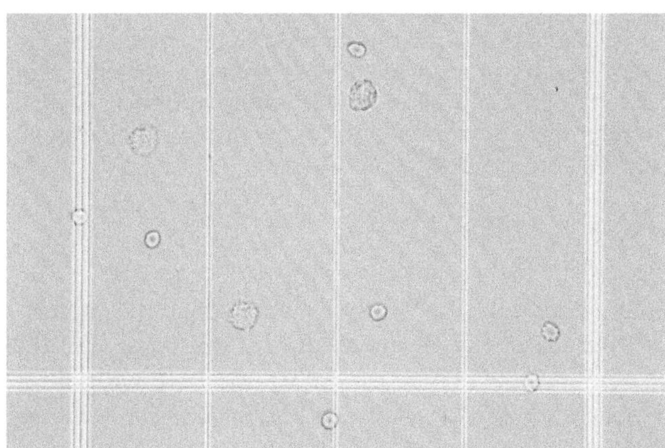

Fig. 11-4 Microscopic recognition of WBCs and RBCs on hemacytometer grid. The large cells with slightly irregular cell margins in each of the three large rectangles in the middle are WBCs. RBCs are smaller, light tan in color, and are round with a dimpled center. (Original magnification X400)

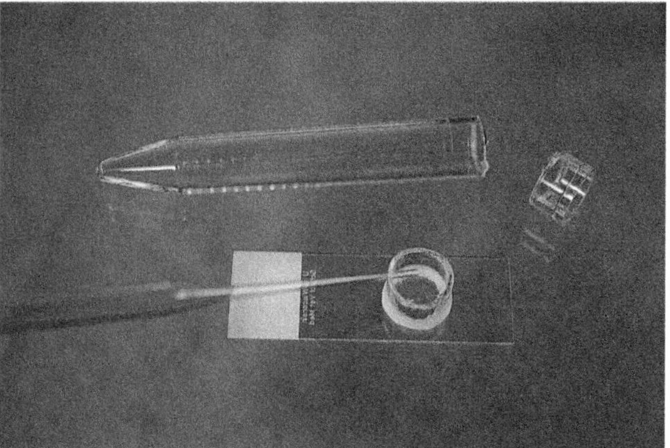

Fig. 11-5 Sedimentation method for concentration of cells in CSF. Severed end of a plastic centrifuge tube is sealed to a glass slide with paraffin. CSF is pipetted into the chamber and allowed to form sediment for 30 minutes.

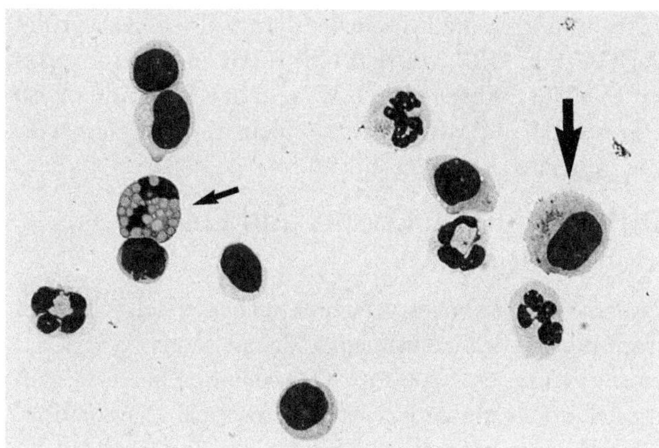

Fig. 11-6 Mixed inflammatory cell response in CSF from a horse with nonseptic meningoencephalitis. Small lymphocytes predominate, with a few neutrophils, one eosinophil *(small arrow)*, and a monocyte *(large arrow)*. (Original magnification X500; Wright's stain)

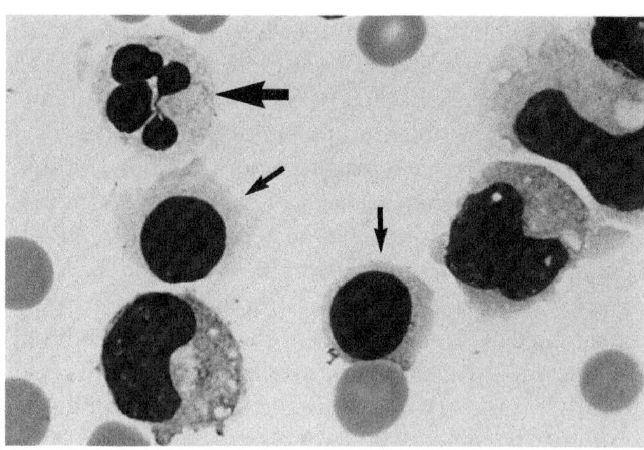

Fig. 11-7 Normal morphology of leukocytes in CSF. Two small lymphocytes *(small arrows)* are surrounded by monocytes and a neutrophil *(large arrow)*. (Wright's stain, X1000)

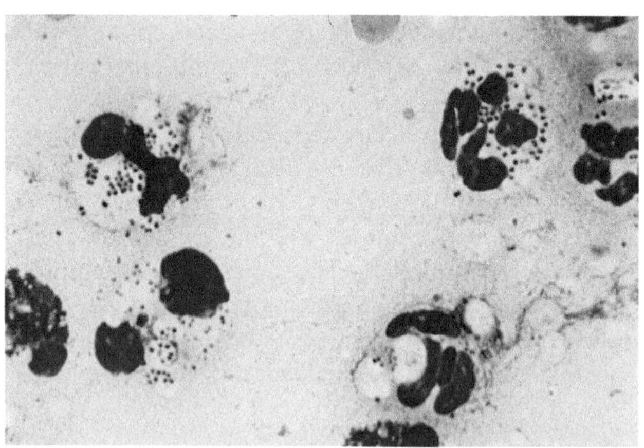

Fig. 11-8 CSF from a foal with septic meningitis. Degenerate neutrophils are present and contain numerous phagocytosed cocci. (Original magnification X1000; Wright's stain)

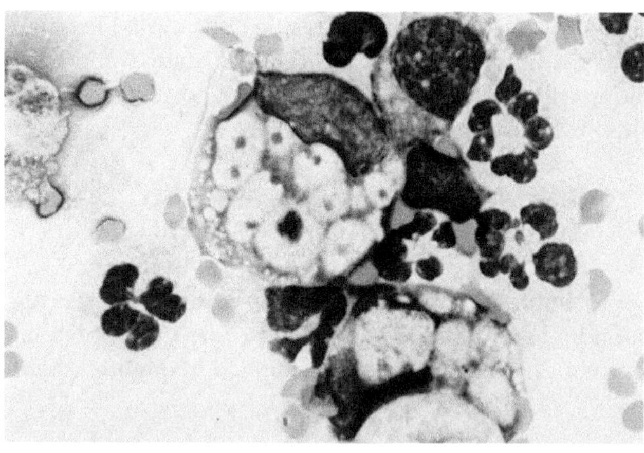

Fig. 11-9 Cytophagia in CSF from a horse with resolving septic meningitis. A mixture of neutrophils, macrophages, and a lymphocyte is present. Macrophages in center and bottom contain phagocytosed cellular debris, which should not be confused with fungal organisms. (Original magnification X1000; Wright's stain)

on glass slides. Addition of protein to the sediment improves cell preservation and slide quality. Air-drilled slides can be stained with Wright's, Giemsa, or Diff-Quik.

Cells can be concentrated by gravity sedimentation using a special apparatus (Fig. 11-5).[3,16] A 2-cm segment is cut from the open end of a 15-ml plastic centrifuge tube using a hot scalpel blade. The smooth end of the cylinder is dipped in melted paraffin or hot petrolatum and placed on a clean glass slide. An aliquot of CSF (0.5 to 1.0 ml) is pipetted into the cylindrical chamber and allowed to form sediment for 30 minutes. After sedimentation the supernatant is gently aspirated, the chamber is dismantled, and the small amount of remaining CSF is carefully absorbed with filter paper or lint-free tissue paper. Slides are allowed to air-dry before staining.

Filtration and cytocentrifugation require specialized equipment available in diagnostic laboratories or teaching hospitals. The cytocentrifuge produces consistent films of fluid specimens by spinning the fluid directly against the glass slide and concentrating the cells in a small circular area on the slide.

TABLE 11-2

CSF Results from Horses with Central Nervous Disease Disease

Disease	Appearance	WBCs (/μl)	RBCs (/μl)	Protein (mg/dl)	Cytologic findings	Other observations
Iatrogenic hemorrhage	Red tinged	8	2300	60	RBCs Few platelets	Clear supernatant
Subarachnoid hemorrhage	Red tinged	10	1749	53	Erythrophagia	Xanthochromic supernatant
Cervical compression	Clear	0	5	59	Normal	
Protozoal myelitis	Slightly cloudy Xanthochromic	80	1900	96	M 90%, L 8% S 2%	AST 25 IU/L CK 1335 IU/L
Verminous encephalomyelitis *(Micronema)*	Clear Xanthochromic	145	135	83	M 2%, L 25% S 68%, E 5%	
Cauda equina neuritis	Slightly cloudy Xanthochromic	6	666	108	M 5%, L 61% S 34%	
Rabies	Clear	88	102	60	M 13%, L 86% S 1%	AST 25 IU/L CK 30 IU/L
Septic meningitis	Slightly cloudy	1870	671	340	M 6%, L 1% S 93%	Bacteria
Herpes myeloencephalitis	Slightly cloudy Xanthochromic	5	1655	108	M 14%, L 57% S 29%	

M, Monocytes or macrophages; *L*, small lymphocytes; *S*, neutrophils; *E*, eosinophils; *AST*, aspartate transaminase; *CK*, creatine kinase.

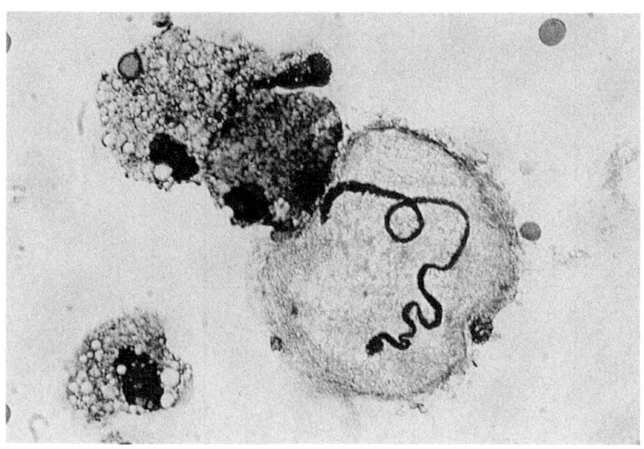

Fig. 11-10 Myelin fragment in CSF from a horse with necrotizing encephalomyelitis. Large spherical structure next to macrophage contains a long spiral fragment of myelin. (Original magnification, X400; Wright's stain)

Membrane filtration requires a filtration apparatus, alcoholic fixation, and Papanicolaou or hematoxylin-eosin staining techniques.[17]

Most of the cells in normal CSF are mononuclear cells (80% to 90%), with a predominance of small lymphocytes and fewer numbers of monocytes and macrophages (Figs. 11-6 and 11-7).[9,13] Neutrophils are occasionally seen. Eosinophils are rare. CSF samples with an increased nucleated cell count *(pleocytosis)* or increased protein value require careful microscopic assessment. Bacteria should be suspected when neutrophilic pleocytosis is present (Fig. 11-8). Fungi, protozoa, or parasite migration should be considered when a mixed pleocytosis with eosinophils is observed.[4] Viral diseases frequently cause a mild mononuclear pleocytosis consisting of lymphocytes and lesser numbers of macrophages.[18] A notable exception is the neutrophilic pleocytosis in the early stages of Eastern equine encephalomyelitis.

Degenerative diseases usually cause a mixed pleocytosis of macrophages, lymphocytes, and neutrophils. When significant numbers of macrophages are identified, the cytoplasm should be examined for pigment and phagocytosed material. *Erythrophagia*, or presence of hemosiderin, indicates hemorrhage. *Cytophagia* by macrophages may be a feature of degenerative diseases or resolving inflammatory process (Fig. 11-9). On rare occasions, myelin fragments from disrupted nerve fibers are noted in the background or undergo phagocytosis by macrophages (Fig. 11-10).

The clinical presentation, neurologic assessment, and range of laboratory findings in equine CNS diseases have been described.[13,17-23] Table 11-2 contains specific examples of CSF alterations in several diseases.

Special Chemistry Assays

Concentrations of sodium, chloride, and magnesium are greater in CSF than in plasma, whereas values for glucose, potassium, and enzymes such as creatine kinase (CK) and aspartate aminotransferase (AST) in CSF are lower than those in plasma.[2,3] These chemical differences result from the active transport mechanisms involved in the formation and absorption of CSF and from the blood-brain and blood-CSF barriers. For correct interpretation, chemical analytes in CSF should be measured concurrently with those in serum. Reference ranges are listed in Table 11-3, but ranges should be generated for each laboratory because methodologies vary.[2,9,11,12]

Glucose, CK, and AST are the most frequently measured values. *Glucose* concentration in CSF varies directly with the plasma concentration but is 30% to 60% lower than plasma.[8,9] Therefore, hyperglycemia and hypoglycemia will raise and lower the CSF glucose concentration accordingly. A reduction in CSF glucose is also observed in horses with marked neutrophilic pleocytosis that is septic or nonseptic. Consumption of glucose by leukocytes and bacteria is a likely mechanism. The value of CSF glucose measurements in the diagnosis of CNS sepsis is usually not worth the expense, since cytologic assessment and bacterial culture are

TABLE 11-3

Reference Values for CSF Chemistry Assays in Horses[2,3]

Assay	Reference
Sodium (mEq/L)	140–150
Potassium (mEq/L)	2.5–3.5
Chloride (mEq/L)	95–123
Calcium (mg/dl)	2.5–6.0
Glucose (mg/dl)	30–70*
Albumin (mg/dl)	34–64
IgG (mg/dl)	3.0–22
CK (IU/L)	0–8*
AST (IU/L)	7–24*

IgG, Immunoglobulin G; *CK*, creatine kinase; *AST*, aspartate aminotransferase.

*For interpretation, CSF value must be compared with concurrent plasma or serum value.

more specific. Enzymes do not permeate the blood-brain or blood-CSF barriers in the normal horse.

CSF activities of CK and AST are very low in normal horses and are the result of gradual release from neural tissue. Increases in these enzymes result from diffusion across an abnormal blood-CSF barriers, necrosis or degeneration of neural tissue, acute inflammation, hemorrhage, and blood or tissue contamination during collection.[1,2,8,12] For interpretation of enzyme results, comparison of CSF and concurrent serum values is necessary, as well as cell counts, protein concentration, and cytologic examination. Increases in CK activity are believed to indicate myelin degeneration, but normal values do not rule out the presence of CNS disease.[8,12] In horses with clinical signs of CNS disease, an increase in CSF CK activity is frequently associated with protozoal myelitis.[24] Other causes may include trauma, idiopathic epilepsy, botulism, articular facet fractures, intervertebral disk protrusion, and toxemia. Severity and extent of disease do not always correlate with enzyme results, but when increases are observed, the prognosis is poor.

REFERENCES

1. De Lahunta: *Veterinary Neuroanatomy and Clinical Neurology*. 2nd ed. Philadelphia, 1983, Saunders, pp 30-52.
2. Bailey and Vernue, in Kaneko: *Clinical Biochemistry of Domestic Animals*. 5th ed. New York, 1989, Academic Press, pp 786-827.
3. Green and Constantinescu: Equine cerebrospinal fluid: analysis. *Compend Contin Educ Pract Vet* 15:288-302, 1993.
4. Mayhew: *Large Animal Neurology: a Handbook for Veterinary Clinicians*. Philadelphia, 1989, Lea & Febiger, pp 49-55.
5. Hayes: Examination of cerebrospinal fluid in the horse. *Vet Clin North Am (Equine Pract)* 3(2):283-291, 1987.
6. Adams and Mayhew: Neurologic diseases. *Vet Clin North Am (Equine Pract)* 1(1):209-234, 1985.
7. Sweeney and Russell: Differences in total protein concentration, nucleated cell count, and red blood cell count among sequential samples of cerebrospinal fluid from horses. *JAVMA* 217:54-57, 2000.
8. Duncan et al, in Oliver, Hoerlein, and Mayhew: *Veterinary Neurology*. Philadelphia, 1987, Saunders, pp 57-64.
9. Mayhew et al: Equine cerebrospinal fluid: reference values of normal horses. *Am J Vet Res* 38:1271-1274, 1977.
10. Bienzle et al: Analysis of cerebrospinal fluid from dogs and cats after 24 and 48 hours of storage. *JAVMA* 216:1761-1764, 2000.
11. Rossdale et al: Biochemical constituents of cerebrospinal fluid in premature and full term foals. *Equine Vet J* 14:134-138, 1982.
12. Smith et al: Central nervous system disease in adult horses. Part I. A data base. *Compend Contin Educ Pract Vet* 9(5):561-569, 1987.
13. Beech: Cytology of equine cerebrospinal fluid. *Vet Pathol* 20:553-562, 1983.
14. Bentz et al: Diagnosing equine protozoal myeloencephalitis: complicating factors. *Compend Contin Educ Pract Vet* 21(10):975-981, 1999.
15. Bernard: Equine protozoal myelitis: laboratory tests and interpretation. *Proc Int Equine Neurol Conf*, 1997, pp 7-10.
16. Jamison and Lumsden: Cerebrospinal fluid analysis in the dog: methodology and interpretation. *Semin Vet Med Surg Small Anim* 3(2):122-132, 1988.
17. Freeman et al: Membrane filtration preparations of cerebrospinal fluid from normal horses and horses with selected neurologic diseases. *Compend Contin Educ Pract Vet* 11(9):1100-1109, 1989.
18. Smith et al: Central nervous system disease in adult horses. Part III. Differential diagnosis and comparison of common disorders. *Compend Contin Educ Pract Vet* 9(10):1042-1053, 1987.
19. Smith et al: Central nervous system disease in adult horses. Part II. Differential diagnosis. *Compend Contin Educ Pract Vet* 9(7):772-780, 1987.
20. Miller and Collatos: Equine degenerative myeloencephalopathy. *Vet Clin North Am (Equine Pract)* 13(1):43-52, 1997.
21. MacKay: Equine protozoal myeloencephalitis. *Vet Clin North Am (Equine Pract)* 13(1):79-96, 1997.
22. Wilson: Equine herpesvirus-1 myeloencephalopathy. *Vet Clin North Am (Equine Pract)* 13(1):53-72, 1997.
23. Yvorchuk-St. Jean: Neuritis of the cauda equina. *Compend Contin Educ Pract Vet* 3(2):421-428, 1987.
24. Furr and Tyler: Cerebrospinal fluid creatine kinase activity in horses with central nervous system disease: 69 cases (1984-1989). *JAVMA* 197:245-248, 1990.

CHAPTER 12

Endometrium

William B. Ley, Wynne A. Digrassie, G. Reed Holyoak, and Steven H. Slusher

Evaluation of a mare's reproductive health is based on the mare's breeding history, reproductive status, and physical examination findings, creating a more complete database from which to make decisions and prognoses. The diagnosis of endometritis should take a progressively invasive approach.

The examination begins with an external appraisal of the mare's tail, external genital conformation, perineum, inside of both hocks, and vulva for evidence of discharge, whether purulent or hemorrhagic. Then the internal reproductive tract is thoroughly examined using rectal palpation and ultrasonography. Rectal palpation is helpful in determining uterine size, symmetry, and tone. Large accumulations of intrauterine fluid can be identified, although small amounts may not be detectable. Signs consistent with pregnancy should be noted. Manual palpation is followed by transrectal ultrasonography of the internal reproductive structures, which is more precise in (1) detecting pregnancy; (2) evaluating uterine and cervical echogenicity, size, and content; (3) determining viability of the fetus, when present; and (4) evaluating for small accumulations of intrauterine fluid. Ensuring that the mare is not pregnant is a critical diagnostic step before performing more invasive procedures for the diagnosis and evaluation of endometritis or endometriosis. Detection of intrauterine fluid accumulation using transrectal ultrasonography is clinically useful because of the positive correlation with the detection of uterine luminal fluid, recovery of inflammatory cells on endometrial cytology, and isolation of pathogenic bacteria from endometrial culture samples.[1,2]

Biopsy and "guarded" (protected) swab samples from the endometrium are then obtained for cytology, aerobic or microaerophilic culture, and histopathology. Whether the practitioner elects to obtain samples for one, two, or all of these tests will depend on the mare's age, breeding history, and current problem.

Sample Collection

Endometrial cytology was reported to be a clinically useful procedure in the veterinary literature as early as 1961.[3] Since then, many other clinical and controlled investigations have reported on cytology's usefulness, interpretation, and validity as a diagnostic procedure for broodmares.[4-24]

The methods for collection of the sample for endometrial cytologic examination range from dry or moistened sterile or nonsterile cotton or calcium alginate swabs, to loop or scraping devices, to low-volume fluid washing or flushing of the uterine lumen. Calcium alginate swabs are preferred over cotton swabs to avoid cotton fiber shedding on the slide.[11] The methodology employed makes little clinical difference as long as (1) the procedure does not harm the endometrium or introduce pathogens to the uterine environment, and (2) the sample collected contains sufficient numbers of endometrial and other cells to enable a reliable cytologic examination. For the practitioner the chosen procedure should be relatively quick and easily performed with common supplies available in the clinic or carried to the farm.

The mare should be prepared with a tail wrap and a perineal scrub using water, cotton, and a mild nondisinfecting soap, then thoroughly rinsed again with clean water and dried with clean paper towels. The practitioner should wear a sterile, shoulder-length, plastic obstetric sleeve, and a sterile, nonbacteriostatic obstetric lubricant should be placed on the back of the gloved hand. The sterile collection device should be guarded by the gloved hand and guided through the vulva, into the vagina, avoiding the urethral opening ventrally, and advanced cranially until the cervix is identified. With the finger(s) the external cervical os should be gently invaded and the full length of one or two fingers inserted through the length of the cervix, stopping at the body of the uterus. The collection device is then carefully guided between the fingers and placed into the uterus.

This basic procedure is used whether a guarded sterile cotton or calcium alginate swab is used to collect samples or whether an artificial insemination or sterile flushing catheter is used for saline wash or lavage to collect the sample. Before the guarded swab is introduced, a thorough vaginal and cervical examination can be performed digitally, thus conserving time and minimizing the number of times the mare's tract is invaded.

It is possible to recover samples simultaneously for both endometrial culture and cytology using the same sterile, guarded, uterine culture device (Accu-Culshure) without risking contamination of the sample for culture, provided a sterile glass slide is used. Other guarded and nonguarded endometrial culture devices with various designs are available. The key point is to guard the swab with the hand or through the design of the collecting instrument to avoid contamination of the cytologic specimen recovered from vulval, vaginal, and cervical cells. Guarded swab devices can also be used with vaginoscopy as an alternative to the sterile sleeved or manual approach.

An alternate method for collection of endometrial cells is a low-volume fluid wash or lavage. After insertion of the sterile insemination pipette into the uterine body, 50 ml of sterile 0.9% sodium chloride solution is rapidly flushed into the uterus using a 60-ml syringe attached to the distal end of the pipette. The practitioner's index finger remains inserted through the cervix to guide and manipulate the tip of the pipette as the fluid is immediately withdrawn by negative pressure applied with the attached syringe. Some side-to-side and dorsal-to-ventral movement is required to find the pockets of fluid for aspiration. In most cases, 1 to 5 ml can be recovered. After recovery the pipette tip is guarded again on exit from the mare, and the total aspirate from the syringe and pipette lumen is placed into a clean or sterile tube or other container for processing.

The washing or flushing method of sample recovery for endometrial cytology may provide a more representative sample of the cells contained within the lumen of the uterus compared with the swab technique.[20] Although this concern may be justifiable in some mares, the guarded swab technique is used more for practical reasons (eg, simultaneous samples for cytology and culture). An endometrial biopsy sample for histopathology can then be collected after the samples for culture and cytology have been obtained, to avoid contaminating them with blood.

Sample Processing

Precleaned, sterile microscope slides are prepared and sterilized inside plastic or cardboard mailing packets. An additional outer envelope sealed before sterilization helps to ensure long-term sterility during transport and storage. If the sample was obtained from a guarded swab with a cotton or calcium alginate tip, the protective sheath is removed, and the tip of the device is gently rolled across the length of the slide in several motions to displace recovered cells onto the sterile slide surface. It is good practice to make two slides for every cytologic examination to allow the practitioner to stain one for immediate evaluation. The second slide serves as a backup slide in case the other is broken or damaged in transport and as an alternate slide to stain using another method. The tip of the same device is then placed into a sterile microbiologic transport medium for preservation of bacterial pathogens that may have been recovered.

When the Accu-Culshure device is used, the tip of the collecting sheath is wiped with an alcohol-moistened gauze or a clean paper towel, and the material from the tip of the device is pushed onto the sterile slide. Another clean slide is used to drag or smear the collected material across a portion of the surface of the receiving slide. The sample for bacterial culture recovered by Accu-Culshure is separated from the area where the sample for cytologic sample is recovered. The portion for microbial culture is then appropriately processed according to the instructions with the device. The slides prepared in this manner are then placed back into their slide mailer boxes for transport to the practitioner's office or mailing to a laboratory. The slides can be allowed to air-dry, or they can be immediately stained using Diff-Quik on the farm or in the clinic's facility.

Samples that are obtained using a saline wash, flush, or lavage technique require more processing than the samples obtained using the guarded swab techniques. The collected fluid sample can be placed into a sterile or clean test tube or placed into a test tube containing 5 ml of 40% ethanol preservative. The fluid samples must be centrifuged and the cytologic smear prepared from the sedimental cells in the bottom of the tubes after centrifugation.

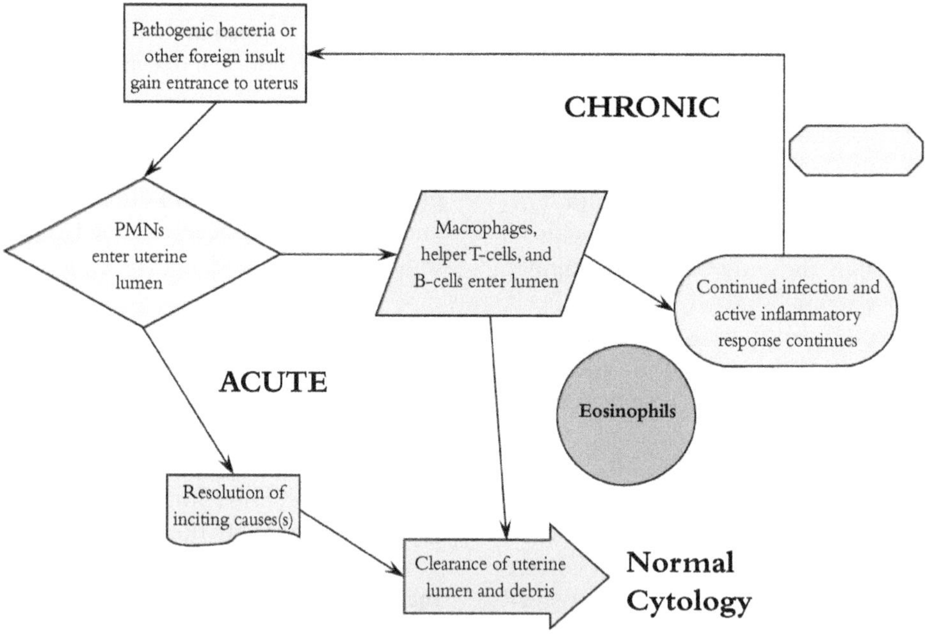

Fig. 12-1 Inflammatory cellular cascade in equine endometrium. *PMNs,* Polymorphonuclear leukocytes.

Staining Methods

Air-dried or ethanol-fixed slides can be stained immediately with modified Wright's or Diff-Quik stain. Air-drying has some trade-offs compared with wet fixation of cytologic specimens. Air-drying preserves cellular material (less loss) but sacrifices cellular detail. Samples that are heavily contaminated by mucus when air-dried will have dark staining of this mucoproteinaceous material that may mask the observation of cellular content on the slide. Wet fixation tends to float some mucoproteins off the slide, preserving cellular detail. When guarded swab recoveries of samples for endometrial cytology have a moderate to heavy mucus contamination, the smeared slides should be immediately stained with Diff-Quik rather than allowing them to air-dry. Alternatively, the mucus-contaminated swab can be placed into a saline or 40% ethanol solution and centrifuged to recover the cellular content of the sample. Diff-Quik provides adequate staining and cellular detail for most routine endometrial cytologic examinations. Alternative stains include rapid Papanicolaou trichrome stain[22] for wet-fixed samples and Gram's-iodine, Wright's, or Wright's-Giemsa stain for air-dried samples.

Evaluation and Interpretation

The primary clinical use of the endometrial cytology examination is to determine the presence or absence of cells indicative of an active inflammatory response in the uterus (Fig. 12-1).[23,25] The cytologic examination should verify or support the need to obtain further tests, such as endometrial culture. Therefore the cytologic examination is time sensitive and should be performed on the farm or the same day as collection in the practitioner's clinic (or other convenient location with bright-field microscopy) to determine the need for submission of the endometrial culture. When performed immediately or soon after recovery, the examination further provides the practitioner with information regarding the mare's response to intrauterine or systemic therapy. The practitioner can then determine the need for further treatment or diagnostic tests while the mare is still under examination. The practitioner should question the clinical significance of the mere isolation of bacteria from a uterine culture that is not supported by the presence of inflammatory cells on the same sample submitted for cytology.[25]

The horse-breeding industry is increasingly using a negative (noninflammatory) endometrial cytology instead of a negative (no significant pathogen isolated) endometrial culture before accepting a mare for natural service or insemination. Too many mares have received unwarranted intrauterine antimicrobial therapy based on a positive endometrial culture without support of inflammatory endometrial cytology, indicative histopathology, evidence of intrauterine fluid accumulation by ultrasonography, or evidence of purulent

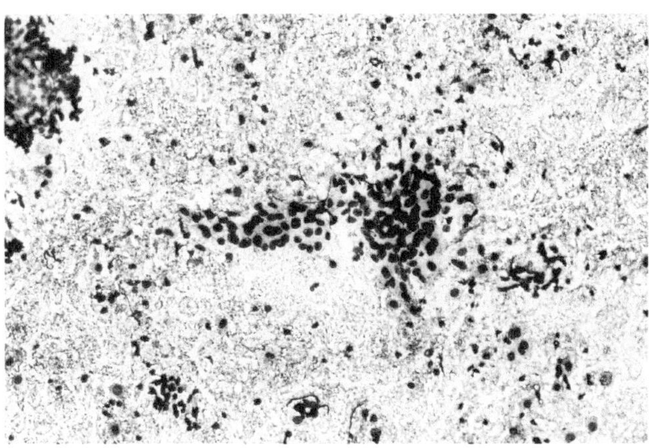

Fig. 12-2 Endometrial cytology from normal mare. (Original magnification X100; Diff-Quik stain)

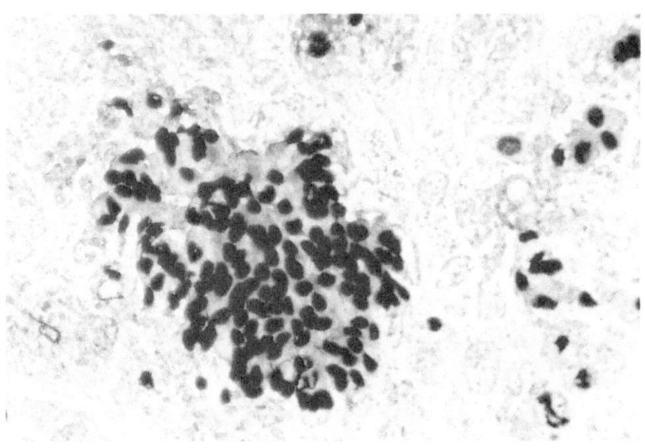

Fig. 12-3 Endometrial cytology from normal mare. (Original magnification X400; Diff-Quik stain)

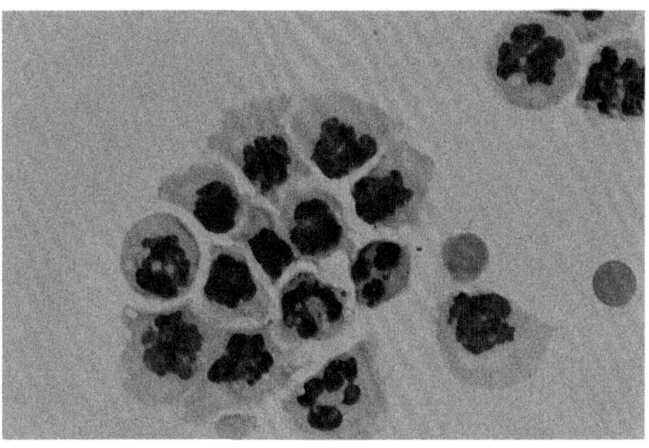

Fig. 12-4 Polymorphonuclear leukocytes on endometrial cytology from a mare infected with *Streptococcus zooepidemicus.* (Original magnification X1000; Diff-Quik stain)

Fig. 12-5 Degenerating polymorphonuclear leukocytes in a mare with chronic active endometritis showing nuclear hypersegmentation and pyknosis. (Original magnification X400; Diff-Quik stain)

vaginal discharge. Correlation between inflammatory endometrial cytology pattern and recovery of pathogenic bacteria from endometrial culture samples has ranged from 76% to 88%.[10,13,14,23] Comparison of acute inflammatory changes between endometrial histopathology and cytology has yielded positive correlations of 70% to 75%.[10,26]

Evaluation of slides should be initiated using low magnification (10X objective) under bright-field microscopy (Fig. 12-2). The slide should be scanned for an initial determination of cell number and pattern. Questions include the following:

- Are sufficient numbers of cells recovered to enable a reasonable interpretation?
- Are the cells evenly dispersed or in clumps or aggregates?
- Are the cells preserved and stained adequately to enable their appropriate identification?
- Is there extraneous material present that might interfere with the identification of cell type (eg, mucoproteinaceous exudate)?
- Are there foreign materials present (eg, cotton fibers, hair, fecal or plant debris, urine crystals, dust)?

After the practitioner has confirmed that the quality of the slide preparation is adequate for the intended purpose, the magnification should be increased to the 40X objective (X400) and the examination continued (Fig. 12-3). Endometrial epithelial cells are typically columnar with or without cilia. They can be observed as individual cells or as part of groups, sheets, or clumps of cells. Some contain mucous globules within the cytoplasm. The nuclei are basal with a dark or stippled chromatin pattern; a singular round nucleolus may be visible in some. Atypical findings in epithelial cells may include increased cytoplasmic

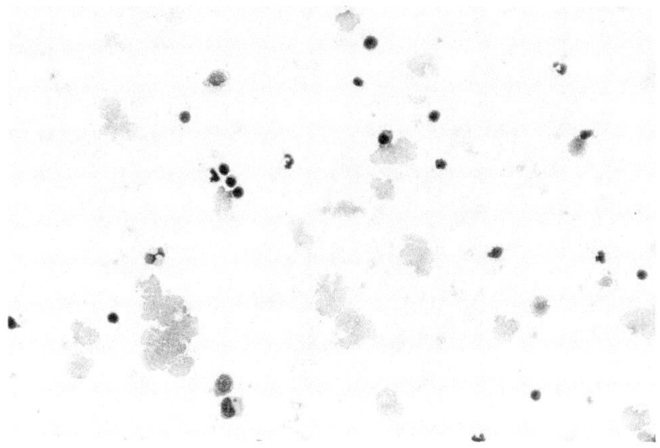

Fig. 12-6 Small mononuclear leukocytes on endometrial cytology. (Original magnification X400; Diff-Quik stain)

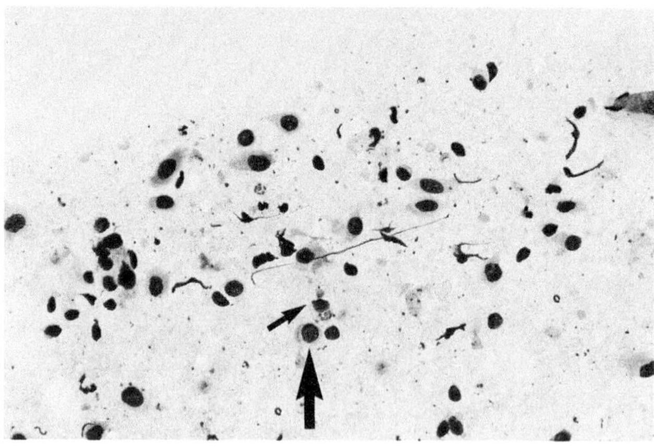

Fig. 12-7 Plasmacyte (*arrow*) on endometrial cytology. (Original magnification X400; Diff-Quik stain)

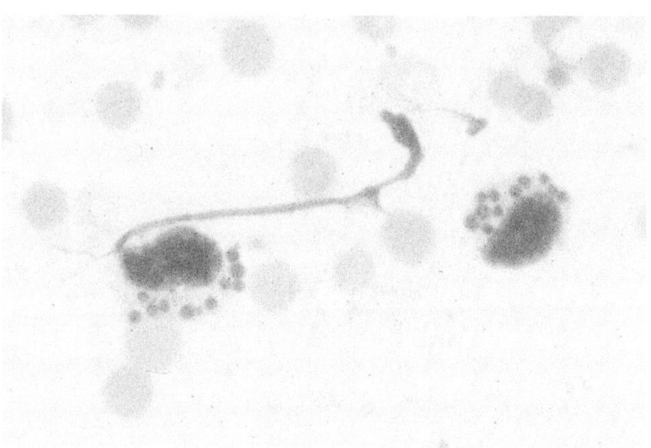

Fig. 12-8 Eosinophils on equine endometrial cytology. (Original magnification X1000; Diff-Quik stain)

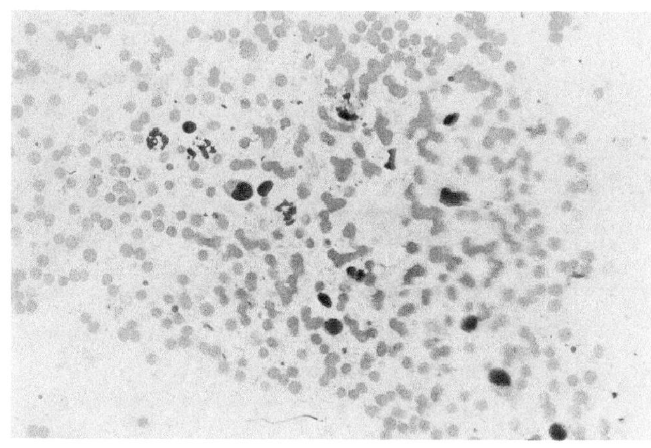

Fig. 12-9 Erythrocytes on endometrial cytology. (Original magnification X400; Diff-Quik stain)

granularity, vacuolization, pyknosis or degeneration of the nucleus, and "giant" cell formation.

The type, number, and cellular quality of inflammatory cells should be noted. *Neutrophils* (*polymorphonuclear leukocytes*, PMNs) may be few in number and well preserved in cellular architecture, or many PMNs may be seen throughout various fields, varying from well preserved to degenerative (Fig. 12-4). PMN nuclear hypersegmentation is a frequent observation in mares that have had an active inflammatory response for more than several days (Fig. 12-5). In acute inflammatory reactions the PMNs are numerous but have relatively nondegenerate nuclei.

Lymphocytes appear as small, relatively dark cells with scant cytoplasm (Fig. 12-6). *Plasma cells* (plasmacytes) are recognized by their eccentric round nuclei, which have a "clock-face" chromatin pattern, and a slightly more abundant and darker blue cytoplasm compared with lymphocytes (Fig. 12-7). Equine *eosinophils* in endometrial cytology are typically larger than PMNs and have faintly pink-staining, large, round intracytoplasmic granules and a lobulated nucleus (Fig. 12-8).

Macrophages may be observed, especially in the resolution phase of endometritis or during spring or fall transition and winter anestrus. Macrophages are typically large, with a foamy, pale-gray to light-blue cytoplasm, and may have vacuoles in the cytoplasm. Some may have bacteria or yeast in the phagosomes. *Red blood cells* (RBCs, erythrocytes) may be observed in postpartum mares, in mares that have recently received an endometrial biopsy, and in some mares with active inflammation or other intrauterine trauma. RBCs are faint staining, light gray to pink, and may appear as "ghost" cells dispersed among the other cells on the microscope slide (Fig. 12-9).

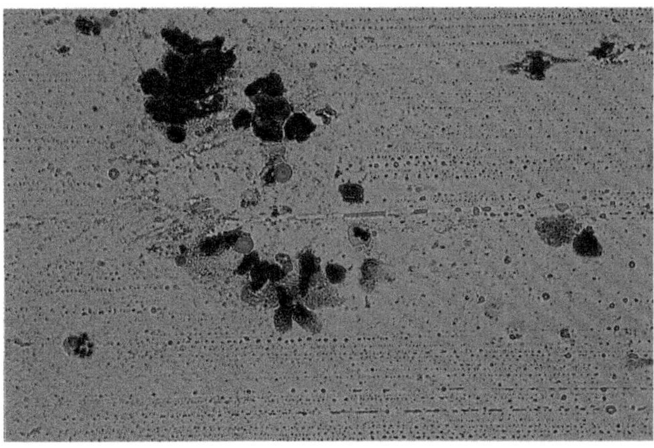

Fig. 12-10 Vaginal squamous epithelial cells on endometrial cytology. (Original magnification X400; Diff-Quik stain)

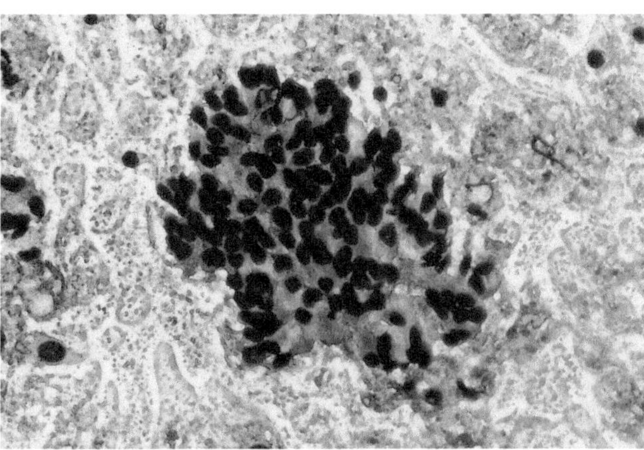

Fig. 12-11 Cervical epithelial cells on endometrial cytology. (Original magnification X400; Diff-Quik stain)

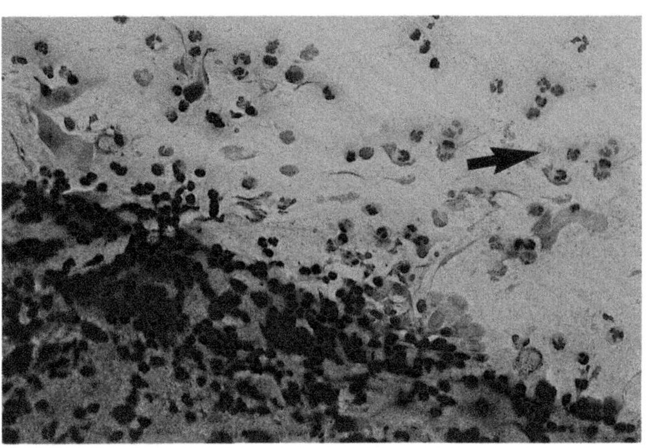

Fig. 12-12 Pyometra on endometrial cytology. (Original magnification X400; Gram's stain)

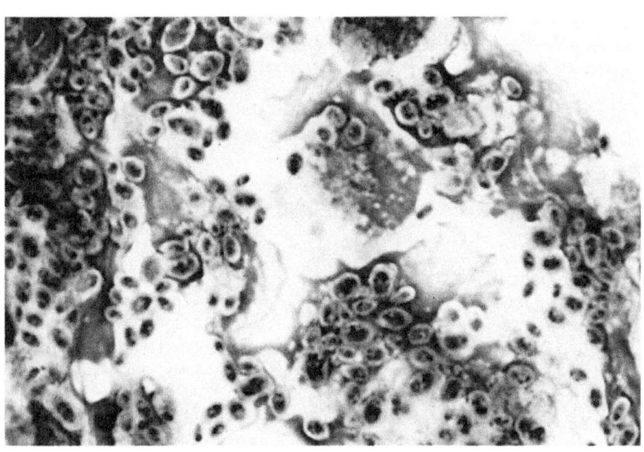

Fig. 12-13 Vegetative yeast forms on endometrial cytology. (Original magnification X1000; Diff-Quik stain)

Vaginal epithelial cells appear as squamous type without nuclei and indicate that the sample was contaminated or collected improperly, since the target area is the uterus, not vagina (Fig. 12-10). *Cervical epithelial cells* are squamous to cuboidal to columnar epithelial type, are smaller and darker staining than endometrial cells, and typically are found in sheets and clumps rather than individually (Fig. 12-11). *Siderophages* are hemosiderin-laden macrophages and are typically encountered during postpartum uterine involution for various periods, up to 30 to 45 days.

Mucus strands may be apparent, interspersed between cells or clumps of cells, and should be more prominent in samples collected during estrus. In normal mares the mucous pattern should be relatively thin and light staining. In abnormal mares, mucus often tends to become thick, heavy, granular, dark staining, and infiltrated with debris or clumps of degenerated cellular material. *Urine crystals* may be encountered and indicate urine pooling in the uterus, cervix, or vagina.

The presence of more than one or two PMNs per five microscopic fields (×400 magnification) indicates an active inflammatory response.[4,9,11,18,24] Because the cellularity of each endometrial smear can vary according to the stage of cycle, collection method, and cytologic smear preparation, the number of PMNs per high-power field is less consistent and reliable than a differential count of 100 or more cells on the microscope slide examined. An endometrial/PMN cell ratio of less than 40:1 or a finding of more than 2% PMNs on the differential cytology count indicates an active inflammatory response[9,18] (Fig. 12-12). The absence of inflammatory cells on the cytologic examination is considered normal. A predominance of eosinophils,

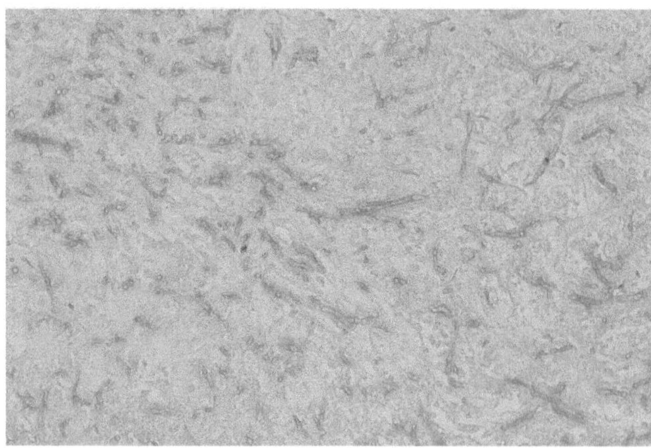

Fig. 12-14 Fungal elements on endometrial histopathology. (Original magnification X400; hematoxylin-eosin stain, green filter)

lymphocytes, and macrophages indicates either a resolving or a chronic endometrial inflammatory response.[18] Pneumovagina has been shown to contribute to a predominance of eosinophils in endometrial cytologic smears.[12]

The diagnosis of *fungal endometritis* may be confirmed by endometrial cytology.[27-29] An inflammatory cell pattern is most often observed, with hyphae or vegetative yeast forms. Yeast are frequently detected using Diff-Quik stain, but the presence of fungal hyphae may be overlooked or undetected (Fig. 12-13). Isolation and identification of the yeast or fungal elements should be used to support the cytologic findings. In some situations it may be necessary to obtain an endometrial biopsy and also stain fixed samples with Gomori's–methenamine silver or periodic acid–Schiff to demonstrate deeper-seated fungal infections[29] (Fig. 12-14).

Summary

Endometrial cytology is most useful to screen for an active inflammatory response in the mare's uterus.[9,18] It is not useful as a guide for indicating chronic infiltrative endometrial inflammation[23,25] or in determining the prognosis for the individual mare to support a pregnancy to full-term gestation.[10] Endometrial biopsy and histopathology to evaluate endometrial glandular architecture and degree of periglandular fibrosis remain the most clinically useful diagnostic tools for these purposes.

REFERENCES

1. McKinnon et al: Diagnostic ultrasonography of the mare's reproductive tract. *J Equine Vet Sci* 8:329-333, 1988.
2. McKinnon et al: Ultrasonographic studies on the reproductive tract of mares after parturition: effect of involution and uterine fluid on pregnancy rates in mares with normal and delayed first postpartum ovulatory cycles. *JAVMA* 192:350-353, 1988.
3. Knudsen and Sollen: Methods for taking samples from the uterus of mares and cows. *Nordisk Vet Med* 13:449-456, 1961.
4. Knudsen: Endometrial cytology as a diagnostic aid in mares. *Cornell Vet* 54:414-422, 1964.
5. Solomon et al: A study of chronic infertility in the mare utilizing uterine biopsy, cytology, and cultural methods. *Proc Am Assoc Equine Pract* 18:55-68, 1972.
6. Gadd: The relationship of bacterial cultures, microscopic smear examination and medical treatment to surgical correction of barren mares. *Proc Am Assoc (Equine Pract)* 21:362-367, 1975.
7. Wingfield and Digby: The technique and clinical application of endometrial cytology in mares. *Equine Vet J* 10:167-170, 1978.
8. Gadd and Bland: The cytology in the cervico-vaginal junction in the broodmare. *Proc Soc Theriogenol* pp 49-54, 1980.
9. Ley: *Endometrial cytology in the mare.* MS thesis, Large Animal Medicine & Surgery, Texas A&M University, College Station, 1981.
10. Wingfield, Digby, and Ricketts: Results of concurrent bacteriological and cytological examinations of the endometrium of mares in routine stud farm practice, 1978-1981. *J Reprod Fertil Suppl* 32:181-185, 1982.
11. Cuoto and Hughes: Technique and interpretation of cervical and endometrial cytology in the mare. *J Equine Vet Sci* 4:265-273, 1984.
12. Slusher et al: Eosinophils in equine uterine cytology and histology specimens. *JAVMA* 184:665-670, 1984.
13. Brook: Cytological and bacteriological examination of the mare's endometrium. *J Equine Vet Sci* 5:16-22, 1985.
14. La Cour and Sprinkle: Relationship of endometrial cytology and fertility in the broodmare. *Vet Clin North Am (Equine Pract)* 7:27-36, 1985.
15. Crickman and Pugh: Equine endometrial cytology: a review of techniques and interpretations. *Vet Med* 81:650-656, 1986.
16. Freeman et al: Equine endometrial cytologic smear patterns. *Comp Contin Educ Pract Vet* 8:S349-S360, 1986.
17. Ley: Additional tips for endometrial cytology. *Vet Med* 86:894, 1986.
18. Bowen et al: Dynamic changes which accompany acute and chronic uterine infections in the mare. *J Reprod Fertil Suppl* 35:675-677, 1987.
19. Saltiel et al: Cervico-endometrial cytology and physiological aspects of the post-partum mare. *J Reprod Fertil Suppl* 35:305-309, 1987.
20. Ball et al: Use of a low-volume uterine flush for microbiologic and cytologic examination of the mare's endometrium. *Theriogenology* 29:1269-1273, 1988.
21. Roszel and Freeman: Equine endometrial cytology. *Vet Clin North Am (Equine Pract)* 4:247-262, 1988.
22. Freeman: A rapid Papanicolaou stain for equine cytologic specimens. *Vet Clin North Am (Equine Pract)* 12:37-41, 1990.
23. Reiswig et al: A comparison of endometrial biopsy, culture and cytology during oestrus and dioestrus in the horse. *Equine Vet J* 25:240-241, 1993.
24. Dascanio et al: How to perform and interpret uterine cytology. *Proc Am Assoc (Equine Pract)* 43:182-186, 1997.
25. Brum-Medici et al: Considerations on the use of ancillary diagnostic aids in the diagnosis of endometritis due to infection in mares. *J Reprod Fertil Suppl* 44:700-703, 1991.
26. Kenney: Cyclic and pathologic changes of the mare endometrium as detected by biopsy, with a note on early embryonic death. *JAVMA* 172:241-262, 1978.
27. Hurtgen and Cummings: Diagnosis and treatment of fungal endometritis in mares. *Proc Soc Theriogenol,* pp 18-22, 1982.
28. Pugh et al: Endometrial candidiasis in five mares. *J Equine Vet Sci* 6:40-43, 1986.
29. Freeman et al: Mycotic infections of the equine uterus. *Vet Clin North Am (Equine Pract)* 8:34-42, 1986.

CHAPTER 13

Semen Quality

William B. Ley, Wynne A. Digrassie, G. Reed Holyoak, and Steven H. Slusher

The Society for Theriogenology has established standards for a stallion's breeding "satisfactoriness" or "soundness" (Fig. 13-1).1 To obtain a satisfactory rating on the examination for breeding soundness, the stallion must (1) be physically capable of mating; (2) possess good libido; (3) have normal external genitalia with scrotal or testicular dimension consistent with good sperm production; (4) test negative for infections and for venereal, bacterial, and viral pathogens; (5) have good semen quality; and (6) have at least 1×10^9 progressively motile, morphologically normal spermatozoa in the second of two ejaculates collected 1 hour apart, preceded by 1 week of sexual rest.[2]

The best semen samples to evaluate for breeding soundness are those that are representative of the stallion's daily sperm output, that is, ejaculates collected after the extragonadal sperm reserve has been depleted.[3] This usually requires 5 to 7 days of daily semen collection. Because this is both time consuming and labor intensive, however, most practitioners instead collect two samples 1 hour apart to evaluate stallion semen quality.

Conventional Methods

Parameters that determine semen quality are similar for the domestic animal species commonly evaluated. Parameters for the horse have been defined, but their individual correlation to fertility are weak to moderate. A "good" spermatozoon must have (1) an intact acrosome, (2) intact plasma membrane, (3) condensed nuclear chromatin, (4) functional mitochondria, and (5) a flagellum allowing the spermatozoon to reach the site of fertilization, undergo capacitation and the acrosomal reaction, penetrate the zona pellucida of the oocyte, and complete the process of fertilization. These parameters define an individual sperm's quality.

Semen quality addresses the parameters of the *population* of spermatozoa present in the ejaculate (or semen sample) as well as the nature of the fluid transport medium (seminal plasma). Minimal parameters of semen quality for the stallion include the (1) gel-free (sperm-rich) volume (milliliters) of the ejaculate, (2) concentration (spermatozoa per milliliter), (3) percentage of progressively motile spermatozoa, and (4) percentage of morphologically normal spermatozoa. Each of these variables can change with the season of the year when the ejaculate was obtained, age of the individual stallion, and frequency of ejaculation for the stallion.

It is critical that semen be collected and handled properly before its laboratory evaluation to prevent artifacts from interfering with interpretation of the sample's quality. Semen collection and sample handling involve the following basic elements:

- The artificial vagina or other collecting device and all surfaces that will come into direct contact with the ejaculate must be warm (37° C) and free from spermicidal agents.
- Collected semen should be transported to the laboratory as quickly as possible, shielding it from direct sunlight, maintaining it at body temperature (37° C), and placing it into a warming bath or incubator at 37° C.

530 Church Street, Suite 700
Nashville, TN 37219
Telephone: 615/244-3060
Facsimile: 615/254-7047

Society for Theriogenology
STALLION BREEDING SOUNDNESS EVALUATION FORM
(Page 1 of 2)

Date: ____________

STALLION INFORMATION

Name: ____________
Age: ______ Breed: ______ Color: ______
Lip Tattoo #: ______ Registration #: ______
Marking/Blends: ____________

Present Breeding Status:
○ Sexually rested ○ Actively breeding ○ At daily sperm output
Intended Use: ____________

OWNER/AGENT

Name: ____________
Address: ____________
Telephone: ______ Fax: ______
Referring Veterinarian: ____________
Telephone: ______ Fax: ______
Veterinary Examiner: ____________
Address: ____________
Telephone: ______ Fax: ______

HISTORY

____

PHYSICAL BREEDING CONDITION

____

EXTERNAL GENITAL EXAMINATION

Method(s) Used:
○ Palpation
○ Ultrasound
○ Other ______

	LEFT	RIGHT
* **Testis:**		
L x W x H (cm):		
Volume (cm³):		
Consistency:		
* **Epididymis:**		
* **Spermatic Cord:**		

* **Prepuce:** ______
* **Penis:** ______
* **Scrotum:** ______
Total Width (cm) ______
* **Other Findings:** ______

INTERNAL GENITAL EXAMINATION

○ Performed
○ Not Performed

Method(s) Used:
○ Palpation
○ Ultrasound
○ Other ______

	LEFT	RIGHT
* **Inguinal Ring(size):**		
* **Vesicular Gland:**		
* **Ampulia:**		
* **Prostatic Lobe:**		

BEHAVIOR AND BREEDING ABILITY

TEMPERAMENT	LIBIDO	ERECTION	MOUNTING	INTROMISSION	EJACULATION

OTHER EXAMINATION FINDINGS

____

ADDITIONAL DIAGNOSTIC TESTS

TEST	DATE PERFORMED	RESULTS

Fig. 13-1 Stallion Breeding Soundness Evaluation Form. (Courtesy Society for Theriogenology.)

Society for Theriogenology

STALLION BREEDING SOUNDNESS EVALUATION FORM

(Page 2 of 2)

Stallion Name: ______________________ Date: ______________

	EJACULATE 1	EJACULATE 2	EJACULATE 3
SEMEN EVALUATION			
Collection Time			
Collection Method			
Number of Mounts/Time to First Mount (min)			
Volume (ml)—gel free/gel			
Gross Appearance			
Seminal Ph/Seminal Osmolarity			
Mobility % (total progressive): ○ raw ○ extended			
Concentration (x 10^9 / ml)—Method use: ________			
Total Number of Sperm (x 10^9)			
SPERM MORPHOLOGY			
○ Buttered Formal Saline ○ Phase Contrast Microscopy ○ Bright Field Microscopy			
○ Stain ________ ○ Other ________			
% Normal Sperm			
% Abnormal Acrosomal Regions/Heads			
% Tailless Heads			
% Proximal Droplets			
% Distal Droplets			
% Abnormally-shaped/Bent Midpieces			
% Bent/Coiled Tails			
Premature (Round) Germ Cells			
Other Cells (WBC, RBC, etc.)			
Total # Sperm x % Morphologically Normal (x 10^9)			
LONGEVITY (VIABILITY) TEST			
Reported as Storage Time (hours)/% Prog. Mobile Sperm			
________ Raw at ____ °C			
________ Extender (10:1) at ____ °C			
________ Extender (10:1) at ____ °C			
________ Extender (25 x 10^9 sperm/ml) at ____ °C			
________ Extender (25 x 10^9 sperm/ml) at ____ °C			
CULTURE AND SENSITIVITY			
Pre-Wash Urethra			
Pre-Wash Penile Shaft			
Pre-Wash Fossa Glandis			
Post-Ejaculate Urethra			
Other ________			
________			
________			

CLASSIFICATION: Based on the intended use of this stallion and interpretation of data resulting from this examination, the above stallion is classified as a/an:

○ Satisfactory Breeding Prospect ○ Questionable Breeding Prospect ○ Unsatisfactory Breeding Prospect

○ See attached letter — Date: ________ Signature: ______________

MEMBER OF SOCIETY FOR THERIOGENOLOGY

Clinic Name: ______________

Fig. 13-1 ***(Continued)***

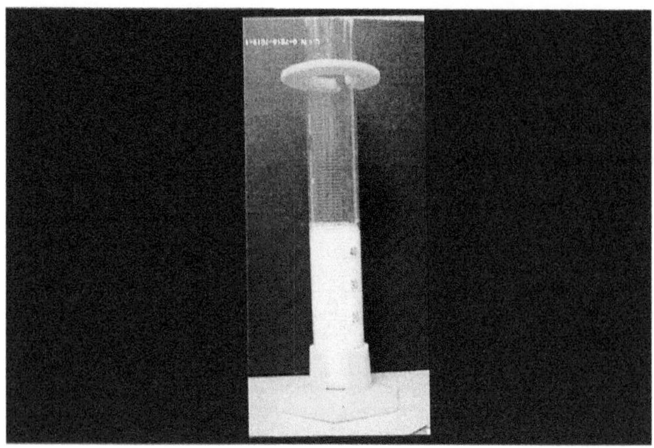

Fig. 13-2 Examination of stallion semen for gel-free volume, color, and opacity.

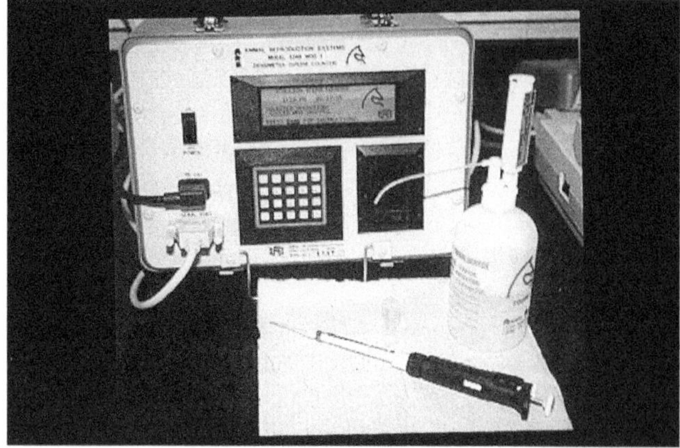

Fig. 13-3 Densimeter for spectrophotometric determination of semen concentration.
(Courtesy Animal Reproduction Systems.)

TABLE 13-1

Range of Normal Values for Stallion Semen Quality

Parameter	Low Normal*	High Normal*
Gel-free volume (ml)	25	150
Gel (ml)	0	100
Progressive motility (%)	30	75
Total motility (%)	40	70
Sperm concentration (million/ml)	30	175
Total sperm per ejaculate (billion)	3.0	12.0
Morphology (% normal)	40	80
Total progressively motile, morphologically normal sperm per ejaculate (billion)	1.0	8.0
pH	7.25	7.65

*Values may vary according to stallion, breed, age, and season of the year at collection.

The *gel fraction* of the ejaculate can be removed either during the semen collection process by appropriate "in-line" filtration (eg, nylon micromesh filter) or after the sample has been collected in the laboratory. The entire ejaculate can be filtered through a sterile, prewarmed funnel that has one or two glass-wool cotton balls placed in the funnel neck to trap the gel from passing through the funnel. Alternatively, the gel in the ejaculate can be aspirated from the ejaculate using a sterile 60-ml syringe. Ejaculate volume (milliliters, gel-free portion) is usually measured in a prewarmed, sterile graduated cylinder (Fig. 13-2). Color and consistency of the ejaculate should be noted to allow estimation of the sperm number and detection of contaminants (eg, urine, blood, purulent exudate). Stallion semen should be an opaque-white color, and any deviation from this may indicate abnormality. Both urine (yellow color) and blood (red color) will damage spermatozoa if left in contact with the ejaculate for longer than 10 to 15 minutes.[4]

The *gel-free portion* of the ejaculate should be split into two parts. One sample is kept as is ("raw," "neat") and should be left in the incubator. The other sample should be mixed with an equal volume of prewarmed semen extender and allowed to equilibrate to room temperature. Milk-based semen extenders for the stallion are available as ready-to-use packages (eg, E-Z Mixin, Animal Reproduction Systems; Kenney Skim Milk Extender, Har-Vet; Skim Milk Extender, Lane). Alternatively, the Modified Kenney Extender can be prepared by mixing 24 g of nonfat dry skim milk solids with 26.5 g of glucose and 40 g of sucrose in sufficient deionized water to obtain 1 L. Antibiotics are optional for use in laboratory settings, but if included, 1 million units of potassium penicillin G and/or 1 g of amikacin sulfate may be added to each liter of skim milk extender.

Concentration and pH

Sperm concentration is measured on the "neat" sample using a Neubauer hemacytometer (American Optical) (Box 13-1), a Makler chamber (Sefi Medical), or most often, photometric methods (Fig. 13-3). A photometric test evaluates optical density of the fluid sample, and therefore raw semen must be used to prevent false readings resulting from particles that may exist in common milk-based extenders.[2,4] Cells other than mature spermatozoa (eg, red cells, neutrophils, round cells) may also falsely elevate the optical density reading. An accurate measurement (number of sperm per milliliter) is essential, since the evaluation of stallion semen quality and breeding soundness is based on *available total sperm numbers* in the ejaculate (gel-free volume × sperm concentration). This value is an estimate of total sperm number per ejaculate and is a crucial parameter in defining stallion semen quality and resultant breeding suitability (Table 13-1). Total sperm count can change depending on the season, frequency of ejaculation, testicular volume, incomplete ejaculation, extragonadal sperm reserves, and intrinsic reproductive tract disease or obstruction.

Seminal pH is measured on the raw sample using a calibrated pH meter within 1 hour of collection. Estimation of this parameter of semen quality using pH paper is not precise. Acidity or alkalinity may alter sperm motility and viability.[2,4] Urine contamination of the ejaculate is usually associated with an abnormally high pH value. Table 13-1 lists normal pH values for stallion semen.

Motility and Morphology

Sperm motility is evaluated using both initial (raw) and diluted (extended) samples.[5] Motility is best analyzed in the laboratory using a drop of raw semen on a prewarmed (37° C) slide under phase-contrast microscopy (×200 to ×400 magnification) with a stage warmer attached to the microscope. Bright-field microscopy is used more often because of the limited number of phase-contrast microscopes owned by practitioners in the field. Visual assessments should include both *total sperm motility*, or percentage of sperm in several microscopic fields exhibiting motility of any form, and *progressive sperm motility*, or percentage of sperm in several microscopic fields moving in a rapid linear fashion. Table 13-1 lists normal ranges.

Estimates of sperm velocity are based on an arbitrary scale of 0 to 4. Many factors can alter the results of motility estimation. As discussed, pH can alter motility, and temperature fluctuations may lead to "cold shock" and lowered motility values. The more concentrated the semen sample, the higher is the subjective assessment of motility. Therefore the recommendation is to evaluate extended semen samples diluted to 25 million sperm/ml to improve accuracy and repeatability of the motility estimate.

Alternate methods of sperm motility evaluation are used. *Computer-assisted sperm analysis* (CASA) yields objective results. Such laboratory-based instruments use computer algorithms based on spermatozoal head movement and dimension.[4,6] Several parameters are analyzed, including total sample motility, individual sperm velocity, flagellar beat frequency, and lateral head displacement.[7] Experiments using CASA have been performed on spermatozoa of humans, bulls, and stallions.[8] In the stallion, CASA was more repeatable than visual methods and videomicrography.[9] Erroneous readings can result because of a high number of intersecting sperm head tracks in concentrated semen samples. CASA motility results have only a weak positive correlation with fertility in stallions.[10] The expense of these instruments limits their use to large reproductive referral centers, infertility clinics, and research institutions.

The gel-free volume of the ejaculate (ml) is multiplied by the concentration (sperm/ml) and the progressive motility (%) in the raw or extended sample to obtain the desired parameter, *total number of progressively motile sperm* in the ejaculate.

Longevity of sperm motility in the semen sample can be evaluated on neat semen equilibrated to room temperature (25° C) for 4 to 12 hours. The longevity estimate may also be performed on extended semen (25 million sperm/ml concentration) at room temperature or equilibrated to refrigeration temperature (5° C) for 12 to 48 hours. An aliquot of either sample should be warmed to 37° C and examined for total and progressive motility at intervals of 1 (room temperature samples) to 8 hours (refrigerated samples). When motility is zero to 10%, the evaluations are complete.

Sperm morphology is typically evaluated with a light (bright-field) microscope at ×1000 magnification (100× objective) on stained microscopic smears of the raw ejaculate. Other methods used for sperm morphology include phase-contrast, differential interference contrast (DIC), and electron microscopy and computed morphometry. Regardless of method used, a *differential count* is made, identifying normal and abnormal sperm types in multiple fields of view and counting a total of 200 cells. The percentage of normal sperm and of each abnormal sperm type is reported. The percentage of morphologically normal spermatozoa is then multiplied by the total number of progressively motile spermatozoa in the ejaculate to provide an estimate of the overall availability of sperm with good characteristics (see Table 13-1). This estimate is the *total number of progressively motile, morphologically normal spermatozoa* that could be used for splitting insemination doses to multiple mares, in cryopreservation, or in determination of breeding "satisfactoriness," as based on the Society for Theriogenology recommendation.

Stains

The most common stain method for stallion semen bright-field microscopic evaluation is *Hancock's stain* (eosin Y–nigrosin stain, live-dead stain) (Fig. 13-4). Alternative stains include eosin B–analine blue (Fig. 13-5), India ink (Fig. 13-6), and Diff-Quik. Special staining for the acrosome can be performed using the

Text continued on p. 197

Box 13-1

Hemacytometer Method for Evaluating Concentration of Stallion Spermatozoa

Sample Dilution

There are three methods of diluting a semen sample before counting on a hemacytometer. The Unopette diluting system contains its own diluent. For the Thoma and "large-volume" methods, a normal saline diluent may be used. For better preservation of the diluted sample, a formaldehyde diluent may be used. It consists of 100 ml of 37% formaldehyde and 9.0 g of sodium chloride (NaCl), adding enough deionized water to result in a volume of 1 L.

Unopette Method

The Unopette system uses a standard disposable blood (RBC) diluting pipette with a predetermined dilution rate of 1:200.

1. The Unopette consists of a reservoir, pipette, and shield.
2. Use the pointed tip of the shield to pierce the thin plastic membrane in the neck of the reservoir, taking care not to spill any diluent.
3. Remove the pipette from the shield and submerge the capillary tube tip into the sample of thoroughly mixed gel-free semen.
4. Allow the semen to fill the capillary tube.
5. Remove the pipette from the sample and use a tissue to wipe the excess semen from the outside of the tube. Do not allow the tissue to contact the open end of the tube as this may cause the sample to "wick" out into the tissue.
6. Squeeze the reservoir and place the capillary end of the pipette into it. Seat the pipette holder in the neck of the reservoir and release the pressure, thereby siphoning the semen into the diluent. Rinse the pipette carefully several times by squeezing the reservoir to force the solution into the overflow chamber but not out of it.
7. Place an index finger over the opening of the pipette and mix solution by gently inverting 10 times.
8. Remove and invert the pipette, replacing it into the reservoir neck. Cap it with the shield.
9. Place the reservoir portion under a stream of hot water for 1 minute to kill the sperm.
10. Discard a few drops before putting the diluted semen on the hemacytometer. The sample is expressed by gently squeezing the reservoir.

Thoma Method

The Thoma RBC pipette, identified with a "101," contains a red mixing bead and gives a 1:100 dilution.

1. Cap the semen container and mix the sample by inverting the container a few times. Remove the cap.
2. Insert the tip of the Thoma pipette into the ejaculate, allowing it to fill to the "1" mark. Be careful not to fill beyond this point, as sperm will adhere to the barrel of the pipette.
3. After wiping the outside of the tip with a tissue, draw the prepared diluent to the "101" mark. Be careful not to fill beyond this point, as it will greatly amplify the error.
4. To mix, gently shake the pipette up and down for 90 seconds. Do not shake the pipette from end to end, as this may force the dilution out of the mixing chamber.
5. Discard a few drops before putting the diluted semen on the hemacytometer. The sample is expelled by gently blowing on the top end of the pipette.

Large-Volume Method

The large-volume method yields a 1:20 dilution and permits measurement of the diluent with larger containers, such as syringes and graduated cylinders. A large-volume pipette (at least 1 ml) is preferred for semen evaluation to facilitate thorough mixing of the diluent and sample.

1. Cap the semen container and mix the gel-free sample by gently inverting the container several times. Remove the cap.
2. Measure 19 ml of the pre-prepared diluent into a test tube.
3. Pipette 1 ml of the semen from its container to the diluent test tube.
4. To ensure that all spermatozoa are rinsed from the pipette, flush the pipette by aspirating and expelling the solution 3 times.
5. Cap the container and mix the solution by gently inverting the container 10 times. Remove the cap.
6. Draw 1 ml of the dilution into a clean pipette. Discard a few drops before putting the diluted sample on the hemacytometer.

Box 13-1 (*Continued*)

Using the Hemacytometer

The sperm count is done on a Bright Line, improved Neubauer hemacytometer. Its shiny counting areas are crossed with microscopic grid lines. It requires use of a hemacytometer cover slip (20 x 26 x 0.4 mm).The cover slip does not rest on the grid area but on the shoulders to either side of the grid. This provides a volume of 0.1 ml for the semen sample in the counting area. The V-shaped indentations on opposing sides of the grid areas are for filling the counting chamber.

The 3 x 3 mm counting grid is divided into 9 primary squares. The 4 corner primary squares are further divided into 16 secondary squares. The center primary square is divided into 25 triple-lined secondary squares. Each of the 25 secondary squares is divided into 20 tertiary squares. It is within this center primary square that all sperm counting is done.

Hemacytometer Preparation

1. Make sure that the grid surface and cover slip are spotlessly clean.
2. Place the cover slip on the shoulders.
3. Touch the tip of the semen dilution pipette to the V-shaped indentation adjacent to the counting grid.
4. Slowly expel the sample and allow it to flow under the cover slip until the counting area is filled. Do not flood the chamber, causing the sample to overflow into the moat.
5. Allow the sample to settle for 3-5 minutes.

Counting

1. Place the hemacytometer on the microscope stage and use the low-power (10X) objective to locate the center primary square of the counting grid.
2. Switch to the high-dry (40X) objective for counting.
3. Count the sperm in 5 secondary squares (triple-lined borders), progressing from corner to diagonal corner of the primary square.
4. Include sperm that touch or cross over the top and left borders of each secondary square, but not those that touch or cross over the bottom and right borders.
5. Record the number of sperm, discard the counted specimen and clean the hemacytometer and cover slip.
6. Repeat the counting procedure 7 more times, for a total of 8 counts. The average of these 8 counts is used in calculating the total number of sperm/ml of semen. Remember to gently mix the diluted solution each time before refilling the counting chamber.

Calculations

1. The concentration of semen is normally expressed as sperm/ml. Sperm concentration is calculated as: sperm/ml = sperm counted x hemacytometer factor x dilution factor.
2. *Hemacytometer Factor*: The 5 secondary squares that were counted represent one fifth of the total area of the 1 x 1 mm center primary counting grid. Assuming that there was an even distribution of sperm across the grid, multiplying the average count by 5 yields the number of sperm contained in the dilution in the 1 x 1 mm space.

   Because the chamber is 0.1 mm deep, multiplying by 10 yields the number of sperm/mm^3/µl.

   To arrive at the number of diluted sperm/cm^3 (1 ml) requires multiplying by 1000 as there are 1000 mm^3/cm^3 (1000 µl/ml).

   To shorten the above calculations, merely multiply the average count (of the 5 secondary squares) by 50,000, which is the *hemacytometer factor*.
3. *Dilution Factor*: This varies with the method used.

   If the Unopette method was used (1:200 dilution), multiply by 200 to arrive at the number of sperm/ml.

   If the Thoma method was used (1:100 dilution), multiply by 100.

   If the large-volume dilution method was used (1:20 dilution), multiply by 20.

Courtesy Oklahoma State University.

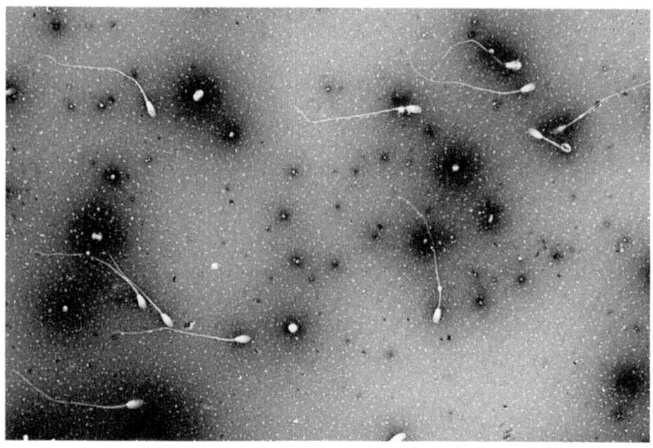

Fig. 13-4 Spermiogram of stallion semen using Hancock's stain.
Most of the cells are white (unstained, or "live"), silhouetted against a purple (nigrosin) background. One cell at upper right is slightly pink staining, indicating it has taken up the eosin fraction of the stain; it would be considered "dead" at staining. (Original magnification X200)

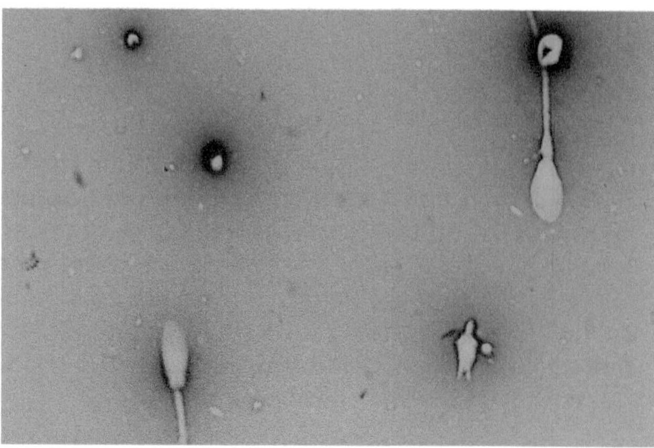

Fig. 13-5 Spermiogram of stallion semen using eosin B–analine blue stain. (Original magnification X1000)

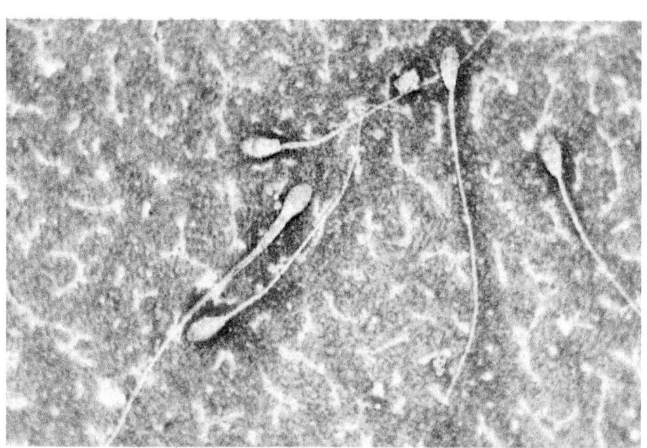

Fig. 13-6 Stallion spermatozoa using India ink preparation.
It is difficult to delineate sufficient cellular architecture to determine normal from abnormal spermatozoa. (Original magnification X1000)

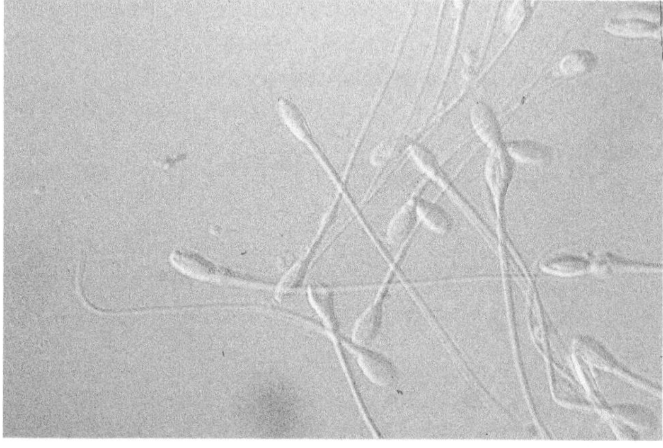

Fig. 13-7 Spermatozoa on differential interference contrast (DIC) microscopy.
The two sperm heads at top have a knobbed acrosomal defect. (Original magnification X1000)

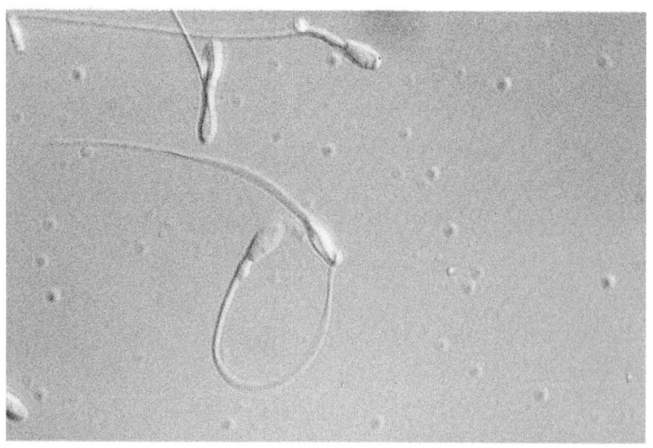

Fig. 13-8 Spermatozoa on DIC microscopy.
The three-dimensional characteristics of each cell are better appreciated. The sperm at upper right has a hairpin bend in the midpiece. The sperm at upper left has a folded acrosomal appearance. Although the cell in the center appears to have a smaller head size, this is an artifact of the wet-mount preparation, viewing the cell on its side rather than on its flat surface, as with the majority of the other cells seen here. The cell to the right of center has a "pseudodroplet," or bunching of the mitochondria in the proximal portion of the midpiece. (Original magnification X1000)

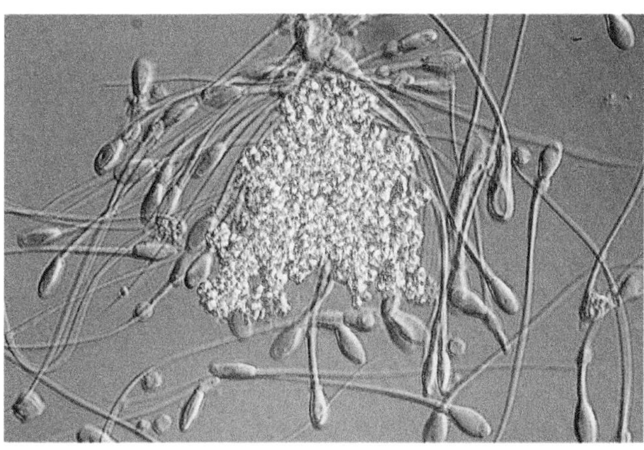

Fig. 13-9 Spermatozoa on DIC microscopy.
Cluster in the center is noncellular material. (Original magnification X1000)

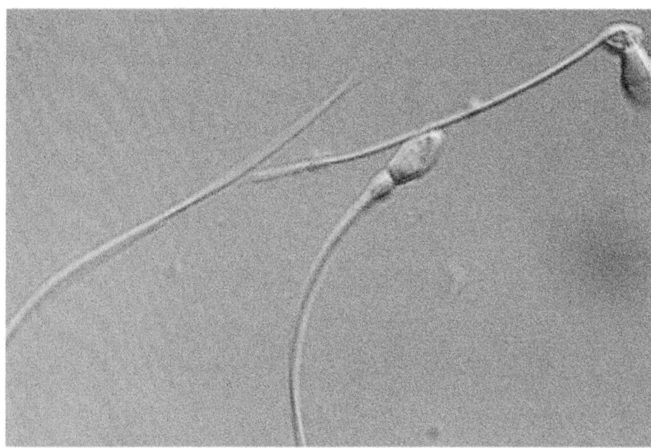

Fig. 13-10 Spermatozoa on DIC microscopy.
This stallion has a predominance of knobbed acrosomal defects and proximal cytoplasmic droplets. (Original magnification X1000)

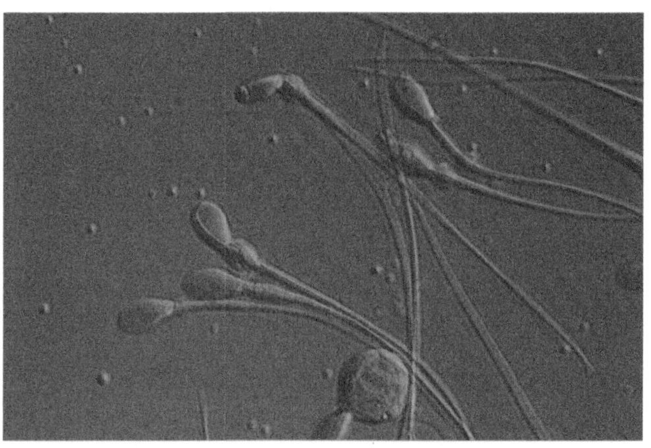

Fig. 13-11 Spermatozoa on DIC microscopy.
Round cell near the bottom is a germinal epithelial cell. (Original magnification X1000; green filter)

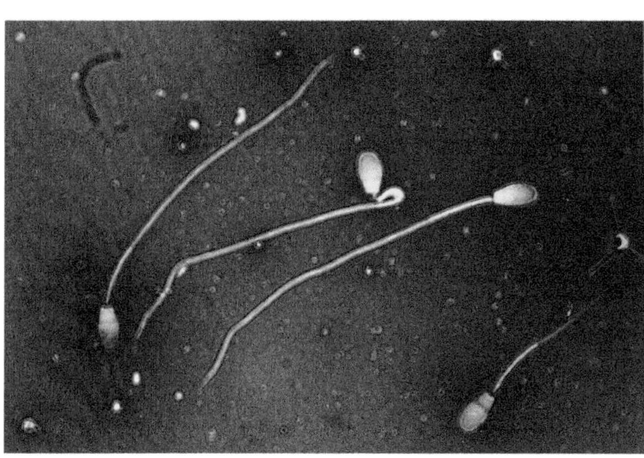

Fig. 13-12 Sperm cell in center has 180-degree bend in midpiece. (Original magnification X1000; Hancock's stain)

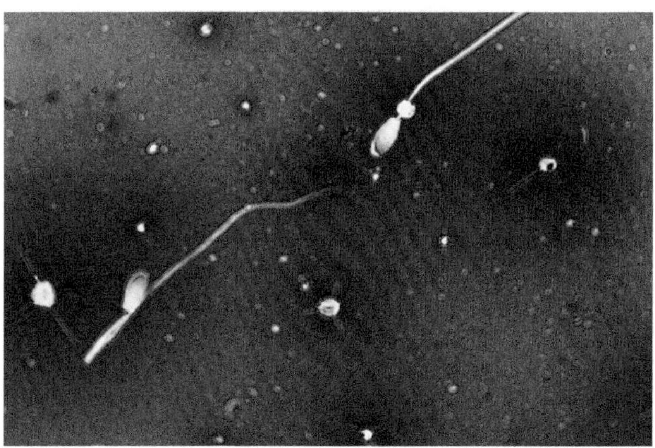

Fig. 13-13 Sperm cell at upper right has proximal cytoplasmic droplet. Cell at lower left has bent or broken midpiece. (Original magnification X1000; Hancock's stain)

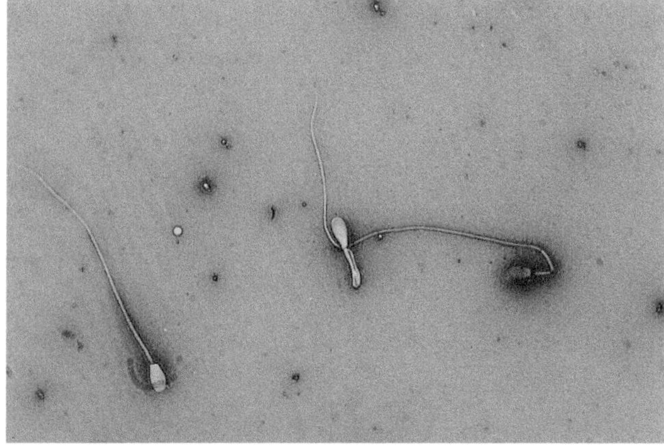

Fig. 13-14 Sperm cell at right has a 90-degree bend or is broken in the midpiece, a minor defect. Cell in the center has a relaxed or double bend in the midpiece, a major defect. (Original magnification X400; Hancock's stain)

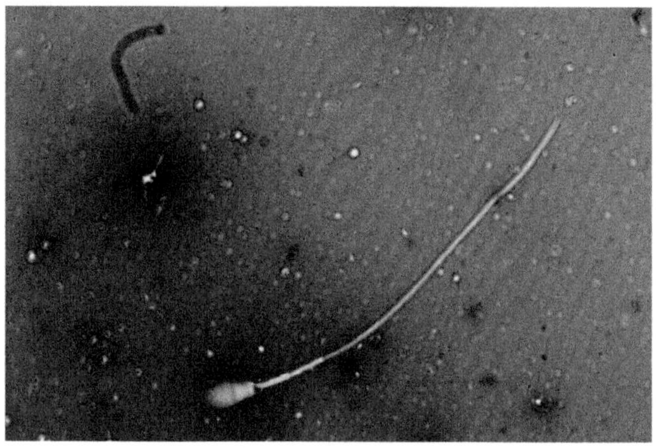

Fig. 13-15 Stallion sperm with abaxial tail attachment to head. (Original magnification X1000; phase contrast, wet mount)

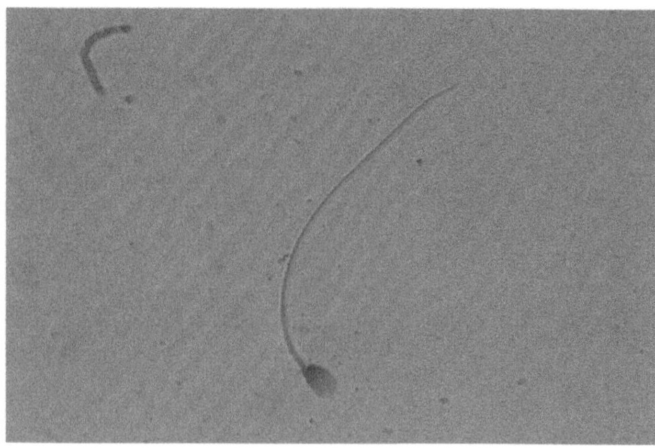

Fig. 13-16 Stallion sperm stained to demonstrate the relatively smaller size of the acrosome on the sperm head. The acrosome is lighter staining, whereas the postacrosomal cap region of the head is darker. (Original magnification X1000; Wells-Awa stain)

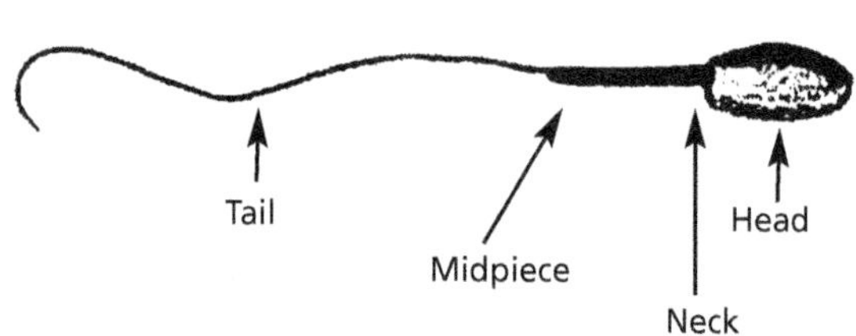

Fig. 13-17 Normal equine spermatozoon. Single sperm,

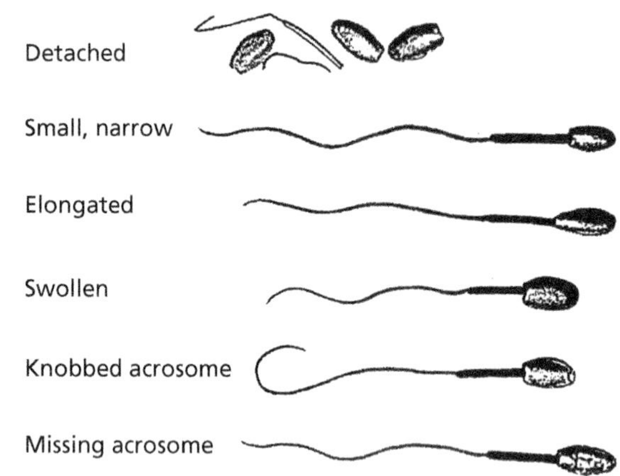

Fig. 13-18 Common abnormalities of equine spermatozoal head.

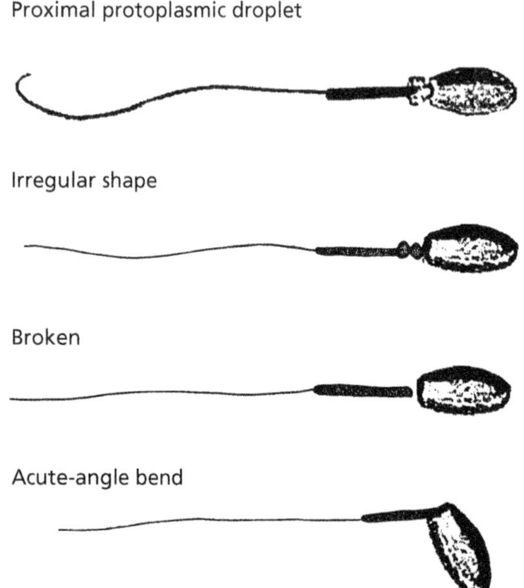

Fig. 13-19 Common abnormalities of equine spermatozoal neck.

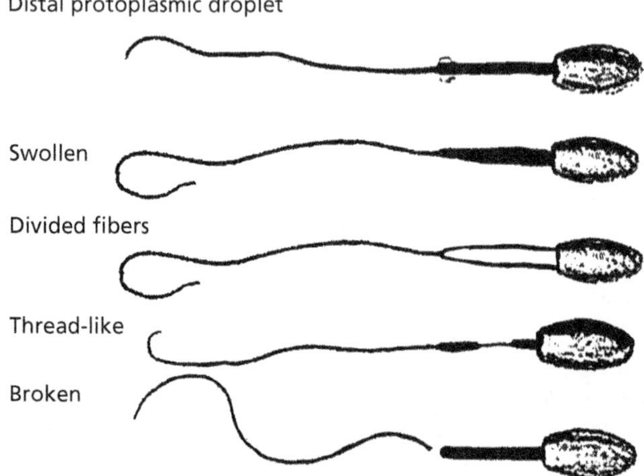

Fig. 13-20 Common abnormalities of equine spermatozoal midpiece.

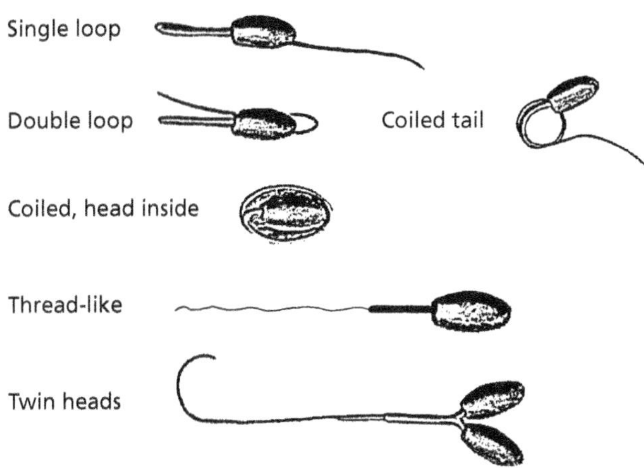

Fig. 13-21 Common abnormalities of equine spermatozoal tail.

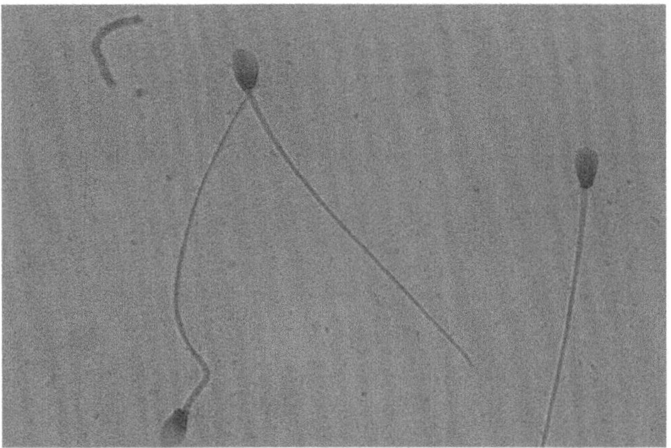

Fig. 13-22 Stallion spermatozoa on Spermac stain demonstrate the lighter-staining acrosome versus the darker-staining postacrosomal cap region of the head. (Original magnification X1000)

Spermac stain. Staining of the nucleus can be performed with the Feulgen stain.[11]

General-purpose cellular stains (eg, Wright's, Giemsa, hematoxylin-eosin) may be used to better delineate germinal and other somatic cells in the semen sample. Sample evaluation using phase-contrast and DIC (Figs. 13-7 to 13-11) microscopy require a wet mount with a buffered formol-saline (0.1%) solution mixed at a 1:1 ratio with raw semen. Some morphology stains have been shown to cause sperm cell abnormalities, especially alterations in head and tail shape.[12]

Morphologic Classification

Sperm morphologic classifications have been established for the stallion.[13,14] Sperm abnormalities may be classified as primary, secondary, and tertiary.[13] *Primary abnormalities* arise within the testicle and involve the sperm head, midpiece (Fig. 13-12), and proximal cytoplasmic droplets[2,4] (Fig. 13-13). *Secondary abnormalities* occur during transport in the excurrent duct system and include detached heads, bent tails (Fig. 13-14), and distal cytoplasmic droplets.[2,4] *Tertiary abnormalities* are induced defects or artifacts caused by improper semen handling after collection.

Some scientists prefer to use a different morphology classification scheme: major versus minor defects.[14] Head and midpiece abnormalities are classified as *major defects* and have been associated with impaired fertility in the bull and stallion. *Minor defects* include bent tails and distal cytoplasmic droplets and probably do not affect fertility significantly.

Sperm morphologic traits can be classified as compensable or uncompensable.[15] *Compensable traits* can be overcome by increasing the inseminated dose of semen (ie, greater sperm number per dose). These traits involve sperm that either do not have the capability to reach the site of fertilization or cannot stimulate the block to polyspermy.[15] Compensable traits include lack of motility (or dead sperm), abnormal plasma membrane integrity, and midpiece or tail abnormalities.[15] *Uncompensable traits* cannot be overcome by increasing the semen dose. The site of fertilization is reached by such sperm, zona penetration occurs, and polyspermy may be blocked. Fertilization cannot be completed, however, or early embryo mortality may be increased. Head abnormalities in this group include nuclear vacuoles and alterations in nuclear chromatin packaging.[15]

Differences in spermatozoal structure that are considered normal in the stallion but abnormal in other species include an asymmetric head, abaxial tail position (Fig. 13-15), and small acrosomal volume[13] (Fig. 13-16).

Currently, most equine reproductive specialists perform a differential count to determine normal or abnormal head, knobbed acrosomes, proximal droplets, swollen or abnormal midpieces, coiled tails, and detached heads (Figs. 13-17 to 13-21). The predominance of a specific defect would then help the evaluator better interpret the effect on the entire population of cells present in the ejaculate, avoiding erroneous assumptions about origin and effect on fertility. Some cell defects (eg, detached heads) can be primary, secondary, and tertiary. Other defects have unknown causes and uncertain effects on semen quality.

Percentage of morphologically normal spermatozoa has a positive correlation with fertility in the stallion.[14] Morphologic abnormalities may indicate biologic stress, trauma, toxin exposure, or cryodamage.[16] However, some breeding trials indicate that although the sperm morphologic examination meets certain minimum criteria for morphologically normal sperm in the representative ejaculate, the stallion's fertility may still be poor.[17] This is particularly true with *frozen-thawed semen*, for which morphologic examination may be within acceptable limits, but pregnancies are not achieved when mares are appropriately inseminated.[4,5] Most reports of poor correlation between percent normal morphology and fertility in stallions have evaluated only small groups of stallions and used a limited number of breedings to mares. A weak positive correlation ($r = 0.34$, $p < 0.01$) was reported between percent morphologically normal spermatozoa and per-cycle fertility estimate in 99 stallions over 2 years.[14]

Using cryopreserved semen, researchers have determined that motility and sperm morphologic evaluation may not sufficiently assess the characteristics that can affect fertility. Researchers are realizing that other parts of the spermatozoa must be assessed and that further tests need to be performed to better evaluate semen quality.[5]

Alternative Methods and Approaches

Acrosome Reaction

The ability of sperm to undergo capacitation and a functional acrosomal reaction at the appropriate time is necessary to achieve zona penetration and can be evaluated in bull and boar semen using DIC microscopy.[18] However, this ability is not as easily evaluated in the stallion.[17] Spermac stain has been used to assess acrosomal integrity with variable success.[5] It causes a green coloration of the intact acrosome to allow better visualization (Fig. 13-22).

A fluorescent chlortetracycline (CTC) stain with five characteristic staining patterns has been used to differentiate between true acrosome-reacted spermatozoa and those undergoing the acrosome reaction.[19] The *zona-free hamster oocyte penetration test* assesses the ability of spermatozoa to complete the acrosome reaction.[20] Some question the validity of this penetration test because all barriers up to the oocyte plasma membrane have been removed.

Plasma Membrane Integrity and Quality

Sperm plasma membrane integrity has been assessed using the *hypo-osmotic swelling* (HOS) *test*. Cells are placed in a hypo-osmotic solution so that water will enter spermatozoa through passive diffusion. If the membrane is intact, the plasma membrane surrounding the flagellum will swell and cause the tail to curl.[21] The HOS test is repeatable, accurate, and compatible with light microscopy. However, it correlates poorly with morphology and motility and does not correlate with the zona-free hamster oocyte penetration test.[22] Results have conflicted as to correlation with stallion fertility.[5]

Seminal Plasma Tests

Certain biochemical tests have been performed to evaluate seminal plasma quality. The interaction between sperm and the contribution of accessory sex glands to the ejaculate is an important function of overall semen quality. Glycerophosphorylcholine (GPC), ergothioneine, citric acid, electrolytes, alkaline phosphatase, aspartate transaminase, and other protein levels have been reported. GPC can be used as an epididymal marker; its presence in the seminal plasma indicates complete versus incomplete ejaculation.[23]

Fluorescent and Cytometric Techniques

Newer technologies are being evaluated for usefulness, repeatability, and correlation between spermatozoal function and fertility. Some of these tests use light or fluorescent microscopy, which is labor intensive and evaluates only a limited number of cells. The flow cytometer is considered a more accurate, quick, and objective tool and is being investigated for multicompartment assessment of spermatozoa.[16,24,25] Fluorescent stains with specificity for certain sperm compartments (*eg*, mitochondria, inner or outer acrosomal membrane, single- or double-stranded DNA) can be used to mark normal or abnormal spermatozoa. With flow cytometry, 10,000 cells per minute can be evaluated, using a laser to activate fluorescent molecules tagged onto individual spermatozoa. Such technology provides quicker results, improves objectivity, and increases the power of statistical tests when related to outcomes of breeding trials. Although not applicable to the field assessment of semen quality, referral centers and veterinary diagnostic laboratories may soon be offering such testing on formalin-preserved, cooled (5° C) and extended-shipped, and cryopreserved semen collected from stallions.

REFERENCES

1. Varner and Society for Theriogenology: Stallion Breeding Soundness Evaluation form. *Proc Soc Theriogenol*, 1992. pp 113-116.
2. Hurtgen: Evaluation of the stallion for breeding soundness. *Vet Clin North Am (Equine Pract)* 8:149-165, 1992.
3. Rousset et al: Assessment of fertility and semen evaluations of stallions. J Reprod Fertil Suppl 35:25-31, 1987.
4. Jasko: Evaluation of stallion semen. *Vet Clin North Am (Equine Pract)* 8:129-148, 1992.
5. Magistrini: Semen evaluation. In Samper: *Equine Breeding Management*, WB Saunders, Philadelphia, 2000. pp 91-108.
6. Braun et al: Effect of seminal plasma on motion characteristics of epididymal and ejaculated stallion spermatozoa during storage at 5 degrees C. DTW Dtsch Tierarztl Wochenschr 101:319-322, 1994.
7. Amann: Can the fertility potential of a seminal sample be predicted accurately? *J Androl* 10:89-98, 1989.
8. Jasko et al: A comparison of two computer-automated semen analysis instruments for the evaluation of sperm motion characteristics in the stallion. *J Androl* 11:453-459, 1990.
9. Varner et al: Use of a computerized system for evaluation of equine spermatozoal motility. *Am J Vet Res* 52:224-230, 1991.
10. Jasko et al: Comparison of spermatozoal movement and semen

characteristics with fertility in stallions: 64 cases (1987-1988). JAVMA 200:979-985, 1992.

11. Card: Detection of abnormal stallion sperm cells by using the Feulgen stain. *Proc Am Assoc (Equine Pract)* 44:176-177, 1998.
12. Dott: Morphology of stallion spermatozoa. *J Reprod Fertil Suppl* 23:41-46, 1975.
13. Bielanski et al: Some characteristics of common abnormal forms of spermatozoa in highly fertile stallions. *J Reprod Fertil Suppl* 32:21-26, 1982.
14. Jasko et al: Determination of the relationship between sperm morphologic classifications and fertility in stallions: 66 cases (1987-1988). *JAVMA* 197:389-394, 1990.
15. Saacke et al: Relationship of semen quality to sperm transport, fertilization, and embryo quality in ruminants. *Theriogenology* 41:45-50, 1994.
16. Graham: Analysis of stallion semen and its relation to fertility. *Vet Clin North Am (Equine Pract)* 12:119-130, 1996.
17. Voss et al: Stallion spermatozoal morphology and motility and their relationships to fertility. *JAVMA* 178:287-289, 1981.
18. Saacke and White: Semen quality tests and their relationship to fertility. *Proc NAAB Tech Conf Artif Insem Reprod* 4:22, 1972.
19. Varner et al: Induction and characterization of acrosome reaction in equine spermatozoa. *Am J Vet Res* 48:1383-1389, 1987.
20. Zhang et al: Acrosome reaction of stallion spermatozoa evaluated with monoclonal antibody and zona-free hamster eggs. *Mol Reprod Dev* 27:152-158, 1990.
21. Nie: Development of a hypoosmotic swelling (HOS) test for stallion semen. *Proc Soc Theriogenol*, 1998. p 146.
22. Chan et al: The relationship between the human sperm hypoosmotic swelling test, routine analysis, and the human sperm zona free hamster ovum penetration test. *Fertil Steril* 44:668-672, 1985.
23. Kosiniak and Bittmar: Analysis of the physiological processes connected with sexual maturation of stallions. *Pol Arch Weter* 27:5-21, 1987.
24. Garner et al: Assessment of spermatozoal function using dual fluorescent staining and flow cytometric analyses. *Biol Reprod* 34:127-138, 1986.
25. Evenson et al: Comparative sperm chromatin structure assay measurements on epiillumination and orthogonal axes flow cytometers. *Cytometry* 19:295-303, 1995.

CHAPTER 14

Peripheral Blood Smears

Kenneth S. Latimer and Pauline M. Rakich

Blood smear examination is an integral part of the complete blood cell count (CBC) and is probably the most important aspect of a routine hematologic examination. A peripheral blood smear is examined (1) to determine the leukocyte differential count, (2) to detect alterations in erythrocyte and leukocyte morphology, and (3) to detect parasites (eg, *Babesia* sp.) and rickettsial inclusions (eg, *Ehrlichia equi*). Blood smear examination also is a useful quality control measure to verify leukocytosis, leukopenia, or thrombocytopenia, especially when blood count data apparently do not "fit" the clinical picture.[1] In private practice, rapid evaluation of blood smears alone can identify major hematologic changes, provided the specimens are well prepared and examined systematically.

This chapter presents basic information and illustrations to allow practitioners to prepare and examine stained blood smears, identify normal blood cells and platelets, perform accurate leukocyte differential counts on sick animals, and recognize clinically important morphologic changes and inclusions within blood cells. Other excellent texts provide more detailed information on blood sample collection and analysis, including blood cell and platelet counts, hemoglobin determination, calculation of red cell indices, and determination of plasma protein and fibrinogen concentrations.[2-6]

Clinical Signs of Hematopoietic Abnormalities

Blood is composed of erythrocytes, leukocytes, platelets and plasma, which contains numerous biologically important proteins. Severe alterations in any of these components can produce clinical signs of disease.

Erythrocytes are primarily involved in oxygen transport. Decreased erythrocyte mass (*anemia*) or decreased erythrocytic functional capacity (*methemoglobinemia*) may result in decreased oxygen transport to body tissues. Clinical signs of anemia include pallor of mucous membranes, exercise intolerance or weakness, tachypnea, tachycardia, and mitral valve murmur secondary to decreased blood viscosity. Hemoglobinuria may be observed in severe intravascular hemolysis. Icterus also may be present but occurs in many other disorders as well, including extravascular hemolysis, anorexia, and liver disease. In methemoglobin-induced disturbances of erythrocytic function, such as following red maple leaf ingestion, the mucous membranes may appear chocolate brown. Oxidative damage to hemoglobin may result in Heinz body formation, with subsequent erythrocyte lysis or phagocytic removal from the blood vascular system.

Clinical signs of disease referable to alterations in leukocyte numbers or function may be vague but frequently include evidence of infection (wounds, abscesses, increased lung sounds, nasal discharge). The most important clinical consequence of leukopenia, usually the result of neutropenia, is bacterial infection. Leukemias may produce nonspecific clinical signs, such as rapid weight loss, or unique signs, such as hemorrhage, paralysis, or lameness involving a single limb. These unique signs may be misleading until a CBC is performed or a blood smear is examined.

Platelets maintain vascular integrity. With severe

thrombocytopenia (<20,000 platelets/μl), petechial hemorrhages may be observed in the mucous membranes and skin.

Hematologic Reference Intervals

Reference intervals, previously known as "normal ranges," are used for comparative purposes to identify patient abnormalities in the CBC.[6] Reference intervals are determined by performing CBCs on a defined (age, breed, gender, reproductive status, physical activity, geographic location) population of clinically healthy horses. Statistical analysis of these data determines a smaller interval within which most test values occur in health, the *reference interval.* These narrower reference intervals allow more rapid detection of sick animals based on examination of laboratory test results.

Table 14-1 presents the reference intervals used to interpret equine hematologic data at the University of Georgia Veterinary Medical Teaching Hospital. These reference intervals reflect general equine practice in Georgia and may not be entirely applicable for specialized practices (exclusively light or draft breeds, racetrack animals, foals) or other areas of the United States, where normal hematologic data may differ slightly.

Blood Smear Preparation

A well-prepared blood smear separates erythrocytes, leukocytes and platelets so they may be identified and examined after staining. Smears of EDTA-anticoagu-

TABLE 14-1

Blood Reference Intervals for Horses*

Erythrocytes

Hematocrit (%)	32–48
Hemoglobin (g/dl)	10–18
Erythrocyte count ($x10^6/\mu l$)	6–12
Reticulocytes (%)	0
MCV (fl)	34–58
MCH (pg)	13–19
MCHC (g/dl)	31–37

Leukocytes

Cell Type	Distribution range (%)	Absolute Range (cells /μl)
Leukocytes	—	6000–12,000
Neutrophils		
Segmented	30–75	3000–6000
Band	0–1	0–100
Lymphocytes	25–60	1500–5000
Monocytes	1–8	0–100
Eosinophils	1–10	0–800
Basophils	0–3	0–300

Platelets

Platelet count ($x10^5/\mu l$)	1–6
Mean platelet volume (fl)	4.1–6.9

Proteins

Plasma protein (refractometry, g/dl)	6.0–8.5
Fibrinogen (heat precipitation, mg/dl)	100–500

*Derived from horses examined at University of Georgia Veterinary Medical Teaching Hospital.
MCV, mean corpuscular volume; *MCH*, mean corpuscular hemoglobin; *MCHC*, *MCH* concentration.

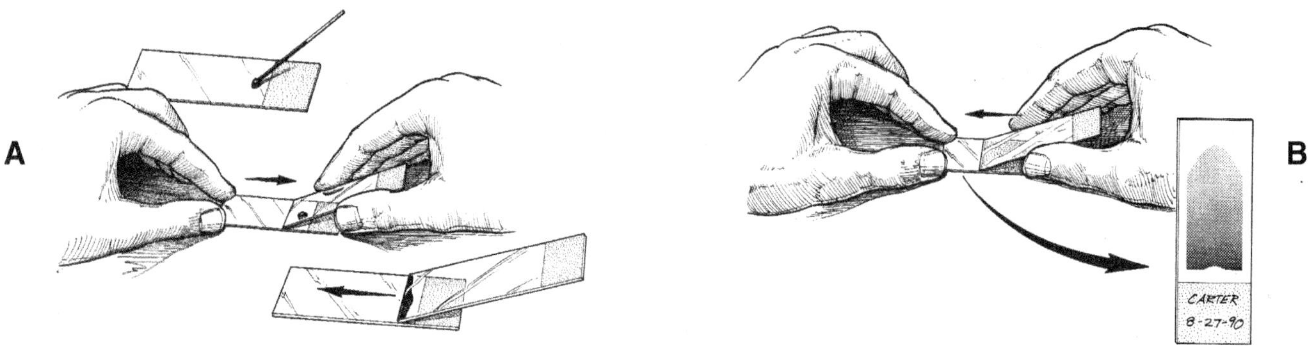

Fig. 14-1 Steps in producing wedge blood smear.
A, Drop of blood is placed near frosted end of slide. Spreader slide is drawn into drop of blood and then advanced. **B,** As spreader slide is rapidly advanced in a smooth motion, the blood smear is completed. A properly prepared blood smear has a distinct feathered edge, a body, and a butt end and is adequately identified.

lated whole blood may be made using 1 × 3–inch frosted-end glass slides (wedge method) or 24 × 24–mm square glass coverslips (coverslip method).[1] Before making smears, the blood sample should be mixed thoroughly because equine erythrocytes sediment rapidly.[3]

Wedge Method

Preparation of acceptable wedge smears requires minimal practice. Wedge smears are made using two clean glass slides (Fig. 14-1).[1] A small drop of blood is placed near the frosted end of one slide using a microhematocrit tube. The second slide (spreader slide) is held between the thumb and forefinger. This slide is held at an angle (about 30 degrees) and drawn backward into the drop of blood. As the blood spreads along the trailing edge of the spreader slide, this slide is advanced in a rapid and smooth motion, carrying the blood with it. The smear is rapidly air dried, labeled in pencil on the frosted end, and stained.

It is not necessary to press down on the spreader slide because its weight alone is sufficient to make a good smear. By altering the angle at which the spreader slide is held, the smear can be made thicker and shorter (>30-degree angle) or longer and thinner (<30-degree angle). If the specimen is "watery" (very anemic blood), the end of the smear slide can be elevated about 45 degrees while the smear is made. This ensures a properly feathered edge without carrying the sample off the end of the slide.

Coverslip Method

Preparation of good coverslip slides requires more manual dexterity and practice than for wedge smears.[1] Coverslip smears are thinner, making blood cell identification easier. Blood cells, especially leukocytes, are more evenly dispersed, resulting in a slightly higher percentage of monocytes on the leukocyte differential count. In contrast, maldistribution of leukocytes may occur in poorly prepared wedge smears, especially along the feathered edge.

Smears are made using two clean square glass coverslips (24 × 24 mm, #1½) (Fig. 14-2). One coverslip is held between the thumb and index finger. Using a microhematocrit tube, a small drop of blood is placed in the center of the coverslip. A second coverslip is quickly dropped onto the blood in a crosswise fashion. The blood spreads rapidly and evenly between the two surfaces. Just before spreading is complete, rays appear along the edges of the rapidly spreading blood, and the coverslips are pulled apart laterally in a single smooth motion. Smears are rapidly air-dried, labeled in pencil along the base of the blood smear, and stained in a routine manner.

Pulling the coverslips apart at the correct moment is critical to produce a thin blood smear without having the coverslips stick together. Proper timing is best learned through practice. Anemic blood samples tend to spread rapidly, whereas polycythemic samples spread more slowly.

Blood Smear Staining

Practitioners should have a basic understanding of hematologic stains and how to troubleshoot common staining problems.[1] With careful attention to detail, high-quality stained blood smears can be produced consistently.

Blood smears are most often stained with Romanowsky stains (Wright's, Giemsa, Leishman's). These stains also are called polychromic stains because three colors (red, blue, purple) are produced. Both classic Wright's stain

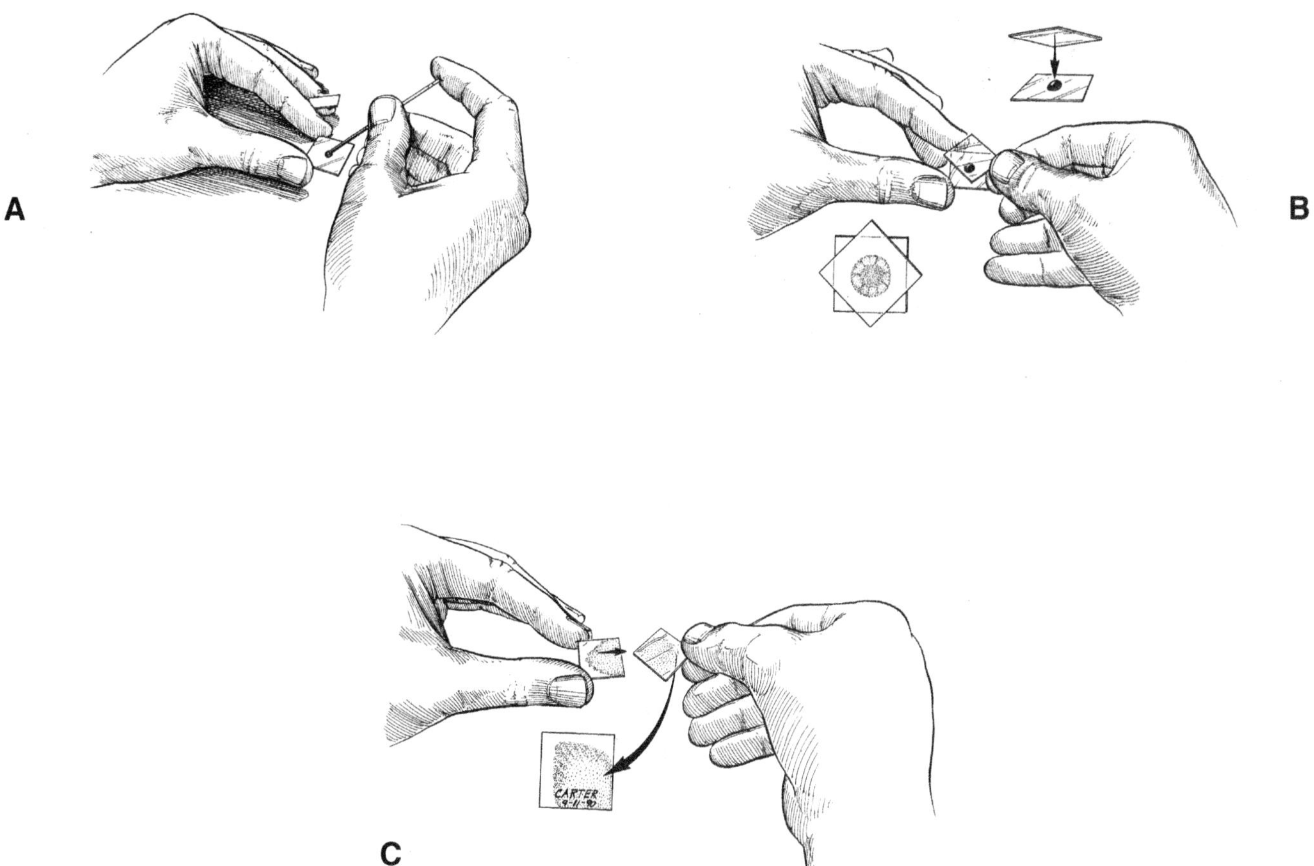

Fig. 14-2 Steps in producing coverslip blood smear.
A, Drop of blood is placed in center of coverslip, using microhematocrit tube. **B,** Second coverslip is placed crosswise over drop of blood, and blood begins to spread. Appearance of radial striations indicates spreading is almost complete. **C,** Coverslips are pulled apart laterally in a smooth, rapid motion when the radial striations appear. The butt of the completed smear is labeled for patient identification.

and Romanowsky-based "quick" stains (eg, Diff-Quik) are often used in private practice settings. These stains are similar but vary slightly in tinctorial properties and staining technique.

Wright's Stain

The blood smear is placed on a staining rack and flooded with Wright's stain. It is incubated for 3 minutes to allow adequate fixation of blood cells and platelets. An equal volume of Wright's buffer is added, and the solutions are mixed by blowing gently on the surface of the stain-buffer mixture. The smear is incubated for 3 more minutes. Staining occurs during this step, and a yellow-green metallic sheen or film develops on the surface of the stain-buffer mixture. At the end of the incubation period, the slide is flooded with tap water to remove the stain-buffer solution. The back of the slide is wiped free of stain residue, and the smear is tilted on end and air-dried. Total staining time is about 6 minutes.

Diff-Quik Stain

Diff-Quik is supplied in three solutions: light blue, red-orange, and blue-purple. Each solution is placed in a separate container or Coplin jar. The staining process begins by dipping the smear in the light blue solution about 5 times to allow adequate fixation of cellular components. The smear is immediately dipped in the red-orange solution about five times to give a red color to certain cellular structures. The smear then is dipped in the blue-purple solution about five times to provide both blue and purple colors. The smear is rinsed

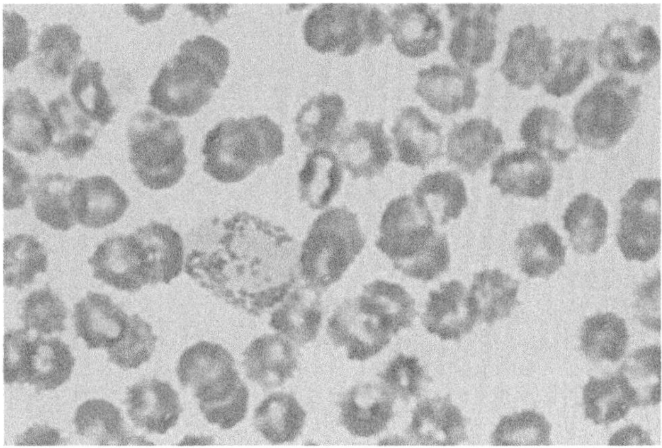

Fig. 14-3 Inadequately stained blood smear. Basophil lacks purple coloration of its nucleus and granules. This smear was salvaged by restaining.

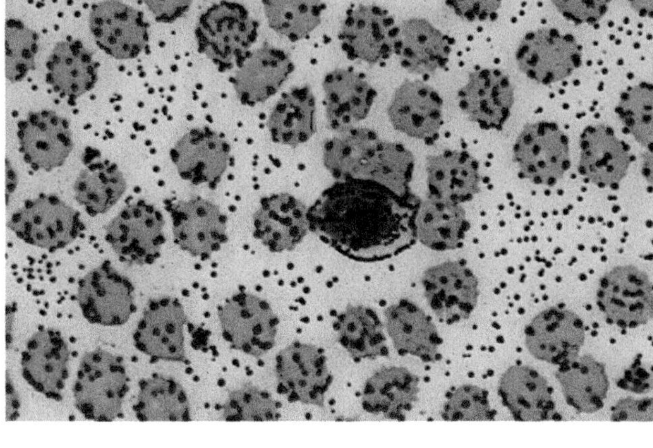

Fig. 14-4 Coarse, globular stain precipitate obscures cellular detail. Precipitate formed when alcohol evaporated from staining solution.

in tap water, stain residue is wiped from the underside of the slide, and the preparation is air-dried on end. Total staining time is approximately 15 seconds.

Troubleshooting Common Problems

Two basic problems are encountered when using Romanowsky stains: inadequate staining of blood cells and platelets and formation of precipitate that tends to obscure cellular and platelet detail.

Inadequate Staining: Inadequate staining is characterized by blood smears in which erythrocytes and eosinophil granules stain bright red and leukocyte nuclei are blue instead of purple (Fig. 14-3). With Wright's stain, this observation usually indicates inadequate staining time or overzealous application of buffer, with subsequent loss of dye solution. Preparations may be salvaged by restaining the smear. To prevent this problem, staining time should be increased, or care should be taken not to apply too much buffer.

With Diff-Quik stain, the problem is caused by inadequate staining time or exhaustion of dyes in the last (blue-purple) solution. The smear may be salvaged by repeating the staining procedure. If staining is still inadequate (purple coloration is not apparent), the last dye solution is exhausted. All solutions should be replaced before restaining the blood smear in question.

Precipitate Formation: Precipitate formation is a problem because it can obscure cellular detail, preventing adequate examination of the blood smear (Figs. 14-4 and 14-5). Smears cannot always be salvaged, but causes of precipitate formation can be corrected rapidly. Problems are more common with Wright's stain than with Diff-Quik stain.

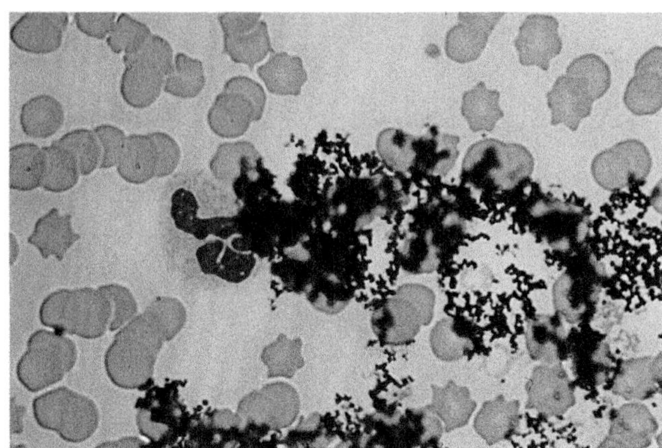

Fig. 14-5 Reticular stain precipitate obscures cellular detail. A metallic film was deposited on the smear as a result of poor washing technique after staining.

A *coarse globular precipitate* forms with Wright's stain if excessive incubation time is allowed after application of the dye solution (Fig. 14-4). The dyes are dissolved in absolute methanol, which eventually evaporates and results in the deposition of a coarse stain precipitate. Therefore the incubation period should be timed carefully to prevent globular precipitate formation.

A *reticular staining precipitate* occurs when the iridescent surface metallic film that develops during Wright's staining is deposited on the slide due to inadequate washing after buffer application (Fig. 14-5). This metallic film obscures cellular detail. Therefore the slides must be rinsed carefully at the end of the staining procedure to prevent precipitate from settling on the surface of the blood smear.

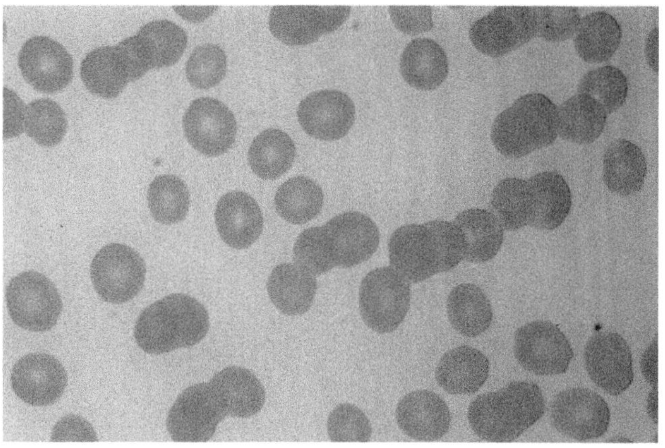

Fig. 14-6 Normal equine erythrocytes exhibit slight central pallor and a tendency toward rouleau formation.

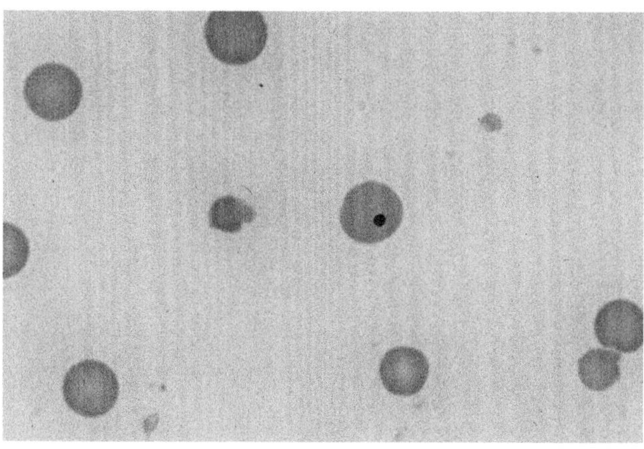

Fig. 14-7 Howell-Jolly body appears as a punctate, dark-purple inclusion in the center erythrocyte.

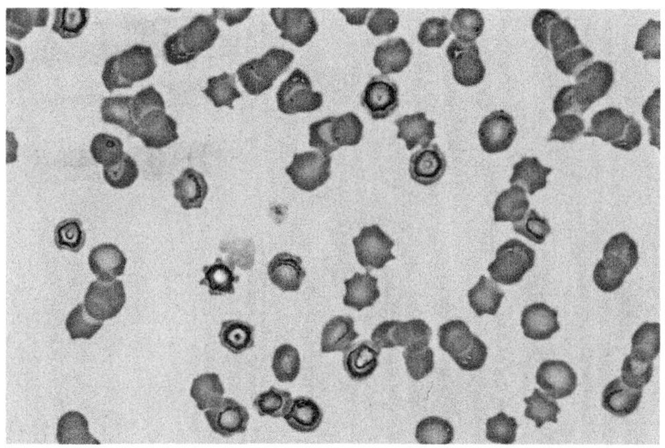

Fig. 14-8 Refractile areas in erythrocytes represent artifacts from incomplete drying of the smear. Scattered erythrocytes are crenated and contain uniformly spaced, pointed membrane projections.

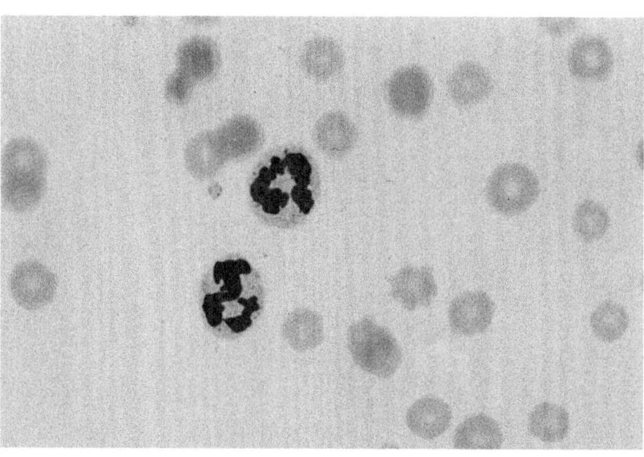

Fig. 14-9 Neutrophils demonstrating nuclear lobulation, a coarse chromatin pattern, and colorless cytoplasm.

Precipitate may also be present in the stock or working dye solutions. With Wright's stain, the stock and working dye solutions should be filtered through Whatman #1 or #2 filter paper into clean storage bottles. With Diff-Quik, the blue-purple solution should be filtered as described earlier into a clean Coplin jar.

Normal Blood Cell Components

Erythrocytes from healthy horses are about 5.7 μm in diameter. These cells stain red and have slight central pallor. Equine erythrocytes sediment rapidly in health, and rouleau formation is observed frequently (Fig. 14-6). *Howell-Jolly bodies* (purple punctate DNA remnants) are observed infrequently in healthy animals and more often in severe anemia (Fig. 14-7). Reticulocytes or polychromatophilic erythrocytes may be observed in bone marrow aspirates but generally are not released into the circulation, even in the presence of severe anemia.

If the blood smear is examined before drying is complete, folds in the erythrocyte membrane may appear refractile (Fig. 14-8). Inexperienced microscopists may mistake this refractile artifact for parasites or a pathologic change. Crenation of erythrocytes may occur if blood smears are allowed to dry slowly or an extremely alkaline pH develops as erythrocytes contact the glass slide ("glass effect"). Crenated erythrocytes are recognized by

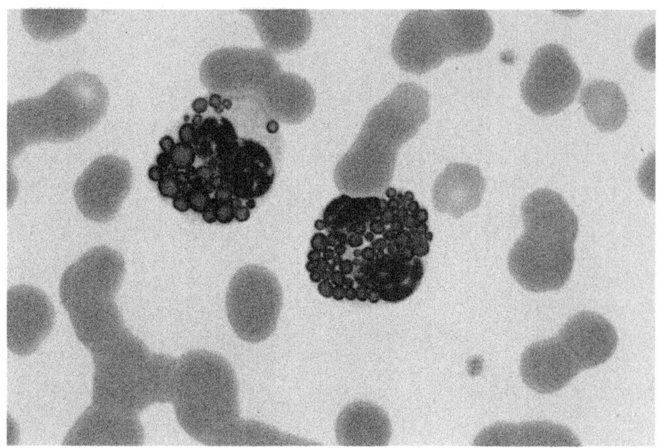

Fig. 14-10 Eosinophils containing uniformly large, round, red cytoplasmic granules. Microscopically, these cells have a raspberry-like appearance.

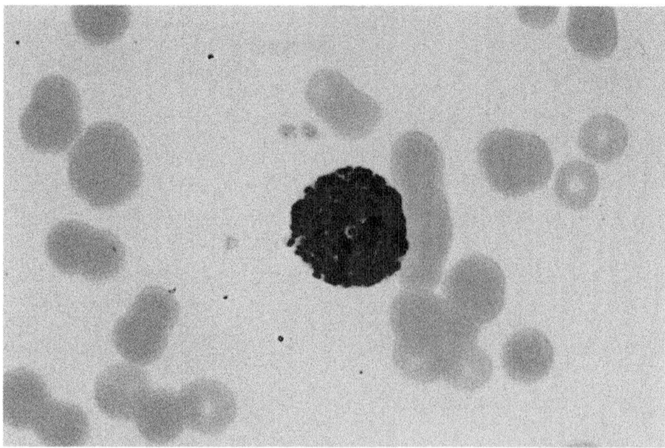

Fig. 14-11 Basophil with a lobulated nucleus and numerous purple cytoplasmic granules, which partially obscure nuclear detail.

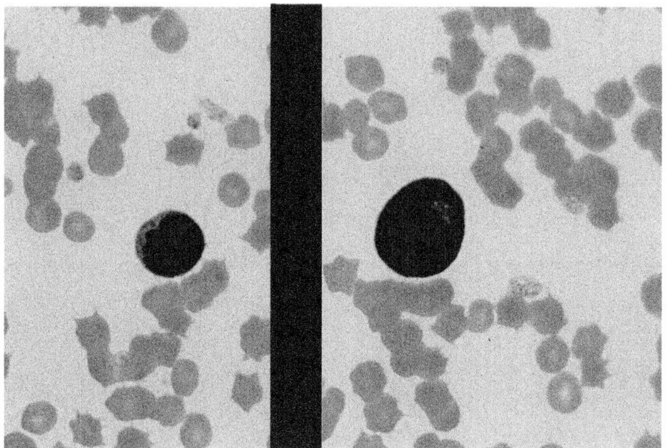

Fig. 14-12 Mature small lymphocyte *(left)* and immunocyte *(right)*.

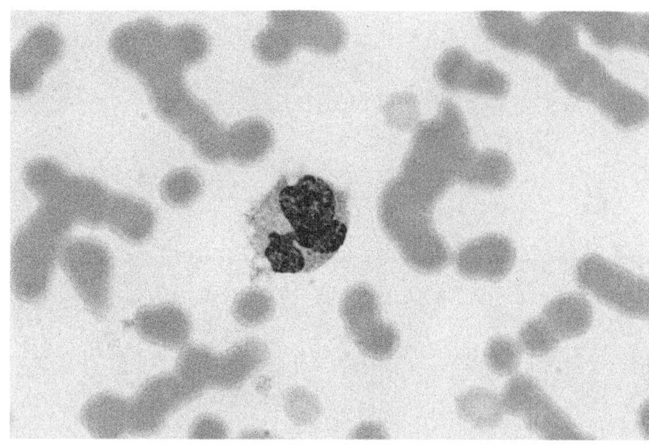

Fig. 14-13 Monocyte with lobulated nucleus, abundant gray cytoplasm, vacuoles, and pseudopodia.

relatively uniformly spaced, blunt-pointed projections of the cell membrane (Fig. 14-8).

Leukocytes are classified as neutrophils, eosinophils, basophils, lymphocytes, or monocytes. Neutrophils are further subclassified as segmenters and bands. Metamyelocytes (juvenile cells), myelocytes, promyelocytes, and myeloblasts (if present) may be subclassified within the neutrophil series if a severe or degenerative left shift is present.

Neutrophils usually have a lobulated nucleus with a coarse chromatin pattern and relatively colorless cytoplasm (Fig. 14-9). The neutrophils from some horses may have indistinct nuclear lobulation, but the chromatin pattern is coarse, and nuclear margins have sharp projections. Documenting a left shift in these animals is slightly more difficult. Neutrophil bands are infrequently observed in health (see later discussion).

Eosinophils are slightly larger than neutrophils and resemble raspberries. Eosinophils have a lobulated nucleus and uniformly large, round, bright-red cytoplasmic granules (Fig. 14-10).

Basophils are slightly larger than neutrophils. These cells have a lobulated nucleus and numerous, fine, dark-purple granules that often obscure nuclear detail (Fig. 14-11).

Mature lymphocytes are intermediate in size between erythrocytes and neutrophils (Fig. 14-12). The nucleus is indented slightly and has a coarse chromatin pattern. The nucleus almost fills the cell; only a thin rim of light-blue cytoplasm may be discerned.

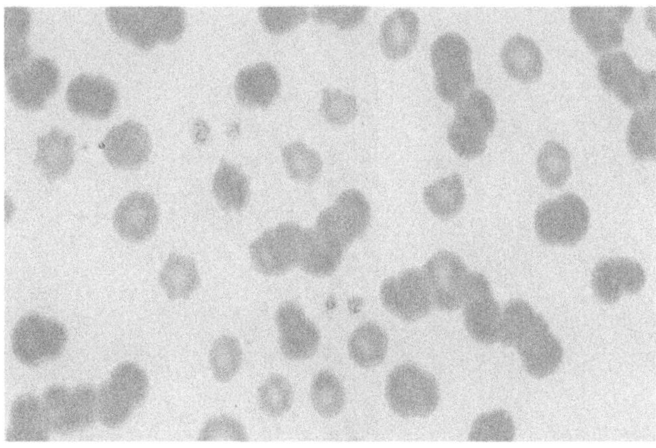

Fig. 14-14 Platelets appear small and often are pale staining in healthy horses.

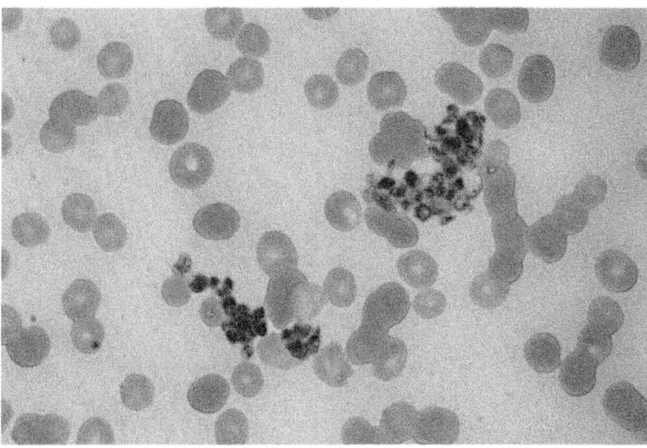

Fig. 14-15 Platelet aggregates of variable size at the feathered edge of the smear indicate poor anticoagulation of the blood sample.

Immunocytes, or *reactive lymphocytes*, are antigenically stimulated lymphocytes (Fig. 14-12). These cells are larger than neutrophils and are recognized readily by their royal-blue cytoplasm, which may contain a pale-staining Golgi zone. The nucleus may have scalloped edges or may assume a cloverleaf configuration. The nuclear chromatin pattern is moderately granular. Nucleolar rings (a slight clearing of the chromatin where the nucleolus is located) are occasionally seen. For purposes of the leukocyte differential count, immunocytes are counted as lymphocytes.

Monocytes are the largest leukocyte in circulating blood (Fig. 14-13). The monocyte's nucleus is variable in shape and may be oval, bilobed, horseshoe shaped, trilobed, or irregular. The nuclear chromatin pattern is less condensed than that of neutrophils. The cytoplasm is abundant and gray. Vacuoles are seen infrequently and are more common with delayed blood smear preparation. Fine, hairlike projections *(pseudopodia)* may be seen along the plasma membrane.

Platelets in horses are smaller and paler staining compared with platelets of other domestic animals (Fig. 14-14). Equine blood smears should be scanned at low power to identify any platelet aggregates along the feathered edge (Fig. 14-15). *Platelet aggregates* indicate poor anticoagulation of the blood sample and result in pseudothrombocytopenia because fewer individual platelets are present to be counted. In rare instances, aggregation may be caused by platelet activation on exposure to EDTA.[7] Repeated platelet counts on anticoagulated blood specimens using sodium citrate or heparin are subsequently within the reference interval.

Blood Smear Examination

Stained blood smears should be examined systematically to ensure that important changes are identified. The entire smear should be scanned at low (10× objective) magnification first. If the smear is improperly stained, this problem may be corrected as outlined earlier. The feathered edge should be examined carefully for platelet aggregates and for unusually large cells, which may indicate neoplasia. After increasing the magnification (45× to 50× objective), the leukocyte count may be estimated by examining the portion of the smear where the leukocyte differential count usually is performed, near the feathered edge where cells are dispersed singly. Finally, at higher (100× objective) magnification, major changes in the leukocyte differential count, blood cell and platelet morphology, and adequacy of platelet numbers are evaluated.

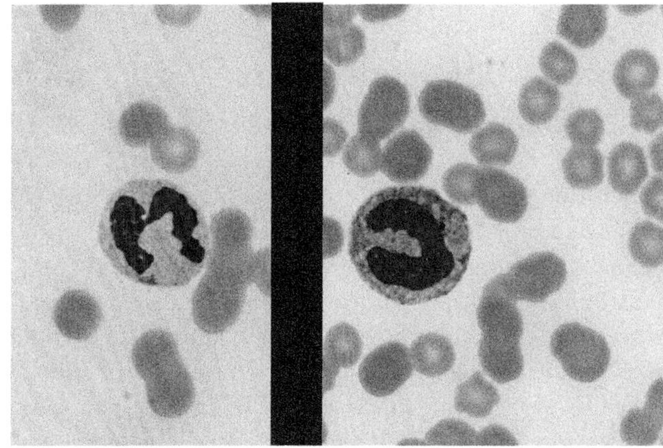

Fig. 14-16 Segmented neutrophil *(left)* exhibits nuclear lobulation, whereas the band neutrophil *(right)* lacks discernible nuclear constrictions.

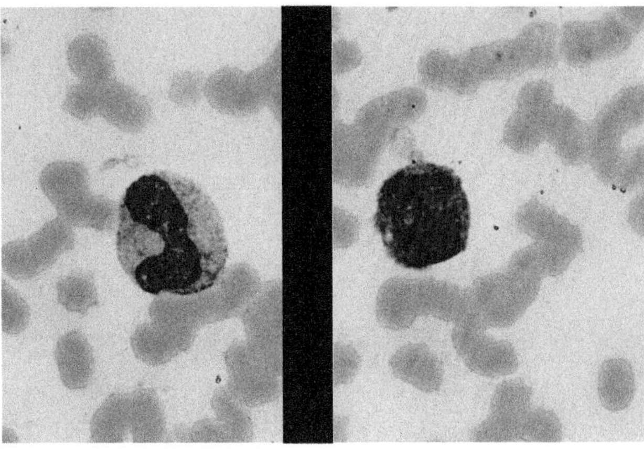

Fig. 14-17 Toxic neutrophil metamyelocyte *(left)* with light-blue cytoplasm and Döhle bodies, and monocyte *(right)* with gray cytoplasm, a distinct vacuole, and pseudopodia.

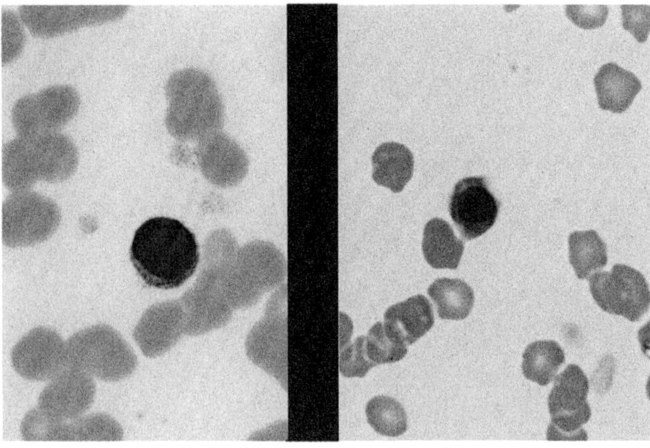

Fig. 14-18 Mature small lymphocyte *(left)* with nucleus almost filling the cytoplasm, compared with a nucleated erythrocyte *(right)* with a smaller, eccentric nucleus and relative abundance of blue-gray cytoplasm.

Leukocyte Differential Count

Several problems consistently arise when performing leukocyte differential counts on sick animals. These difficulties may be overcome with practice in blood smear examination.

Distinguishing and quantitating segmented and band neutrophils are important to determine if a left shift is present. However, identification of segmenters and bands may be difficult, especially in healthy animals with indistinct nuclear lobulation. *Segmented neutrophils* generally have a more coarse chromatin pattern and nuclear constrictions that exceed one-half the width of the nucleus (Fig. 14-16). *Band neutrophils* have parallel sides, and nuclear constrictions are minimal (ie, less than one-half the width of the nucleus) if present.

Differentiating *toxic neutrophils*, especially bands and metamyelocytes, from monocytes may also be challenging (Fig. 14-17). Certain criteria may be useful. The cytoplasm of toxic neutrophils stains light blue, appears foamy, and may contain Döhle bodies (see Neutrophil Morphology). In contrast, the cytoplasm of monocytes stains a darker blue-gray and may have distinct, variably sized, clear vacuoles. Monocytes also may have pseudopodia along the cell membrane. If a left shift and toxic changes of neutrophils can be recognized, it is generally of little consequence if one or two cells in a 100-cell leukocyte differential count are misidentified as toxic neutrophil metamyelocytes or monocytes. If necessary, additional CBCs can be performed to evaluate these hematologic changes.

Distinguishing small lymphocytes from nucleated erythrocytes is occasionally a problem (Fig. 14-18). Both cells are about the same overall size. The lymphocyte's nucleus almost entirely fills the cytoplasm, whereas the nucleus of a metarubricyte is small and eccentric with a very dense chromatin pattern. Mature lymphocytes have a thin rim of light-blue cytoplasm, whereas nucleated erythrocytes have moderately abundant blue-gray to gray-orange cytoplasm.

Identification of immunocytes (reactive lymphocytes) may be confusing to novice microscopists performing leukocyte differential counts. These cells may be mistaken for monocytes, misidentified as neoplastic lymphocytes, or simply may defy classification (see earlier discussion and Fig. 14-12). The presence of immunocytes is noted when assessing leukocyte morphology.

Erythrocyte Morphology

Alterations in erythrocyte values may be broadly classified as polycythemia (packed cell volume >48%) or anemia (packed cell volume <32%). The patient's hydration status and plasma protein concentration (as determined by refractometry) must be considered when evaluating polycythemia or anemia. Algorithms can assist in diagnosing polycythemic and anemic states (Figs. 14-19 and 14-20).

Evaluation of erythrocyte morphology can help determine the underlying mechanism of anemia. Because horses rarely release reticulocytes into the blood, determining whether the anemia is regenerative or nonregenerative may be difficult.[4,6,8] Basic information related to plasma protein concentration, iron status, and cytologic examination of bone marrow may be helpful.

Howell-Jolly Bodies and Nucleated Erythrocytes: Although Howell-Jolly bodies (see Fig. 14-7) may be observed infrequently in health, these structures and nucleated erythrocytes (see Fig. 14-18) are observed more often during severe anemia. Increased numbers of

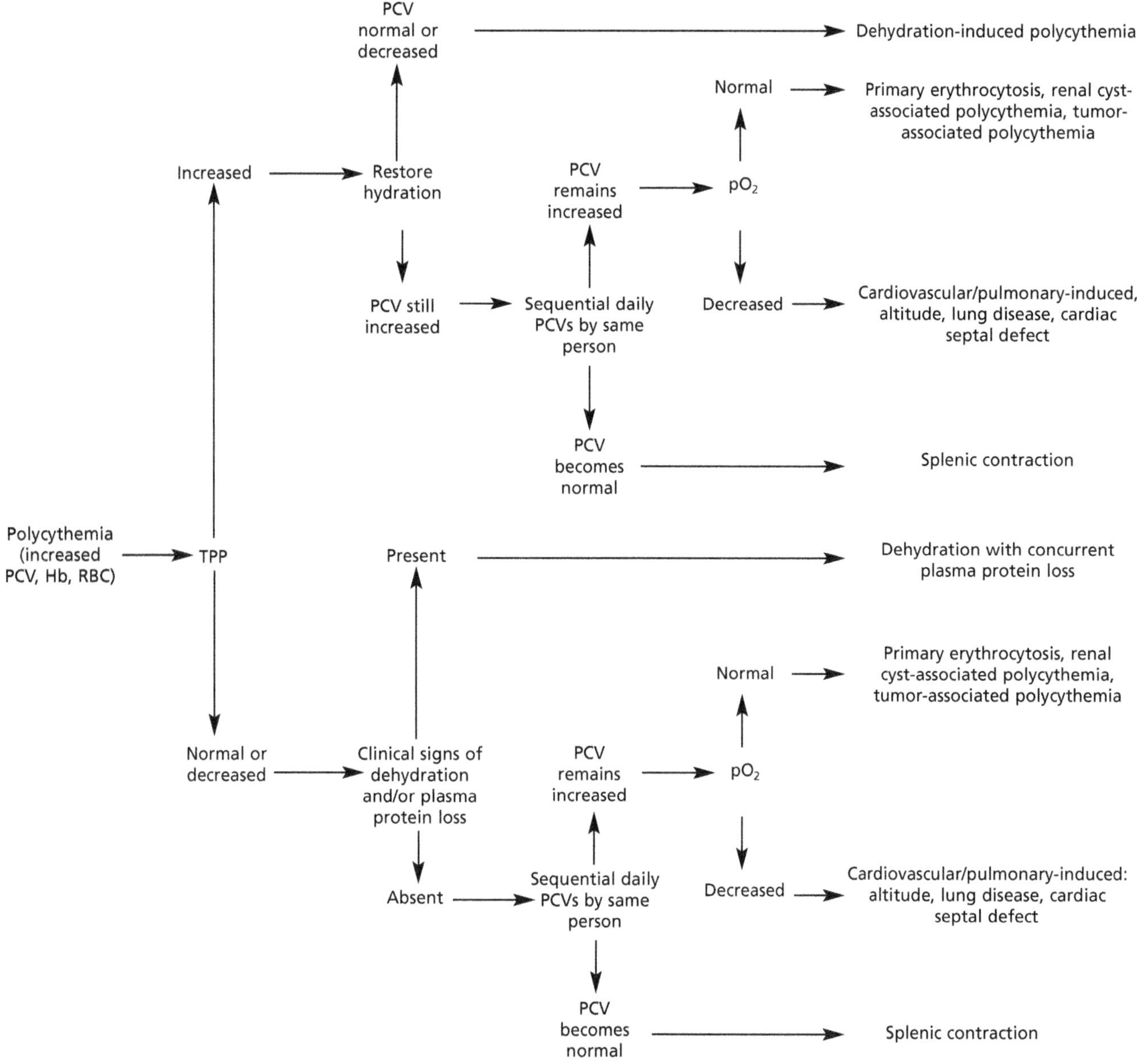

Fig. 14-19 Algorithm to assist in diagnosis of polycythemia.
PCV, Packed cell volume; *Hb*, hemoglobin; *RBC*, red blood cell count; *TPP*, total plasma protein; pO_2, partial pressure of oxygen. (From Tyler et al: *Vet Clin North Am [Equine Pract]* 3:461-484, 1987.)

Howell-Jolly bodies and nucleated erythrocytes may suggest erythrocyte regeneration, but bone marrow evaluation and serial packed cell volumes are necessary to document a regenerative response.

Microcytosis: Small erythrocytes that retain a variable degree of central pallor are called *microcytes* (Fig. 14-21). Microcytosis, with *hypochromia* (increased central pallor of erythrocytes) and *poikilocytosis* (misshapen erythrocytes), suggests iron deficiency.[4] Microcytosis may be associated with chronic blood loss from parasitism, gastrointestinal neoplasia, or severe gastrointestinal ulceration. As iron stores are depleted, less iron is available for hemoglobin production.

A *critical hemoglobin concentration* is necessary to arrest erythrocyte mitotic activity in the bone marrow. With decreased hemoglobin production, erythrocyte precursors undergo additional mitoses before the critical hemoglobin concentration is achieved to inhibit mitosis. The result is an increased number of smaller erythrocytes. An impression of iron deficiency may be confirmed by demonstrating hypoferremia, with a normal to

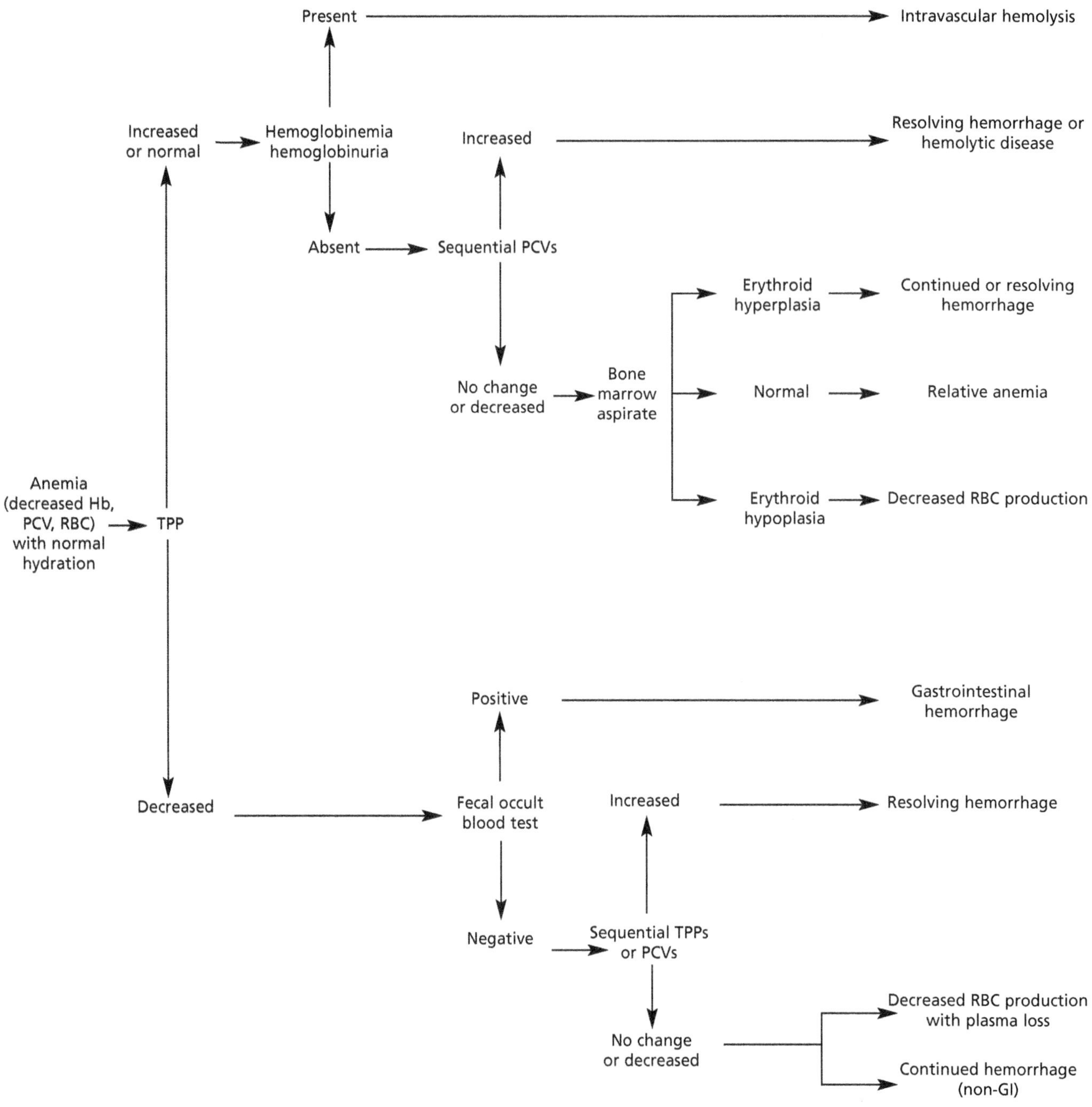

Fig. 14-20 Algorithm to assist in diagnosis of anemia.
PCV, Packed cell volume; *Hb*, hemoglobin; *RBC*, red blood cell count; *TPP*, total plasma protein. (From Tyler et al: *Vet Clin North Am [Equine Pract]* 3:461-484, 1987.)

increased total iron-binding capacity or decreased ferritin concentration in serum specimens. Alternatively, decreased iron stores may be apparent in Perl's-stained bone marrow smears.[4]

Erythrocyte Fragmentation: Erythrocyte fragmention is indicated by observing misshapen erythrocytes (*poikilocytes*), especially *schistocytes* (erythrocyte fragments with two to four angular or pointed projections) and *keratocytes* (helmet cells), within stained blood smears.[4] Poikilocytes appear slightly elongated with pointed ends (Fig. 14-22). Fragmentation of erythrocytes is associated with endothelial damage and fibrin deposition during infection, inflammation, or neoplasia in highly vascular organs, including the lung, liver, spleen, kidneys, bone marrow, and placenta (during third trimester of pregnancy).[4]

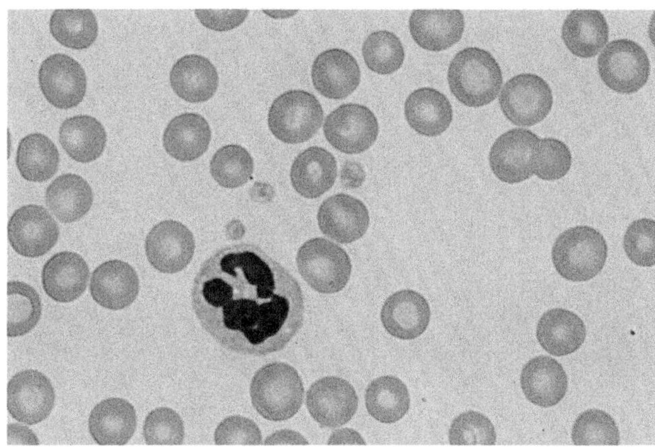

Fig. 14-21 Blood smear from a foal with iron deficiency anemia shows microcytes with increased central pallor.

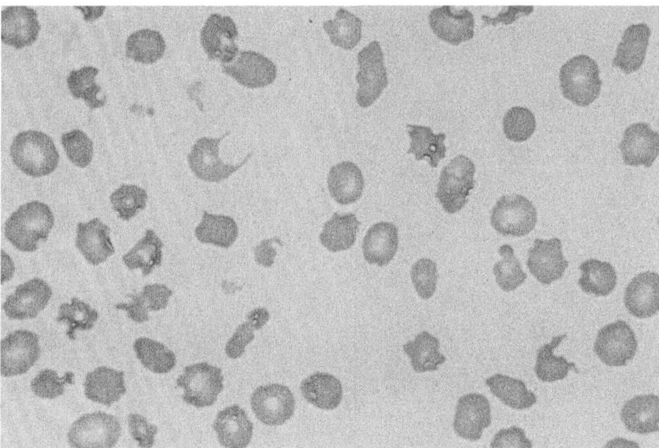

Fig. 14-22 Blood smear containing schistocytes, suggesting microangiopathic injury of erythrocytes. (Courtesy Dr. Rick Cowell.)

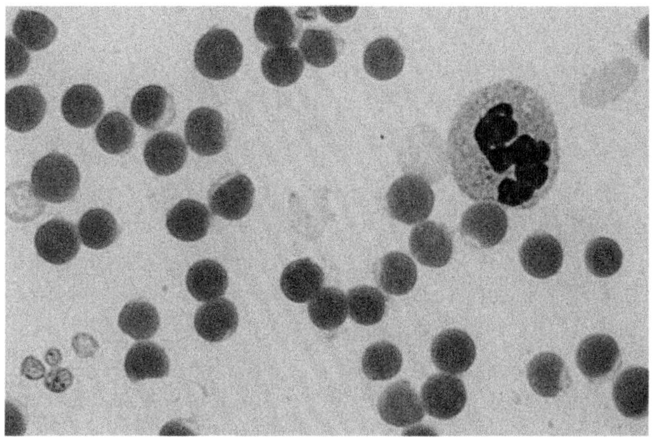

Fig. 14-23 Eccentric erythrocytes (hemighosts), characterized by partial absence of hemoglobin. These cells indicate an early stage of oxidative damage. An erythrocyte "ghost" also appears at left center.

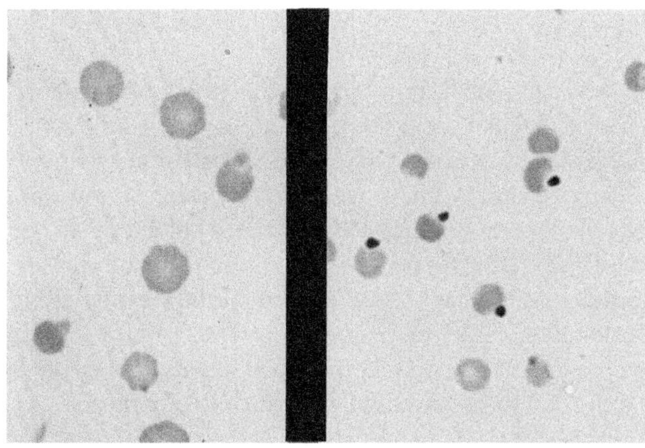

Fig. 14-24 Heinz bodies in a blood smear from a horse after phenothiazine deworming. *Left,* Heinz bodies appear pink and protrude from cell margins (Wright's stain). *Right,* Heinz bodies are more apparent and stain dark blue (new methylene blue stain).

Erythrocyte Oxidative Damage: Oxidative damage to erythrocytes may be associated with membrane lipid peroxidation, denaturation of hemoglobin, or a change in the valence state of the iron atom. Historically, oxidative damage of equine erythrocytes has involved the administration of phenothiazine anthelmintics or ingestion of wild onions or wilted red maple leaves.[9-12] Early oxidative damage is associated with scattered erythrocytes with a unique appearance, called *eccentrocytes* or *hemighosts.* All these damaged erythrocytes have an intact but partially cross-linked cell membrane. Areas of membrane cross-linking are devoid of hemoglobin, giving the erythrocyte an eccentric appearance (Fig. 14-23).

Heinz bodies (denatured aggregates of hemoglobin) are more obvious when present. In Wright's-stained blood smears, Heinz bodies often project from the cell margin, presenting a "light bulb" appearance. On Wright's stain, Heinz bodies stain pinkish red (similar to normal hemoglobin) but also may appear slightly lighter in color (Fig. 14-24). When blood smears are prepared with new methylene blue stain (0.5% dye in normal saline), Heinz bodies are readily observed as dark-blue dots (Fig. 14-24). Blood smears with extensive Heinz body formation may contain scattered erythrocyte "ghosts," which result from erythrolysis, with preservation of the cellular membrane but loss of hemoglobin.

Spherocytes: Spherocytes are small round erythrocytes that lack discernible central pallor (Fig. 14-25). They are observed infrequently in equine blood smears because equine erythrocytes only have slight

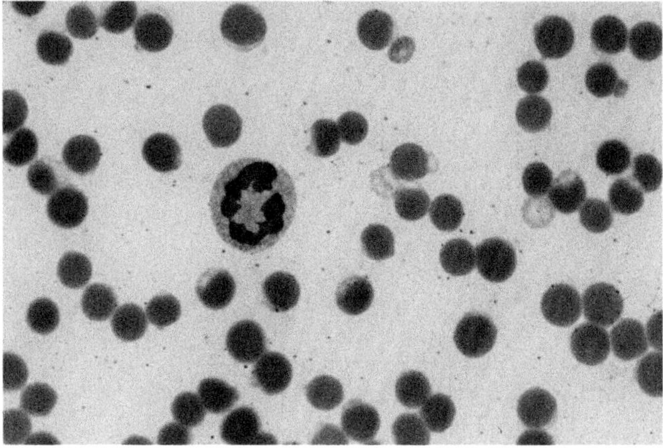

Fig. 14-25 Spherocytes and eccentrocytes in blood from a horse with red maple toxicity. Note the lack of central pallor in spherocytes.

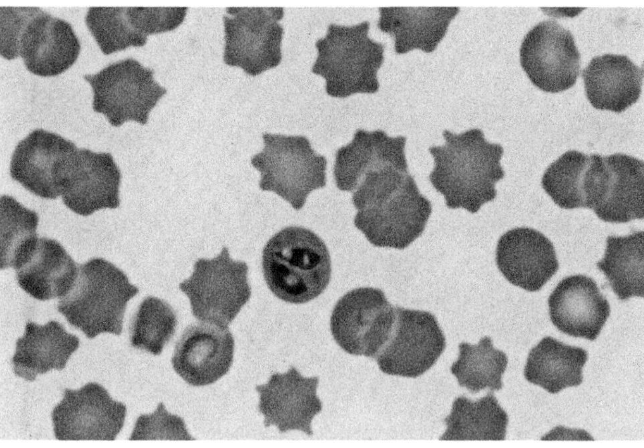

Fig. 14-26 Erythrocyte containing *Babesia caballi* piroplasms. The organisms stain purple and are teardrop shaped.

central pallor in health. Spherocytes result from partial removal of red cell membrane by the monocyte-macrophage system, while the cytoplasmic volume remains essentially unchanged. After membrane removal, the biconcave erythrocytes assume a globoid shape. Membrane may be removed secondary to antibody or complement attachment (as in immune-mediated hemolytic anemia) or by pitting of Heinz bodies (as in red maple leaf toxicity). The medical history may suggest the possibility of plant ingestion or drug administration. Immune-mediated hemolysis can be verified by Coombs' (antiglobulin) testing using species-specific antiserum.

Basophilic Stippling: Basophilic stippling is characterized by fine blue-gray speckles within erythrocytes, as observed in Romanowsky-stained blood smears. Basophilic stippling may be seen in erythrocytes from horses with lead poisoning, but identification of this change depends greatly on technique (eg, use of anticoagulants, rapidity of blood smear drying).[13,14] Additionally, normoblastosis (metarubricytosis, or increased numbers of nucleated erythrocytes) and Howell-Jolly bodies may be observed as more consistent features of lead poisoning.[14]

Parasites: *Babesia caballi* and *Babesia equi* are the only erythrocytic parasites of clinical significance in North American horses.[15] These protozoans may cause severe anemia, but only a small proportion of red blood cells may be parasitized. Organisms are most often observed when 0.1% or more of the erythrocyte population is infected. Organisms are teardrop shaped, with one to four organisms per cell (Fig. 14-26). In the absence of documented parasitemia, serologic tests may confirm a diagnosis of babesiosis.[4,6]

Leukocyte Alterations in Disease

Leukocyte numbers and morphology may be altered in various diseases. Initial impressions of altered total and differential leukocyte counts may be detected by rapid inspection of the blood smear. These qualitative impressions are subjective and should be verified by quantitative CBC data when possible.

The leukocyte count may be estimated by examining the area of the smear where the differential count is performed. The average number of white blood cells (WBCs) in 10 fields of view is determined using the 45× or 50× objective and is multiplied by 1500 to 2000. An estimate of less than 6000 WBCs/μl suggests leukopenia, whereas an estimate greater than 12,000 WBCs/μl suggests leukocytosis. These subjective estimates should be confirmed by quantitative counts when time permits.

Higher magnification provides an "impression" of major changes in the leukocyte differential count. An actual 100- or 200-cell tabulation of cell types generally is not necessary. Such impressions include neutrophilia, neutropenia, presence or absence of a left shift, lymphocytosis, lymphopenia, eosinophilia, eosinopenia, and basophilia. Box 14-1 lists common differential diagnoses for these findings.

Other common morphologic changes in neutrophils, as determined by examining the stained blood smear, are discussed next. Changes involving other leukocyte types are rare and are not presented here, except for those encountered in leukemias.

Neutrophil Morphology

Morphologic alterations of neutrophils in disease usually are associated with a left shift and toxic changes. In rare

Box 14-1 Differential Diagnosis of Altered Leukocyte Counts

Neutrophilia

Physiologic causes: fear, excitement, brief but strenuous exercise
Corticosteroid-associated causes: drugs, severe stress
Inflammation: (various causes)
Infection: bacterial, viral, fungal
Granulocytic leukemia (very rare)

Neutropenia

Defective neutrophil production in bone marrow: drugs, irradiation, bone marrow necrosis (bacterial), myelophthisis, myelofibrosis, osteopetrosis, disseminated granulomatous inflammation, neoplasia

Excessive tissue demand for neutrophils: septicemia/endotoxemia (salmonellosis, foal septicemia), severe bacterial infections, blister beetle toxicosis, cecal perforation, colic, chronic enteritis, monocytic ehrlichiosis (Potomac horse fever), phenylbutazone toxicity, immune-mediated neutropenia

Lymphocytosis

Physiologic causes: especially high-strung light breeds
Chronic infection: bacterial, viral
Postvaccination sequela
Lymphosarcoma/Lymphocytic leukemia: unusual to rare

Lymphopenia

Corticosteroid-associated: drugs, severe stress
Acute infection: bacterial, viral
Combined immunodeficiency: especially Arabian horses

Monocytosis

Suppuration, tissue necrosis
Hemolysis, hemorrhage
Pyogranulomatous inflammation
Nonhematopoietic neoplasia
Monocytic/myelomonocytic leukemia (very rare)

Eosinophilia

Parasitism: subtle in foals
Inflammatory/hypersensitivity reactions
Hypereosinophilic syndromes
Eosinophilic myeloproliferative disease, leukemia (rare)

Eosinopenia

Corticosteroid-associated causes: drugs, severe stress
Acute infection (any cause)

Basophilia

Intestinal disease, including parasitism

instances, cytoplasmic inclusions that are specific for rickettsial infection may be observed.

Left Shift: A left shift consists of increased numbers of bands and juvenile neutrophils in the peripheral blood (Fig. 14-27). If the total neutrophil count is within the reference interval or increased, a clinically important left shift exists if band or juvenile numbers are 300/μl or greater. If neutropenia exists, a significant left shift is present if these forms compose 10% or more of the neutrophil population.

Band neutrophils often have an S- or U-shaped nucleus with a less condensed chromatin pattern than that of

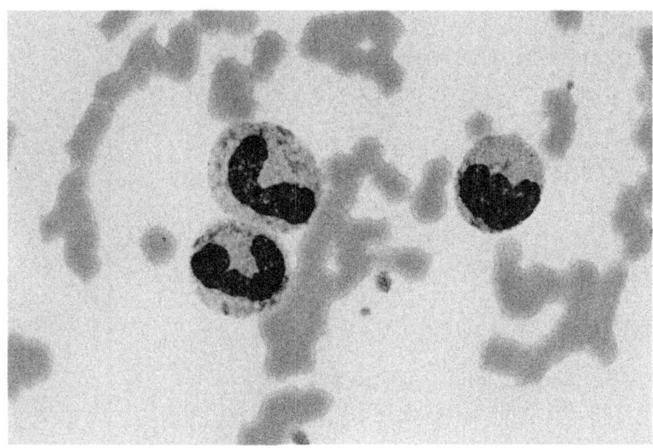

Fig. 14-27 Band and juvenile neutrophils *(left shift)* in the blood of a horse with a severe bacterial infection. Cytoplasmic basophilia and Döhle bodies indicate toxic change.

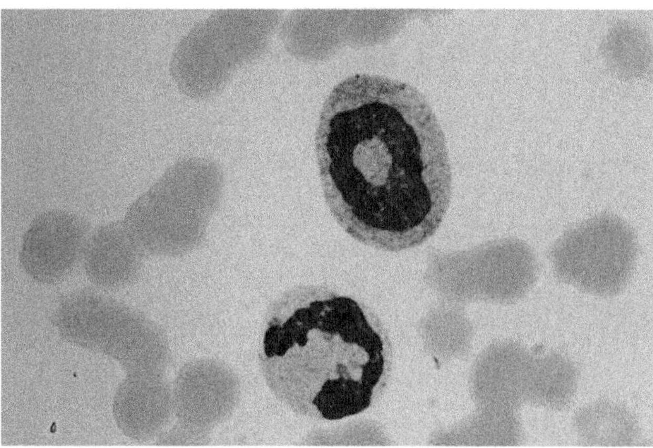

Fig. 14-28 Enlarged toxic neutrophil with ring-shaped nucleus in the blood of a horse with salmonellosis. A segmented neutrophil is seen below the toxic neutrophil.

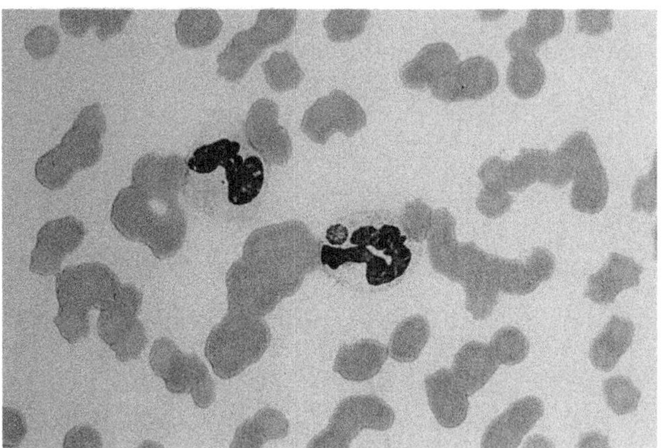

Fig. 14-29 *Ehrlichia equi* morula in cytoplasm of neutrophil at right. (Courtesy Dr. John Harvey.)

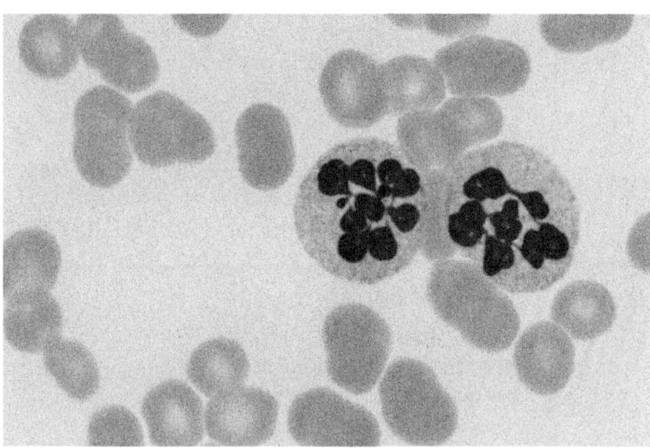

Fig. 14-30 Idiopathic nuclear hypersegmentation of neutrophils. (Courtesy Dr. K.W. Prasse.)

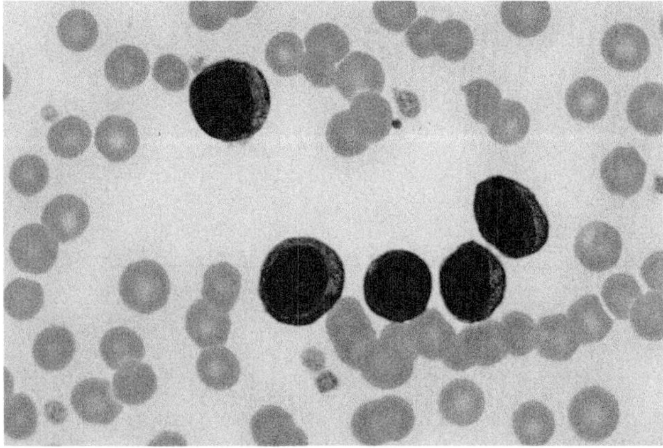

Fig. 14-31 Blood smear from a horse with chronic lymphocytic leukemia shows small cell size and a mature chromatin pattern. (Courtesy Dr. Bernard Feldman.)

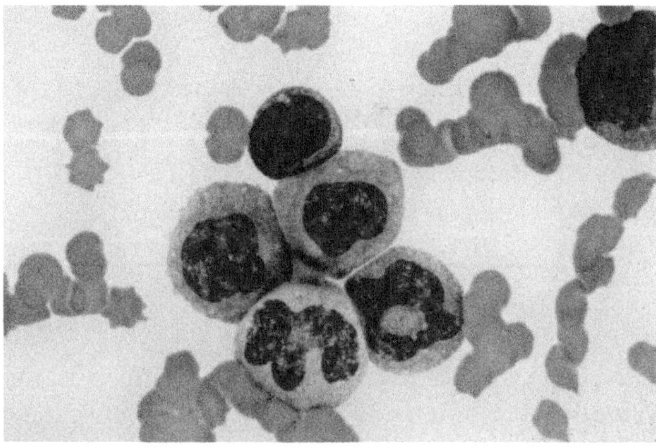

Fig. 14-32 Blood smear from a horse with myelomonocytic leukemia shows a blast cell and differentiating monocytes and neutrophils. (Courtesy Dr. Julia Blue.)

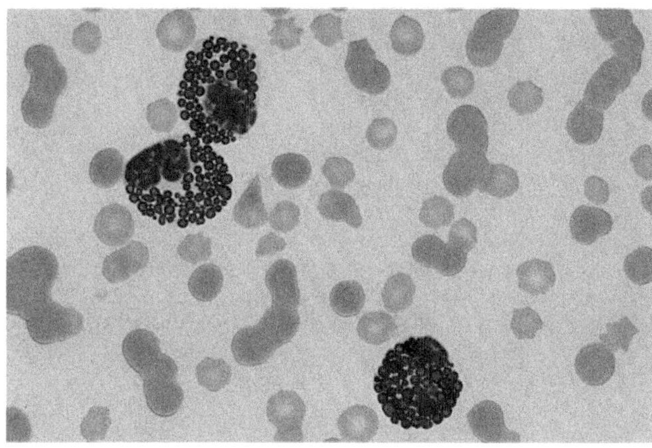

Fig. 14-33 In this blood smear from a horse with eosinophilic myeloproliferative disease, cell nuclei are hyposegmented.

segmented neutrophils (see Fig. 14-16). Indentations in the nucleus do not exceed 50% of the width, suggesting a lack of nuclear segmentation. In horses that lack distinct nuclear lobulation of neutrophils in health, band neutrophils are identified by a less condensed chromatin pattern and blunting of nuclear membrane projections.

Toxic Changes: Toxic changes of neutrophils typically include cytoplasmic basophilia, foamy cytoplasmic vacuolation, and *Döhle bodies* (small blue-gray angular particles near the cell margin) (Fig. 14-27).[2,3] *Toxic granulation* (increased pinkish purple cytoplasmic granularity) is another manifestation of toxic change but is observed infrequently in equine blood smears. These changes suggest severe systemic inflammation, endotoxemia, infection, or drug toxicity. Disappearance of toxic change is a favorable prognostic sign, with cytoplasmic basophilia being the last manifestation of toxic change to resolve during convalescence. In severe infections, such as acute salmonellosis, toxic neutrophils may appear swollen and nuclei may assume unusual configurations, such as ring shapes (Fig. 14-28).

Rickettsial Morulae: *Ehrlichia equi* infection may be diagnosed by finding gray, mulberry-like rickettsial morulae within the neutrophil cytoplasm (Fig. 14-29).[16] Morulae are present during clinical illness and may be found within circulating neutrophils in severe cases of the disease. Absence of morulae, however, does not exclude the diagnosis. If equine ehrlichiosis is a differential diagnosis, determination of acute and convalescent antibody titers may assist in definitive diagnosis.

Neutrophil Nuclear Hypersegmentation: Idiopathic neutrophil hypersegmentation has been reported in one horse.[17] Almost all the neutrophils appeared hypersegmented and sometimes contained more than 11 nuclear lobes (Fig. 14-30). This interesting hematologic abnormality does not appear to be clinically significant and may be congenital in origin.

Neutrophil nuclear hypersegmentation is observed more frequently as a sequel to *corticosteroid* administration or endogenous *cortisol* release. Under the influence of corticosteroids, neutrophils circulate longer in the blood and undergo progressive nuclear lobulation with age.[6] In corticosteroid-associated hypersegmentation, only a few cells are affected in any given smear.

Leukemias and Myeloproliferative Diseases

Leukemias and myeloproliferative diseases have been reported infrequently in horses.[18-23] Leukemia involves neoplastic proliferation of hematopoietic cell lines, including granulocytes, monocytes, lymphocytes, erythrocytes, and megakaryocytes. Unregulated proliferation of cell lines may occur singly or in combination. Myeloproliferative diseases are characterized by disturbed cellular maturation. Leukopenia or leukocytosis may occur and eventually culminate in overt leukemia. Generally, Romanowsky-stained blood and bone marrow smears allow diagnosis of well differentiated leukemia with recognizable cellular morphology, but these smears cannot distinguish poorly differentiated leukemia of one immature blast cell line from another. This distinction, however, may be made in larger veterinary centers by application of cytochemical stains and by electron microscopic examination of cellular ultrastructure.

Leukemia may be suspected on blood smear examination by finding blast cells, disturbed cellular maturation, and occasionally, dramatic increases in the cell count (Figs. 14-31 to 14-33). Bone marrow aspiration may help confirm the diagnosis. Because leukemias and myeloproliferative diseases are relatively rare in horses, consultation with veterinary hematologists and oncologists may facilitate diagnosis and case management.

REFERENCES

1. Latimer: *VPP 537-L Laboratory Manual of Clinical Pathology Techniques*. 4th ed. Athens, 1990, University of Georgia.
2. Feldman, Zinkl, and Jain: *Schalm's Veterinary Hematology*. 5th ed. Philadelphia, 2000, Lippincott Williams & Wilkins.
3. Schalm: *Manual of Equine Hematology*. Santa Barbara, 1984, Veterinary Practice Publishing.
4. Tyler et al: Hematologic values in horses and interpretation of hematologic data. Vet Clin North Am (Equine Pract) 3:461-484, 1987.
5. Lassen and Swardson: Hematology and hemostasis in the horse: normal functions and common abnormalities. *Vet Clin North Am (Equine Pract)* 11:351-389, 1995.
6. Latimer and Mahaffey, in Colahan et al: Equine Medicine and Surgery. 5th ed. St Louis, 1999, Mosby, pp 1973-1981, 1989-2001, 2025-2031.
7. Hinchcliff et al: Diagnosis of EDTA-dependent pseudothrombocytopenia in a horse. JAVMA 203:1715-1716, 1993.
8. Blue et al: Immune-mediated hemolytic anemia induced by penicillin in horses. Cornell Vet 77:263-276, 1987.
9. McSherry et al: The hematology of phenothiazine poisoning in horses. Can Vet J 7:3-12, 1966.

10. Pierce et al: Acute hemolytic anemia caused by wild onion poisoning in horses. JAVMA 160:323-327, 1972.
11. George et al: Heinz body anemia and methemoglobinemia in ponies given red maple *(Acer rubrum)* leaves. *Vet Pathol* 19:521-533, 1982.
12. Tennant et al: Acute hemolytic anemia, methemoglobinemia, and Heinz body formation associated with ingestion of red maple leaves by horses. JAVMA 179:143-150, 1981.
13. George and Duncan: The hematology of lead poisoning in man and animals. *Vet Clin Pathol* 8:23-30, 1979.
14. Burrows and Borchard: Experimental lead toxicosis in ponies: comparison of the effects of smelter effluent-contaminated hay and lead acetate. *Am J Vet Res* 43:2129-2133, 1982.
15. Simpson et al: Comparative morphologic features of *Babesia caballi* and *Babesia equi*. *Am J Vet Res* 28:1693-1697, 1967.
16. Madigan: Equine ehrlichiosis. *Vet Clin North Am* (*Equine Pract*) 9:423-428, 1993.
17. Prasse et al: Idiopathic hypersegmentation of neutrophils in a horse. *JAVMA* 178:303-305, 1981.
18. Latimer, in Colahan et al: *Equine Medicine and Surgery*. 5th ed. St Louis, 1999, Mosby, pp 2031-2034.
19. Edwards et al: Plasma cell myeloma in the horse: a case report and literature review. *J Vet Intern Med* 7:169-176, 1993.
20. Monteith and Cole: Monocytic leukemia in a horse. *Can Vet J* 36:765-766, 1995.
21. Buechner-Maxwell et al: Intravascular leukostasis and systemic aspergillosis in a horse with subleukemic acute myelomonocytic leukemia. *J Vet Intern Med* 8:258-263, 1994.
22. Ringger et al: Acute myelogenous leukaemia in a mare. *Aust Vet J* 75:329-331, 1997.
23. Clark et al: Myeloblatic leukaemia in a Morgan horse mare. *Equine Vet J* 31:446-448, 1999.

CHAPTER 15

Bone Marrow

Kenneth S. Latimer and Claire B. Andreasen

Bone marrow is the major hematopoietic organ of the body and is responsible for production of erythrocytes, platelets, granulocytes, monocytes, and a small number of lymphocytes. Most blood lymphocytes, however, are derived from the secondary or peripheral lymphoid tissues, including tonsil, lymph nodes, gut-associated lymphoid tissue, bronchial-associated lymphoid tissue, and spleen.

Almost all bones of the body are involved in hematopoiesis at birth. In the neonate, isolated hematopoietic activity also may be present within the spleen and liver. As adulthood approaches, hematopoietic activity is generally restricted to the proximal long bones and axial skeleton (vertebrae, sternebrae, pelvis, ribs).[1] Hematopoietic activity may resume within the diaphyses of long bones, spleen, and liver in response to a profound increase in blood cell demand, such as in equine infectious anemia, or to unregulated blood cell production, such as in primary erythrocytosis (polycythemia vera) or leukemia.[2,3]

Bone Marrow Aspiration

Bone marrow aspiration biopsy is a valuable adjunct in evaluating diseases of hematopoietic tissues. Primary indications for bone marrow examination include anemia, persistent leukopenia, leukocyte cytoplasmic and nuclear maturation abnormalities, persistent thrombocytopenia, unexplained pancytopenia, suspected hematologic neoplasia, and suspicion of bone marrow necrosis or infiltrative disease, including stromal proliferation, infectious agents, or metastatic neoplasia.[1,4]

Contraindications

Bone marrow aspiration biopsy is a relatively innocuous procedure in horses. Excessive hemorrhage is theoretically possible after bone marrow aspiration, but this is extremely rare.[4] If severe thrombocytopenia (<20,000 platelets/μl), clotting factor deficiencies, or disseminated intravascular coagulation is present, any hemorrhage usually can be corrected by applying direct pressure to the aspiration site for 4 to 5 minutes.[1] When aspirating marrow from sternebrae, the needle should be placed carefully to prevent cardiac puncture. One horse died after sternal bone marrow aspiration because of left ventricular laceration and subsequent cardiac tamponade. Monoclonal gammopathy and defective hemostasis in this horse probably contributed to development of cardiac tamponade.[5] Iatrogenic infection is theoretically possible but is unlikely when the aspiration site is properly prepared and aseptic technique is followed.[4]

Specimen Collection

Marrow aspiration is simply tissue aspiration through cortical bone. Bone marrow can be collected from the sternum, ribs, or ilium using an 18-gauge spinal needle. The aspiration site should be clipped, cleaned with surgical disinfectant, and locally anesthetized with 2% lidocaine. Both the subcutis and the periosteum should be infiltrated with the local anesthesia solution.

A small stab incision is made in the skin with a #11 scalpel blade. The needle is inserted until the periosteum is penetrated and marked resistance encountered. The cortical bone is penetrated by applying steady pressure while

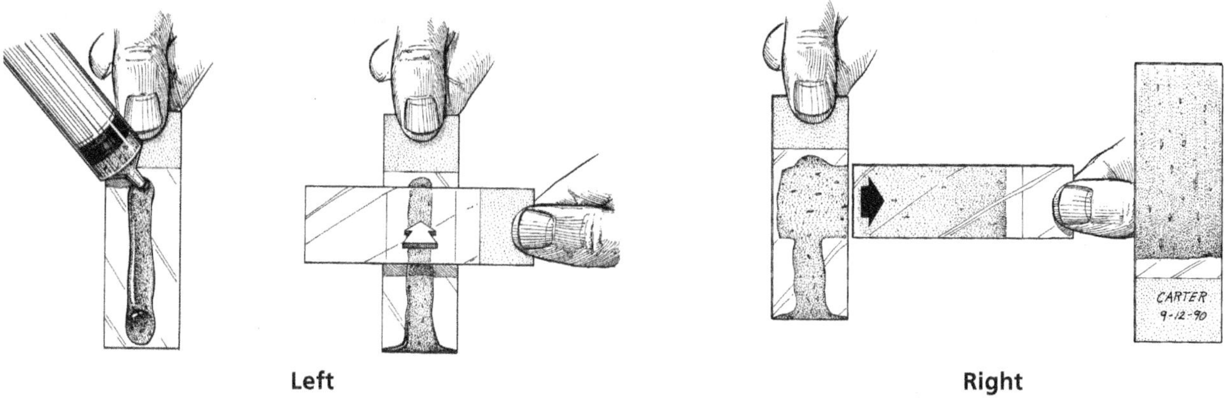

Fig. 15-1 Bone marrow squash preparation. *Left,* Marrow is expelled onto a slide held vertically. Marrow particles adhere as blood flows downward. A second slide (smear slide) is held at a right angle to the first slide. *Right,* Smears are made by pressing gently and pulling the second slide laterally. The completed smear is labeled, air-dried, and stained.

rotating the spinal needle. The extent of bone penetration and effort required to obtain bone marrow depend on the site of aspiration and the animal's age. Generally, 1 to 2 cm of penetration of the tuber coxae are sufficient in the adult, and similar sites in the foal require less penetration. Cortical bone is more resistant to needle penetration in adults, and considerably less effort is required to penetrate cortical bone in foals.

Once the spinal needle is properly seated in the marrow cavity, the stylet is removed from the needle, and bone marrow is aspirated into a 12-ml syringe containing 1 to 2 drops of 10% disodium ethylenediaminetetraacetate (EDTA) or 1 to 2 ml of a 2% EDTA solution. Strong suction usually is necessary to aspirate bone marrow; the syringe plunger can be withdrawn to the 10-ml mark with little damage to hematopoietic cells. About 0.2 ml (2 to 4 drops) of marrow are aspirated into the syringe. If marrow cannot be aspirated, the stylet is replaced, and the needle is repositioned slightly (proximally or distally) depending on clinical judgment. Another attempt to aspirate bone marrow is then made. When marrow aspiration is complete, the syringe may be detached, and the specimen and anticoagulant are mixed with a swirling motion. If small bone marrow particles can be observed along the barrel of the syringe, the spinal needle is removed.

Occasionally, bone marrow may be collected at necropsy. Specimens must be obtained within 30 minutes of death because subsequent cellular degeneration may preclude adequate examination. Bone marrow is most easily and quickly obtained by cracking a rib, carefully removing cortical bone fragments, and gently recovering the gelatinous marrow. The marrow specimen can subsequently be used to prepare cytologic touch imprints or smears, after which the remaining marrow can be preserved in 10% neutral-buffered formalin solution for histologic evaluation.

Specimen Preparation and Staining

A few drops of marrow suspension are expelled onto a slide that is held vertically (Fig. 15-1). Marrow particles adhere, whereas blood flows down the slide. Squash preparations are made by holding a second slide at a right angle to the first slide and pressing gently while pulling the second slide laterally (Fig. 15-1). Alternatively, the marrow may be expelled into a Petri dish, where particles may be selected with a Pasteur pipette. Particles are placed on a slide, and squash preparations are made as described earlier. For marrow core biopsies, the core can be rolled gently between two slides to produce cytologic specimens before tissue fixation. For necropsy specimens, a small portion of marrow is used to prepare cytologic touch imprints or squash preparations.

Once air-dried, bone marrow specimens may be stained by the classic Wright's stain technique or rapid modification of the Wright's stain procedure using Diff-Quik stain. With the classic Wright's stain, the staining and buffering times should be extended to 5 minutes each because of increased cellularity of the preparations. With the Diff-Quik procedure, bone marrow smears should be dipped in each solution a total of 10 to 20 times to account for increased cellularity. Under low microscopic magnification (10× objective), red, blue, and purple colors should be apparent. Lack of purple color, especially in cell nuclei, indicates insufficient staining. The preparation can be salvaged by repeating the staining procedure on the original smear until the desired tinctorial properties are

TABLE 15-1

Bone Marrow Reference Intervals for Horses

Cell Type	Range (%)	Mean (%)
Myeloid (Granulocytic) Series		
Myeloblasts	0–5	1.0
Promyelocytes (progranulocytes)	0.5–3.5	1.7
Neutrophils		
Myelocytes	1.0–7.5	3.2
Metamyelocytes	1.5–15.0	5.6
Bands	6.0–6.5	15.7
Segmenters	3.0–16.5	8.4
Eosinophils (total)	0.0–5.0	1.8
Basophils (total)	0.0–1.0	0.3
Total myeloid cells	26.5–45.0	35.7
Erythroid Series		
Rubriblasts, prorubricytes	0.0–2.0	0.7
Rubricytes, metarubricytes	29.5–89.5	55.0
Total erythroid cells	47.0–69.0	58.0
M/E Ratio	0.48–0.91	0.71
Other Cells		
Lymphocytes	1.5–8.5	3.5
Plasma cells	0.0–2.0	0.6
Monocytes, macrophages	0.0–1.0	0.2
Mitotic figures	0.0–3.5	0.8

achieved. (See Chapter 14 for more information on staining procedures and problems.)

Bone Marrow Evaluation

Adequate evaluation of bone marrow aspirates requires familiarity with normal blood cell development and knowledge of the patient's current complete blood count (CBC) data.[6,7] Familiarity with normal blood cell development is necessary to discern abnormalities in blood cell maturation and morphology rapidly, as well as detect unusual cell populations in a bone marrow aspirate. Knowledge of current blood cell data is mandatory to interpret bone marrow response in various disease states. For example, an impression of an increased myeloid/erythroid (M/E) ratio in the presence of nonregenerative anemia and a normal leukogram suggests erythroid hypoplasia, whereas the impression of an increased M/E ratio in the presence of neutrophilia and a normal packed cell volume suggests granulocytic hyperplasia.

Bone marrow evaluation can be accomplished by subjective assessment of the marrow aspirate in most cases. In a clinical setting, calculation of a precise M/E ratio based on a 500-cell differential count is laborious and often of limited value. Therefore, cursory interpretation of bone marrow specimens should be directed toward an impression of the changes consistent with available clinical findings and CBC data. However, bone marrow reference intervals for horses are included for practitioners who want to perform 500-cell differential counts and calculate M/E ratios (Table 15-1).

Marrow sample evaluation involves subjective assessment of particle cellularity; megakaryocyte numbers and maturity; and erythroid and myeloid development, maturation, and morphology. In addition, the presence of lymphoid cells, macrophages, stromal cells, and

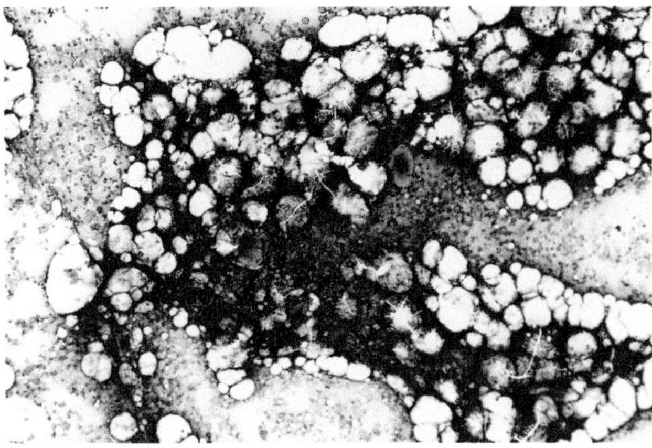

Fig. 15-2 Normocellular bone marrow particle consisting of 50% fat (clear spaces) and 50% hematopoietic cells.

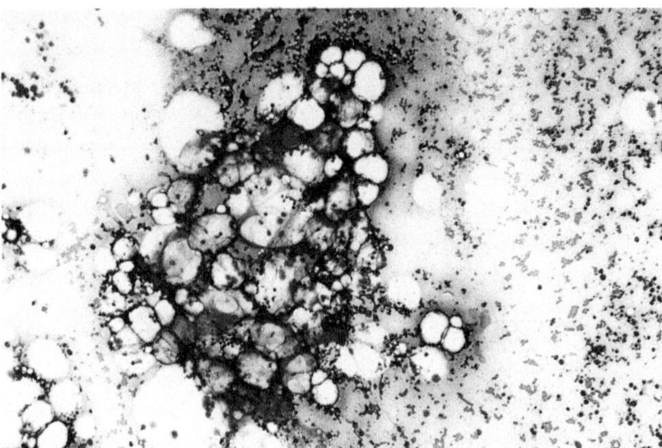

Fig. 15-3 Hypocellular bone marrow particle with abundant fat (>50%) and few hematopoietic cells.

unusual cell populations should be addressed. Examination should proceed in a systematic manner so important changes are not overlooked. Generally, particle cellularity, megakaryocyte numbers, and megakaryocyte maturation are evaluated at lower magnification using the 4× to 20× microscope objectives. Erythroid and myeloid maturation and other critical examinations of cell morphology should be done using the 45× to 50× and 100× microscope objectives.

Particle Cellularity

Precise evaluation of bone marrow cellularity requires histologic examination of bone marrow core biopsies taken from a site of active hematopoiesis or disease. Bone marrow core biopsy is not performed routinely in many private practices, so marrow cellularity is assessed cytologically using stained marrow smears and the 10× microscope objective. Bone marrow particles in cytologic preparations consist of *fat* (appearing as clear spaces or balloon-like adipocytes) and clusters of *hematopoietic cells*, in which dense aggregates of cells stain dark bluish purple. *Normocellular* particles observed in healthy adult horses consist of 50% fat and 50% cells (Fig. 15-2). *Hypocellular* particles consist mainly of fat (Fig. 15-3), and *hypercellular* particles are composed of dense cellular aggregates (Fig. 15-4). Hypocellular bone marrow particles suggest decreased hematopoiesis. In contrast, hypercellular particles suggest increased hematopoiesis (normal or abnormal response), infiltrative disease, or primary or metastatic neoplasia. Examination of the cellular composition of the marrow at higher magnification determines which of these conditions exists.

Megakaryocyte Number and Maturity

Adequate numbers of mature megakaryocytes are necessary for normal platelet production. Megakaryocytes are the largest cells usually encountered in marrow aspirates. Osteoclasts, although large, are infrequently observed and are distinctly multinucleate. Megakaryocytes are about 100 μm in diameter, contain abundant cytoplasm, and have a lobulated nucleus. Immature megakaryocytes are smaller, contain fewer nuclear lobulations, and have blue granular cytoplasm (Fig. 15-5). Mature megakaryocytes are larger, have increased nuclear lobulations, and contain pink granular cytoplasm (Fig. 15-6).

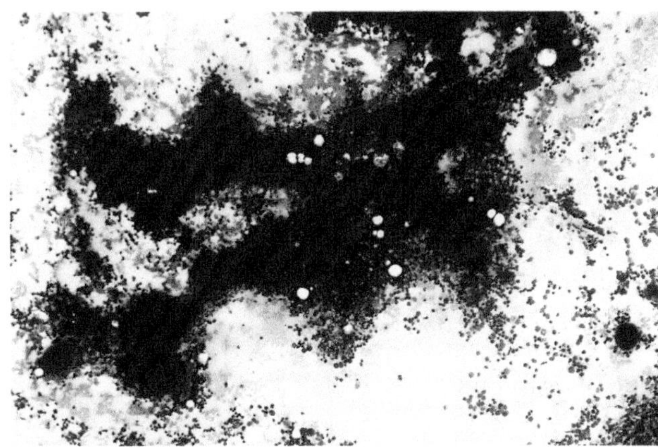

Fig. 15-4 Hypercellular bone marrow particle containing increased proportion of hematopoietic cells and very little fat.

In health, one to several megakaryocytes may be observed per 10× objective field of view. Megakaryocytes are most often noticeable within or around bone marrow particles but also may be scattered singly throughout the smear. An absence of megakaryocytes in conjunction with thrombocytopenia suggests decreased platelet production. Frequent to increased numbers of megakaryocytes in conjunction

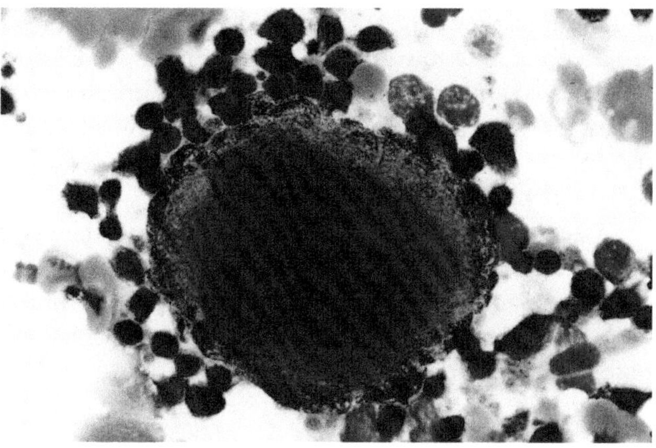

Fig. 15-5 Immature megakaryocyte containing fewer nuclear lobulations and blue granular cytoplasm.

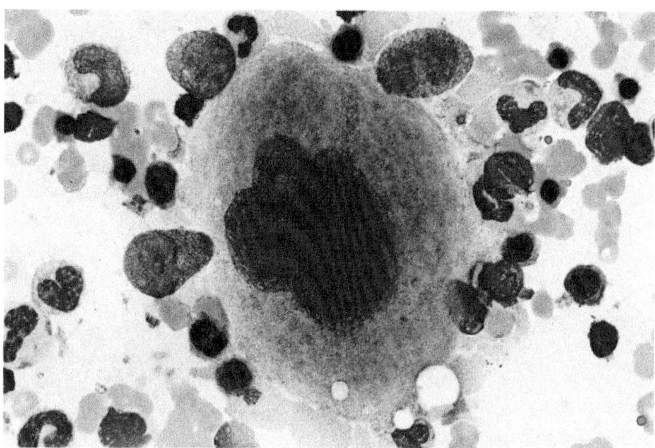

Fig. 15-6 Mature megakaryocyte with many nuclear lobulations and abundant pink granular cytoplasm.

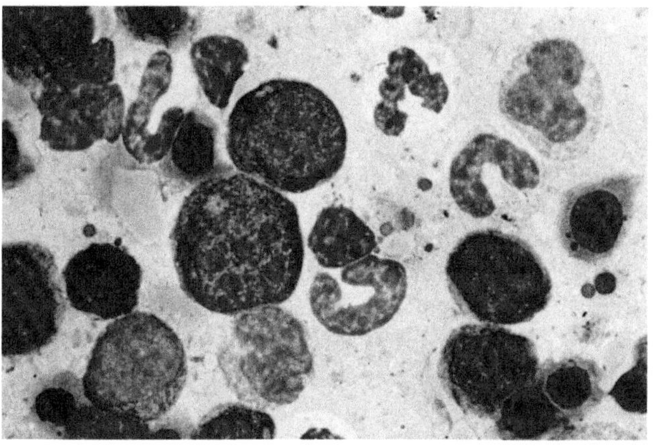

Fig. 15-7 Bone marrow smear from an anemic horse with erythroid hyperplasia. Rubriblasts, prorubricytes, and rubricytes predominate.

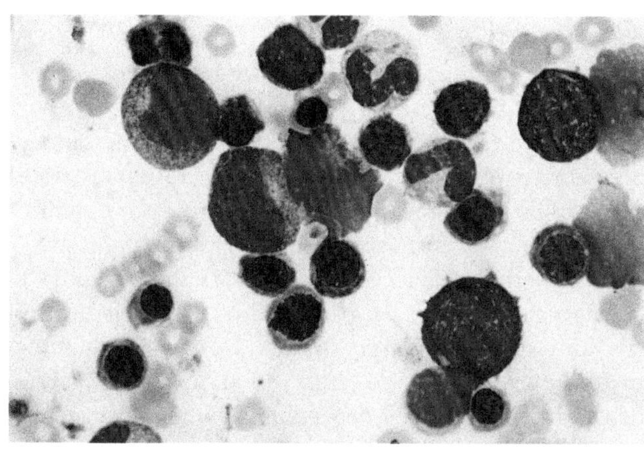

Fig. 15-8 Bone marrow smear from an anemic horse with erythroid hyperplasia contains many rubricytes and metarubricytes. Polychromatophilic erythrocytes are present in the background.

with thrombocytopenia suggest platelet consumption or destruction.

Erythroid Series

In Health: As erythroid cells mature, cell size decreases, the nuclear chromatin pattern becomes progressively more dense until the nucleus is extruded, and cytoplasmic color changes from blue to gray to red-orange as the ribosomes of young cells produce hemoglobin for oxygen transport. Maturation is orderly and sequential, progressing through the following stages: rubriblast, prorubricyte, rubricyte, metarubricyte, polychromatophilic erythrocyte (reticulocyte), and mature erythrocyte. In health, about 5% of the erythroid population consists of prorubricytes and rubriblasts. The remaining 95% of the erythroid series consists of rubricytes and metarubricytes.

Rubriblasts are relatively large cells with a centrally located round nucleus, fine chromatin pattern, one or two prominent nucleoli, and a thin rim of royal-blue, slightly granular cytoplasm. A pale-staining Golgi zone may be observed in the cytoplasm adjacent to the nucleus (Fig. 15-7).

Prorubricytes are similar in appearance to rubriblasts except that their nuclear chromatin is slightly more granular. Nucleoli are not apparent (Fig. 15-7).

Rubricytes vary in size according to time elapsed since mitosis and degree of maturity. Recent daughter cells and more mature rubricytes are smaller. More mature rubricytes have progressively condensed chromatin patterns, but the nucleus is centrally located (Figs. 15-8 and 15-9).

Metarubricytes have a very condensed chromatin pattern, the "ink dot" nucleus. The nucleus is often centrally to

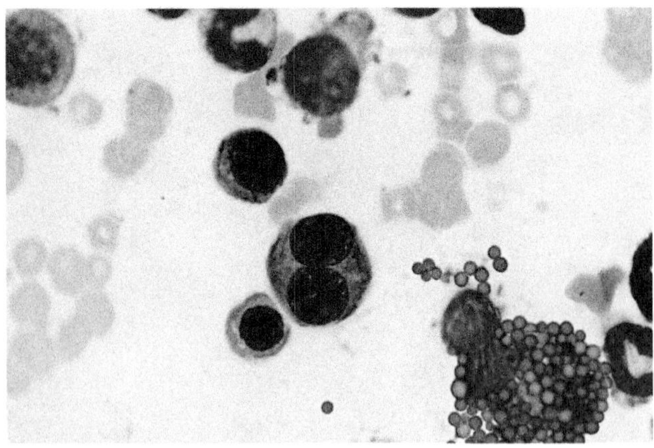

Fig. 15-9 Bone marrow smear from a horse with nonregenerative anemia and mild leukopenia. Binucleate erythrocytes suggest abnormal red cell production.

eccentrically located and the cytoplasmic color may vary from light blue-gray to grayish orange (Fig. 15-9).

Polychromatophilic erythrocytes in Romanowsky-stained bone marrow smears are anucleate erythrocytes with a uniformly blue-gray to gray-orange cytoplasm, depending on the concentration of hemoglobin (Fig. 15-8). In new methylene blue–stained smears, these cells have an aggregate or reticular pattern due to aggregation of ribosomes and are called *reticulocytes*. Thus, polychromatophilic erythrocyte and reticulocyte are terms describing the same cell, depending on which stain is used to identify it.

Mature erythrocytes are anucleate, may contain very slight central pallor, and stain red-orange because of an abundance of hemoglobin. Rarely, these cells may contain a small, round remnant of nuclear material that stains deep purple, called a Howell-Jolly body (see Chapter 14).

In Disease: The basic question in evaluating the erythroid series is to determine whether anemia is regenerative or nonregenerative. Basic laboratory information includes the packed cell volume, appearance of the erythrocytes on the stained blood smear, and total plasma protein concentration (see Fig. 14-20).

In cases of *regenerative anemia* the M/E ratio is decreased due to a preponderance of erythroid cells (see Figs. 15-7 and 15-8). Most of these cells are rubricytes and metarubricytes, but a slight shift to immaturity (>5% of the erythroid cells are prorubricytes or younger) may be observed. Romanowsky-stained bone marrow smears have a greater proportion of polychromatophilic erythrocytes in the background; these cells appear as reticulocytes in new methylene blue–stained marrow smears. Also, the number of Howell-Jolly bodies may be increased.

In summary, evidence of erythroid regeneration is present in a bone marrow aspiration biopsy if the M/E ratio is decreased, more than 5% of anucleate erythrocytes appear as polychromatophilic cells after Romanowsky staining, or more than 5% reticulocytes are observed after new methylene blue staining.

In *nonregenerative anemia*, numbers of cells in the erythroid series are decreased or these cells are infrequently observed. Generally, most of these cells appear as late rubricytes or metarubricytes; prorubricytes and rubricytes are observed rarely.

Erythroid neoplasia is extremely rare in horses, although one case of primary erythrocytosis (polycythemia vera) has been observed.[3] Bone marrow examination in primary erythrocytosis is unrewarding, as erythroid cells mature normally despite unregulated red blood cell production. Erythrocyte maturation abnormalities, such as binucleate erythrocytes or asynchronous nuclear to cytoplasmic maturation, rarely are observed (see Fig. 15-9). Likewise, myeloproliferative diseases are rare in horses.

Leukocytic Series

Granulocytic Series in Health: Granulocytic cells include neutrophils, eosinophils, basophils, and their precursors. In Romanowsky-stained bone marrow smears, the more mature cells are recognized by the staining reactions of their specific or secondary granules. Neutrophil granules are colorless or neutral, eosinophil granules are red-orange, and basophil granules are purple. Specific granules are first discerned by light microscopy at the myelocyte stage of development. Cell development and maturation follow an orderly process in the following sequence: myeloblast, promyelocyte (progranulocyte), myelocyte, metamyelocyte, band, and segmenter.

In health, 85% or more of the granulocytes (especially neutrophils) are metamyelocytes, bands, or segmenters. The remaining cells are promyelocytes or myeloblasts. The following discussion presents identifying features of these cells during sequential maturation in the bone marrow.

Myeloblasts are relatively large cells with a round central nucleus, fine chromatin pattern, and one or more nucleoli (Fig. 15-10). The thin rim of blue cytoplasm is devoid of discernible granules.

Promyelocytes (progranulocytes) have slightly more condensed chromatin and nucleoli are inapparent (Figs. 15-10 and 15-11). The light-blue cytoplasm contains scattered primary granules that stain pinkish purple. In contrast to the chunky specific granules in cells of the basophilic series, the granules within promyelocytes are very fine.

Myelocytes have a round to oval nucleus and lack visible nucleoli. The chromatin pattern is more con-

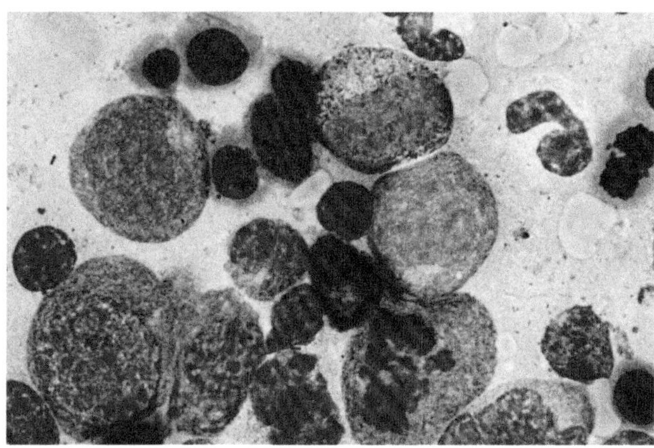

Fig. 15-10 Bone marrow smear from a horse with granulocytic hyperplasia in response to infection. Myeloblasts, promyelocytes, and band neutrophils are present.

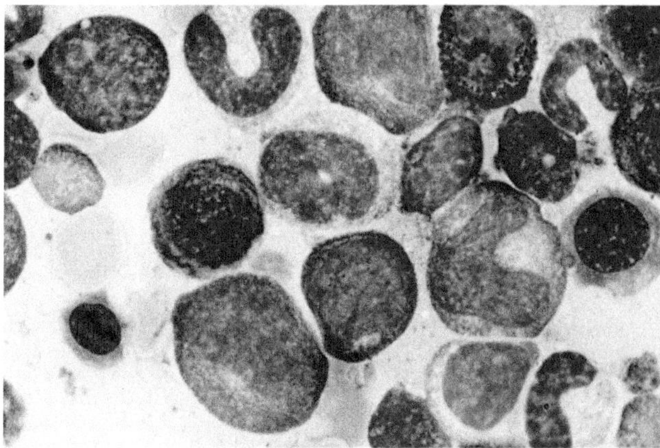

Fig. 15-11 Bone marrow smear from a horse with granulocytic hyperplasia. A myeloblast, promyelocyte, and metamyelocyte *(center)* are surrounded by band neutrophils, rubricytes, and a basophilic metamyelocyte.

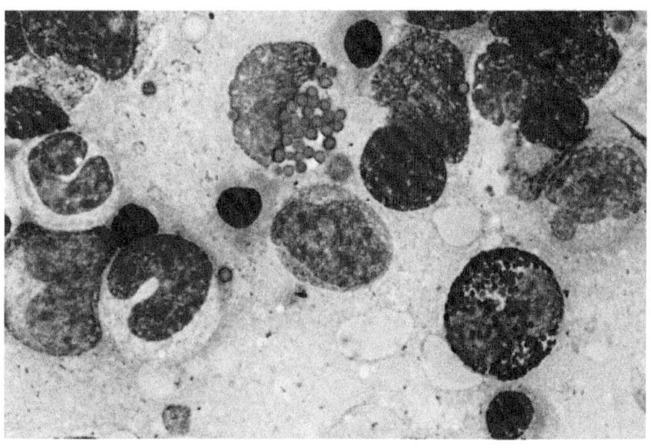

Fig. 15-12 Basophilic metamyelocyte and ruptured eosinophil precursor demonstrate the size of specific basophil and eosinophil granules.

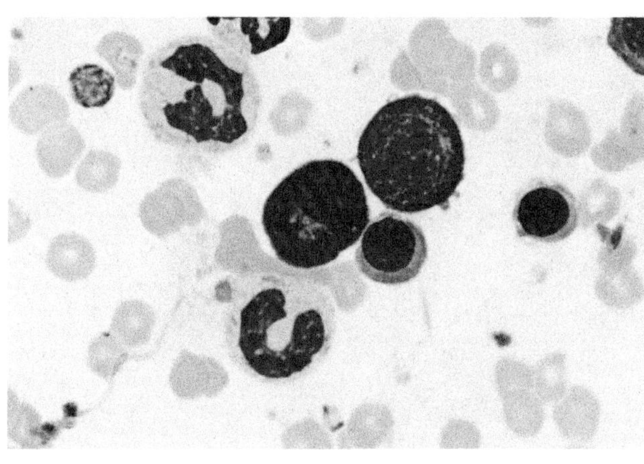

Fig. 15-13 Band and segmented neutrophils are admixed with rubricytes and a single plasma cell.

densed than that of promyelocytes. The tinctorial properties of the specific (secondary) granules allow classification of myelocytes and all subsequent stages of development as members of the neutrophilic, eosinophilic, or basophilic series (Fig. 15-12).

Metamyelocytes have a slightly indented nucleus with bulbous ends that may assume a dumbbell appearance (Figs. 15-10 and 15-11). The cytoplasm may retain a pale-blue cast.

Band neutrophils have an S- or U-shaped nucleus with parallel sides and moderately condensed chromatin (Fig. 15-13). Nuclear indentations, if present, are less than 50% of the width of the nucleus.

Segmented neutrophils usually have a lobulated nucleus (Fig. 15-13), although nuclei of segmenters in some horses may be poorly lobulated. In these animals, jagged nuclear margins may be observed in the absence of distinct lobulation. Nuclear indentations, if present, exceed 50% of the nuclear width.

Granulocytic Series in Disease: With severe systemic *inflammation*, *infection* (endotoxemia, bacteremia), or marrow *toxins*, changes in the bone marrow may precede those in the blood by 3 to 5 days. An example would be a horse with acute salmonellosis and neutropenia. If the bone marrow is preparing to respond to the increased tissue demand for neutrophils, bone marrow aspirates would display granulocytic hyperplasia (Figs. 15-10 and 15-11). Further, the storage pool of segmenters and bands may be depleted, suggesting a

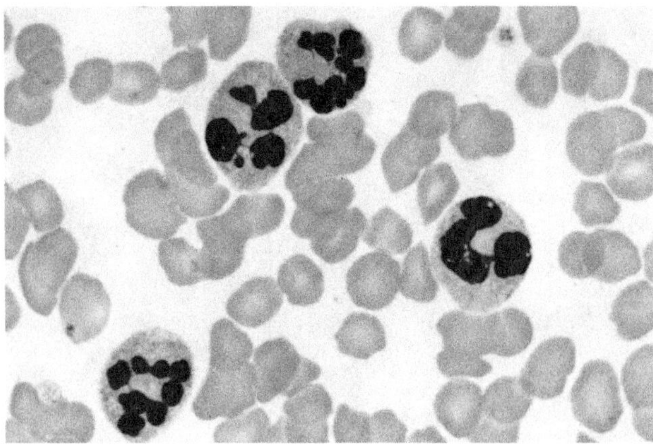

Fig. 15-14 Bone marrow smear from horse with idiopathic neutrophil hypersegmentation. Neutrophils show progressive segmentation. (Courtesy Dr. K.W. Praase.)

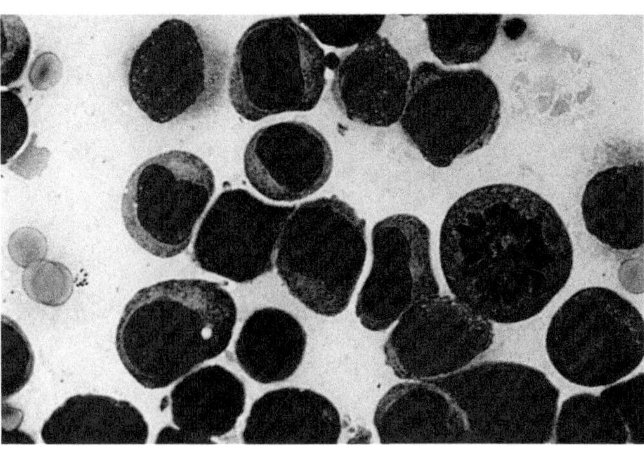

Fig. 15-15 Bone marrow smear from a horse with myelomonocytic leukemia. Developing blast cells exhibit some degree of nuclear indentation. Mitotic figure is also present. (Courtesy Dr. Julia Blue.)

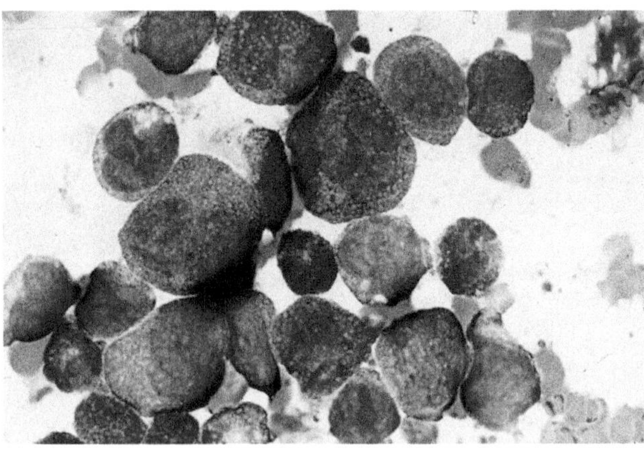

Fig. 15-16 Bone marrow smear from a horse with eosinophilic myeloproliferative disease. Maturing blasts and promyelocytes exhibit small, round eosinophilic granules. Normally, blasts and promyelocytes do not contain specific granules. (Courtesy Dr. Debra Deem Morris.)

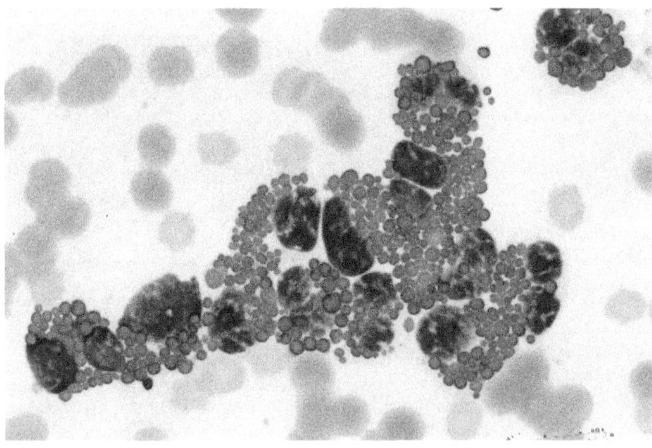

Fig. 15-17 Bone marrow smear from a horse with hypereosinophilic syndrome. Eosinophilic myelocytes to segmented neutrophils display prominent granule formation.

shift to immaturity, in which myeloid precursors are proliferating to expand neutrophil production. In such states, cells of the neutrophilic series may exhibit toxic changes (cytoplasmic basophilia, cytoplasmic vacuolation, Döhle bodies, toxic granulation) and nuclear maturation abnormalities (ring-shaped nuclei) may be observed (see Chapter 14).

In cases of *pancytopenia*, myeloid precursors (especially neutrophil precursors) may be depleted. Causes of pancytopenia include drugs, toxins, and ionizing radiation, but the precise cause of pancytopenia may be obscure in some instances.[8-10]

Bone marrow necrosis may result from bacterial toxin production. Marrow aspirates from neutropenic animals may stain poorly, and cells may lyse easily or may appear extremely degenerate. A bone marrow core biopsy is often necessary to confirm a subjective impression of bone marrow necrosis.

Idiopathic hypersegmentation of neutrophil nuclei has been observed in a horse.[11] Most neutrophils in the blood were hypersegmented, sometimes containing more than 11 nuclear lobes. Neutrophil maturation proceeds to nuclear hypersegmentation within the bone marrow (Fig. 15-14; see also Fig. 14-30). Neutrophil hypersegmentation appears benign because a predisposition to infection has not been recorded. Although its hereditary nature is unknown, neutrophil nuclear hypersegmentation may prove to be of congenital origin when other cases are reported.

Nonlymphoid leukemias have been reported rarely in horses.[1,12-16] Leukemia is an unregulated production of hematopoietic cells within the bone marrow. Suspicion of a leukemic state is the result of finding increased numbers of blast and immature cells in the blood, which may be accompanied by cell lines showing variable degrees of maturation. Alternatively, the presence of an extremely large number of more mature cells, such as neutrophils, may arouse suspicion of leukemia.

Bone marrow aspirates are highly cellular, with an increased number of blasts. With diligent examination, the specific cell line may be discerned. These findings have been reported for granulocytic, monocytic and myelomonocytic (a mixture of neutrophils and monocytes) leukemias in horses (Fig. 15-15).[1,12-16] Eosinophilic leukemia/myeloproliferative disease also has been reported, but it is difficult if not impossible to distinguish from idiopathic hypereosinophilic syndromes (Figs. 15-16 and 15-17).[17,18] Some leukemias, such as those involving stem cells and blasts, may be difficult to diagnose without cytochemical staining or ultrastructural examination of the neoplastic cell line.[1,7,12] Consultation with a veterinary hematologist or oncologist may be necessary to diagnose some leukemias.

Other Cells in Health: Other cells encountered less frequently in bone marrow smears from healthy horses include lymphocytes, bone marrow stem cells, plasma cells, monocytes, macrophages, mitotic figures, osteoblasts, and osteoclasts.

Lymphocytes are small cells that are intermediate in size between erythrocytes and neutrophils. They have a slightly indented nucleus that almost fills the cytoplasm. The nuclear chromatin pattern is very dense. A thin rim of light-blue cytoplasm may be discerned. Lymphocytes may constitute 2% to 9% of the bone marrow nucleated cell population. *Bone marrow stem cells* are morphologically indistinguishable from small lymphocytes in Wright-stained bone marrow smears. Lymphocytes and bone marrow stem cells are more conspicuous in cases of marked pancytopenia.

Plasma cells (plamacytes) have a round, eccentric nucleus with a coarse, patchy chromatin pattern (Fig. 15-13). Cytoplasm is abundant, dark blue, and often contains a Golgi zone. These features allow the microscopist to distinguish this cell from a rubricyte. Plasma cells constitute less than 2% of the nucleated cell population of normal bone marrow aspirates, but plasma cell numbers may be increased somewhat during antigenic stimulation.

Monocytes and *macrophages* are recognized by an oval to lobate nucleus, lacy chromatin pattern, and abundant gray cytoplasm. Monocytes may have pseudopodia, and macrophages may contain hemosiderin or cellular debris (Fig. 15-18). These cells account for 1% or less of the marrow nucleated cell population. In health, monocytes are infrequently observed because a maturation and storage pool for these cells does not exist in the bone marrow as it does for neutrophils. Therefore, monocytes are only recognized readily in cases of profound neutropenia, especially when compensatory monocytosis is noted in the leukogram.

Mitotic figures are characterized by ribbon-like chromosomes, bluish cytoplasm, and distinct cell membranes (Fig. 15-19). Mitotic figures account for 4% or less of the entire nucleated bone marrow cell population. Considerable hematopoietic cell turnover occurs in health, and cell turnover may increase in disease states. The presence of mitotic activity is expected, and mitotic figures do not invariably signify neoplasia.

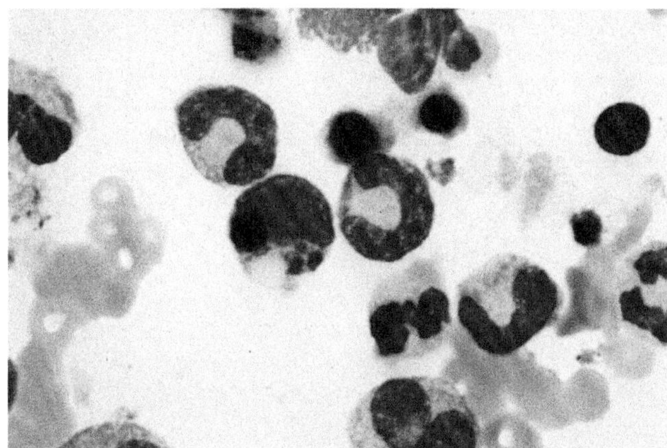

Fig. 15-18 Bone marrow macrophage *(center)* contains phagocytosed nuclear material and golden-brown hemosiderin particles.

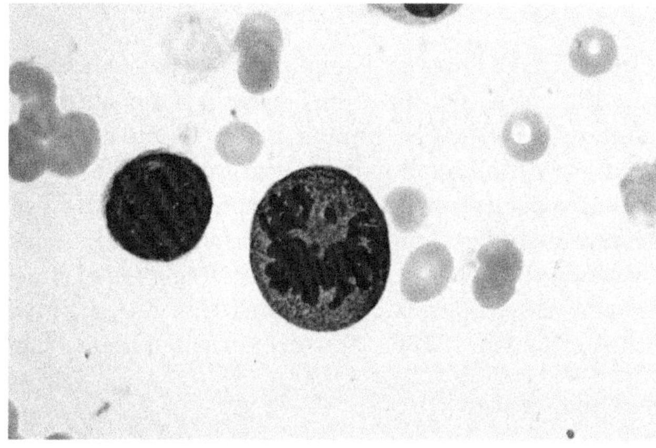

Fig. 15-19 Mitotic figure and rubricyte in bone marrow smear.

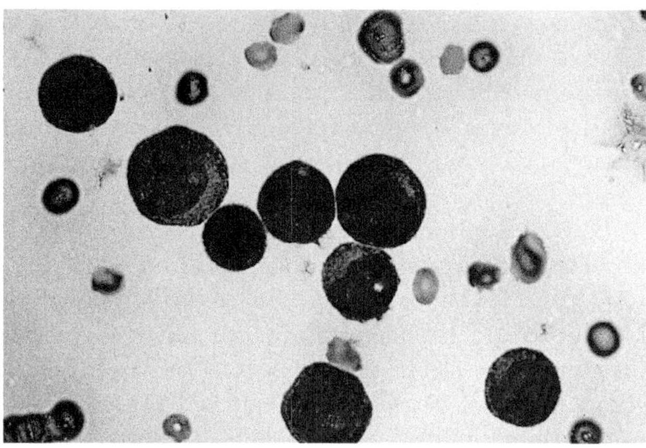

Fig. 15-20 Bone marrow smear from horse with disseminated lymphosarcoma. Most of the cells are medium- to large-sized, immature lymphocytes. A single small, well-differentiated lymphocyte is present for size comparison.

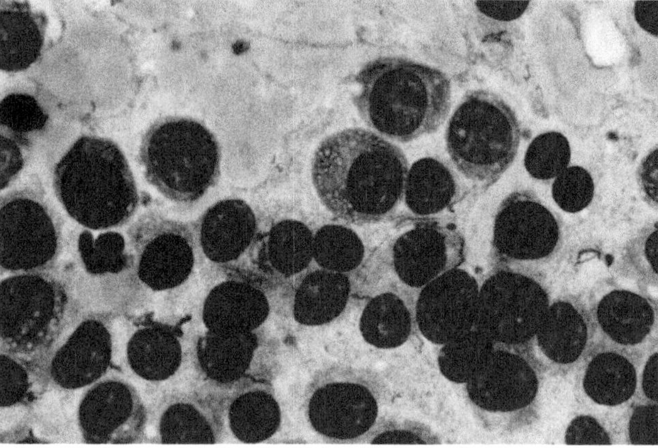

Fig. 15-21 Bone marrow smear from horse with plasmacyte myeloma. Lymphoid cells show distinct plasmacytoid differentiation.

Other Cells in Disease: Lymphoid neoplasia is encountered infrequently, but in such cases marrow aspirates contain a relatively homogeneous population of cells.[1,5,7,12,19] In lymphosarcoma with marrow involvement, neoplastic lymphocytes may appear large, with a fine chromatin pattern, multiple nucleoli, and blue granular cytoplasm that often contains a pale-staining Golgi zone (Fig. 15-20). In plasma-cell myeloma/leukemia, marrow aspirates contain 15% to 20% recognizable plasma cells (Fig. 15-21). In addition, monoclonal gammopathy, Bence Jones proteinuria, and osteolysis may be present.[19]

Stromal reactions may be difficult to recognize cytologically, although increased fibroblasts, osteoblasts, or osteoclasts may be visualized on rare occasions. Bone marrow core biopsies are the preferred specimen to diagnose such disorders as myelofibrosis, osteopetrosis, and necrosis.

REFERENCES

1. Latimer and Mahaffey, in Colahan et al: Equine Medicine and Surgery. 5th ed. St Louis, 1999, Mosby, pp 1973-1981, 1989-2001, 2025-2031.
2. Valli and Parry, in Jubb et al: Pathology of Domestic Animals. 4th ed. Academic Press, New York, 1993. pp 101-265.
3. Beech et al: Erythrocytosis in a horse. JAVMA 184:986-989, 1984.
4. Cowell, Tyler, and Meinkoth: *Diagnostic Cytology and Hematology of the Dog and Cat.* 2nd ed. St Louis, 1999, Mosby, pp 284-304.
5. Jacobs et al: Monoclonal gammopathy in a horse with defective hemostasis. Vet Pathol 20:643-647, 1983.
6. Schalm: *Manual of Equine Hematology.* Santa Barbara, Calif, 1984, Veterinary Practice Publishing.
7. Feldman, Zinkl, and Jain: *Schalm's Veterinary Hematology.* 5th ed. Philadelphia, 2000, Lippincott Williams & Wilkins.
8. Brown: Physiologic responses to exercise of irradiated and nonirradiated Shetland ponies: a five year study. *Am J Vet Res* 36:645-652, 1975.
9. Bello et al: Effects of the immunosuppressant methotrexate in ponies. Am J Vet Res 34:1291-1297, 1973.
10. Berggren: Aplastic anemia in a horse. *JAVMA* 179:1400-1402, 1981.
11. Prasse et al: Idiopathic hypersegmentation of neutrophils in a horse. JAVMA 178:303-305, 1981.
12. McClure: Leukoproliferative disorders in horses. *Vet Clin North Am Equine Pract* 16:165-182, 2000.
13. Searcy and Orr: Chronic granulocytic leukemia in a horse. *Can Vet J* 22:148-151, 1981.
14. Ringger et al: Acute myelogenous leukaemia in a mare. Aust Vet J 75:329-331, 1997.
15. Monteith and Cole: Monocytic leukemia in a horse. *Can Vet J* 36:765-766, 1995.
16. Buechner-Maxwell et al: Intravascular leukostasis and systemic aspergillosis in a horse with subleukemic acute myelomonocytic leukemia. J Vet Intern Med 8:258-263, 1994.
17. Morris et al: Eosinophilic myeloproliferative disorder in a horse. JAVMA 185:993-996, 1984.
18. Latimer et al: Extreme eosinophilia with disseminated eosinophilic granulomatous disease in a horse. Vet Clin Pathol 25:23-26, 1996.
19. Edwards et al: Plasma cell myeloma in the horse: a case report and literature review. J Vet Intern Med 7:169-176, 1993.

Color Plates

Plate 1

1A. Nondegenerate neutrophil. Note the tightly clumped, dark-staining (basophilic) nuclear chromatin. (Wright's stain, original magnification 250X)

1B. A hypersegmented neutrophil *(arrow)*. Hypersegmentation is an age-related change. (Wright's stain, original magnification 250X)

1C. Toxic band neutrophils. Toxic changes develop in neutrophils during their production in the bone marrow and are caused by inflammation. (Wright's stain, original magnification 250X)

1D. Neutrophils showing hydropic degeneration (degenerative neutrophils). Hydropic degeneration develops in neutrophils after they have migrated from the blood into an area of inflammation. It is caused by such toxins as endotoxin. Note that the nuclear chromatin is spread out, fills up more of the cytoplasm, and stains more eosinophilic than that of the nondegenerate neutrophil. Bacterial rods *(arrows)* are present within the cytoplasm of some of the neutrophils. A pyknotic cell with round, somewhat eosinophilic spheres of nuclear chromatin is also present *(double arrow)*. (Wright's stain, original magnification 250X)

1E. Plasma cell *(arrow)*, characterized by an eccentric round nucleus with abundant deep blue cytoplasm and a prominent clear Golgi apparatus, and small lymphocytes. (Wright's stain, original magnification 250X)

1F. Lymphoblasts, characterized by a moderate amount of bluish cytoplasm and finely stippled nuclear chromatin and visible nucleolus. (Wright's stain, original magnification 250X)

1G. A reactive lymphocyte, characterized by an increased amount of bluish cytoplasm. (Wright's stain, original magnification 250X)

1H. A reactive lymphocyte. (Wright's stain, original magnification 250X)

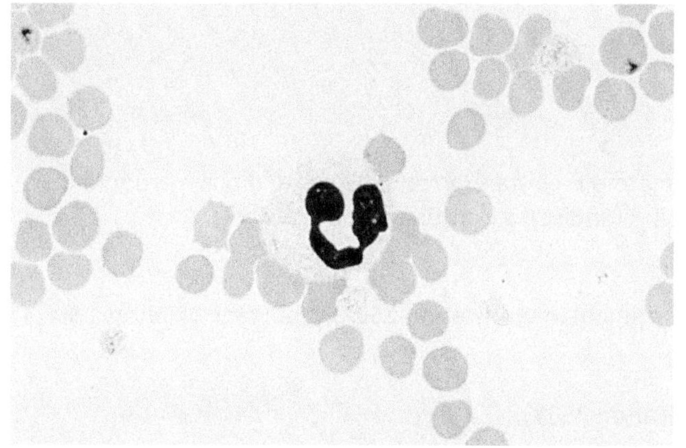

Plate 1A

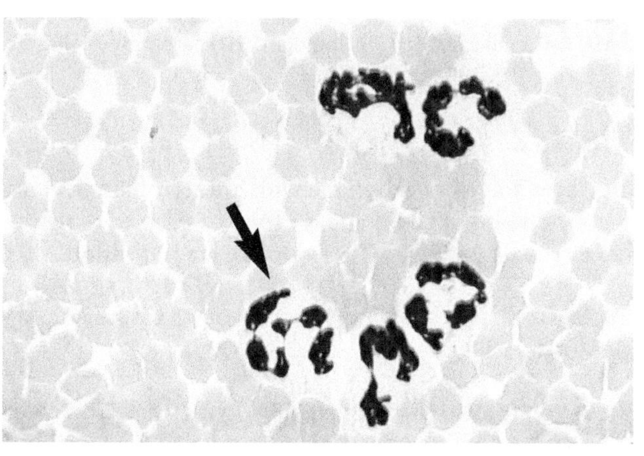

Plate 1B

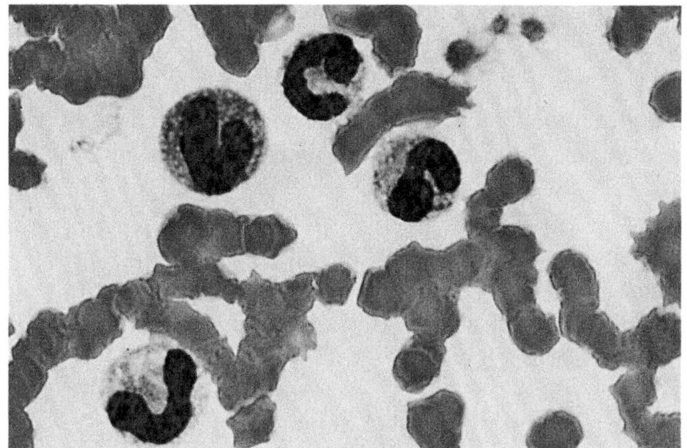

Plate 1C

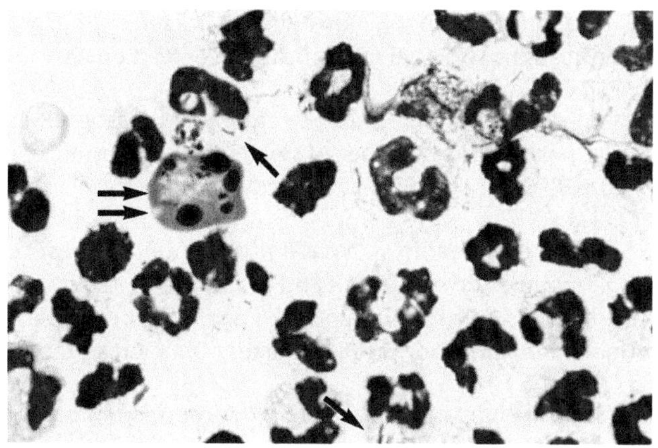

Plate 1D

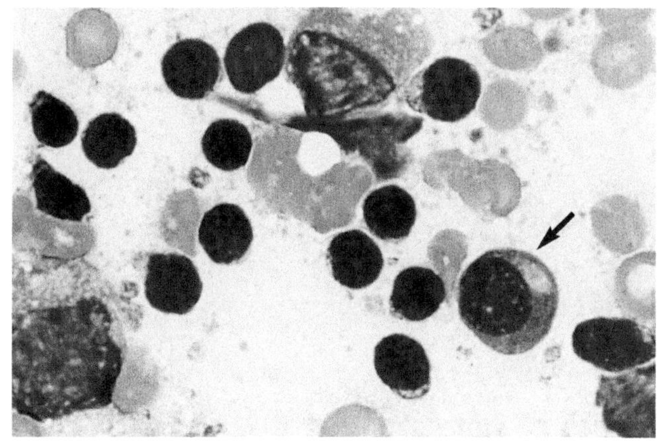

Plate 1E

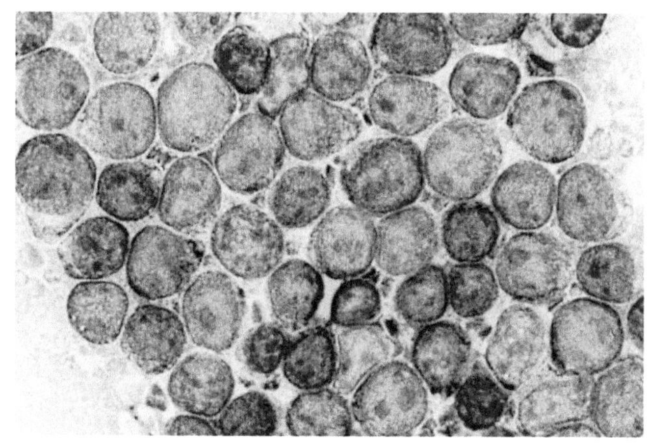

Plate 1F

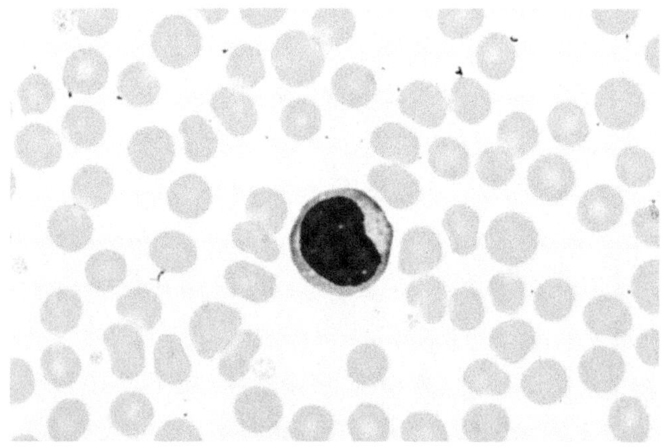

Figure 1G

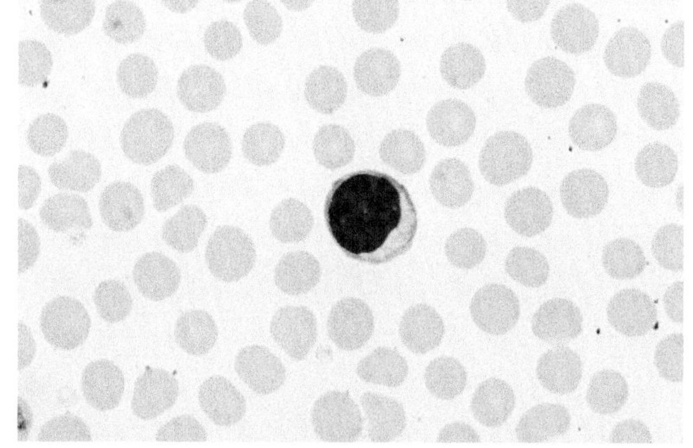

Plate 1H

Plate 2

2A. Large foamy macrophage with intracytoplasmic golden, hematoidin crystals *(arrows)*. Hematoidin is a product of erythrocyte breakdown and is often referred to as tissue bilirubin. It indicates intratissue or intracavity hemorrhage. (Wright's stain, original magnification 250X)

2B. Macrophages showing erythrophagocytosis. (Wright's stain, original magnification 250X) (Courtesy Oklahoma State University, Stillwater.)

2C. An epitheloid macrophage. (Wright's stain, original magnification 250X)

2D. Foamy macrophages from peritoneal fluid. (Wright's stain, original magnification 100X)

2E. The equine eosinophil *(arrow)* is characterized by large, round, eosinophilic (red) intracytoplasmic granules. (Wright's stain, original magnification 250X) (Courtesy Oklahoma State University, Stillwater.)

2F. An eosinophil, two lymphocytes, and two basophils *(arrows)*. Equine basophils are characterized by a segmented nucleus and a large number of small intracytoplasmic basophilic granules. (Wright's stain, original magnification 330X) (Courtesy Oklahoma State University, Stillwater.)

2G. Sediment smear from a nasal flush contains a mast cell *(arrow)* and a goblet cell *(double arrow)*. Mast cells have a single, round to oval nucleus and moderate to large numbers of small, red-purple intracytoplasmic granules. Goblet cells have a single roundish nucleus and large but variably sized, red to blue intracytoplasmic granules. (Wright's stain, original magnification 330X) (Courtesy Oklahoma State University, Stillwater.)

2H. Several endospores *(arrow)* of *Rhinosporidium* in an aspirate of a nasal mass. (Wright's stain, original magnification 250X) (Courtesy Oklahoma State University, Stillwater.)

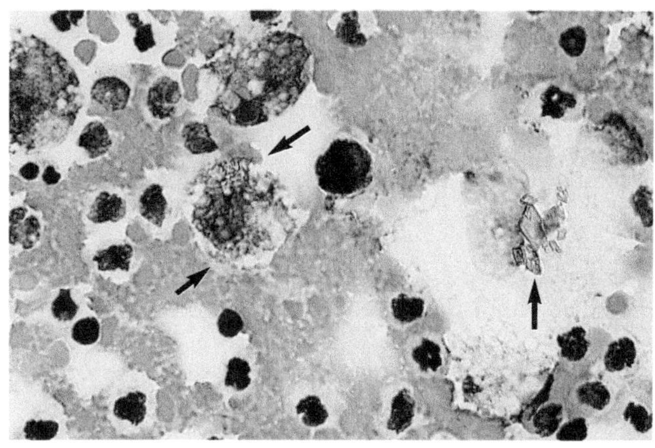

Plate 2A

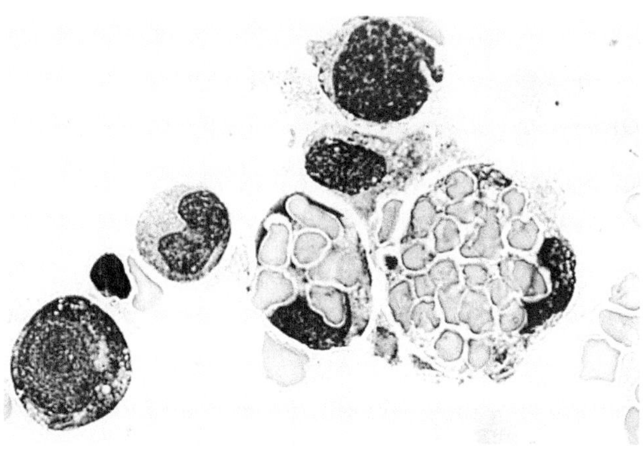

Plate 2B

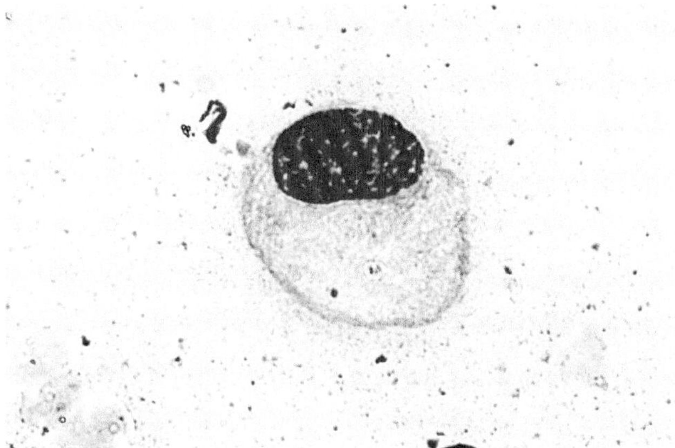

Plate 2C

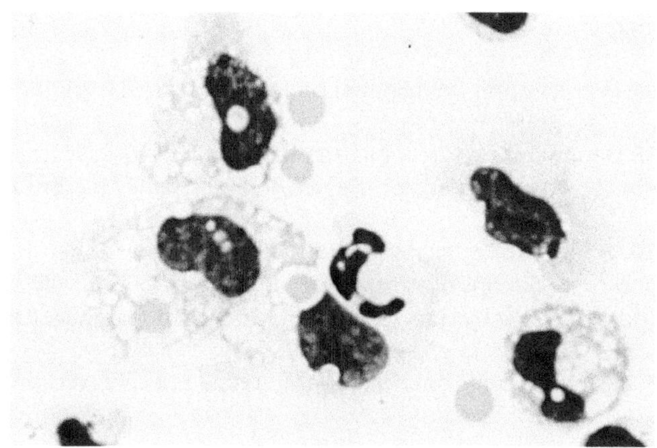

Plate 2D

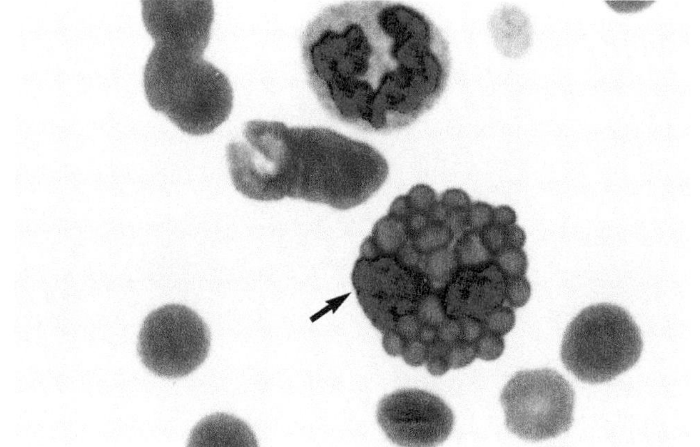

Plate 2E

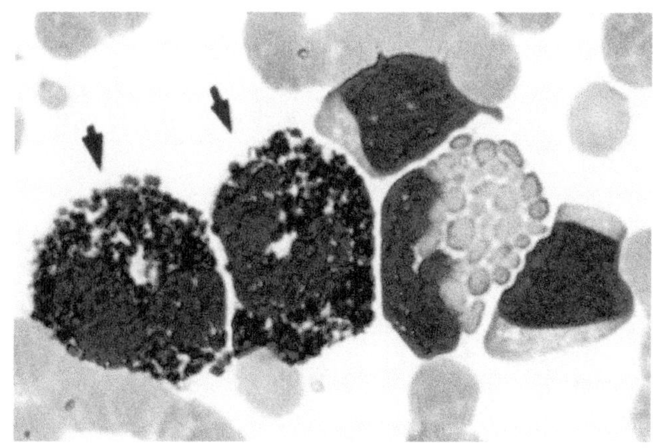

Plate 2F

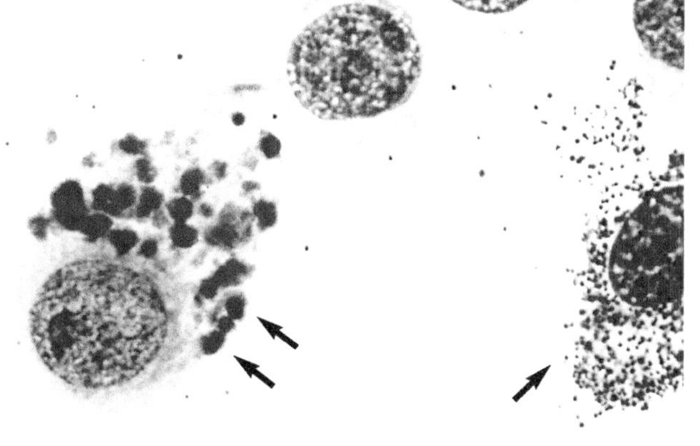

Plate 2G

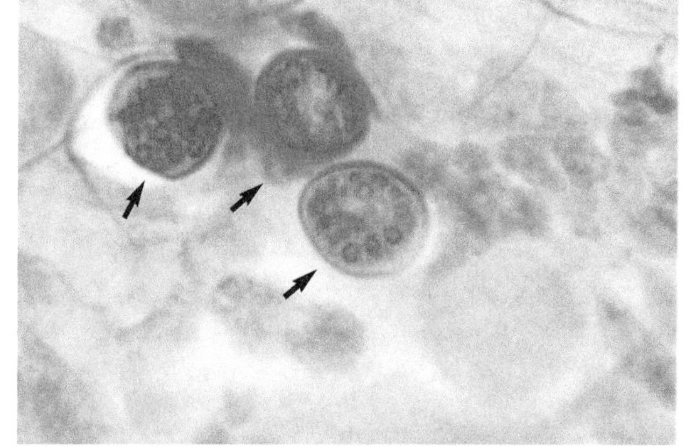

Plate 2H

Plate 3

3A. Purulent inflammation is characterized by the predominance of neutrophils. Many of the neutrophils in this slide are degenerative. (Diff-Quik stain, original magnification 125X)

3B. Pyogranulomatous inflammation. A *Blastomyces dermatitidis* organism *(arrow)* is in the center of the field. Neutrophils, macrophages, and an inflammatory giant cell are present. (Wright's stain, original magnification 250X)

3C. Eosinophilic inflammation is characterized by large numbers of eosinophils. The eosinophils in this slide are readily recognized by their intracytoplasmic round eosinophilic granules. (Wright's stain, original magnification 250X)

3D. *Left,* Numerous small, bipolar bacterial rods are present extracellularly. (Wright's stain, original magnification 250X) *Right,* Several degenerate neutrophils. One neutrophil contains phagocytized bacterial rods. (Wright's stain, original magnification 330X)

3E. A neutrophil containing phagocytized cocci. (Wright's stain, original magnification 250X)

3F. Degenerate neutrophils and bacteria. The long filamentous bacterial rods that stain somewhat blue with reddish dots are characteristic of the Actinomyces family *(arrows).* (Wright's stain, original magnification 250X)

3G. A large superficial squamous cell with many adherent *Simonsiella* bacteria on its surface and a few bacterial rods and cocci. *Simonsiella* organisms appear microscopically as a single large bacterium but are actually several bacterial rods lying side by side, giving the striated appearance. (Wright's stain, original magnification 250X)

3H. A neutrophil containing phagocytized bacilli. (Wright's stain, original magnification 250X)

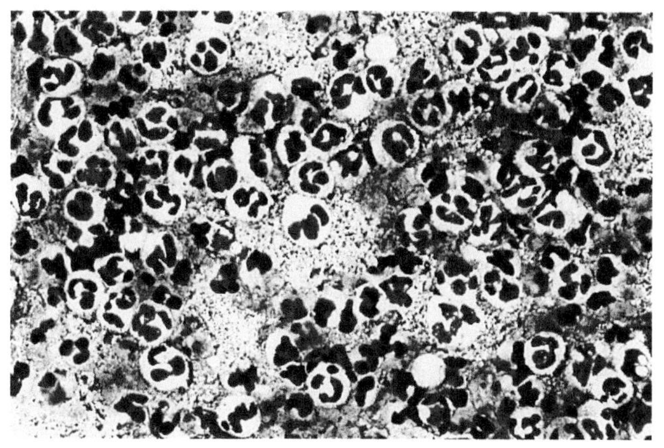

Plate 3A

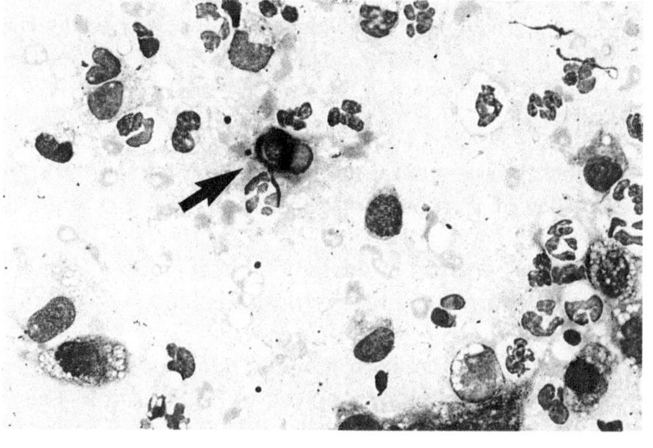

Plate 3B

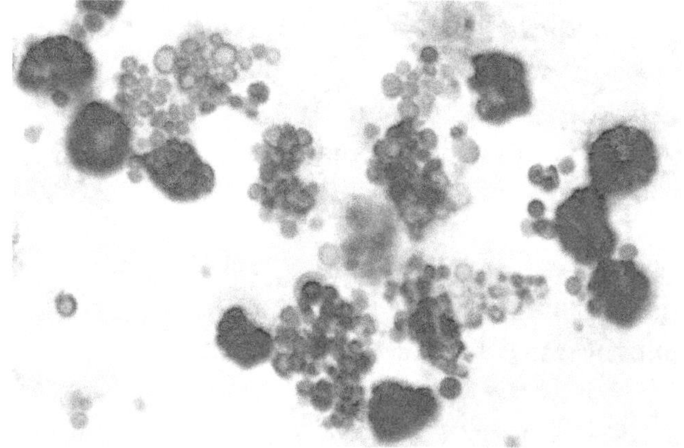

Plate 3C

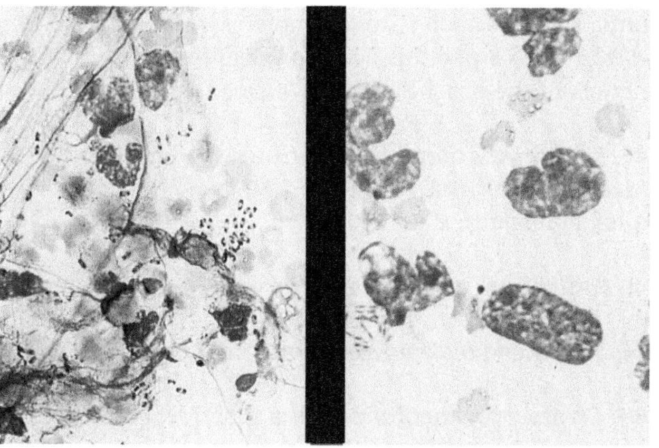

Plate 3D

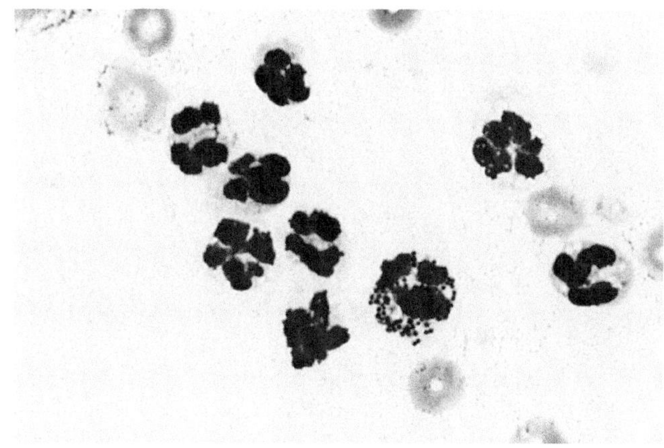

Plate 3E

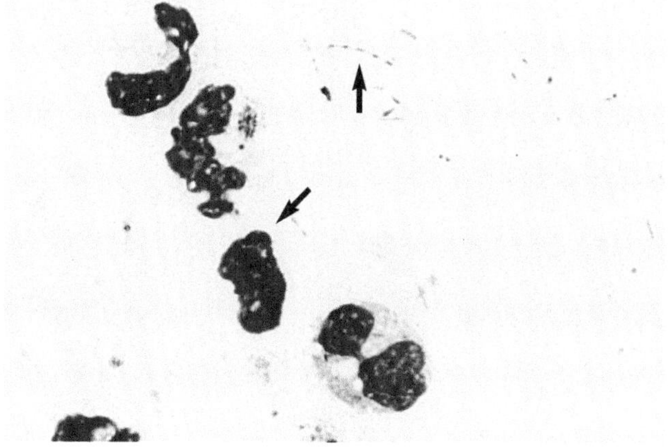

Plate 3F

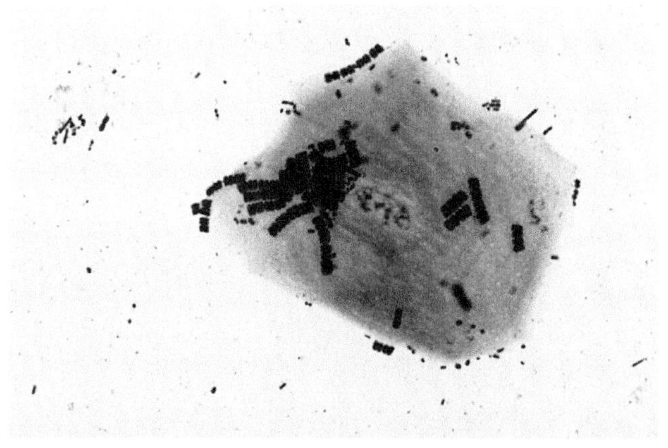

Plate 3G

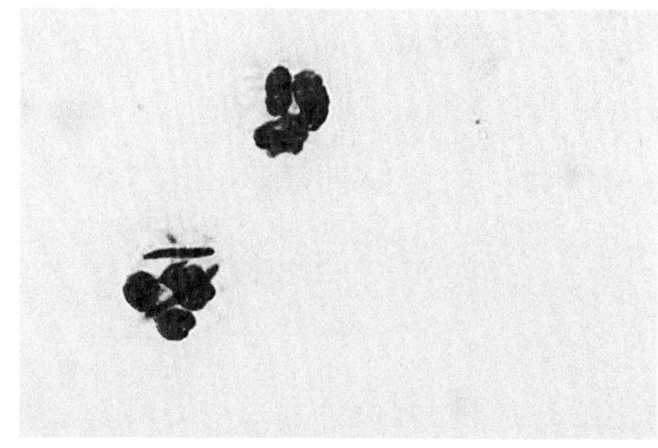

Plate 3H

Plate 4

4A. Macrophages containing nonstaining bacterial rods identified as clear streaks through the cell *(arrow)* are suggestive of *Mycobacterium* infection. (Wright's stain, original magnification 400X)

4B. Acid-fast stain from the same animal as in 4A, showing the reddish filamentous *Mycobacterium* organisms. (Wright's stain, original magnification 250X)

4C. A large macrophage containing numerous *Histoplasma* organisms is shown. *Histoplasma* organisms are small (1 to 4 μ in diameter), round to oval, yeast-like organisms. They have a dark blue/purple-staining nucleus surrounded by a very thin, clear halo. (Wright's stain, original magnification 250X)

4D. A neutrophil containing numerous *Sporothrix schenckii* organisms is in the center of the field. *Sporothrix schenckii* organisms are small (1 to 4 μ in diameter) and round to oblong, with a thin, clear halo. They are about the same size as *Histoplasma* organisms. They can be differentiated by identifying the fusiform or oblong (cigar) shape that some, but not all, of the organisms have. (Wright's stain, original magnification 250X)

4E. *Blastomyces dermatitidis (arrows)* is a bluish, spherical, thick-walled, yeast-like organism in Romanowsky-stained smears. The organisms are 8 to 20 μ in diameter. Occasionally a single broad-based bud may be present. (Wright's stain, original magnification 250X)

4F. *Blastomyces dermatitidis* organisms in a macrophage *(arrows)*. (Wright's stain, original magnification 250X)

4G. A budding *Blastomyces dermatitidis* organism *(arrow)*. (Wright's stain, original magnification 100X)

4H. *Cryptococcus neoformans* is a spherical, yeast-like organism that frequently has a thick, clear-staining, mucoid capsule. The organism with its capsule ranges in size from 8 to 40 μ. Occasionally a single narrow-based bud may be present. Numerous budding and nonbudding *Cryptococcus neoformans* organisms with prominent nonstaining capsules are shown. (Wright's stain, original magnification 250X)

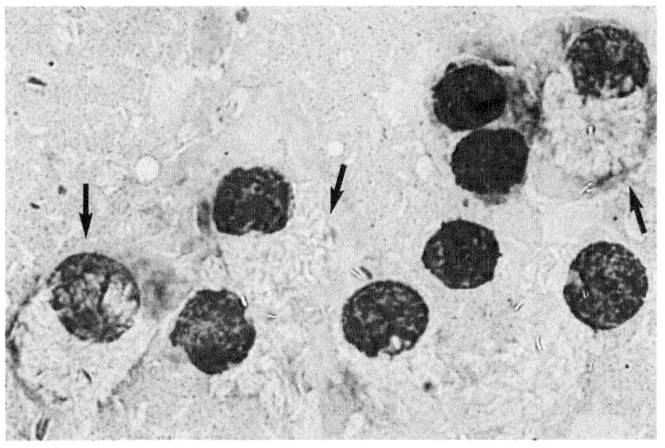

Plate 4A

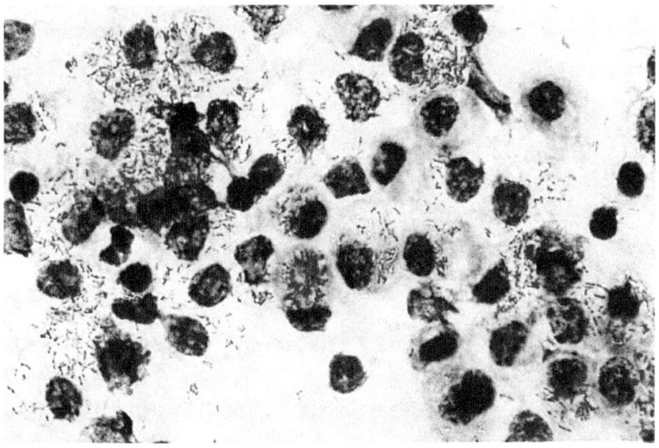

Plate 4B

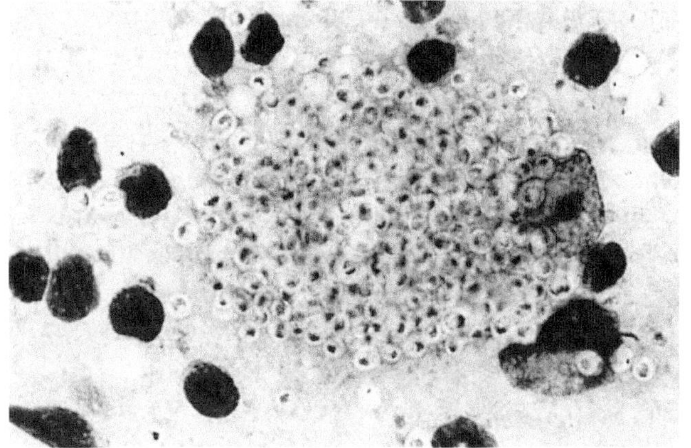

Plate 4C

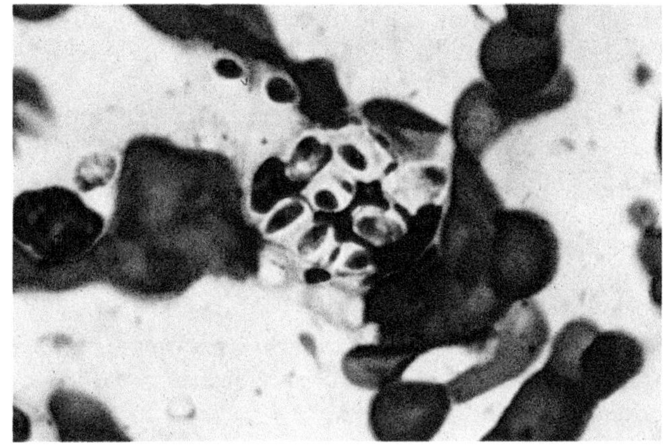

Plate 4D

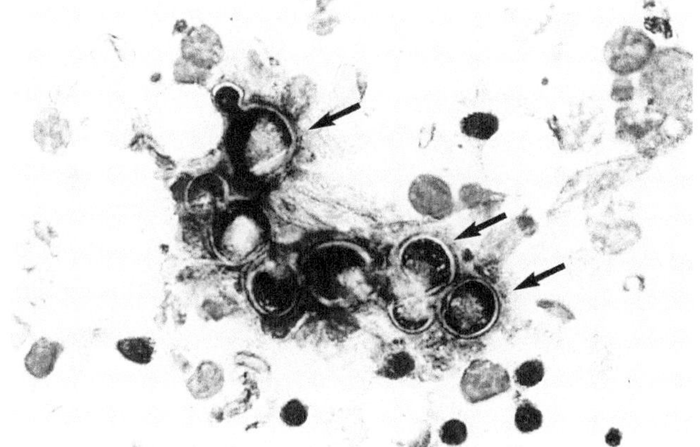

Plate 4E

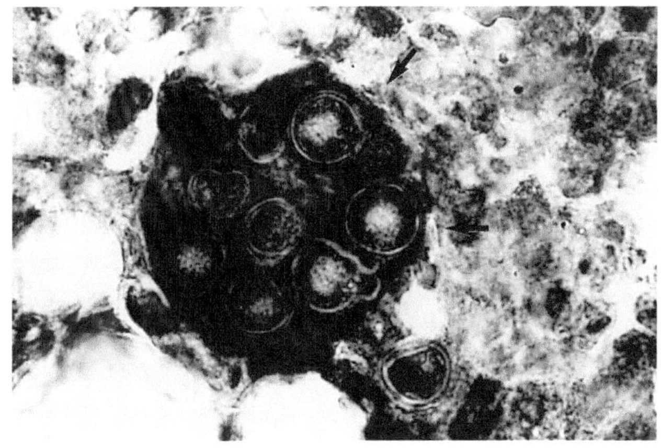

Plate 4F

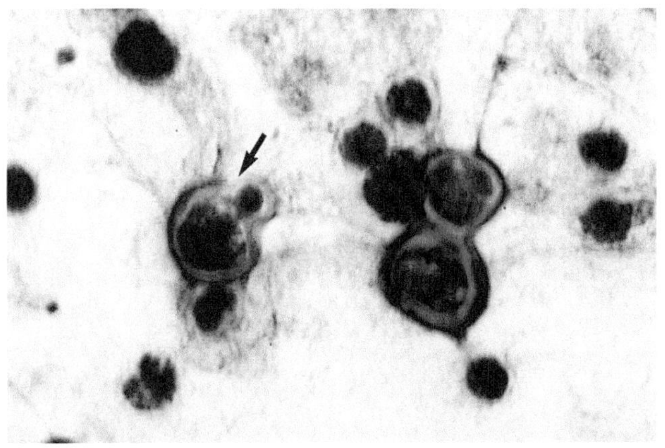

Plate 4G

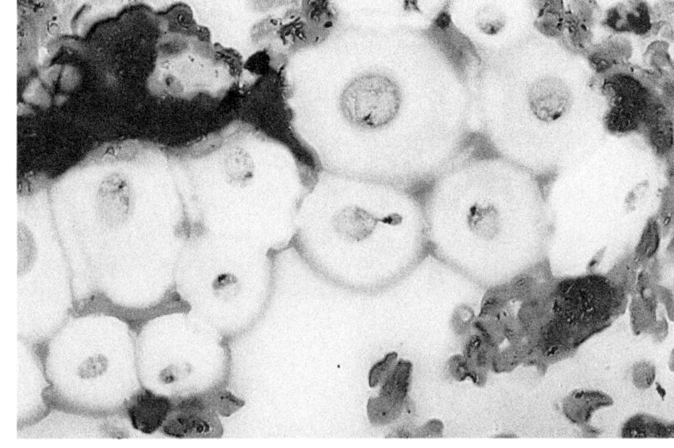

Plate 4H

Plate 5

5A. *Coccidioides immitis* organisms are large, double-contoured, blue-staining spherical bodies (10 to 100 μ in diameter). Occasionally, endospores varying from 2 to 5 μ in diameter may be seen within some of the larger spherules. (Wright's stain, original magnification 125X)

5B. Numerous fungal hyphae are present. The many macrophages and neutrophils indicate a pyogranulomatous response. (Wright's stain, original magnification 250X)

5C. The negative image of a nonstaining fungal hyphae can be seen in the background. Some fungi do not stain with the routine Romanowsky stains. However, most stain with new methylene blue. (Wright's stain, original magnification 250X)

5D. *Ehrlichia* morula within the cytoplasm of a neutrophil. (Wright's stain, original magnification 250X) (Courtesy Oklahoma State University, Stillwater.)

5E. *Babesia* organisms within an RBC. (Wright's stain) (Courtesy Oklahoma State University, Stillwater.)

5F. Lung imprint. A *Pneumoncystis carinii (arrow)* is shown. *Pneumoncystis carinii* cysts are 5 to 10 μ in diameter and usually contain 4 to 8 intracystic bodies 1 to 2 μ in diameter. With Romanowsky stains, intact cysts are distinctive in appearance, but the free trophozoites are difficult to differentiate from debris. (Wright's stain, original magnification 250X)

5G. Numerous *Leishmania donovani* organisms *(arrows)*. *Leishmania donovani* organisms are small and round to oval. They have clear to very light blue cytoplasm, an oval nucleus, and small, dark, ventral kinetoplast. (Wright's stain, original magnification 330X)

5H. This liver impression shows a hepatocyte containing *Bacillus piliformis* (Tyzzer's disease) *(arrow)*. (Wright's stain, original magnification 250X) (Courtesy Oklahoma State University, Stillwater.)

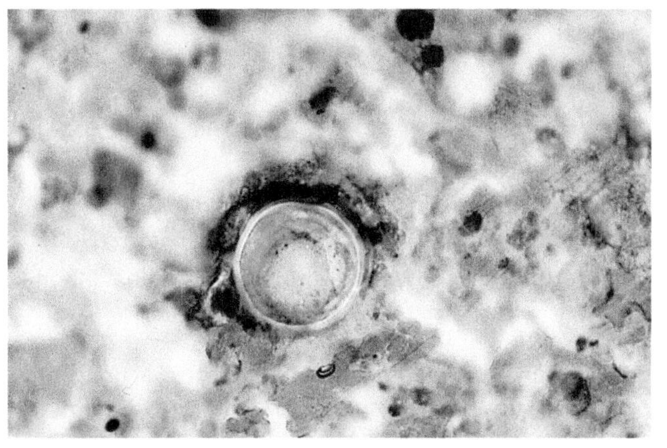

Plate 5A

Plate 5B

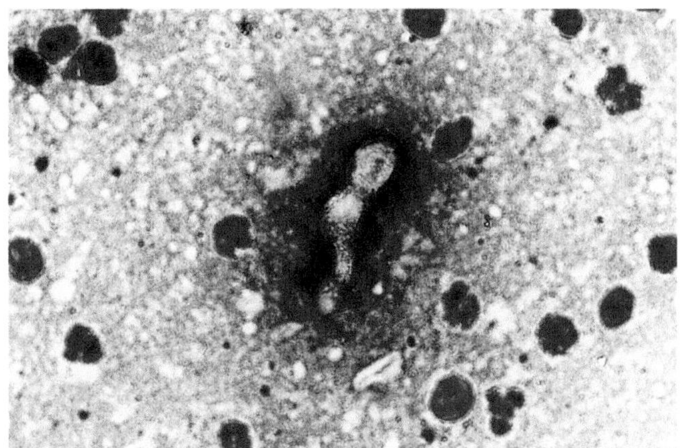

Plate 5C

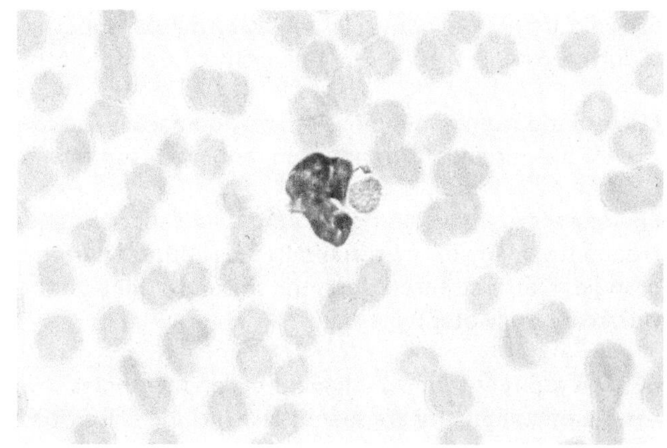

Plate 5D

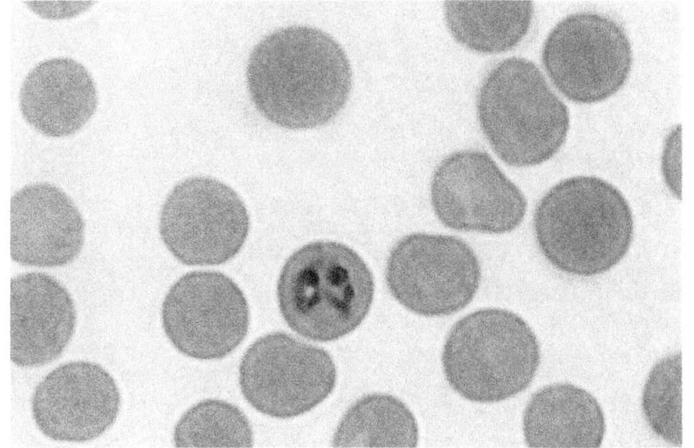

Plate 5E

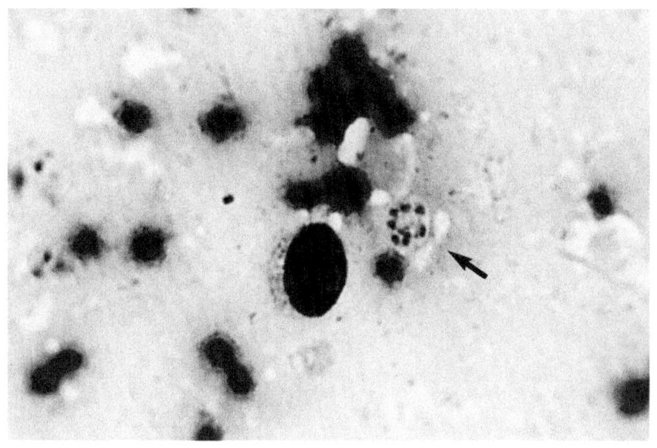

Plate 5F

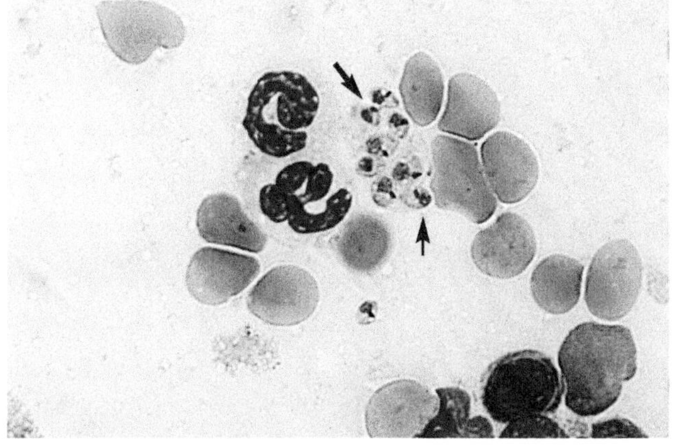

Plate 5G

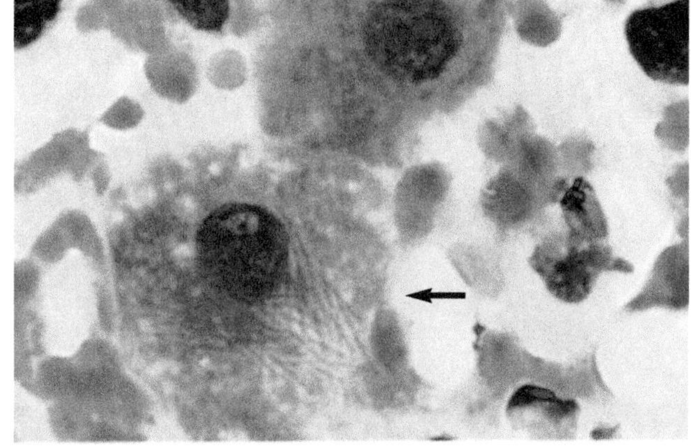

Plate 5H

Plate 6

6A. Several large carcinoma cells. (Wright's stain, original magnification 250X) (Courtesy Oklahoma State University, Stillwater.)

6B. Aspirate from a sebaceous adenoma. A cluster or acinus of sebaceous cells is shown. (Wright's stain, original magnification 250X)

6C. A cluster of malignant glandular epithelial cells is shown. Note the acinar arrangement and numerous vacuoles suggesting glandular origin. Also notice the coarse chromatin pattern, anisocytosis, anisokaryosis, and prominent large nucleoli. One of the cells has a nucleolus that is larger than the RBC present. (Wright's stain, original magnification 125X)

6D. Four basal squamous cells and three mature superficial squamous cells. (Wright's stain, original magnification 100X) (Courtesy Dr. C.B. Andreason, University of Georgia, Athens.)

6E. Aspirate from a squamous-cell carcinoma. Several squamous epithelial cells with nuclear/cytoplasmic asynchrony and visible nucleoli. (Wright's stain, original magnification 132X)

6F. Melanocytes have a single, round to oval nucleus and a small to abundant amount of green-black pigment. Frequently, many of the tissue cells are ruptured during aspiration and/or smear preparation, resulting in many melanin granules scattered throughout the smear. (Wright's stain, original magnification 250X) (Courtesy Oklahoma State University, Stillwater.)

6G. This aspirate from a malignant melanoma shows several melanoma cells containing melanin pigment. Numerous criteria of malignancy are seen. These include anisocytosis; coarse chromatin; increased nucleus: cytoplasm ratio; and prominent, variably sized, and angular nucleoli. (Wright's stain, original magnification 250X)

6H. This aspirate from a lipoma contains numerous fat cells. They are large and round, with pyknotic nuclei and clear cytoplasm. (Wright's stain, original magnification 25X)

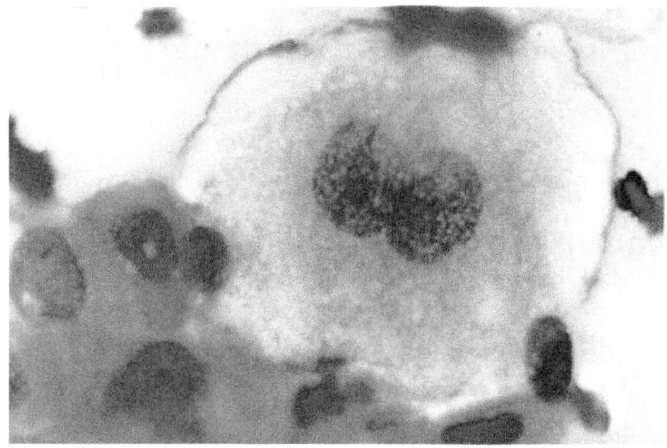

Plate 6A

Plate 6B

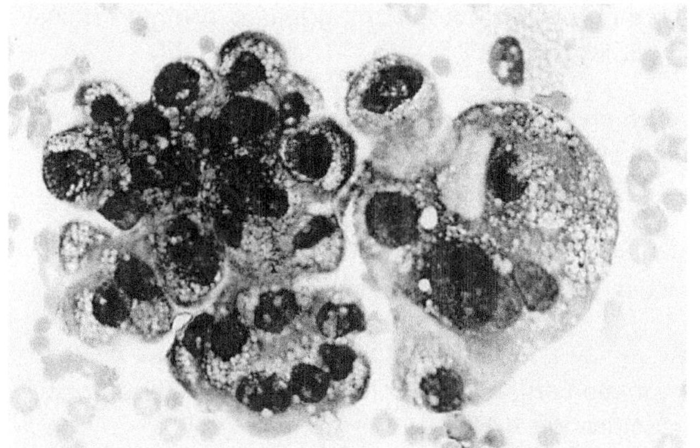

Plate 6C

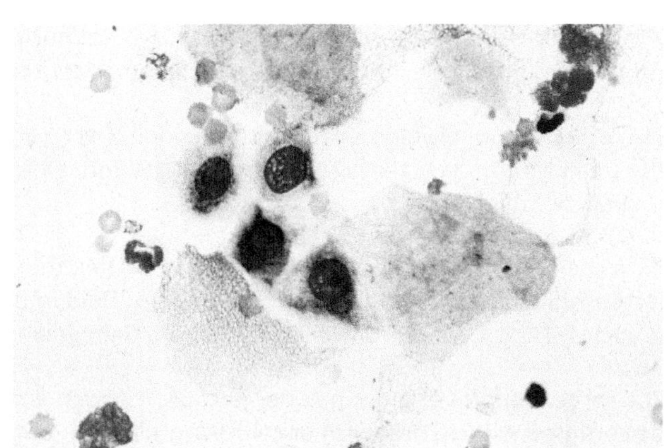

Plate 6D

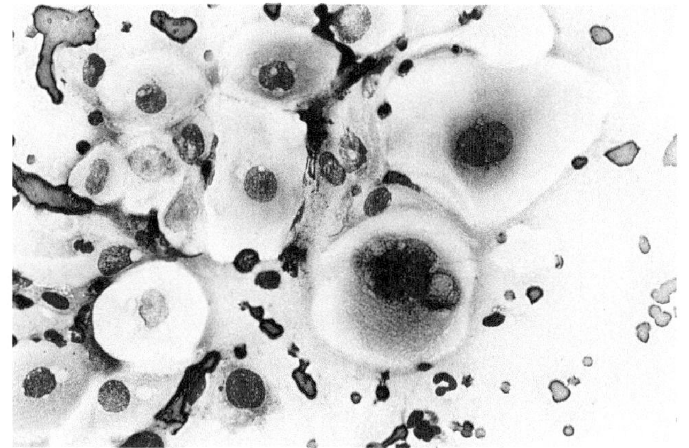

Plate 6E

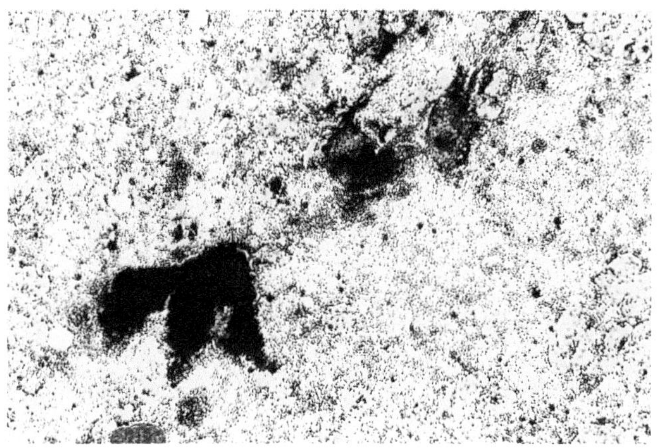

Plate 6F

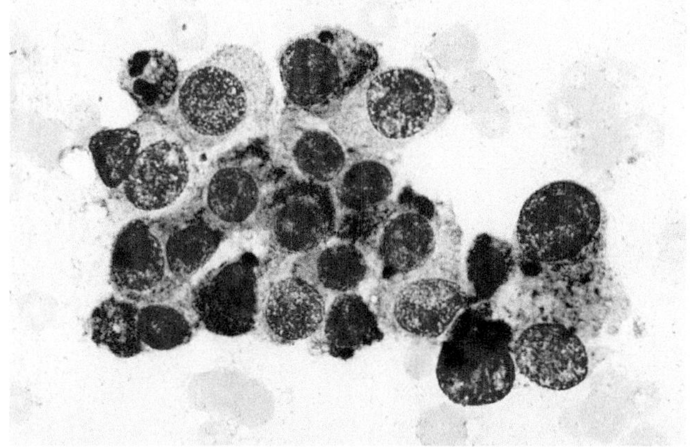

Plate 6G

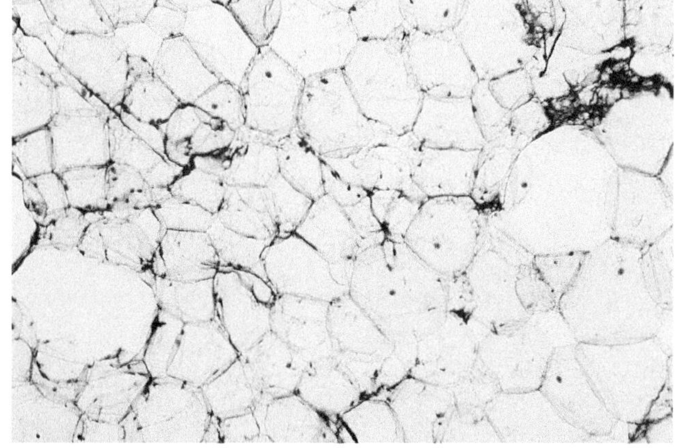

Plate 6H

Plate 7

7A. Fibrocytes have long slender nuclei, with long slender tails of cytoplasm streaming away from the nuclei. (Wright's stain, original magnification 250X)

7B. Aspirate from a hemangioma shows several spindle-shaped cells. Note how the nuclei of the hemangioma cells appear very thin and capable of folding over upon themselves. (Wright's stain, original magnification 250X) (Courtesy Oklahoma State University, Stillwater.)

7C. Aspirate from a malignant spindle-cell tumor. Spindle cells show criteria of malignancy including anisocytosis; coarse chromatin; prominent, variably sized, and occasionally angular nucleoli; and increased nucleus: cytoplasm ratio. (Wright's stain, original magnification 250X)

7D. Mast cells are recognized by their round to oval nucleus and red-purple intracytoplasmic granules. (Wright's stain, original magnification 100X) (Courtesy Oklahoma State University, Stillwater.)

7E. Aspirate from a lymphomatous lymph node. Over 50% of the lymphoid cells are lymphoblasts. They are larger than the small lymphocytes that are also present. (Wright's stain, original magnification 330X) (Courtesy Oklahoma State University, Stillwater.)

7F. A sheet of mesothelial cells. Mesothelial cells line the abdominal and thoracic cavities and can be accidentally collected while obtaining aspirates from organs or fluid in these cavities. (Wright's stain, original magnification 100X) (Courtesy Dr. D.J. Meyer, University of Florida, Gainesville.)

7G. Three granules of glove powder *(arrows)*. Glove powder is a common artifact on cytologic smears and should not be confused with an organism or cell. (Wright's stain, original magnification 100X)

7H. Bone marrow aspirate. A capillary is shown stretching across the photomicrograph. (Wright's stain, original magnification 25X)

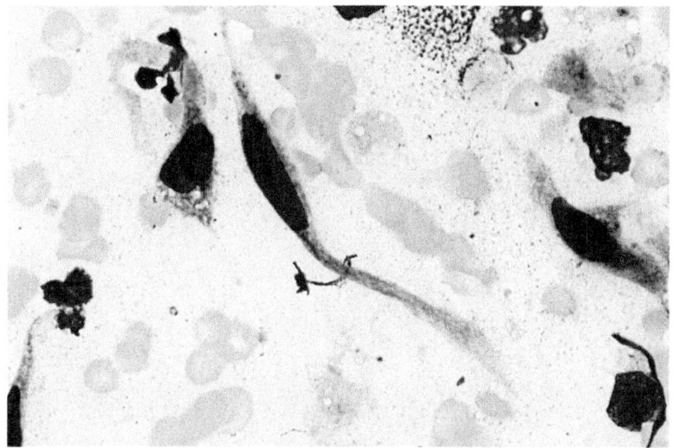
Plate 7A

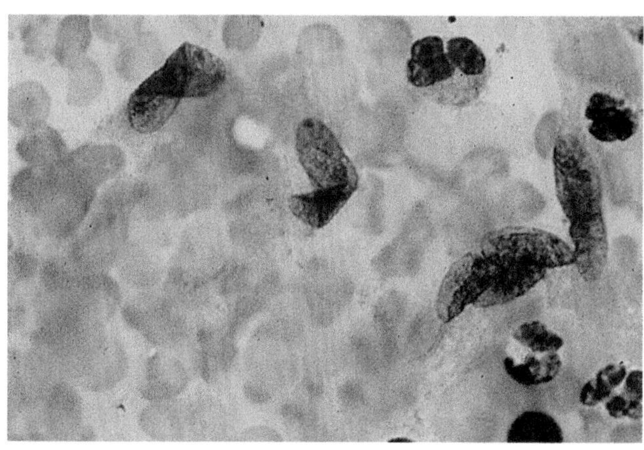
Plate 7B

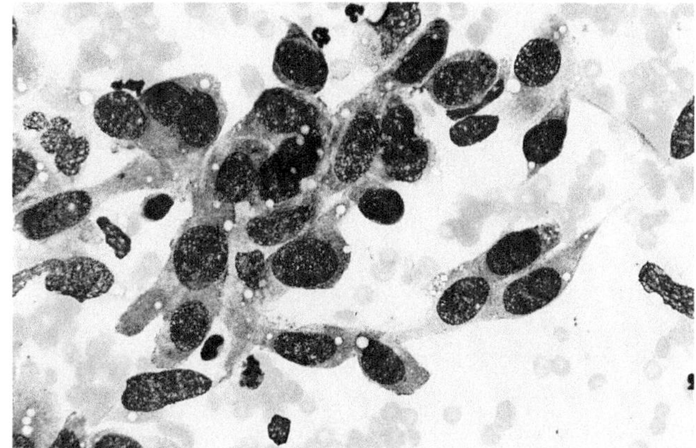
Plate 7C

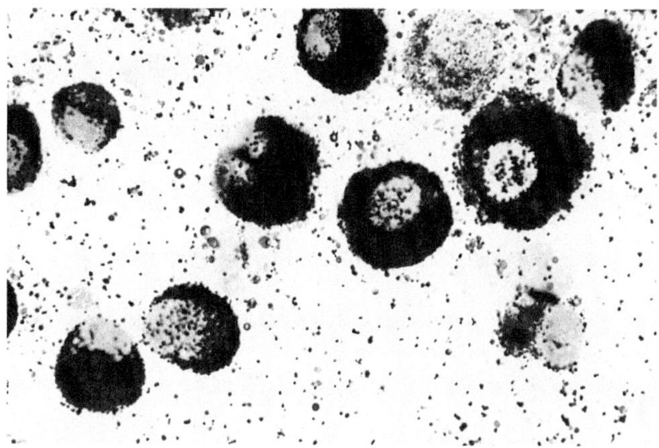
Plate 7D

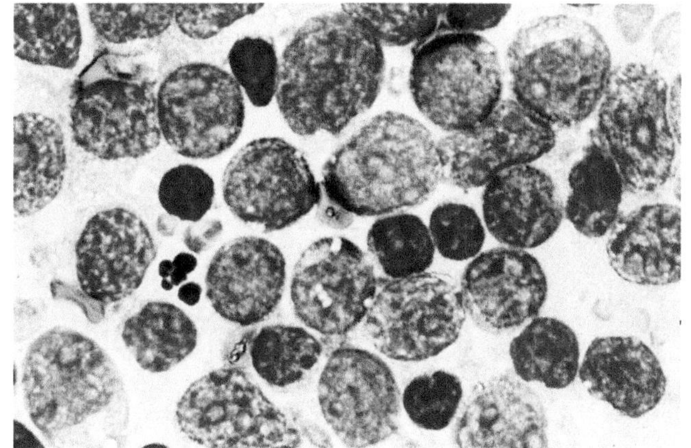
Plate 7E

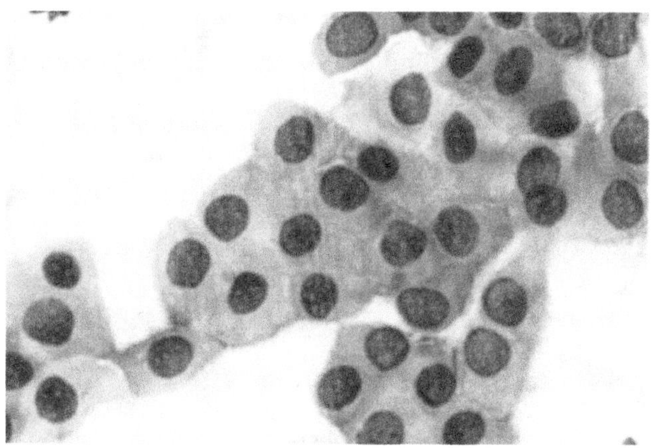
Plate 7F

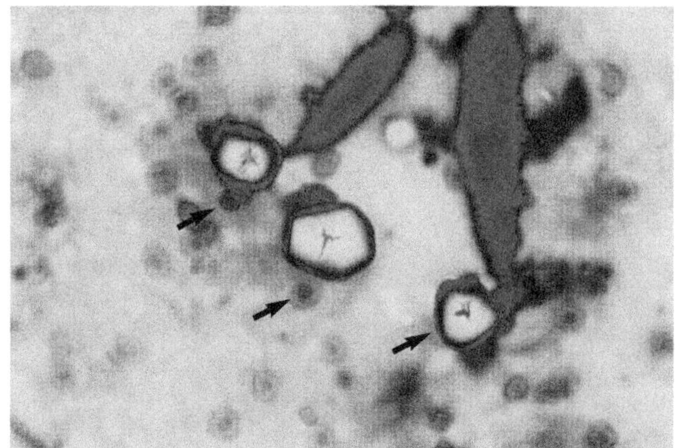
Plate 7G

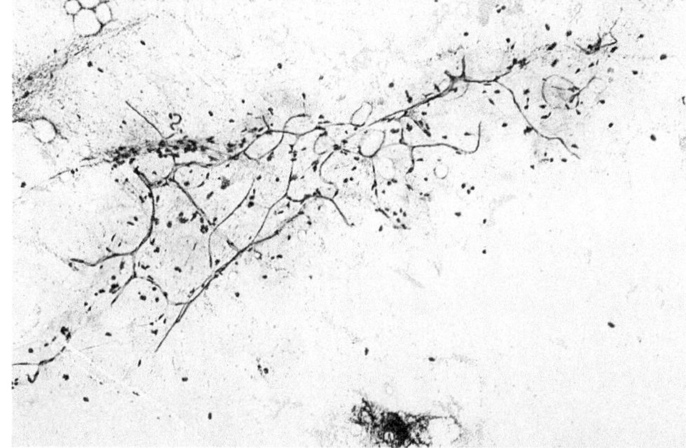
Plate 7H

Index

C

D

F

J

K

L

M

N

O

P

Q

R

S

V

W

X

Y

Z

Printed and bound by CPI Group (UK) Ltd, Croydon, CR0 4YY

08/06/2025

01896880-0003